Find videos for
Pediatric Audiology, Second Edition
online at MediaCenter.thieme.com!

To access additional material or resources available with this book, please visit http://www.thieme.com/bonuscontent. After completing a short form to verify your purchase, you will be provided with the instructions and access codes necessary to retrieve any bonus content.

Videos available online:

1. An Introduction to Testing Techniques
2. Behavioral Observation Audiometry: Introduction
3. Behavioral Observation Audiometry: Testing
4. Visual Reinforcement Audiometry: Introduction
5. Visual Reinforcement Audiometry: Testing
6. Conditioned Play Audiometry: Introduction
7. Conditioned Play Audiometry: Testing
8. Speech Play Audiometry: Introduction
9. Speech Play Audiometry: Testing
10. Cochlear Implant Surgery
11. Special Features: Behavioral Observation Audiometry without Audio Commentary

Total length of videos: 1 hour, 40 minutes

	WINDOWS	MAC	TABLET
Recommended Browser(s) **	Microsoft Internet Explorer 8.0 or later, Firefox 3.x	Firefox 3.x, Safari 4.x	HTML5 mobile browser. iPad — Safari. Opera Mobile — Tablet PCs preferred.
	** all browsers should have JavaScript enabled		
Flash Player Plug-in	Flash Player 9 or Higher* * Mac users: ATI Rage 128 GPU does not support full-screen mode with hardware scaling		Tablet PCs with Android OS support Flash 10.1
Minimum Hardware Configurations	Intel® Pentium® II 450 MHz, AMD Athlon™ 600 MHz or faster processor (or equivalent) 512 MB of RAM	PowerPC® G3 500 MHz or faster processor Intel Core™ Duo 1.33 GHz or faster processor 512MB of RAM	Minimum CPU powered at 800MHz 256MB DDR2 of RAM
Recommended for optimal usage experience	Monitor resolutions: • Normal (4:3) 1024×768 or Higher • Widescreen (16:9) 1280×720 or Higher • Widescreen (16:10) 1440×900 or Higher DSL/Cable internet connection at a minimum speed of 384.0 Kbps or faster WiFi 802.11 b/g preferred.		7-inch and 10-inch tablets on maximum resolution. WiFi connection is required.

Pediatric Audiology
Diagnosis, Technology, and Management

Second Edition

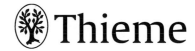

Pediatric Audiology
Diagnosis, Technology, and Management

Second Edition

Jane R. Madell, CCC-A/SLP, LSLS Cert. AVT
Director
Pediatric Audiology Consulting
New York, New York

Carol Flexer, PhD, CCC-A, LSLS Cert. AVT
Distinguished Professor Emeritus, Audiology
School of Speech-Language Pathology and Audiology
The University of Akron
Akron, Ohio

Thieme
New York · Stuttgart

MW

Thieme Medical Publishers, Inc.
333 Seventh Ave.
New York, NY 10001

Executive Editor: Tim Hiscock
Managing Editor: Elizabeth D'Ambrosio
Senior Vice President, Editorial and Electronic Product Development: Cornelia Schulze
Production Editor: Kenneth L. Chumbley
International Production Director: Andreas Schabert
Vice President, Finance and Accounts: Sarah Vanderbilt
President: Brian D. Scanlan
Compositor: Prairie Papers Inc.
Printer: Sheridan Books

Library of Congress Cataloging-in-Publication Data

Pediatric audiology : diagnosis, technology, and management / [edited by] Jane R. Madell, Carol Flexer.—2nd ed.
  p. ; cm.
 Includes bibliographical references and index.
 ISBN 978-1-60406-844-3 (alk. paper)—ISBN 978-1-60406-845-0 (eISBN)
 I. Madell, Jane Reger. II. Flexer, Carol Ann.
 [DNLM: 1. Hearing Disorders—diagnosis. 2. Child. 3. Correction of Hearing Impairment. 4. Education of Hearing Disabled. 5. Hearing Tests. 6. Infant. WV 271]
 RF291.5.C45
 618.92'09789—dc23

2013015940

Printed in the United States of America

5 4 3 2 1

ISBN 978-1-60406-844-3

Also available as an ebook:
eISBN 978-1-60404-845-0

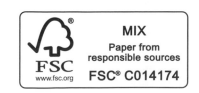

3/17/14

Contents

Video Contents

An Introduction to Testing Techniques with Jane R. Madell, PhD

Behavioral Observation Audiometry
    Introduction
    Testing

Visual Reinforcement Audiometry
    Introduction
    Testing

Conditioned Play Audiometry
    Introduction
    Testing

Speech Audiometry
    Introduction
    Testing

Cochlear Implant Surgery with Dr. George Alexiades

Special Features
    Behavioral Observation Audiometry without Audio Commentary

Foreword

With this book, two master clinicians are expressing what has become a tremendous evolution—almost a revolution—in pediatric audiology. It seems only yesterday that we were still struggling to identify children with hearing loss as early as possible, when the terms *auditory neuropathy* and *auditory dysynchony* were not part of our vocabulary, when *connexin 26* was the province only of obscure geneticists, when cochlear implants were still controversial, when no one had any idea how to habilitate a newborn baby, and when Jane R. Madell and I started our struggle to keep behavioral observation and visual reinforcement audiometry (VRA) in the audiology stream of consciousness.

Jane R. Madell and Carol Flexer are aware of the need for constant updates of the rapidly evolving technology in the field, as well as the new understandings of genetics, early education, and surgical advances. In addition to drawing on their own extensive and distinguished experiences, they have assembled contributors who are most knowledgeable in specific areas of pediatric audiology. Speaking for myself, I can't get enough information about all the advances that have appeared, seemingly overnight.

It begins with the sophisticated maturation of newborn hearing screening, with all the developments attendant on this aspect of the revolution (e.g., knowledge of diseases, genetics, medical treatment, and assessments, which mark the identification and diagnosis of a hearing disorder in the infant), and follows with all the ensuing activities that make for a successful program in identification and management of the child with hearing loss from birth. School children and teenagers are not neglected in this comprehensive report.

This vision of an ideal audiologic world is presented by two people who know whereof they speak. Jane R. Madell has forever fought the good fight for appropriate hearing aid and cochlear implant fittings for children, for behavioral testing of babies, and for audiologists to foster a one-on-one relationship with the children they test. She shares my insistence that all the electronic and electrophysiological applications for children's testing are only the beginning of the acquaintance one must establish with a child experiencing hearing loss. You can learn a great deal of pertinent information for habilitation by watching and playing with the child.

Carol Flexer has also fought the good fight for the child with hearing loss. She has concentrated on the auditory experience in speech and language training. Her book, *Developing Listening and Talking, Birth to Six*, expresses her message that children with hearing loss can best learn speech and language through listening with well-fitted, appropriate hearing aids. Cochlear implants are also included in the emphasis on auditory development, and a chapter in this book is devoted to that experience. She has always represented what's best in audiology.

I can't think of anything they've missed in this presentation of what's new and relevant in pediatric audiology, It's going to be a great read.

Marion P. Downs, DrHS
Professor Emerita
Department of Otolaryngology
University of Colorado School of Medicine
Denver, Colorado

Preface

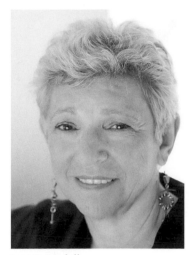
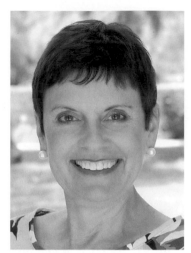

Jane R. Madell   Carol Flexer

This second edition is intended as a text for AuD and PhD courses in pediatric and educational audiology and also as a field guide for audiologists working in pediatric and educational audiology settings. This is a practical *how-to* book about the diagnosis and technological and educational management of infants and children with hearing disorders.

Accordingly, this text is divided into four sections:

- Hearing Loss: Essential Information
- Diagnosing Hearing Disorders in Infants and Children
- Hearing Access Technologies for Infants and Children
- Educational and Clinical Management of Hearing Loss in Children

Each chapter offers a wealth of information, and all are written by experts in specific target areas. We have also drawn on our over 80 collective years of experience as pediatric and educational audiologists to enrich this book.

We want students to keep this book as a reference when they graduate. In addition, we hope that practicing audiologists will be able to use this book as a reference when they are approaching techniques that are new to them or when they are performing behavioral diagnostic procedures that may be used only occasionally.

Even though this book cannot possibly explain every aspect of pediatric and educational audiology in detail, it can provide basic information, augmented by extensive resources, on how to move to the next level of diagnosis and management. In addition, this book includes a practical component: a DVD that demonstrates test techniques to assist both students and practicing audiologists in improving their clinical skills regarding behavioral and functional assessments of infants and children of all ages.

Other professionals working in related fields may also be interested in this book, such as speech-language pathologists, listening and spoken language specialists including auditory-verbal therapists (LSLS Cert. AVT) and auditory verbal educators (LSLS Cert. AVEd), teachers of children who are deaf or hard of hearing, otolaryngologists, pediatricians, and families of children with hearing loss.

Jane R. Madell
Carol Flexer

Acknowledgments

This second edition is a labor of love (in addition to a lot of hard work). It allows us to discuss, in detail, work that is near and dear to our hearts, and to which we have contributed over 80 collective years of experience as pediatric and educational audiologists.

This book would not have been written without an amazing group of chapter authors who generously contributed their time and knowledge. We are most grateful for their collegiality and expertise; it has been a privilege to work with them.

We must thank our families who have, for many years, learned to put up with us not always being around to do mom things because we were doing audiology things. (We began our careers at a time when lots of moms were still staying home and not attempting to have a career outside the home.) We thank our amazingly supportive husbands, Rob Madell and Pete Flexer, our equally amazing children, Jody, Josh, Heather, Hillari, and David, our children in-laws, James, Dawn, Joe, Josh, and Hilary, and the most special group of grandchildren, Eva, Rose, Trixie, Yehuda, Rachel, Yishai, Libby, Tikva, Rebekah, Binyamin, Jak, Yonah, and Flossy and those still to come (from whom we continue to learn every day.)

We could not have accomplished this work were it not for the wonderful audiologists, auditory therapists, educators, and physicians who came before us and set the stage for work with young children—the women and men who taught us to believe that anything was possible and that a hearing loss should not stop anyone from being whatever he or she wants to be.

We would know much less than we know were it not for all the very special families who have given us the privilege of allowing us to work with them day after day, and the students who taught us as we taught them. Thanks to Dan Projansky who made the DVD possible. And finally, we want to thank our publisher, Thieme, and editors Elizabeth D'Ambrosio and Kenny Chumbley, who helped us find our way.

We dedicate this book to all of them.

Jane R. Madell
Carol Flexer

Contributors

George Alexiades, MD, PC, FACS
Co-Director of Residency Education
Associate Professor
Department of Otolaryngology
The New York Eye and Ear Infirmary
New York, New York

Arthur Boothroyd
Distinguished Professor Emeritus
City University of New York
San Diego, California

Susan Cheffo (deceased)
Director of Educational Services
Cochlear Implant Program
Beth Israel Medical Center
New York, New York

Teresa Ching, PhD
Senior Research Scientist
National Acoustic Laboratories
Australian Hearing Hub
Macquarie University
Macquarie Park, Australia

Lisa Vaughan Christensen, AuD
Doctor of Audiology
Arkansas School for the Deaf
Little Rock, Arkansas

Harvey Dillon, PhD
Director
National Acoustic Laboratories
Sydney, Australia

Kris English, PhD
Professor of Audiology
School of Health Professions
The University of Akron
Akron, Ohio

M. Patrick Feeney, PhD
Director
VA RR&D National Center for Rehabilitative Auditory
  Research
Portland Veterans Affairs Medical Center
Department of Otolaryngology–Head and Neck
  Surgery
Oregon Health and Science University
Portland, Oregon

Carol Flexer, PhD, CCC-A, LSLS Cert. AVT
Distinguished Professor Emeritus, Audiology
School of Speech-Language Pathology and
  Audiology
The University of Akron
Akron, Ohio

Richard Gans, PhD
Founder and Executive Director
American Institute of Balance
Largo, Florida

René H. Gifford, PhD
Assistant Professor, Hearing and Speech Sciences
Director, Cochlear Implant Program
Associate Director, Pediatric Audiology
Vanderbilt Bill Wilkerson Center
Nashville, Tennessee

Maryanne Golding
National Acoustic Laboratories
Macquarie Park, Australia

Joan G. Hewitt, AuD
Pediatric Audiologist
Project TALK/Pediatric Hearing Specialists
Encinitas, California

Rebecca Hodges, MS, CGC
Certified Genetic Counselor
Department of General Surgery
Familial Cancer Risk Assessment Center
Burlington, Massachusetts

Ronald A. Hoffman, MD, MHCM
Co-Director, Cochlear Implant Center
New York Eye and Ear Infirmary
Professor of Clinical Otolaryngology
New York Medical College
New York, New York

Garima Kamo, BA
Founder
Grako LLE
Parent of hearing impaired child
Cary, North Carolina

Andrea Kelly
Professional Leader
Auckland District Health Board
Honorary Research Fellow
University of Auckland
Grafton, New Zealand

Rebecca Kooper, AuD
Educational Audiologist
Long Beach, New York

Katherine A. Lafferty, MS, CGC
Licensed Genetic Counselor
Laboratory for Molecular Medicine
Partners HealthCare Center for Personalized Genetic
    Medicine
Cambridge, Massachusetts

Lisa M. Lamson, AuD
Project Manager
Pediatric Audiology Research Lab
Syracuse University
Syracuse, New York

Jane R. Madell, CCC-A/SLP, LSLS Cert. AVT
Director
Pediatric Audiology Consulting
New York, New York

Karen Muñoz, EdD
Associate Professor, Audiology
Communicative Disorders and Deaf Education
Utah State University
Logan, Utah

Marilyn W. Neault, PhD, PASC, CISC
Director
Habilitative Audiology Program
Boston Children's Hospital
Boston, Massachusetts

Beth A. Prieve, MS, PhD
Professor
Department of Communication Sciences and
    Disorders
Syracuse University
Syracuse, New York

Suzanne C. Purdy, MSc, PhD, DipAud
Professor and Head of Speech Science
School of Psychology
The University of Auckland
Auckland, New Zealand

Virginia Ramachandran, AuD, PhD
Senior Staff Audiologist and Research Coordinator
Department of Otolaryngology–Head and Neck
    Surgery
Henry Ford Hospital
Detroit, Michigan

Heidi L. Rehm, PhD
Assistant Professor
Department of Pathology
Harvard Medical School
Boston, Massachusetts

Ellen A. Rhoades, EdS
Auditory-Verbal International Consultant
Plantation, Florida

Jackson Roush, PhD
Professor and Director
Division of Speech and Hearing Sciences
University of North Carolina School of Medicine
Chapel Hill, North Carolina

Sylvia Rotfleisch, MSc(A)
Certified Auditory Verbal Therapist
HEAR to Talk
Los Angeles, California

Chris A. Sanford, PhD
Assistant Professor
Department of Communication Sciences and
    Disorders
Idaho State University
Pocatello, Idaho

Joseph Smaldino, PhD, CCC-A
Professor
Department of Communication Sciences and
    Disorders
Illinois State University
Normal, Illinois

Donna L. Sorkin, MA
Executive Director
American Cochlear Implant Alliance
McLean, Virginia

Brad A. Stach, PhD
Director
Division of Audiology
Department of Otolaryngology–Head and Neck
  Surgery
Henry Ford Hospital
Detroit, Michigan

Arlene Stredler-Brown, MA
Director
The Keystone Project
Adjunct Faculty
University of British Columbia
Vancouver, Canada
Fellow, National Leadership Consortium on Sensory
  Disabilities
Department of Speech, Language, and Hearing
  Sciences
University of Colorado
Boulder, Colorado

Karl R. White, PhD
Director
National Center for Hearing Assessment and
  Management
Emma Eccles Jones Endowed Chair in Early
  Childhood Education
Professor of Psychology
Utah State University
Logan, Utah

Gail M. Whitelaw, PhD
Clinic Director
The Ohio State University Speech-Language-Hearing
  Clinic
Department of Speech and Hearing Science
The Ohio State University
Columbus, Ohio

Elizabeth Ying, MA, CCC-SLP
Director of Hearing Habilitation
The Ear Institute
Children's Hearing Center
New York Eye and Ear Infirmary's Ear Institute
New York, New York

Part I
Hearing Loss: Essential Information

Chapter 1

Why Hearing Is Important in Children

Carol Flexer and Jane R. Madell

Key Points

- Because of technology and brain neuroplasticity, everything we used to know and believe to be true about hearing loss has changed.

- The problem with hearing loss is that it keeps sound from reaching the brain; the purpose of hearing aids and cochlear implants is to access, stimulate, and grow auditory neural connections throughout the brain as the foundation for spoken language, reading, and academics.

- There is a distinction between hearing and listening.

- Today's child who is "deaf" without using technology may function like a child with a mild to moderate hearing loss when provided with hearing aids or a cochlear implant because critical neural connections have been developed through meaningful auditory stimulation.

- Because about 95% of children with hearing loss are born to hearing and speaking families, listening and talking likely will be desired outcomes for the vast majority of families we serve; those outcomes require vigilant, consistent, and caring audiologic management.

Approximately 12,000 new babies with hearing loss are identified every year, according to the National Institute on Deafness and Other Communication Disorders. In addition, estimates are that another 4,000 to 6,000 infants and young children between birth and 3 years of age who passed the newborn screening test acquire late-onset hearing loss. Therefore, ~ 16,000 to 18,000 new babies and toddlers are identified with hearing loss per year, making hearing loss the most common birth defect.

Numerous studies over the decades have demonstrated that when hearing loss of any degree is not adequately diagnosed and treated, it can negatively affect the speech, language, academic, emotional, and psychosocial development of young children. Therefore, the secondary effects of hearing loss, rather than the hearing loss itself, adversely affect a child's development.

Recently, there has been a surge of information and technology about testing and managing hearing loss in infants and children. The impetus for this surge has been newborn hearing screening. As a result of identifying and treating hearing loss in neonates, we now are dealing with a vastly different population of children with hearing loss, a population that never existed before. With this new population, whose hearing loss is identified at birth, the secondary developmental and communicative deficits of hearing loss that were so common just a few years ago can be prevented. What has happened in the field of hearing loss is revolutionary, and the pediatric audiologist is in the linchpin position.

How does the pediatric audiologist of today diagnose and treat this new population of babies and children with hearing loss and their families? How does audiology, as a (health) diagnosing and treating profession, collaborate with other health-care providers, early interventionists, speech-language pathologists, teachers, and, of course, families in providing quality services? The first step is to recognize that because of technology and brain neuroplasticity, everything that we used to know and believe to be true about hearing loss has changed.

This chapter will begin at the beginning: with a discussion of the changing world for pediatric audiologists. Next, auditory neural development will be explored, along with a discussion of neuroplasticity. A new context for the word "deaf" will be posited, and the chapter will end with a discussion of the acoustic filter model of hearing loss.

◆ Factors Changing the Practice of Pediatric Audiology

The popular book about change, *Who Moved My Cheese?* by Spencer Johnson, M.D. (1998), is particularly meaningful in the world of hearing loss. Changes brought about through technology and early hearing detection and intervention (EHDI) programs have permitted outcomes of listening and talking only dreamed of a few years ago. It is important to realize that the new outcomes available today do not invalidate the treatment decisions made by pediatric audiologists in the past. Audiologists did what was necessary with what was available at the time. For example, until the 1970s, children with bilateral hearing loss were routinely fitted with only one hearing aid.

With increased knowledge, we can now offer better services. Audiologists today do the best that can be done in today's world. Tomorrow's world will bring new possibilities, and we will need to "move with the cheese." Our job as pediatric audiologists is to prepare today's babies to be take-charge adults in the world of 2030, 2040, and 2050 . . . , not in the world of 1970 or 1990 or even 2016. Because information and knowledge are the currencies of today's cultures, listening, speaking, reading, writing, and electronic technologies must be made available to our babies and children to the fullest degree possible.

◆ Relationship of Auditory Neural Development and Speech and Reading Skills

The problem with hearing loss is that it keeps sound from reaching the brain. The purpose of hearing aids and cochlear implants is to access, stimulate, and grow auditory neural connections throughout the brain as the foundation for spoken language, reading, and academics (Boons et al, 2012; Gordon, Papsin, & Harrison, 2004).

There is substantial evidence that "hearing" is indeed the most effective modality for the teaching of spoken language (speech), reading, and cognitive skills (Boons et al, 2012; Geers, Strube, Strube, Tobey, Pisoni, & Moog, 2011; Sloutsky & Napolitano, 2003; Tallal, 2004; 2005; Werker, 2006). Furthermore, with today's amplification technologies, including cochlear implants, and early identification and intervention, auditory brain access is available to babies with even the most profound deafness. This brain access allows the use of a developmental model of intervention that prevents the negative developmental outcomes of hearing loss that were so common a few years ago.

◆ Brain Development, Neuroplasticity, and Treatment of Hearing Loss in Children

Studies of brain development show that sensory stimulation of the auditory centers of the brain is critical and, indeed, influences the actual organization of auditory brain pathways (Boothroyd, 1997; Berlin & Weyand, 2003; Chermak, Bellis, & Musiek, 2007; Kraus & Anderson, 2012). The fact is, the brain can organize itself only around the stimuli that it receives. If complete acoustic events are received, then that is how the brain will be organized. Conversely, if hearing loss filters some or all speech sounds from reaching auditory centers of the brain, then the brain will be organized differently. "When we want to remember (or learn) something we have heard, we must hear it clearly because memory can be only as clear as its original signal . . . muddy in, muddy out" (Doidge, 2007, p. 68). Signal enhancement, such as that provided by amplification technology, is really about brain stimulation, with subsequent development of auditory-neural pathways.

Neural imaging has demonstrated that areas in the primary and secondary auditory cortex are most active when a child listens and reads. That is, phonologic or phonemic awareness, which is the explicit awareness of the speech sound structure of language units, forms the basis for the development of literacy skills (Kraus & Hornickel, 2010; Pugh, 2005; Robertson, 2009; Strickland & Shanahan, 2004; Tallal, 2004). Clearly, anything we can do to access and "program" those critical and powerful auditory centers of the brain with acoustic detail will expand children's abilities to listen and learn spoken language. As McConkey Robbins, Koch, Osberger, Zimmerman-Phillips, and Kishon-Rabin (2004) contend, early and ongoing auditory intervention is essential.

Important neural deficits caused by prolonged lack of auditory stimulation have been identified in the higher auditory centers of the brain; auditory stimulation directly influences speech perception and language processing in humans (Kretzmer, Meltzer, Haenggeli, & Ryugo, 2004; Sharma, Nash, & Dorman, 2009; Shaywitz & Shaywitz, 2004). In order for auditory pathways to mature, acoustic stimulation must occur early and often, because normal maturation of central auditory pathways is a precondition for the normal development of speech and language skills in children. Research also suggests that children receiving implants very early (around 1 year of age) may benefit more from the relatively greater plasticity of the auditory pathways than will children who are implanted later in the developmentally sensitive period (Boons et al, 2012; Sharma et al, 2005; Sharma et al, 2009). Sharma's ongoing results suggest that rapid changes in P1 latencies and changes in response morphology are not unique to electrical stimulation, but rather reflect the response of a deprived sensory system to new stimulation. Gordon and coworkers (Gordon, Papsin, & Harrison, 2003; Gordon et al, 2004) concurred and reported that activity in the auditory pathways to the level of the midbrain can be provoked by stimulation from a cochlear implant. The hypothesis that early implantation appears to activate changes in central auditory pathways is supported by evidence provided by Gordon and colleagues.

To summarize, neuroplasticity is greatest during the first three and a half years of life. The younger the infant, the greater is the neuroplasticity (Sharma, Dorman, & Spahr, 2002; Sharma et al, 2004, 2005, 2009). Rapid infant brain growth requires prompt intervention, typically including amplification and a program to promote auditory skill development. In the absence of sound, the brain reorganizes itself to receive input from other senses, primarily vision; this process, called cross-modal reorganization, reduces auditory neural capacity. Early (in the first year of life) amplification or implantation stimulates a brain that is in the initial process of organizing itself and is therefore more receptive to auditory input, resulting in greater auditory capacity. Furthermore, early implantation synchronizes activity in the cortical layers.

◆ New Context for the Word "Deaf"

In this day and age, hearing aids and/or cochlear implants and FM technology can provide access to the entire speech spectrum to infants and children with even the most profound hearing losses as long as they have an intact cochlea. Indeed, there is no degree of hearing loss that prohibits access to sound if cochlear implants are available. Degree of hearing loss as a limiting factor in auditory acuity is now an "old" acoustic conversation. That is, when one uses the word "deaf," the implication is that one has no access to sound, period. The word "deaf" in 1970 occurred in a very different context than the word "deaf" used today. Today's child who is "deaf" without using technology may function like a child with a mild to moderate hearing loss when he or she is using hearing aids or a cochlear implant because critical neural connections have been developed through meaningful auditory stimulation. Therefore, the words used today to express hearing loss may need to be reconsidered. For this new generation of children with hearing loss, the degree of hearing loss ought not determine their functional outcome; performance *with* technology is what will determine functional outcome. These are the new hearing children.

◆ Hearing versus Listening

There is a distinction between hearing and listening. Hearing is acoustic access to the brain; it includes improving the signal-to-noise ratio by managing the environment and using hearing technology. Listening, on the other hand, is focusing and attending to the acoustic events that are available to the child (Beck & Flexer, 2011).

Sequencing is important. Hearing must be made available by audiologists before *listening* can be taught by parents, early interventionists, speech-language pathologists, auditory-verbal therapists, teachers, and, of course, audiologists. That is, one can reasonably focus on developing listening skills and strategies only after acoustic events have been made available to the brain—not before.

◆ The Invisible Acoustic Filter Effect of Hearing Loss

Hearing loss of any type or degree that occurs in infancy or childhood can interfere with the development of a child's spoken language, reading and writing skills, and academic performance (Davis, 1990; Ling, 2002). That is, hearing loss can be described as an invisible acoustic filter that distorts, smears, or eliminates incoming sounds, especially sounds from a distance—even a short distance. The negative effects of a hearing loss may be apparent, but the hearing loss itself is invisible and easily ignored or underestimated.

As human beings we are neurologically "wired" to develop spoken language (speech) and reading skills through the central auditory system. Most people think that reading is a visual skill, but recent research on brain mapping shows that primary reading centers of the brain are located in the auditory cortex—in the auditory portions of the brain (Chermak et al, 2007; Kraus & Hornickel, 2010; Pugh, Sandak, & Frost, 2006; Tallal, 2005). That is why many children who are born with hearing losses, and who do not have access to auditory input when they are very young (through hearing aids or cochlear implants and auditory teaching), tend to have a great deal of difficulty reading, even though their vision is fine (Robertson, 2009). Therefore, the earlier and more efficiently a pediatric audiologist can enable a child's access to meaningful sound, with subsequent direction of the child's attention to sound, the better opportunity that child will have to develop spoken language, literacy, and academic skills (American Academy of Audiology, 2012). With the technology and early auditory intervention available today, a child with a hearing loss *can* have the same opportunity as a typical hearing child to develop spoken language, reading, and academic skills.

◆ Summary

Pediatric audiologists have a key role in determining the future opportunities of a child with a hearing loss. Sound has to reach the brain before auditory-based learning can occur. All hearing losses in infants and children involve developmental and educational issues requiring audiologic intervention. Some hearing problems also involve medical issues. Parents and other family members have to be made to understand the importance of auditory learning for language and literacy development so that they can take an active part in building their children's skills. The purposes of audiologic environmental and technological management strategies are to enhance the reception of clear and intact acoustic signals to access, develop, and organize the auditory centers of the brain.

Pitfall

- Without clear detection of the entire speech spectrum, higher levels of auditory processing are not possible, and a baby or child's listening, spoken language, and literacy outcomes will be compromised.

The pediatric audiologist has a critical role in educating families and therefore needs to be ever mindful of the desired outcomes expressed by the family.

The family's vision for how they want their child to communicate serves as the guide for the technological and treatment recommendations that are made. Because ~ 95% of children with hearing loss are born to hearing and speaking families, listening and talking likely will be desired outcomes for the vast majority of families we serve. Those outcomes require vigilant, consistent, and caring audiologic management.

In this day and age, the degree of hearing loss does not determine the functional outcome for infants and children who are young enough to have brain neural plasticity; these children's auditory brain centers can be accessed, stimulated, and developed through the early use of amplification or cochlear implant technologies and appropriate specialized intervention.

Someone once said, "Neglect the future, and no one will thank you for managing the present." Our job as pediatric audiologists is to be visionary. How we audiologically diagnose and treat babies from the beginning, and educate their families, lays the neurologic foundation for the child's entire life.

Discussion Questions

1. What is the relationship between hearing and listening?
2. How does auditory neuroplasticity relate to early fitting of hearing aids and/or cochlear implants?
3. What is the context for the word "deaf" in this day and age?
4. How does the family's desired outcome for their child influence the services provided by a pediatric audiologist?

References

American Academy of Audiology. (2012). Guidelines for the Assessment of Hearing in Infants and Young Children. Retrieved from the American Academy of Audiology website, http://www.audiology.org/resources/documentlibrary/Documents/201208_AudGuideAssessHear_youth.pdf

Beck, D., & Flexer, C. (2011). Listening is where hearing meets brain . . . in children and adults. The Hearing Review, 18(2), 30–35.

Berlin, C. I., & Weyand, T. G. (2003). The brain and sensory plasticity: Language acquisition and hearing. Clifton Park, NY: Thomson Delmar Learning.

Boons, T., Brokx, J. P., Dhooge, I., Frijns, J. H., Peeraer, L., Vermeulen, A., . . . van Wieringen, A. (2012, Sep–Oct). Predictors of spoken language development following pediatric cochlear implantation. Ear and Hearing, 33(5), 617–639.

Boothroyd, A. (1997). Auditory development of the hearing child. Scandinavian Audiology. Supplementum, 46, 9–16.

Chermak, G. D., Bellis, J. B., & Musiek, F. E. (2007). Neurobiology, cognitive science, and intervention. In G. D. Chermak & F. E. Musiek (Eds.), Handbook of central auditory processing disorder: Comprehensive intervention volume II, pp. 3–28. San Diego: Plural Publishing Inc.

Davis, J. (1990). Our forgotten children: Hard-of-hearing pupils in the schools. Bethesda, MD: Self Help for Hard of Hearing People.

Doidge, N. (2007). The BRAIN that changes itself. London, England: Penguin Books, Ltd.

Geers, A. E., Strube, M. J., Tobey, E. A., Pisoni, D. B., & Moog, J. S. (2011, Feb). Epilogue: factors contributing to long-term outcomes of cochlear implantation in early childhood. Ear and Hearing, 32(1, Suppl), 84S–92S.

Gordon, K. A., Papsin, B. C., & Harrison, R. V. (2003, Dec). Activity-dependent developmental plasticity of the auditory brain stem in children who use cochlear implants. Ear and Hearing, 24(6), 485–500.

Gordon, K. A., Papsin, B. C., & Harrison, R. V. (2004). Thalamocortical activity and plasticity in children using cochlear implants. International Congress Series, 1273, 76–79.

Johnson, S. (1998). Who moved my cheese? New York: Putnam's Sons.

Kraus, N., & Anderson, S. (2012). Hearing matters: Hearing with our brains. The Hearing Journal, 65(9), 48.

Kraus, N., & Hornickel, J. (2010, Sep 21). Biological markers of reading and speech-in-noise perception in the auditory system. The ASHA Leader. Retrieved from http://www.asha.org/Publications/leader/2010/100921/Biological-Markers.htm

Kretzmer, E. A., Meltzer, N. E., Haenggeli, C. A., & Ryugo, D. K. (2004, May). An animal model for cochlear implants. Archives of Otolaryngology–Head & Neck Surgery, 130(5), 499–508.

Ling, D. (2002). Speech and the hearing impaired child. Washington, DC: Alexander Graham Bell Association of the Deaf and Hard of Hearing.

Pugh, K. (2005). Neuroimaging studies of reading and reading disability: Establishing brain/behavior relations. Paper presented at the Literacy and Language Conference at the Speech, Language, and Learning Center, Beth Israel Medical Center, New York City, November 30, 2005.

Pugh, K., Sandak, R., & Frost, S. J. (2006). Neurobiological investigations of skilled and impaired reading. In D. Dickinson & S. Neuman (Eds.), Handbook of early literacy research, Vol. 2. New York: Guilford.

Robertson, L. (2009). Literacy and deafness: Listening and spoken language. San Diego, CA: Plural.

McConkey Robbins, A., Koch, D. B., Osberger, M. J., Zimmerman-Phillips, S., & Kishon-Rabin, L. (2004, May). Effect of age at cochlear implantation on auditory skill development in infants and toddlers. Archives of Otolaryngology–Head & Neck Surgery, 130(5), 570–574.

Sharma, A., Dorman, M. F., & Spahr, A. J. (2002, Dec). A sensitive period for the development of the central auditory system in children with cochlear implants: implications for age of implantation. Ear and Hearing, 23(6), 532–539.

Sharma, A., Tobey, E., Dorman, M., Bharadwaj, S., Martin, K., Gilley, P., et al. (2004, May). Central auditory maturation and babbling development in infants with cochlear implants. Archives of Otolaryngology–Head & Neck Surgery, 130(5), 511–516.

Sharma, A., Martin, K., Roland, P., Bauer, P., Sweeney, M. H., Gilley, P., & Kunkel, F. (2005, Sep). P1 latency as a biomarker for central auditory development in children with hearing impairment. Journal of the American Academy of Audiology, 16(8), 564–573.

Sharma, A., Nash, A. A., & Dorman, M. (2009, Jul-Aug). Cortical development, plasticity and re-organization in children with cochlear implants. Journal of Communication Disorders, 42(4), 272–279.

Shaywitz, S. E., & Shaywitz, B. A. (2004). Disability and the brain. Educational Leadership, 61, 7–11.

Sloutsky, V. M., & Napolitano, A. C. (2003, May-Jun). Is a picture worth a thousand words? Preference for auditory modality in young children. Child Development, 74(3), 822–833.

Strickland, D. S., & Shanahan, T. (2004). Laying the groundwork for literacy. Educational Leadership, 61, 74–77.

Tallal, P. (2004, Sep). Improving language and literacy is a matter of time. Nature Reviews. Neuroscience, 5(9), 721–728.

Tallal, P. (2005). Improving language and literacy. Paper presented at the Literacy and Language Conference at the Speech, Language, and Learning Center, Beth Israel Medical Center, New York City, November 30, 2005.

Werker, J. (2006). Infant speech perception and early language acquisition. Paper presented at the 4th Widex Congress of Paediatric Audiology, Ottawa, Canada, May 19–21, 2006.

Chapter 2

Hearing Disorders in Children

Brad A. Stach and Virginia Ramachandran

Key Points

- There are many pathological conditions that cause hearing disorders in childhood, including disease, trauma, and developmental disturbance.
- Some hearing disorders are unique to childhood; others impact children to a greater or lesser extent than they do adults.
- Conductive hearing disorder results from problems involving structures of the outer and middle ear, including congenital anomalies and otitis media and its complications.
- Sensory hearing disorder results from problems involving the cochlea, including congenital inner-ear anomalies, maternal infections, such as cytomegalovirus and toxoplasmosis, and acquired infections, such as meningitis and mumps.
- Neural hearing disorder results from problems involving the auditory nervous system, including neoplasms and hypoxia.
- The impact of hearing disorder on speech and language development varies as a function of degree, type, configuration, and stability of hearing loss and when in the course of development hearing loss occurs.

A hearing disorder results from a disruption in function of structures that transmit an acoustic signal from the outer ear to the point of perception in the brain. Many pathologic conditions, including disease, trauma, and developmental disturbance, cause hearing disorders during childhood. In most cases, the impacts on hearing sensitivity and suprathreshold perception are predictable from the nature of the pathology.

Hearing disorders are customarily classified according to the nature of the interruption in sound transmission. Conductive hearing disorder results from a problem with transmission of mechanical energy to the cochlea, involving the structures of the outer and middle ear. Sensory hearing disorder results from a problem with the transduction of hydraulic energy to electrical energy, involving the cochlea. Neural hearing disorder results from a problem with the transmission of the electrical signal to and throughout the brain, involving the eighth cranial nerve and the central auditory nervous system pathways.

The prevalence of hearing disorders in children is relatively high compared with other childhood disorders. As many as 3 in 1000 infants are born with congenital bilateral sensorineural hearing loss. The number with significant, permanent sensorineural hearing loss in at least one ear is closer to 8 in 1000 infants. Combining these incidences with transient conductive disorder, as many as 15 in 1000 infants have some degree of hearing disorder. By the time children reach school age, from 10 to 15% fail hearing screenings, in most cases because of the residual effects of middle ear disorder.

Some hearing disorders are unique to childhood; others affect children to a greater or lesser extent than they do adults. Several factors, including type of disorder, severity, and time of onset, interact to determine the impact of childhood hearing disorder on speech and language development. Disorders that fluctuate or are transient tend to have a more subtle impact on overall hearing ability than do permanent disorders. Similarly, disorders that are unilateral are likely to have far less impact than those that are bilateral. In general, the more severe the hearing disorder, the more likely it will be to affect normal speech and language acquisition. Interacting with type and severity of the disorder is the age of onset. Some hearing disorders are present at birth, or are congenital; others occur after birth, or are acquired. Onset of hearing disorder is also often described in relation to birth. A hearing disorder can occur before (prenatal), during (perinatal), or after (postnatal) birth.

◆ Embryological Development

Prenatal disorders are typically caused by abnormal embryological development. The auditory system arises from two of the three germ cell layers that differentiate shortly after fertilization. The outer and inner ear systems develop primarily from the ectodermal tissues; the middle ear components from the mesodermal layer. Development of the auditory system begins in the third week of gestation. At 7–8 weeks, the semicircular canals are formed. The cochlea is adult-like by 25 weeks of gestation, while the middle ear continues to develop until the end of gestation. The auditory system develops alongside all other body systems, and developmental abnormalities that affect one body system can readily impact the developmental sequence of other systems. Genetic anomalies can cause embryological abnormalities, as can factors external to the developing fetus, such as drugs and alcohol. The timing of development of auditory system structures is highly specific, and the relative timing of genetic or environmental insults is critical to the ultimate anatomic and functional outcomes. Depending on the causative factor and its timing, other body systems that are undergoing similarly critical development may also be affected, resulting in a constellation of symptoms, known as a syndrome. See Northern and Downs (2002), Lambert and Canalis (2000), Hill (2011), and Jones and Jones (2011) for review.

The remainder of this chapter will focus on the characteristics of hearing disorders related to specific exogenous etiologies, which have factors that are not necessarily intrinsic to the genetic makeup of the individual. Endogenous conditions, which are inherited, are discussed in Chapter 3.

◆ Conductive Hearing Disorders

Nature of Conductive Hearing Disorders

Conductive hearing loss is caused by attenuation of sound as it travels from the outer ear to the cochlea. The roles of the outer ears and ear canals in the collection and enhancement of sound are necessarily reduced by a conductive disorder. When the middle ear mechanism is involved, its important function as an impedance-matching transformer of acoustic air pressure waves to fluid motion in the cochlea is likewise disrupted. As a rule, a pathologic condition that affects the physical mass of the outer and middle ear mechanism will reduce sensitivity to higher-frequency sound; one that affects the stiffness will reduce sensitivity to lower-frequency sound. The net effect will be attenuation across the frequency range of hearing.

Because conductive hearing loss acts primarily as an attenuator of sound, it has little or no impact on suprathreshold hearing. Perception of loudness, differential thresholds for pitch and loudness, temporal processing, and speech recognition ability are all normal at suprathreshold levels.

Conductive hearing disorders in children are most commonly acquired and transient. Most respond well to medical management and have negligible impact on long-term auditory function. There are two notable exceptions. First, congenital disorders, which are primarily caused by structural deformities or anomalies, can cause significant conductive hearing loss and may not be readily treatable until the child is older and skull growth is complete. Second, some children with recurrent middle ear disorder and resultant fluctuating hearing sensitivity appear to be prone to suprathreshold hearing disorder and language/learning problems, presumably because of the inconsistency of auditory input during the critical period of language development (Uclés, Alonso, Aznar, & Lapresta, 2012; Thornton, Chevallier, Koka, Lupo, & Tollin, 2012).

Causes of Conductive Hearing Disorders

Some common causes of conductive hearing loss are listed in **Table 2.1**.

Acquired Prenatal Conductive Disorders

Outer Ear Anomalies

Atresia is the absence of an opening of the ear or external auditory meatus (for reviews, see Declau, Cremers, & Van de Heyning, 1999; Lambert & Dodson, 1996). It is not uncommon, occurring in ~ 1 in 5,800 to 10,000 births. Bony atresia is the congenital absence of the ear canal caused by a wall of bone separating the external ear from the middle ear. Membranous atresia is the absence of a canal caused by a dense soft

Table 2.1 Some causes of conductive hearing disorder

Acquired prenatal disorders	Acquired postnatal disorders
Atresia	Otitis media with effusion
Middle ear anomalies	Tympanic membrane perforation
	Cholesteatoma
	Excessive cerumen
	Otitis externa

tissue plug obstructing the canal. Atresia is unilateral in ~ 70 to 85% of cases. Atresia can cause maximum conductive hearing loss (~ 60 dB) depending on the density of the blockage.

Other congenital anomalies of the ear canal and outer ear can also cause conductive disorders. An abnormally small or malformed ear is known as microtia. Although microtia does not necessarily cause hearing disorder, it is often associated with abnormalities of the ear canal, including stenosis or narrowing of the ear canal. Stenosis may or may not cause a hearing disorder, but it can cause additional complications, including excessive cerumen accumulation and even cholesteatoma formation.

Middle Ear Anomalies

Abnormalities of the ear canal and auricula are often associated with middle ear anomalies (Declau et al, 1999), although they can occur in isolation. Middle ear anomalies include ossicular dysplasia, fenestral malformations, and congenital cholesteatoma. Ossicular dysplasia can result in fixation, deformity, and disarticulation of the bones, especially the incus and stapes. In congenital stapes fixation, the stapes footplate is fixed into the bony wall of the cochlea at the oval window. Lack of oval window development is an example of fenestral malformation. Congenital cholesteatoma is a cyst that is present in the middle ear space without any evidence of causative factors such as otitis media.

Causes of Prenatal Outer and Middle Ear Anomalies

Congenital outer and middle ear anomalies are often a result of genetic causes. Genetic causes of hearing loss in the pediatric population are addressed in Chapter 3 of this text. In many cases, these anomalies may be one of a constellation of symptoms occurring as part of a syndrome or sequence. Often, prenatal outer and middle ear anomalies may occur with other craniofacial anomalies and/or sensorineural hearing loss. Some of the more common syndromes associated with prenatal outer and middle ear anomalies are Treacher-Collins syndrome (Granström and Tjellström, 1992; Marres, 2002), branchio-oculo-facial (BOF) syndrome (Carter et al, 2012; Raveh, Papsin, & Forte, 2000; Rodríguez Soriano, 2003), Hutchinson-Gilford progeria syndrome (Guardiani et al, 2011), Down syndrome (Kaf, 2011), Townes-Brocks syndrome (Sudo et al, 2010), lacrimo-auriculodental-digital (LADD) syndrome (McKenna, Burke, & Mellan, 2009), oculoauricularvertebral dysplasia (Goldenhar syndrome) (Skarzyński, Porowski, & Podskarbi-Fayette, 2009), Klippel-Feil syndrome (Yildirim, Arslanoğlu, Mahiroğullari, Sahan, & Ozkan, 2008), Cornelia de Lange syndrome (Kim, Kim, Lee, Lee, &

Kim, 2008), and CHARGE (coloboma of the eye, heart anomaly, choanal atresia, retardation, genital and ear anomalies) syndrome (Blake and Prasad, 2006).

Acquired Postnatal Conductive Disorders

Otitis Media with Effusion

Otitis media is a general term to describe inflammation of the middle ear mucous membrane and tympanic membrane (for reviews, see Bluestone, 1998; Shekelle, Takata, & Chan, 2003; Smith & Danner, 2006). Otitis media is the most common diagnosis in patients who make office visits to physicians in the United States. Estimates are that 76 to 95% of all children have one episode of otitis media by 6 years of age. The prevalence is highest during the first 2 years and declines with age. Approximately 60% of those children who have otitis media before the age of 1 year will have six or more bouts within the ensuing 2 years (Gribben, Salkeld, Hoare, & Jones, 2012).

The growing use of pneumococcal conjugate vaccines holds promise for reducing rates of otitis media. (El-Makhzangy, Ismail, Galal, Sobhy, & Hegazy, 2012; Gisselsson-Solén, Melhus, & Hermansson, 2011; Kellner, 2011; Principi, Baggi, & Esposito, 2012). The most commonly associated microbial contributions to otitis media are *Haemophilus influenzae* and *Streptococcus pneumoniae*, with *Moraxella catarrhalis* and others contributing to a lesser extent (Khoramrooz et al, 2012). Vaccination has been associated with a decrease in the percentage of cases of otitis media due to *H. influenzae* and a resultant increase in the relative number of cases of *S. pneumoniae* (Sierra et al, 2011; Coker et al, 2010).

Risk factors for otitis media include young age, Native American or Inuit heritage, anatomic defects, exposure to smoke in the household, male sex, crowded living conditions, poor sanitation, inadequate medical care, eating in prone position, obesity, and day care (Csákányi, Czinner, Spangler, Rogers, & Katona, 2012; Kuhle, Kirk, Ohinmaa, Urschitz, & Veugelers, 2012; Lok, Anteunis, Meesters, Chenault, & Haggard, 2012; Morrissey, 2012). There is also increasing evidence of genetic susceptibility to otitis media (Hafrén, Kentala, Einarsdottir, Kere, & Mattila, 2012; Rye, Blackwell, & Jamieson, 2012).

Otitis media is usually caused by eustachian tube dysfunction secondary to upper respiratory tract infection. Swelling of the nasopharynx results in failure of the eustachian tube to protect, clear, and equalize the pressure of the middle ear space, permitting reflux of infectious secretions from the nasopharynx into the middle ear.

Otitis media is usually defined by the presence or absence of effusion in the middle ear space, the type of effusion, and the time course of the disorder. *Otitis media with effusion* (OME) is the common term used to describe the disorder. The fluid may be referred to as serous (thin, watery, sterile), suppurative (containing pus), purulent (suppurative), mucoid (thick, viscid), and sanguineous (containing blood). Adhesive otitis media involves severe retraction of the tympanic membrane into the middle ear space.

Acute otitis media with effusion is the term describing rapid onset of symptoms of middle ear inflammation, including redness of the tympanic membrane and otalgia. It is usually referred to as acute if it lasts fewer than 3 weeks; subacute if it lasts fewer than 3 months. Middle ear effusion is signaled by bulging and limited mobility of the tympanic membrane, otorrhea, or a fluid level behind the tympanic membrane. Other nonspecific symptoms in an infant or toddler may include fever, excessive crying, or pulling on the ears. Vertigo, dizziness, and imbalance are also common in children with otitis media (McCaslin, Jacobson, & Gruenwald, 2011). Recurrent acute OME consists of repeated episodes of acute otitis media with normal middle ear examinations between episodes. Persistent middle ear effusion is an asymptomatic effusion that persists following treatment for acute OME. The term *chronic* OME is used to describe a condition that lasts longer than 3 months. Chronic suppurative otitis media is a chronic infection of the middle ear and mastoid with a perforation of the tympanic membrane and otorrhea.

OME may resolve spontaneously or may require treatment with antibiotics or pressure-equalization tubes, with varying effects on recurrence rates (Cheong & Hussain, 2012; Kujala et al, 2012). Hearing loss fluctuates with the presence or absence of fluid. Untreated OME can lead to several complications, including cholesterol granuloma, adhesive otitis media, facial paralysis, labyrinthitis, acute mastoiditis, petrositis, meningitis, sigmoid sinus thrombosis, extradural abscess, brain abscess, otic hydrocephalus, and sensorineural hearing loss. In rare cases, especially in developing regions of the world, otitis media can result in death (Monasta et al, 2012).

Among the more common complications are tympanic membrane perforation, tympanosclerosis, and cholesteatoma (Slattery & House, 1998).

Complications of Otitis Media with Effusion

The tympanic membrane may become perforated as a result of OME because of increased pressure from fluid in the middle ear space, or it may be perforated from barotrauma, trauma, myringotomy, or tympanostomy tube placement (Slattery & House, 1998). Although perforations generally heal spontaneously, they may require surgical intervention to repair the damaged membrane. Drainage from perforation may cause a secondary infection of the external auditory canal or auricula. A perforation may or may not result in hearing loss, depending on its size and location.

Tympanosclerosis is a degeneration of collagenous fibrous tissues of the tympanic membrane and is a common sequela of OME, occurring in ~ 10% of cases (Hunter & Margolis, 1997; Slattery & House, 1998). Calcification or ossification may occur and spread to the ossicles in rare cases. Tympanosclerosis can often be observed as a horseshoe-shaped plaque on the tympanic membrane. Tympanosclerosis is not associated with significant hearing loss unless it also involves the ossicular chain.

Cholesteatomas are cysts that contain keratinizing squamous epithelium and are found in the middle ear, mastoid, external auditory canal, or petrous bone (for reviews, see Bennett, Warren, Jackson, & Kaylie, 2006; Semaan & Megerian, 2006; Sie, 1996). Congenital cholesteatomas are present behind an intact tympanic membrane with no history of significant otitis media or eustachian tube dysfunction. Acquired cholesteatomas are more common and are usually a consequence of chronic otitis media. Cholesteatomas can be destructive as they grow and compete for space with the normal structures of the areas they occupy. Conductive hearing loss varies as a function of the structures involved. Average air–bone gaps are estimated to be 30 to 38 dB. Allowed to grow unchecked, a cholesteatoma can erode the middle ear ossicles and cause ossicular discontinuity, creating additional conductive hearing loss. In advanced cases, sensorineural hearing loss can also occur because of cochlear erosion.

Excessive Cerumen

Excessive cerumen is an accumulation of ear wax in the ear canal (for reviews, see Roeser & Ballachanda, 1997; Roeser & Roland, 1992). Impacted cerumen completely occludes the ear canal. Excessive cerumen occurs in ~ 10% of children, and it may have an even greater incidence, up to 28 to 36%, in children with developmental delays. Children who have a history of cerumen impaction are also more likely to have more otitis media with effusion and a higher rate of associated sensorineural hearing loss (Olusanya, 2003). A high-frequency conductive hearing loss can occur when the ear canal is 80 to 95% occluded. A low-frequency conductive loss occurs with total occlusion of the ear canal.

Otitis Externa

Otitis externa is the broad term for inflammation or infection of the external auditory canal and auricula (for reviews, see Bojrab, Bruderly, & Abdulrazzak, 1996; Osguthorpe & Nielsen, 2006; Rosenfeld et al, 2006). Otitis externa rarely causes hearing disorder, except in cases where it causes stenosis of the external auditory meatus. Acute diffuse otitis externa, also known as swimmer's ear, is one example of otitis externa. It is a bacterial infection that causes itching, tenderness, and pain and may include hearing loss and aural fullness as the external auditory canal decreases in size with swelling. Several fungal, viral, and bacterial infections of the external ear have been reported; rarely, though, do they result in hearing disorder. Complications of otitis externa may include ear canal stenosis, myringitis, and tympanic membrane perforation. Ototoxicity from topical otic preparations for treatment of external otitis can also occur.

Table 2.2 Some causes of sensory hearing disorder

Acquired prenatal disorders	Acquired perinatal and postnatal disorders
Inner ear anomalies	PPHN/ECMO
Cytomegalovirus	Meningitis
Syphilis	Autoimmune inner-ear disorder
Rubella	
Toxoplasmosis	Mumps
	Measles
	Ototoxicity

◆ Sensory Hearing Disorders

Nature of Sensory Hearing Disorders

Sensory, or sensorineural, hearing disorder is caused by a failure in the cochlear transduction of sound from the mechanical vibrations of the middle ear to neural impulses in the eighth cranial nerve. Sensory disorders can occur from any number of changes in cochlear structure and function, but the most vulnerable structures seem to be the outer hair cells of the organ of Corti, which are responsible for the exquisite sensitivity and fine-tuning of the cochlea.

Hearing sensitivity loss is the hallmark of a sensory disorder and ranges from mild to profound. Sensorineural hearing loss is usually permanent, although it can fluctuate in some cases and may be treatable in others. Depending on the cause, the loss may also be progressive.

Disorders of cochlear processes result in reduced sensitivity of the cochlear receptor cells, reduced frequency resolution, and reduced dynamic range. These complex changes in cochlear function can have a significant negative impact on suprathreshold hearing. The cause of most congenital hearing loss is genetic and is described in Chapter 3.

Causes of Sensory Hearing Disorders

Some common causes of sensory hearing disorder are listed in **Table 2.2**.

Acquired Prenatal Sensory Disorders

Inner Ear Anomalies

Inner ear malformations occur when development of the membranous and/or bony labyrinth is arrested during fetal development (Reilly, Lalwani, & Jackler, 1998). Although in many cases the arrest of development is genetic, some cases are the result of teratogenic influences during pregnancy (Irving &

Ruben, 1998), including viral infections such as rubella, drugs such as thalidomide, and fetal radiation exposure.

Inner ear malformations can be divided into those in which both the osseous and membranous labyrinths are abnormal and those in which only the membranous labyrinth is abnormal. The former anomalies are better understood because they can be readily identified with scanning techniques, although magnetic resonance imaging (MRI) has become a useful tool for imaging of the soft tissue structures as well (Huang, Zdanski, & Castillo, 2012; Joshi, Navlekar, Kishore, Reddy, & Kumar, 2012).

Included in the malformations of both membranous and osseous labyrinths are complete labyrinthine aplasia (Michel deformity), common cavity defect, cochlear aplasia and hypoplasia, and Mondini defect (Reilly et al, 1998). Michel deformity is a very rare malformation characterized by complete absence of membranous and osseous inner ear structures, resulting in total deafness. Common-cavity malformation comprises about one-fourth of all cochlear malformations (Casselman et al, 2001). It is a membranous and osseous malformation in which the cochlea is not differentiated from the vestibule, usually resulting in substantial hearing loss. Cochlear aplasia is a rare malformation consisting of complete absence of the membranous and osseous cochlea and no auditory function, but presence of semicircular canals and vestibule. Cochlear hypoplasia is a malformation in which less than one full turn of the cochlea is developed. Cochlear hypoplasia accounts for ~ 15% of cochlear malformations. Mondini malformation, an incomplete partition of the cochlea, is a relatively common inner ear malformation in which the cochlea contains only ~ 1.5 turns, and the osseous spiral lamina is partially or completely absent. The resulting hearing loss is highly variable.

Other abnormalities of both the osseous and membranous labyrinth include anomalies of the semicircular canals, the internal auditory canals, and the cochlear and vestibular aqueducts. One example of the latter is large vestibular aqueduct syndrome, a malformation of the temporal bone that is associated with early-onset hearing loss and vestibular disorders. Hearing loss is usually progressive, profound, and bilateral (Cox & MacDonald, 1996). Large vestibular aqueduct syndrome is often associated with Mondini malformation.

Included in malformations limited to the membranous labyrinth are complete membranous labyrinth dysplasia (Bing Siebenmann) and two forms of partial dysplasia, cochleosaccular dysplasia (Scheibe aplasia) and cochlear basal turn dysplasia (Alexander aplasia). The Bing Siebenmann malformation is a rare malformation that results in complete lack of development of the membranous labyrinth. Scheibe aplasia is a common inner ear abnormality in which there is failure of the organ of Corti to develop fully, collapse of the cochlear duct, adherence of the vestibular membrane to the limbus, and degeneration of the stria vascularis. Alexander aplasia is an abnormal development of the basal turn of the cochlea, with typical development in the remainder of the cochlea, resulting in low-frequency residual hearing.

In recent years, there has been greater success with cochlear implantation in cases of deafness caused by these deformities, despite the unusual anatomy (Jeong & Kim, 2012; Sennaroglu, 2010).

Cytomegalovirus

Cytomegalovirus (CMV) is the largest known member of the human herpesvirus family and is the most common fetal viral illness (for review, see Fowler & Boppana, 2006; Gaytant, Steegers, Semmekrot, Merkus, & Galama, 2002; Pass, 2005; Pass, Fowler, Boppana, Britt, & Stagno, 2006). Congenital infection is the result of transplacental transmission of CMV and is known as cytomegalic inclusion disease. Sensorineural hearing loss is the most common clinical finding of congenital CMV. Other findings include microcephaly, petechiae (small purple spots on a body surface), intrauterine growth retardation, enlargement of the liver and spleen, and inflammation of the choroid and retina (chorioretinitis). Hearing loss is of variable severity and can be bilateral or unilateral. The most commonly found configuration is flat (Dahle et al, 2000). Threshold fluctuations are common (more than 20% of cases), and hearing loss is often progressive (more than 15%). Petechiae and intrauterine growth retardation in symptomatic neonates are factors that independently predict hearing loss (Rivera et al, 2002). Approximately 10 to 15% of congenitally infected infants are symptomatic at birth. Children with symptomatic congenital CMV are at greater risk for hearing impairment (22–65%) than those with asymptomatic infection (6–23%), and hearing loss tends to appear earlier and with greater severity in these patients (Fowler & Boppana, 2006).

Recent studies suggest that certain antiviral medications or hyperimmunoglobulin therapies may have a protective effect against hearing loss if administered in the prenatal or neonatal periods (Buonsenso et al, 2012; del Rosal et al, 2012; Stronati, Lombardi, Garofoli, Villani, & Regazzi, 2013; Japanese Congenital Cytomegalovirus Infection Immunoglobulin Fetal Therapy Study Group, 2012; Visentin et al, 2012).

Congenital Syphilis

Congenital syphilis is a bacterial infection that is transmitted from mother to fetus in utero or through contact with a genital lesion during delivery (for review, see Ingall, Sanchez, & Baker, 2006; Irving & Ruben, 1998; Pletcher & Cheung, 2003). The disease occurs in 11.2 cases per 100,000 live births (Centers for Disease Control and Prevention, 2004). Congenital syphilis is categorized by its time of occurrence into early and late stages. In early congenital syphilis, occurring within the first 2 years of life, severity can range from severe multiorgan involvement to minor symptoms. Although rarely observed in the United States, late congenital syphilis includes the set of symptoms known as Hutchinson's triad: small, notched teeth; hearing loss; and interstitial keratitis. Typical hearing loss is a rapid symmetric progression from high-frequency sensory loss to complete bilateral deafness. Hearing loss can also involve neural or conductive components. Vestibular function may also be severely affected. The Hennebert sign, in which nystagmus is observed as a result of pressure applied to the external auditory canal, is often found in otosyphilis.

Maternal Rubella

Maternal rubella occurs when an infected mother transmits the rubella virus to the fetus (for review, see Banatvala & Brown, 2004; Cooper & Alford, 2006; Irving & Ruben, 1998). Expression of symptoms of maternal rubella infection, called congenital rubella syndrome or Gregg syndrome, includes a wide variety of defects, usually affecting hearing, vision, and heart function, and often involving mental retardation and microcephaly. Subclinical infections are more common than those that are symptomatic at birth. However, 70% of infants who are asymptomatic at birth will develop symptoms within the first 5 years of life. Hearing loss is the most common manifestation of congenital rubella, occurring in up to 80% of infected children. Hearing loss ranges from unilateral mild loss to bilateral profound deafness; severe bilateral losses are more common. Configuration of the hearing loss is usually flat, and hearing sensitivity may be asymmetric. Children with normal pure tone thresholds may demonstrate abnormal auditory brainstem responses (Niedzielska, Katska, & Szymula, 2000). Once transmission has occurred, fetal infection is chronic. Infection tends to persist throughout fetal life and after birth and to continue to cause pathology in the child.

Toxoplasmosis

Toxoplasmosis is an infection caused by the parasite *Toxoplasma gondii* (for review, see Jones, Lopez, Wilson, Schulkin, & Gibbs, 2001; Rorman, Zamir, Rilkis, & Ben-David, 2006). The parasite can be transmitted to humans by ingestion of raw or inadequately cooked infected meat or foods that have come in contact with infected meat, ingestion of parasites that cats have passed in their feces, or transplacental transmission of the infection from a woman to her fetus. Despite increasing probability of infection with pregnancy progression, consequences are more severe when fetal infection occurs in early stages of pregnancy. Although most newborns (70 to 90%) infected with congenital toxoplasmosis are asymptomatic at birth, up to 80% of these children develop sequelae later in life. Those who are symptomatic often have a classic triad of chorioretinitis, intracranial calcifications, and hydrocephalus. The disease course may also include cognitive abnormalities of variable severity, seizures, or learning disabilities with onset after several months or years. Auditory disorder can occur from mastoid and cochlear inflammation and involvement of the auditory brainstem. The resulting disorder is a sensory or neural hearing loss that may range from mild unilateral loss (Wilson, Remington, Stagno, & Reynolds, 1980) to bilateral deafness (Sever et al, 1988).

Acquired Perinatal and Postnatal Sensory Disorders

Persistent Pulmonary Hypertension of the Newborn/Extracorporeal Membrane Oxygenation

Persistent pulmonary hypertension of the newborn (PPHN), also known as persistent fetal circulation, is a condition wherein the infant's blood flow bypasses the lungs, thereby eliminating oxygen supply to the organs of the body (for review, see Perreault, 2006; Verklan, 2006). PPHN is associated with perinatal respiratory problems such as meconium aspiration or pneumonia. Sensorineural hearing loss is a common complication of PPHN and has been found in from 32% (Kawashiro, Tsuchihashi, Koga, Kawano, & Itoh, 1996) to 37% of surviving children. Hearing loss ranges from high-frequency unilateral loss to severe to profound bilateral loss and is progressive in many cases.

PPHN is treated by administration of oxygen or oxygen and nitric oxide via a mechanical ventilator.

Extracorporeal membrane oxygenation (ECMO) is a treatment for PPHN that involves diverting blood from the heart and lungs to an external bypass where oxygen and carbon dioxide are exchanged before the blood reenters the body. When ECMO is applied as part of respiratory management, it has been associated with hearing loss in up to 75% of cases (Kawashiro et al, 1996; Lasky, Wiorek, & Becker, 1998; Mann & Adams, 1998). Hearing loss is often progressive.

Meningitis

Meningitis is an inflammation of the membranes that surround the brain and spinal cord. There are three types of meningitis: bacterial, aseptic, and viral. The greatest frequency of hearing loss occurs in cases of bacterial meningitis (Bao & Wong, 1998); estimates range from 5 to 35% of cases. Other common signs and symptoms of bacterial meningitis include fever, seizures, neck stiffness, and altered mental status. (For reviews, see Chávez-Bueno & McCracken, 2005, Sáez-Llorens & McCracken, 2003.) Vestibular function may be compromised as well (Wiener-Vacher, Obeid, & Abou-Elew, 2012). Hearing disorder ranges from mild to profound sensitivity loss or total deafness, may be unilateral or bilateral, and may be progressive. Most involvement is thought to be cochlear, but central auditory involvement may occur in some individuals (Bedford et al, 2001; Cherukupally & Eavey, 2004; Hodgson et al, 2001; Hugosson et al, 1997; Koomen et al, 2003; Kutz, Simon, Chennupati, Giannoni, & Manolidis, 2006). Hearing loss is usually permanent, although there have been reports of some recovery of hearing over time in some individuals (Bao & Wong, 1998). Cochlear osteoneogenesis, or bony growth in the cochlea, may occur following meningitis, complicating possible cochlear implantation (Dodds, Tyszkiewicz, & Ramsden, 1997; Fishman & Holliday, 2000). The use of magnetic resonance imaging may have utility in predicting hearing loss prior to onset and prior to ossification, which may have a positive impact on treatment planning (Kopelovich, Germiller, Laury, Shah, & Pollock, 2011). There have been reports of meningitis following cochlear implantation, especially with use of a positioner during implantation (Callanan & Poje, 2004). However, there is a strong association between cochlear deformities, particularly Michel deformity, and meningitis that may be independent of cochlear implantation (Anandi, Tullu, Bhatia, & Agrawal, 2012; Lien et al, 2011).

Autoimmune Inner Ear Disease

Autoimmune inner ear disease (AIED) is a syndrome of potentially reversible, bilateral, rapidly progressive, and often fluctuating sensory hearing loss that may be associated with vestibular symptoms mimicking Meniere's disease (for review, see Bovo, Aimoni, & Martini, 2006; Harris, 1998; Matteson et al, 2003; Ryan, Harris, & Keithley, 2002). Symptoms are thought to be consequences of immune-mediated inflammation in the inner ear. The disorder may be specific to the ear or may occur as a manifestation of a systemic immune-mediated inflammatory disorder, such as rheumatoid arthritis, systemic lupus erythematosus, inflammatory bowel disease, polyarteritis nodosa, or Cogan syndrome. Hearing sensitivity is generally responsive to immunosuppressive drugs, such as steroids. AIED is associated with sensory hearing loss that is generally bilateral, asymmetric, and rapidly progressive.

Viral Infections

Mumps is a viral infection that attacks a variety of organs, especially the salivary glands (for a review of mumps and hearing loss, see McKenna, 1997). Although the incidence in the United States of hearing loss associated with mumps is low because of vaccination, it continues to occur in other areas of the world (Kawashima et al, 2005), and outbreaks have occurred in the United States as recently as 2006 (Centers for Disease Control and Prevention, 2006). Infection following vaccination for mumps has also been known to occur (Asatryan, et al, 2008). Mumps has historically been the most common cause associated with unilateral acquired sensorineural hearing loss in children. The typical pattern of sensory hearing loss is unilateral and profound, with sudden onset. Endolymphatic hydrops (Meniere disease) is also a common manifestation of mumps virus.

Measles is a highly contagious viral illness that characteristically causes symptoms of rash, cough, fever, conjunctivitis, photophobia, and Koplik spots (white spots on the membranous surfaces of the mouth) (McKenna, 1997; Rima & Duprex, 2006). Hearing loss is a common complication of measles. Before vaccination in the United States became widespread, measles accounted for 5 to 10% of all cases of profound, bilateral sensorineural hearing loss. Measles is still a significant cause of hearing loss and deafness in other parts of the world (Lasisi, Ayodele, & Ijaduola, 2006). Sensory hearing loss from measles virus is typically severe, permanent, and bilateral, although milder hearing loss can occur. Conductive hearing loss from otitis media is also a common complication of measles, which may be due to immunosuppression following viral infection. Localized measles virus in the otic capsule is also hypothesized to be a causative factor in later development of otosclerosis (Karosi & Sziklai, 2010; Markou & Goudakos, 2009; Neidermeyer & Arnold, 2008; Schrauwen & Van Camp, 2010).

Ototoxicity

Ototoxicity is hearing loss from the toxic effects of drugs on the inner ear (Irving & Ruben, 1998; Rol & Cohen, 1998; Roland, 2004; Rybak & Whitworth, 2005). Aminoglycoside antibiotics (streptomycin, gentamicin, dihydrostreptomycin, neomycin, kanamycin, erythromycin, and vancomycin), loop diuretics (furosemide), antineoplastic agents (cisplatin), salicylates, and antimalarial drugs (quinine) can all damage the cochlea. Effects relate to the level of the drug in the system, synergistic effects of these drugs in combination, potentiation of effect caused by coexisting renal disease, and hereditary susceptibility in the case of aminoglycosides. Children and neonates are considered to be at lower risk for ototoxicity than are adults in most cases. One exception is cisplatin-induced hearing loss, which has a higher incidence and increased severity in children, causing hearing loss in ~ 60% of pediatric cases (Brock et al, 2012). Cisplatin ototoxicity may also have additional risk factors, including sex, age (Yancey et al, 2012), and genetic susceptibility (Oldenburg, Fosså, & Ikdahl, 2008; Ross et al, 2009). Hearing loss from ototoxicity is generally symmetric sensory loss that progresses from higher to lower frequencies with increased drug exposure. Because of this pattern, monitoring for ototoxicity via distortion-product otoacoustic emissions may be particularly valuable for children (Bhagat et al, 2010). Some hearing loss also involves neural components with certain drug classes.

◆ Neural Hearing Disorders

Nature of Neural Hearing Disorders

Neural hearing disorders tend to be divided into two groups: retrocochlear disorders and auditory processing disorders. When a disorder is caused by an active, measurable disease process, such as a neoplasm, or from damage caused by trauma or stroke, it is often referred to as a retrocochlear disorder. That is, retrocochlear disorders result from structural lesions of the nervous system. Neural hearing disorders in children from retrocochlear pathology are relatively rare. When they do occur, the hearing disorder is characterized by patterns of abnormality consistent with those found in adults with similar lesions (Bergman, Costeff, Koren, Koifman, & Reshef, 1984; Goodglass, 1967; Jerger, 1987). Children with intra- and extraaxial neoplasms have abnormal, degraded monotic speech perception, and those with temporal lobe lesions have abnormal dichotic speech perception. Although most children and adults tend to exhibit similar patterns of abnormality, some children with central nervous system lesions may have auditory deficits that are more generalized and less severe than in adults with similar lesions (Woods, 1984). Regardless, the morbidity and mortality of tumors in young children is significantly greater than in adults.

When an impairment is due to developmental disorder or delay, it is often referred to as an auditory processing disorder (APD). That is, APDs result from functional lesions of the nervous system. The term APD is also used to describe the functional consequence of a retrocochlear disorder.

The most common symptom of neural hearing disorder is difficulty extracting a signal of interest from a background of noise. Although the basis for the disorder is not always clear, it most often results in an inability to structure auditory space appropriately. This spatial hearing deficit usually translates into difficulty hearing in noise, which becomes particularly obvious in a classroom setting. Another common symptom is difficulty localizing a sound source, especially in the presence of background noise. Perhaps as a consequence of these symptoms, children and their parents and teachers are also likely to describe behaviors such as inattentiveness and distractibility. Auditory processing disorders are discussed in detail in Chapter 16.

Causes of Neural Hearing Disorder

Some common causes of neural hearing disorder are listed in **Table 2.3**.

Auditory Neuropathy Spectrum Disorder

Auditory neuropathy spectrum disorder is a term that is used to describe disorders that are operationally defined based on a constellation of clinical findings. That constellation varies necessarily as a function of age. In older children, auditory neuropathy is defined by an absent auditory brainstem response (ABR), poor speech perception, varying levels of hearing sensitivity loss, absence of acoustic reflexes, and a preservation of some cochlear function as evidenced

Table 2.3 Some causes of neural hearing disorder

Causes of neural disorders
Neoplasms
Hydrocephalus
Hypoxia
Hyperbilirubinemia

by the preservation of otoacoustic emissions (OAEs) and/or cochlear microphonics. In infants, auditory neuropathy is defined by absent ABR and preserved OAEs and/or cochlear microphonics (Hayes & Sininger, 2008).

It is becoming apparent that the term *auditory neuropathy*, as it is defined clinically, may represent at least two fairly different disorders, one sensory and the other neural (Rapin & Gravel, 2006). The auditory neuropathy of sensory origin—AN(S)—is probably a sensory hearing disorder that represents a transduction problem, with the failure of the cochlea to transmit signals to the auditory nerve. The most likely origin of AN(S) is the inner hair cells, a concept that has been reported both in patient populations (Konrádsson, 1996; Loundon et al, 2005) and in animal models (Harrison, 1998). Preservation of the otoacoustic emissions and cochlear microphonics represents normal function of outer hair cells without any inner hair cells to sensitize. In cases of AN(S), the absence of an ABR is a reflection of the sensitivity loss of the system and accurately predicts substantial hearing loss. Hearing loss from AN(S) acts like any other sensitivity loss in terms of its influence on speech and language acquisition and its amenability to hearing aids and cochlear implants.

Auditory neuropathy of neural origin—AN(N)—was first described as a specific disorder of the auditory nerve that results in a loss of synchrony of neural firing (Starr, Picton, Sininger, Hood, & Berlin, 1996). Because of the nature of the disorder, it is also referred to as auditory dys-synchrony (Berlin, Hood, & Rose, 2001). The cause of auditory neuropathy is often unknown, although it may be observed in cases of syndromic peripheral pathologies (e.g., Friedreich ataxia, Charcot-Marie-Tooth syndrome). The age of onset is usually before 10 years. Hearing sensitivity loss ranges from normal to profound and is most often flat or reverse-sloped in configuration. Hearing loss often fluctuates and is progressive in some children. Speech perception is often substantially poorer than what would be expected from the audiogram (Sininger & Oba, 2001). AN(N) may not be as amenable to conventional amplification and implant treatment as AN(S).

Other Neural Hearing Disorders

Neoplasm

Unlike those in adults, tumors of the posterior fossa in children are less likely to be acoustic schwannoma and more likely to be intrinsic tumors, such as gliomas and medulloblastomas (for review, see Angeli & Brackmann, 1998). These benign tumors of the cerebellopontine angle affect the auditory system when they impinge on the eighth cranial nerve. The most common form of acoustic tumor in children is that found in association with neurofibromatosis type 2 (NF2). NF2 is characterized by bilateral cochleovestibular schwannomas. The schwannomas are faster-growing and more virulent than the unilateral type. This is an autosomal dominant disease and is associated with other intracranial tumors. Hearing loss in NF2 is not particularly different from that due to a unilateral type of schwannoma, except that it is bilateral and often progresses more rapidly.

Hydrocephalus

The cause of neural hearing disorders in children has also been attributed to more diffuse sources, including hydrocephalus, hypoxia, and hyperbilirubinemia. In hydrocephalus, the most common finding is one of neuromaturational delay of the auditory system as measured on the ABR. This is usually due to enlarged ventricles and is not associated with permanent changes in auditory function.

Hypoxia

Hypoxia is a deficiency in the amount of oxygen in the body. Hearing disorder is often associated with hypoxia, although the effects of respiratory distress in neonates are difficult to separate from other possible factors, such as kernicterus, treatment with ototoxic medications, and low birth weight (Roizen, 2003; Yoshikawa, Ikeda, Kudo, & Kobayashi, 2004). Disorders of auditory neural function are often diffuse, although progressive sensorineural hearing loss can occur as a result.

Hyperbilirubinemia

Hyperbilirubinemia is an excess of bilirubin in the blood that can be caused by many factors (for review, see Shapiro, 2003). Hyperbilirubinemia is associated with auditory neuropathy and other neural hearing disorders. The clinical spectrum of bilirubin-induced auditory toxicity ranges from transient auditory dysfunction to permanent sensory hearing loss. Audiometric findings include predominantly high-frequency bilateral and symmetric hearing loss with recruitment and abnormal loudness growth. Auditory nerve and generalized auditory brainstem dysfunction may occur (Amin, 2004; Sharma et al, 2006). Other more diffuse APDs have also been associated with hyperbilirubinemia.

Discussion Questions

1. What are the differences in expectations for suprathreshold hearing among conductive, sensory, and neural hearing loss?

2. What are some possible effects on speech and language development from acquired conductive hearing losses, such as otitis media with effusion?

3. What diseases and disorders may cause progressive hearing loss in childhood? How might knowledge about the possibility of a progressive hearing loss influence assessment and follow-up decisions?

4. What types of drugs cause ototoxicity? How might monitoring of hearing during treatment with ototoxic medication contribute to preservation of hearing?

5. How are the two types of neural hearing disorders—retrocochlear disorders and auditory processing disorders—different from one another?

References

Angeli, S. I., & Brackmann, D. E. (1998). Posterior fossa tumors in children. In A. K. Lalwani and K. M. Grundfast (Eds.), Pediatric otology and neurotology (pp. 489–504). Philadelphia, PA: Lippincott-Raven.

Amin, S. B. (2004). Clinical assessment of bilirubin-induced neurotoxicity in premature infants. Seminars in Perinatology, 28(5), 340–347.

Anandi, S., Tullu, M. S., Bhatia, S., & Agrawal, M. (2012). Mondini dysplasia as a cause for recurrent bacterial meningitis: an early diagnosis. Journal of Child Neurology, 27(8), 1052–1055.

Asatryan, A., Pool, V., Chen, R. T., Kohl, K. S., Davis, R. L., & Iskander, J. K.; VAERS team (2008). Live attenuated measles and mumps viral strain-containing vaccines and hearing loss: Vaccine Adverse Event Reporting System (VAERS), United States, 1990–2003. Vaccine, 26(9), 1166–1172.

Banatvala, J. E., & Brown, D. W. G. (2004). Rubella. Lancet, 363(9415), 1127–1137.

Bao, X., & Wong, V. (1998). Brainstem auditory-evoked potential evaluation in children with meningitis. Pediatric Neurology, 19(2), 109–112.

Bedford, H., de Louvois, J., Halket, S., Peckham, C., Hurley, R., & Harvey, D. (2001). Meningitis in infancy in England and Wales: follow up at age 5 years. BMJ (Clinical Research Ed.), 323(7312), 533–536.

Bennett, M., Warren, F., Jackson, G. C., & Kaylie, D. (2006). Congenital cholesteatoma: theories, facts, and 53 patients. Otolaryngologic Clinics of North America, 39(6), 1081–1094.

Bergman, M., Costeff, H., Koren, V., Koifman, N., & Reshef, A. (1984). Auditory perception in early lateralized brain damage. Cortex, 20(2), 233–242.

Berlin, C., Hood, L., & Rose, K. (2001). On renaming auditory neuropathy as auditory dys-synchrony. Audiology Today, 13, 15–17.

Bhagat, S. P., Bass, J. K., White, S. T., Qaddoumi, I., Wilson, M. W., Wu, J., & Rodriguez-Galindo, C. (2010). Monitoring carboplatin ototoxicity with distortion-product otoacoustic emissions in children with retinoblastoma. International Journal of Pediatric Otorhinolaryngology, 74(10), 1156–1163.

Blake, K. D., & Prasad, C. (2006). CHARGE syndrome. Orphanet Journal of Rare Diseases, 1, 34.

Bluestone, C. D. (1998). Otitis media: a spectrum of diseases. In A. K. Lalwani and K. M. Grundfast (Eds.), Pediatric otology and neurotology (pp. 233–240). Philadelphia, PA: Lippincott-Raven.

Bojrab, D. I., Bruderly, T., & Abdulrazzak, Y. (1996). Otitis externa. Otolaryngologic Clinics of North America, 29(5), 761–782.

Bovo, R., Aimoni, C., & Martini, A. (2006). Immune-mediated inner ear disease. Acta Oto-Laryngologica, 126(10), 1012–1021.

Brock, P. R., Knight, K. R., Freyer, D. R., Campbell, K. C., Steyger, P. S., Blakley, B. W., . . . Neuwelt, E. A. (2012). Platinum-induced ototoxicity in children: a consensus review on mechanisms, predisposition, and protection, including a new International Society of Pediatric Oncology Boston ototoxicity scale. Journal of Clinical Oncology, 30(19), 2408–2417.

Buonsenso, D., Serranti, D., Gargiullo, L., Ceccarelli, M., Ranno, O., & Valentini, P. (2012). Congenital cytomegalovirus infection: current strategies and future perspectives. European Review for Medical and Pharmacological Sciences, 16(7), 919–935.

Callanan, V., & Poje, C. (2004). Cochlear implantation and meningitis. International Journal of Pediatric Otorhinolaryngology, 68(5), 545–550.

Carter, M. T., Blaser, S., Papsin, B., Meschino, W., Reardon, W., Klatt, R., . . . Chitayat, D. (2012). Middle and inner ear malformations in mutation-proven branchio-oculo-facial (BOF) syndrome: case series and review of the literature. American Journal of Medical Genetics. Part A, 158A(8), 1977–1981.

Casselman, J. W., Offeciers, E. F., De Foer, B., Govaerts, P., Kuhweide, R., & Somers, T. (2001). CT and MR imaging of congenital abnormalities of the inner ear and internal auditory canal. European Journal of Radiology, 40(2), 94–104.

Centers for Disease Control and Prevention. (2004). Congenital syphilis—United States, 2002. Morbidity & Mortality Weekly Report, 53, 716–719.

Centers for Disease Control and Prevention. (2006). Brief report: update: mumps activity–United States, January 1–October 7, 2006. Morbidity & Mortality Weekly Report, 55, 1152–1153.

Chávez-Bueno, S., & McCracken, G. H., Jr. (2005). Bacterial meningitis in children. Pediatric Clinics of North America, 52(3), 795–810.

Cheong, K. H., & Hussain, S. S. (2012). Management of recurrent acute otitis media in children: systematic review of the effect of different interventions on otitis media recurrence, recurrence frequency and total recurrence time. The Journal of Laryngology and Otology, 126(9), 874–885.

Cherukupally, S. R., & Eavey, R. (2004). Vaccine-preventable pediatric postmeningitic sensorineural hearing loss in southern India. Otolaryngology—Head and Neck Surgery, 130(3), 339–343.

Coker, T. R., Chan, L. S., Newberry, S. J., Limbos, M. A., Suttorp, M. J., Shekelle, P. G., & Takata, G. S. (2010). Diagnosis, microbial epidemiology, and antibiotic treatment of acute otitis media in children: a systematic review. Journal of the American Medical Association, 304(19), 2161–2169.

Cooper, L. Z., & Alford, C. A. (2006). Rubella. In J. S. Remington, J. O. Klein, C. B. Wilson, & C. J. Baker (Eds.), Infectious diseases of the fetus and newborn infant (pp. 893–926). Philadelphia, PA: Elsevier Saunders.

Cox, L. C., & MacDonald, C. B. (1996). Large vestibular aqueduct syndrome: a tutorial and three case studies. Journal of the American Academy of Audiology, 7(2), 71–76.

Csákányi, Z., Czinner, A., Spangler, J., Rogers, T., & Katona, G. (2012). Relationship of environmental tobacco smoke to otitis media (OM) in children. International Journal of Pediatric Otorhinolaryngology, 76(7), 989–993.

Dahle, A. J., Fowler, K. B., Wright, J. D., Boppana, S. B., Britt, W. J., & Pass, R. F. (2000). Longitudinal investigation of hearing disorders in children with congenital cytomegalovirus. Journal of the American Academy of Audiology, 11(5), 283–290.

Declau, F., Cremers, C., & Van de Heyning, P.; Study Group on Otological Malformations and Hearing Impairment (1999). Diagnosis and management strategies in congenital atresia of the external auditory canal. British Journal of Audiology, 33(5), 313–327.

del Rosal, T., Baquero-Artigao, F., Blázquez, D., Noguera-Julian, A., Moreno-Pérez, D., Reyes, A., & Vilas, J. (2012). Treatment of symptomatic congenital cytomegalovirus infection beyond the neonatal period. Journal of Clinical Virology, 55(1), 72–74.

Dodds, A., Tyszkiewicz, E., & Ramsden, R. (1997). Cochlear implantation after bacterial meningitis: the dangers of delay. Archives of Disease in Childhood, 76(2), 139–140.

El-Makhzangy, A. M., Ismail, N. M., Galal, S. B., Sobhy, T. S., & Hegazy, A. A. (2012). Can vaccination against pneumococci prevent otitis media with effusion? European Archives of Oto-Rhino-Laryngology, 269(9), 2021–2026.

Fishman, A. J., & Holliday, R. A. (2000). Principles of cochlear implant imaging. In S. B. Waltzman & N. L. Cohen (Eds.), Cochlear implants (pp. 79–107). New York, NY: Thieme Medical Publishers, Inc.

Fowler, K. B., & Boppana, S. B. (2006). Congenital cytomegalovirus (CMV) infection and hearing deficit. Journal of Clinical Virology, 35(2), 226–231.

Gaytant, M. A., Steegers, E. A. P., Semmekrot, B. A., Merkus, H. M., & Galama, J. M. D. (2002). Congenital cytomegalovirus infection: review of the epidemiology and outcome. Obstetrical & Gynecological Survey, 57(4), 245–256.

Gisselsson-Solén, M., Melhus, A., & Hermansson, A. (2011). Pneumococcal vaccination in children at risk of developing recurrent acute otitis media—a randomized trial. Acta Paediatrica (Oslo, Norway), 100(10), 1354–1358.

Goodglass, H. (1967). Binaural digit presentation and early lateral brain damage. Cortex, 3, 295–306.

Granström, G., & Tjellström, A. (1992). Ear deformities in mandibulofacial dysostosis. Acta Oto-Laryngologica. Supplementum, 493(Supplement), 113–117.

Gribben, B., Salkeld, L. J., Hoare, S., & Jones, H. F. (2012). The incidence of acute otitis media in New Zealand children under five years of age in the primary care setting. Journal of Primary Health Care, 4(3), 205–212.

Guardiani, E., Zalewski, C., Brewer, C., Merideth, M., Introne, W., Smith, A. C., . . . Kim, H. J. (2011). Otologic and audiologic manifestations of Hutchinson-Gilford progeria syndrome. The Laryngoscope, 121(10), 2250–2255.

Hafrén, L., Kentala, E., Einarsdottir, E., Kere, J., & Mattila, P. S. (2012). Current knowledge of the genetics of otitis media. Current Allergy and Asthma Reports, 12(6), 582–589.

Harris, J. P. (1998). Autoimmune inner ear diseases. In A. K. Lalwani & K. M. Grundfast (Eds.), Pediatric otology and neurotology (pp. 405–419). Philadelphia, PA: Lippincott-Raven.

Harrison, R. V. (1998). An animal model of auditory neuropathy. Ear and Hearing, 19(5), 355–361.

Hayes, D., & Sininger, Y. S. (2008). Guidelines for identification and management of infants and young children with auditory neuropathy spectrum disorder. Aurora, CO: The Children's Hospital.

Hill, M. (2011). Embryology of the ear. In R. Seewald & A. M. Tharpe (Eds.), Comprehensive handbook of pediatric audiology (pp. 3–22). San Diego, CA: Plural.

Hodgson, A., Smith, T., Gagneux, S., Akumah, I., Adjuik, M., Pluschke, G., . . . Genton, B. (2001). Survival and sequelae of meningococcal meningitis in Ghana. International Journal of Epidemiology, 30(6), 1440–1446.

Huang, B. Y., Zdanski, C., & Castillo, M. (2012). Pediatric sensorineural hearing loss, part 1: Practical aspects for neuroradiologists. AJNR. American Journal of Neuroradiology, 33(2), 211–217.

Hugosson, S., Carlsson, E., Borg, E., Brorson, L. O., Langeroth, G., & Olcén, P. (1997). Audiovestibular and neuropsychological outcome of adults who had recovered from childhood bacterial meningitis. International Journal of Pediatric Otorhinolaryngology, 42(2), 149–167.

Hunter, L. L., & Margolis, R. H. (1997). Effects of tympanic membrane abnormalities on auditory function. Journal of the American Academy of Audiology, 8(6), 431–446.

Ingall, D., Sanchez, P. J., & Baker, C. J. (2006). Syphilis. In J. S. Remington, J. O. Klein, C. B. Wilson, & C. J. Baker (Eds.), Infectious diseases of the fetus and newborn infant (pp. 545–580). Philadelphia, PA: Elsevier Saunders.

Irving, R. M., & Ruben, R. J. (1998). The acquired hearing losses of childhood. In A. K. Lalwani & K. M. Grundfast (Eds.), Pediatric otology and neurotology (pp. 375–385). Philadelphia, PA: Lippincott-Raven.

Japanese Congenital Cytomegalovirus Infection Immunoglobulin Fetal Therapy Study Group. (2012). A trial of immunoglobulin fetal therapy for symptomatic congenital cytomegalovirus infection. Journal of Reproductive Immunology, 95(1–2), 73–79.

Jeong, S. W., & Kim, L. S. (2012). Cochlear implantation in children with cochlear aplasia. Acta Oto-Laryngologica, 132(9), 910–915.

Jerger, S. (1987). Validation of the pediatric speech intelligibility test in children with central nervous system lesions. Audiology, 26(5), 298–311.

Jones, S. M., & Jones, T. A. (2011). Genetics, embryology, and development of auditory and vestibular systems. San Diego, CA: Plural.

Jones, J. L., Lopez, A., Wilson, M., Schulkin, J., & Gibbs, R. (2001). Congenital toxoplasmosis: a review. Obstetrical & Gynecological Survey, 56(5), 296–305.

Joshi, V. M., Navlekar, S. K., Kishore, G. R., Reddy, K. J., & Kumar, E. C. (2012). CT and MR imaging of the inner ear and brain in children with congenital sensorineural hearing loss. Radiographics, 32(3), 683–698.

Kaf, W. A. (2011). Wideband energy reflectance findings in presence of normal tympanogram in children with Down's syndrome. International Journal of Pediatric Otorhinolaryngology, 75(2), 219–226.

Karosi, T., & Sziklai, I. (2010). Etiopathogenesis of otosclerosis. European Archives of Oto-Rhino-Laryngology, 267(9), 1337–1349.

Kawashima, Y., Ihara, K., Nakamura, M., Nakashima, T., Fukuda, S., & Kitamura, K. (2005). Epidemiological study of mumps deafness in Japan. Auris, Nasus, Larynx, 32(2), 125–128.

Kawashiro, N., Tsuchihashi, N., Koga, K., Kawano, T., & Itoh, Y. (1996). Delayed post-neonatal intensive care unit hearing disturbance. International Journal of Pediatric Otorhinolaryngology, 34(1–2), 35–43.

Kellner, J. (2011). Update on the success of the pneumococcal conjugate vaccine. Paediatrics and Child Health (Oxford), 16(4), 233–240.

Khoramrooz, S. S., Mirsalehian, A., Emaneini, M., Jabalameli, F., Aligholi, M., Saedi, B., . . . Razmpa, E. (2012). Frequency of *Alloicoccus otitidis*, *Streptococcus pneumoniae*, *Moraxella catarrhalis* and *Haemophilus influenzae* in children with otitis media with effusion (OME) in Iranian patients. Auris, Nasus, Larynx, 39(4), 369–373.

Kim, J., Kim, E. Y., Lee, J. S., Lee, W. S., & Kim, H. N. (2008). Temporal bone CT findings in Cornelia de Lange syndrome. AJNR. American Journal of Neuroradiology, 29(3), 569–573.

Konrádsson, K. S. (1996). Bilaterally preserved otoacoustic emissions in four children with profound idiopathic unilateral sensorineural hearing loss. Audiology, 35(4), 217–227.

Koomen, I., Grobbee, D. E., Roord, J. J., Donders, R., Jennekens-Schinkel, A., & van Furth, A. M. (2003). Hearing loss at school age in survivors of bacterial meningitis: assessment, incidence, and prediction. Pediatrics, 112(5), 1049–1053.

Kopelovich, J. C., Germiller, J. A., Laury, A. M., Shah, S. S., & Pollock, A. N. (2011). Early prediction of postmeningitic hearing loss in children using magnetic resonance imaging. Archives of Otolaryngology–Head & Neck Surgery, 137(5), 441–447.

Kuhle, S., Kirk, S. F., Ohinmaa, A., Urschitz, M. S., & Veugelers, P. J. (2012). The association between childhood overweight and obesity and otitis media. Pediatric Obesity, 7(2), 151–157.

Kujala, T., Alho, O. P., Luotonen, J., Kristo, A., Uhari, M., Renko, M., . . . Koivunen, P. (2012). Tympanostomy with and without adenoidectomy for the prevention of recurrences of acute otitis media: a randomized controlled trial. The Pediatric Infectious Disease Journal, 31(6), 565–569.

Kutz, J. W., Simon, L. M., Chennupati, S. K., Giannoni, C. M., & Manolidis, S. (2006). Clinical predictors for hearing loss in children with bacterial meningitis. Archives of Otolaryngology–Head & Neck Surgery, 132(9), 941–945.

Lambert, P. R., & Canalis, R. F. (2000). Anatomy and embryology of the auditory and vestibular systems. In R. F. Canalis & P. R. Lambert (Eds.), The ear: comprehensive otology (pp. 17–66). Philadelphia: Lippincott Williams and Wilkins.

Lambert, P. R., & Dodson, E. E. (1996). Congenital malformations of the external auditory canal. Otolaryngologic Clinics of North America, 29(5), 741–760.

Lasisi, O. A., Ayodele, J. K., & Ijaduola, G. T. A. (2006). Challenges in management of childhood sensorineural hearing loss in sub-Saharan Africa, Nigeria. International Journal of Pediatric Otorhinolaryngology, 70(4), 625–629.

Lasky, R. E., Wiorek, L., & Becker, T. R. (1998). Hearing loss in survivors of neonatal extracorporeal membrane oxygenation (ECMO) therapy and high-frequency oscillatory (HFO) therapy. Journal of the American Academy of Audiology, 9(1), 47–58.

Lien, T. H., Fu, C. M., Hsu, C. J., Lu, L., Peng, S. S., & Chang, L. Y. (2011). Recurrent bacterial meningitis associated with Mondini dysplasia. Pediatrics and Neonatology, 52(5), 294–296.

Lok, W., Anteunis, L. J., Meesters, C., Chenault, M. N., & Haggard, M. P. (2012). Risk factors for failing the hearing screen due to otitis media in Dutch infants. European Archives of Oto-Rhino-Laryngology, 269(12), 2485–2496.

Loundon, N., Marcolla, A., Roux, I., Rouillon, I., Denoyelle, F., Feldmann, D., . . . Garabedian, E. N. (2005). Auditory neuropathy or endocochlear hearing loss? Otology & Neurotology, 26(4), 748–754.

Mann, T., & Adams, K. (1998). Sensorineural hearing loss in ECMO survivors. Extracorporeal membraneous oxygenation. Journal of the American Academy of Audiology, 9(5), 367–370.

Markou, K., & Goudakos, J. (2009). An overview of the etiology of otosclerosis. European Archives of Oto-Rhino-Laryngology, 266(1), 25–35.

Marres, H. A. (2002). Hearing loss in the Treacher-Collins syndrome. Advances in Oto-Rhino-Laryngology, 61, 209–215.

Matteson, E. L., Fabry, D. A., Strome, S. E., Driscoll, C. L., Beatty, C. W., & McDonald, T. J. (2003). Autoimmune inner ear disease: diagnostic and therapeutic approaches in a multidisciplinary setting. Journal of the American Academy of Audiology, 14(4), 225–230.

McCaslin, D. L., Jacobson, G. P., & Gruenwald, J. M. (2011). The predominant forms of vertigo in children and their associated findings on balance function testing. Otolaryngologic Clinics of North America, 44(2), 291–307, vii.

McKenna, G. J., Burke, F. M., & Mellan, K. (2009). Case report: Presentation of lacrimo-auriculodento-digital (LADD) syndrome in a young female patient. European Archives of Paediatric Dentistry; Official Journal of the European Academy of Paediatric Dentistry, 10(Suppl 1), 35–39.

McKenna, M. J. (1997, Dec). Measles, mumps, and sensorineural hearing loss. Annals of the New York Academy of Sciences, 830, 291–298.

Monasta, L., Ronfani, L., Marchetti, F., Montico, M., Vecchi Brumatti, L., Bavcar, A., . . . , Tamburlini, G. (2012). Burden of disease caused by otitis media: systematic review and global estimates. Public Library of Science One, 7(4), e36226. doi: 10.1371/journal.pone.0036226.

Morrissey, T. W. (2012). Multiple child care arrangements and common communicable illnesses in children aged 3 to 54 months. Maternal and Child Health Journal, (Aug 31) [Epub ahead of print].

Neidermeyer, H. P., & Arnold, W. (2008). Otosclerosis and measles virus—association or causation? ORL: Journal of Otorhinolaryngology and Its Related Specialties, 70(1), 63–69.

Niedzielska, G., Katska, E., & Szymula, D. (2000). Hearing defects in children born of mothers suffering from rubella in the first trimester of pregnancy. International Journal of Pediatric Otorhinolaryngology, 54(1), 1–5.

Northern, J. L., & Downs, M. P. (2002). Hearing in children (5th ed). Philadelphia, PA: Lippincott Williams and Wilkins.

Oldenburg, J., Fosså, S. D., & Ikdahl, T. (2008). Genetic variants associated with cisplatin-induced ototoxicity. Pharmacogenomics, 9(10), 1521–1530.

Olusanya, B. O. (2003). Hearing impairment in children with impacted cerumen. Annals of Tropical Paediatrics, 23(2), 121–128.

Osguthorpe, J. D., & Nielsen, D. R. (2006). Otitis externa: Review and clinical update. American Family Physician, 74(9), 1510–1516.

Pass, R. F. (2005). Congenital cytomegalovirus infection and hearing loss. Herpes, 12(2), 50–55.

Pass, R. F., Fowler, K. B., Boppana, S. B., Britt, W. J., & Stagno, S. (2006). Congenital cytomegalovirus infection following first trimester maternal infection: symptoms at birth and outcome. Journal of Clinical Virology, 35(2), 216–220.

Perreault, T. (2006). Persistent pulmonary hypertension of the newborn. Paediatric Respiratory Reviews, 7S, S175–S176.

Pletcher, S. D., & Cheung, S. W. (2003). Syphilis and otolaryngology. Otolaryngologic Clinics of North America, 36(4), 595–605, vi.

Principi, N., Baggi, E., & Esposito, S. (2012). Prevention of acute otitis media using currently available vaccines. Future Microbiology, 7(4), 457–465.

Rapin, I., & Gravel, J. S. (2006). Auditory neuropathy: a biologically inappropriate label unless acoustic nerve involvement is documented. Journal of the American Academy of Audiology, 17(2), 147–150.

Raveh, E., Papsin, B. C., & Forte, V. (2000). Branchio-oculo-facial syndrome. International Journal of Pediatric Otorhinolaryngology, 53(2), 149–156.

Reilly, P. G., Lalwani, A. K., & Jackler, R. K. (1998). Congenital anomalies of the inner ear. In A. K. Lalwani & K. M. Grundfast (Eds.), Pediatric otology and neurotology (pp. 201–210). Philadelphia, PA: Lippincott-Raven.

Rima, B. K., & Duprex, W. P. (2006). Morbilliviruses and human disease. The Journal of Pathology, 208(2), 199–214.

Rivera, L. B., Boppana, S. B., Fowler, K. B., Britt, W. J., Stagno, S., & Pass, R. F. (2002). Predictors of hearing loss in children with symptomatic congenital cytomegalovirus infection. Pediatrics, 110(4), 762–767.

Rodríguez Soriano, J. (2003). Branchio-oto-renal syndrome. Journal of Nephrology, 16(4), 603–605.

Roeser, R. J., & Ballachanda, B. B. (1997). Physiology, pathophysiology, and anthropology/epidemiology of human earcanal secretions. Journal of the American Academy of Audiology, 8(6), 391–400.

Roeser, R. J., & Roland, P. S. (1992). What audiologists must know about cerumen and cerumen management. American Journal of Audiology, 1, 27–35.

Roizen, N. J. (2003). Nongenetic causes of hearing loss. Mental Retardation and Developmental Disabilities Research Reviews, 9(2), 120–127.

Rol, J. T., Jr, & Cohen, N. L. (1998). Vestibular and auditory ototoxicity. In C. W. Cummings (Ed.), Otolaryngology—head and neck surgery (3rd ed., pp. 3186–3197). St. Louis, MO: Mosby Year Book.

Roland, P. S. (2004). New developments in our understanding of ototoxicity. Ear, Nose, and Throat Journal, 83(9, Suppl 4), 15–16, discussion 16–17.

Rorman, E., Zamir, C. S., Rilkis, I., & Ben-David, H. (2006). Congenital toxoplasmosis—prenatal aspects of Toxoplasma gondii infection. Reproductive Toxicology (Elmsford, N.Y.), 21(4), 458–472.

Rosenfeld, R. M., Brown, L., Cannon, C. R., Dolor, R. J., Ganiats, T. G., Hannley, M., . . . American Academy of Otolaryngology–Head and Neck Surgery Foundation (2006). Clinical practice guideline: acute otitis externa. Otolaryngology - Head and Neck Surgery, 134(4, Suppl), S4–S23.

Ross, C. J., Katzov-Eckert, H., Dubé, M. P., Brooks, B., Rassekh, S. R., Barhdadi, A., . . . Hayden, M. R.; CPNDS Consortium (2009). Genetic variants in TPMT and COMT are associated with hearing loss in children receiving cisplatin chemotherapy. Nature Genetics, 41(12), 1345–1349.

Ryan, A. F., Harris, J. P., & Keithley, E. M. (2002). Immune-mediated hearing loss: basic mechanisms and options for therapy. Acta Oto-Laryngologica. Supplementum, (548), 38–43.

Rybak, L. P., & Whitworth, C. A. (2005). Ototoxicity: therapeutic opportunities. Drug Discovery Today, 10(19), 1313–1321.

Rye, M. S., Blackwell, J. M., & Jamieson, S. E. (2012). Genetic susceptibility to otitis media in childhood. The Laryngoscope, 122(3), 665–675.

Sáez-Llorens, X., & McCracken, G. H., Jr. (2003). Bacterial meningitis in children. Lancet, 361(9375), 2139–2148.

Schrauwen, I., & Van Camp, G. (2010). The etiology of otosclerosis: a combination of genes and environment. The Laryngoscope, 120(6), 1195–1202.

Semaan, M. T., & Megerian, C. A. (2006). The pathophysiology of cholesteatoma. Otolaryngologic Clinics of North America, 39(6), 1143–1159.

Sennaroglu, L. (2010). Cochlear implantation in inner ear malformations—a review article. Cochlear Implants International, 11(1), 4–41.

Sever, J. L., Ellenberg, J. H., Ley, A. C., Madden, D. L., Fuccillo, D. A., Tzan, N. R., & Edmonds, D.M. (1988). Toxoplasmosis: maternal and pediatric findings in 23,000 pregnancies. Pediatrics, 82(2), 181–192.

Shapiro, S. M. (2003). Bilirubin toxicity in the developing nervous system. Pediatric Neurology, 29(5), 410–421.

Sharma, P., Chhangani, N. P., Meena, K. R., Jora, R., Sharma, N., & Gupta, B. D. (2006). Brainstem evoked response audiometry (BAER) in neonates with hyperbilirubinemia. Indian Journal of Pediatrics, 73(5), 413–416.

Shekelle, P., Takata, G., & Chan, L. S.(2003). Diagnosis, natural history and late effects of otitis media with effusion. Summary, Evidence report/technology assessment No. 55 (No. 02-E025). Rockville, MD: Agency for Healthcare Research & Quality.

Sie, K. C. Y. (1996). Cholesteatoma in children. Pediatric Clinics of North America, 43(6), 1245–1252.

Sierra, A., Lopez, P., Zapata, M. A., Vanegas, B., Castrejon, M. M., Deantonio, R., . . . Colindres, R. E. (2011). Non-typeable Haemophilus influenzae and Streptococcus pneumoniae as primary causes of acute otitis media in Colombian children: a prospective study. BMC Infectious Diseases, 11, 4.

Sininger, Y., & Oba, S. (2001). Patients with auditory neuropathy: who are they and what can they hear? In Y. Sininger & A. Starr (Eds.), Auditory neuropathy (pp. 15–36). San Diego, CA: Singular Thomson Learning.

Skarzyński, H., Porowski, M., & Podskarbi-Fayette, R. (2009). Treatment of otological features of the oculoauriculovertebral dysplasia (Goldenhar syndrome). International Journal of Pediatric Otorhinolaryngology, 73(7), 915–921.

Slattery, W. H. I., & House, J. W. (1998). Complications of otitis media. In A. K. Lalwani & K. M. Grundfast (Eds.), Pediatric otology and neurotology (pp. 251–263). Philadelphia, PA: Lippincott-Raven.

Smith, J. A., & Danner, C. J. (2006). Complications of chronic otitis media and cholesteatoma. Otolaryngologic Clinics of North America, 39(6), 1237–1255.

Starr, A., Picton, T. W., Sininger, Y., Hood, L. J., & Berlin, C. I. (1996). Auditory neuropathy. Brain, 119(Pt 3), 741–753.

Stronati, M., Lombardi, G., Garofoli, F., Villani, P., & Regazzi, M. (2013). Pharmacokinetics, pharmacodynamics and clinical use of valganciclovir in newborns with symptomatic congenital cytomegalovirus infection. Current Drug Metabolism, 14(2), 208–215.

Sudo, Y., Numakura, C., Abe, A., Aiba, S., Matsunaga, A., & Hayasaka, K. (2010). Phenotypic variability in a family with Townes-Brocks syndrome. Journal of Human Genetics, 55(8), 550–551.

Thornton, J. L., Chevallier, K. M., Koka, K., Lupo, J. E., & Tollin, D. J. (2012). The conductive hearing loss due to an experimentally induced middle ear effusion alters the interaural level and time difference cues to sound location. Journal of the Association for Research in Otolaryngology, 13(5), 641–654.

Uclés, P., Alonso, M. F., Aznar, E., & Lapresta, C. (2012). The importance of right otitis media in childhood language disorders. International Journal of Otolaryngology, 2012, 818927. doi: 10.1155/2012/818927

Verklan, M. T. (2006). Persistent pulmonary hypertension of the newborn: not a honeymoon anymore. The Journal of Perinatal & Neonatal Nursing, 20(1), 108–112.

Visentin, S., Manara, R., Milanese, L., Da Roit, A., Forner, G., Salviato, E., . . . Gussetti, N. (2012). Early primary cytomegalovirus infection in pregnancy: maternal hyperimmunoglobulin therapy improves outcomes among infants at 1 year of age. Clinical Infectious Diseases, 55(4), 497–503.

Wiener-Vacher, S. R., Obeid, R., & Abou-Elew, M. (2012). Vestibular impairment after bacterial meningitis delays infant posturomotor development. The Journal of Pediatrics, 161(2), 246–251, e1.

Wilson, C. B., Remington, J. S., Stagno, S., & Reynolds, D. W. (1980). Development of adverse sequelae in children born with subclinical congenital Toxoplasma infection. Pediatrics, 66(5), 767–774.

Woods, B. T. (1984). Dichotic listening ear preference after childhood cerebral lesions. Neuropsychologia, 22(3), 303–310.

Yancey, A., Harris, M. S., Egbelakin, A., Gilbert, J., Pisoni, D. B., & Renbarger, J. (2012). Risk factors for cisplatin-associated ototoxicity in pediatric oncology patients. Pediatric Blood & Cancer, 59(1), 144–148.

Yildirim, N., Arslanoğlu, A., Mahiroğullari, M., Sahan, M., & Ozkan, H. (2008). Klippel-Feil syndrome and associated ear anomalies. American Journal of Otolaryngology, 29(5), 319–325.

Yoshikawa, S., Ikeda, K., Kudo, T., & Kobayashi, T. (2004). The effects of hypoxia, premature birth, infection, ototoxic drugs, circulatory system and congenital disease on neonatal hearing loss. Auris, Nasus, Larynx, 31(4), 361–368.

Chapter 3

Genetics of Hearing Loss

Katherine A. Lafferty, Rebecca Hodges, and Heidi L. Rehm

Key Points

- More than half of childhood hearing loss is genetic.

- Any child with sensorineural hearing loss (SNHL) should have a genetic evaluation.

- Approximately 70% of genetic SNHL is nonsyndromic.

- In most cases of genetic hearing loss, there is no family history.

- The most common cause of congenital nonsyndromic SNHL is mutations in the *GJB2* (connexin 26) gene.

- Symptoms like vision loss, thyroid problems, fainting episodes, pigmentary abnormalities, and hematuria may be indications that hearing loss is part of a genetic syndrome.

- Clinical genetic testing is available for several genes associated with syndromic and nonsyndromic hearing loss.

- Genetic counseling is highly recommended for individuals and families before and after pursuing genetic testing for hearing loss.

The prevalence of congenital (present at birth) hearing loss is estimated at 1.4 in 1000 births and 3.5 per 1000 by adolescence, making it the most frequently occurring birth defect (Centers for Disease Control and Prevention [CDC], 2010; Morton & Nance, 2006). Genetic causes contribute to a child's hearing loss in ~ 50% of cases (Gorlin, Toriello, & Cohen, 1995; Morton, 1991). Our understanding of the genes that play critical roles in hearing and deafness has grown exponentially. Approximately half of nonsyndromic recessive hearing loss is caused by mutations in the *GJB2* gene, which encodes the connexin 26 protein (Cx26). Genetic testing for *GJB2* mutations has been available for many years and has substantially increased the likelihood of obtaining an etiology for congenital hearing loss. The ability to diagnose the cause of

hearing loss has an impact on the medical decisions made by patients, their families, and their physicians. Knowledge gained from a genetic evaluation and appropriate genetic testing can simplify the diagnosis, prognosis, recurrence risk estimates, and treatment decisions offered by the physician. Furthermore, this information helps individuals understand the cause and heritability of their hearing losses.

◆ Basic Genetics and Inheritance Patterns

Genetic information is packaged inside virtually every cell of the body in structures called chromosomes. There are 23 pairs of chromosomes in each cell. One chromosome of each pair is inherited from the mother and the other from the father. Genes are segments of the chromosome that provide the body with instructions for growth, development, and function. Just as there are two copies of each chromosome (one from each parent), there are also two copies of every gene. The two copies may differ from each other; the different versions are called variants. When something happens to a gene to change it into a new variant, it is said to undergo a mutation. A genetic condition is the result of a variant in a gene that alters the body's instructions from the way they normally work. Some genetic conditions arise when only one copy of a gene is altered. This is referred to as a dominant genetic condition, as the altered gene "dominates" over the other (normal) copy. Other genetic conditions, referred to as recessive, arise only when both copies of a gene are the same variant. If something is said to be "inherited," it means it is passed on from one or both parents to the child, though parents or other family members may not be clinically affected. **Figs. 3.1, 3.2, 3.3,** and **3.4** discuss these forms of inheritance. Inheritance on any chromosome other than the sex chromosomes is said to be autosomal.

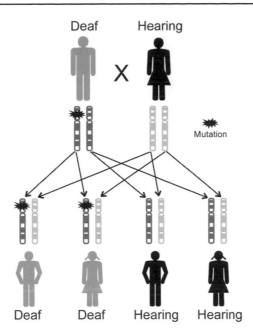

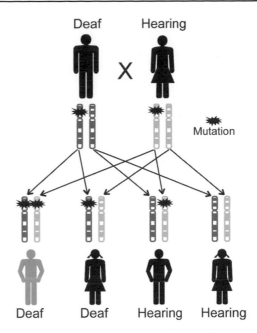

Fig. 3.1 Dominant inheritance. When a mutation is passed in a dominant way, it means that only one copy of the gene needs to have the mutation to cause the resulting condition. The changed condition also appears in each generation (e.g., grandparent, parent, child). Therefore, if a person has one parent with the dominant mutation, he or she will have the condition (e.g. hearing loss). That also means that *every* child of that person will have a 50% (or 1 in 2) chance of having the mutation and therefore the condition.

Fig. 3.2 Recessive inheritance. Mutations in both copies of a gene (one from each parent) are required to cause a recessive genetic condition such as a hearing loss. Individuals with just one recessive mutation are called carriers and are not affected by the condiiton. If each parent has one recessive mutation, each child has a 25% (or 1 in 4) chance of having the condition and a 50% chance of being an unaffected carrier. Hearing loss that is inherited in a recessive pattern often appears without any family history.

◆ Causes of Permanent Hearing Loss

There are many causes of permanent hearing loss, which can be broadly grouped into genetic and non-genetic etiologies. Historical estimates indicate that approximately half of children identified with a permanent hearing loss have a genetic cause and the other half have an environmental or unknown cause (Toriello, Reardon, & Gorlin, 2004). Genetic causes of hearing loss may be classified as syndromic or non-syndromic. Approximately one third of genetic hearing loss is syndromic, indicating that it is associated with additional medical problems. In contrast, the majority of children with genetic hearing loss have no other associated medical problems. In these cases, the loss is classified as nonsyndromic.

Genetic hearing loss can also be subdivided by mode of inheritance: ~ 77% of cases of hereditary hearing losses are recessive, 22% are dominant, and 1% are X-linked (Morton, 1991). In addition, a small fraction (less than 1%) represents those families with mitochondrial inheritance, in which the trait is passed through the maternal lineage. These patterns of inheritance are discussed in **Figs. 3.1, 3.2, 3.3,** and **3.4,** and the breakdown of different forms of hearing loss is illustrated in **Fig. 3.5**. In all cases of genetic, or "inherited," hearing loss, the genetic variant is present in every cell of a child at birth. However, in many cases, particularly for gene variants with dominant inheritance, the hearing loss may not begin until late childhood or adulthood.

Because a large proportion (77%) of nonsyndromic genetic hearing loss is recessive, where each parent is a carrier of a mutation but has normal hearing, there are many instances when a couple with no family history of hearing loss will give birth to a child with hearing loss. At least 90% of children born with a hearing loss are born to parents with normal hearing (Mitchell & Karchmer, 2004). The underlying cause of hearing loss in these cases can be especially difficult to determine, because the loss may be either genetic or acquired. It is therefore important to be aware of nongenetic causes of hearing impairment, which are discussed in other chapters. Recognition of nongenetic causes is critical, for in some cases there are interventions that can either resolve the hearing loss or stop its progression.

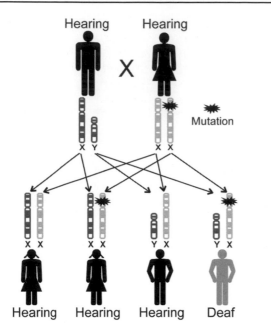

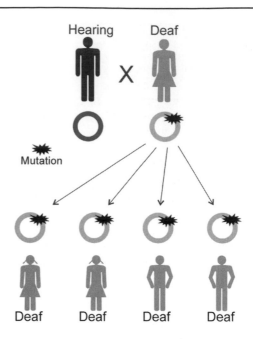

Fig. 3.3 X-linked inheritance. The X and Y chromosomes are called sex chromosomes because they determine what sex the person is. Women have two X chromosomes; men have one X and one Y chromosome. If a mutation is said to be X-linked, it means it occurs only on the X chromosome. Since women have two X chromosomes, if one X chromosome has a recessive mutation, the second chromosome can provide a functioning copy of the gene, and the condition will often not develop. In men, the Y chromosome cannot provide a normal copy of the gene, so the condition will occur. Therefore, hearing loss resulting from X-linked mutations is usually seen only in males. If the mother has the mutation on one copy of her X chromosomes, each female child has a 50% chance of being a carrier (but will not have hearing loss) and each male child will have a 50% chance of having hearing loss.

Fig. 3.4 Mitochondrial inheritance. Mitochondrial genes are found inside the mitochondria, which are found within each of our cells. Unlike most of our genes, which are passed on by each parent, mitochondria are passed on by the mother only. This means that if the mother has hearing loss mutation in one of her mitochondrial genes, she will pass it on to all of her children, and they may have hearing loss. If the father has a hearing loss mutation in one of his mitochondrial genes, he will not pass it on to any of his children, and thus they will not have hearing loss.

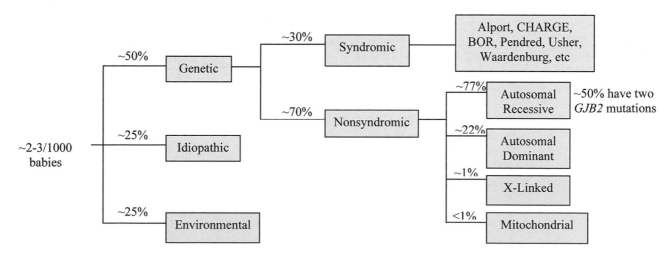

Fig. 3.5 Breakdown of etiologies of hearing loss.

Pitfall

- Unfortunately, diagnosis of the etiology of hearing loss remains difficult even if environmental causes have been ruled out, as the current paucity of molecular diagnostic tests makes it difficult to conclude positively that a patient's hearing loss has genetic origins. In addition, even when an environmental risk factor is present, a definitive association with hearing loss can be difficult.

As such, a genetics evaluation is a very important part of the child's workup and is recommended for all children with sensorineural hearing loss (SNHL) (Genetic Evaluation of Congenital Hearing Loss Expert Panel, 2002). With the advent of newborn hearing screens, essential guidelines for genetic screening and evaluations have been established by such groups as the American College of Medical Genetics and Genomics (ACMG) (2002). Approaches used by clinical geneticists and genetic counselors to aid in a genetics evaluation include review of the family history as well as pregnancy and neonatal histories. A complete review of the child's medical and developmental histories and a complete physical and dysmorphology examination are necessary to identify specific risk factors as well as clinical findings that may indicate a syndromic form of hearing loss.

Currently, more than 500 genes have been identified and found to be associated with syndromic and nonsyndromic forms of hearing loss (OMIM, 2012), and more are expected to be discovered as time goes on. The number of single-gene or gene panel tests that are available has been growing as our knowledge of the genetics of hearing loss grows. Families and physicians can discuss the importance of a genetic diagnosis in the context of each patient and family. A confirmed molecular diagnosis may be less critical in an example of syndromic hearing loss, where other defining symptoms enable an accurate clinical diagnosis. However, for nonsyndromic hearing loss, as well as in instances when the signs and symptoms of a particular syndrome do not begin until after birth, such as retinitis pigmentosa in Usher syndrome and thyroid abnormalities in Pendred syndrome, the use of genetic testing can aid in determining the causative gene and mode of inheritance and predict the development of any associated clinical findings.

◆ Nonsyndromic Genetic Hearing Loss

Most genetic hearing loss is nonsyndromic. In these cases, the only clinical finding is hearing loss, except that some patients may have accompanying vestibu-

lar symptoms. Although hearing loss and vestibular dysfunction do not always occur together, the existence of many disorders involving both the auditory and vestibular systems reflects their close anatomic proximity, structural similarity, and common developmental origin. Unfortunately, the diagnosis of vestibular problems is often challenging, especially at young ages.

Pearl

- An early clue to vestibular problems can be a delay in walking (Angeli, 2003).

One of the difficulties in studying nonsyndromic hearing loss, and discovering the underlying genetic causes, is the immense genetic heterogeneity in nonsyndromic forms of hearing loss. Although subtle pathologic differences may allow clinical differentiation between certain subtypes of nonsyndromic hearing loss, there is still a plethora of genes whose dysfunction can result in highly similar clinical presentations. In fact, mapping efforts have located more than 120 independent loci (gene locations) for nonsyndromic hearing loss (Van Camp & Smith, 2012). In the reference compilations (OMIM, 2012; Van Camp & Smith, 2012) each locus is labeled "DFN" followed by "A" for dominant inheritance, "B" for recessive, or no additional letter (in OMIM) or "X" (in the Hereditary Hearing Loss page) for X-linked. A unique number is then added to the locus designation to indicate the sequential order in which the genes were mapped.

Pearl

- In general, autosomal recessive forms of hearing loss are usually prelingual, and autosomal dominant ones often result in progressive, postlingual hearing loss. This likely reflects the fact that most recessive disorders represent a complete loss of a gene's function, whereas dominant disorders may represent an interaction between the activity of the normal gene product and the activity of the mutant product.

The responsible gene has been identified in 63 of these nonsyndromic loci, covering 27 forms of autosomal dominant hearing loss, 40 forms of autosomal recessive hearing loss, 3 forms of X-linked recessive hearing loss, and 2 forms of mitochondrial hearing loss. The discrepancy in these numbers reflects the fact that different mutations in some of these genes can cause both recessive and dominant forms of hearing loss. For a full summary of hearing loss loci, refer to the frequently updated Hereditary Hearing Loss home page, which contains tables summarizing the details of these nonsyndromic loci, as well as a wealth of other information for the research community and others interested in hereditary hearing loss (Van Camp & Smith, 2012).

Connexin Hearing Loss

DFNB1 was the first recessive hearing loss locus identified in 1994, and the responsible gene, *GJB2*, encodes the gap junction b2 protein, known as connexin 26. Mutations in the *GJB2* gene are the most common cause of SNHL, responsible for 12 to 24% of permanent childhood SNHL (Putcha et al, 2007). This gene represents a common cause of hearing loss across the world, though different regions have distinct common mutations. For instance, two frameshift mutations, 35delG and 167delT, are more commonly identified in Caucasians (carrier rate 2.5% in the United States) and Ashkenazi Jews (4%), respectively. A third frameshift mutation, 235delC, is prevalent in Asians, with a carrier frequency of 1%. A database of most published mutations can be found online at the Connexins and Deafness Web site (Smith & Van Camp, 2005; Calvo, Gasparini, & Estivill, 2007).

Hearing loss caused by *GJB2* mutations is typically congenital, though roughly 4% are now thought to be delayed in onset (Norris et al, 2006). The severity of hearing loss ranges from mild to profound; certain mutations, such as M34T and V37I, are associated with a milder hearing loss (ranging from normal to moderate) (Snoeckx et al, 2005). In addition, more than 50% of individuals with *GJB2*-related hearing loss will show progression of varying degrees (Kenna et al, 2010). Despite all this information, there can be variability in the presentation of hearing loss from person to person, or even within a family, with the same genetic variants. Therefore, this information is helpful in providing possible prognosis for a child, but it is not completely predictive.

On some occasions, mutations in the connexin 26 gene can be inherited in an autosomal dominant rather than a recessive pattern. Dominant sensorineural hearing loss caused by *GJB2* mutations is generally early-onset, moderate to severe, and frequently progressive. Some of these dominant mutations can also cause syndromic rather than nonsyndromic hearing loss, in which patients have variable types of skin findings, such as Vohwinkel or keratitis-ichthyosis-deafness (KID) syndrome.

In addition to *GJB2*, other gap junction genes also play a role in the development of hearing loss, such as *GJB6*, encoding the connexin 30 protein. Located directly adjacent to the *GJB2* gene, the *GJB6* gene is located in a region that is known to be deleted in some patients with a single *GJB2* mutation. In the United States, only 1% of individuals with hearing loss have this mutation, and it almost always is present in combination with a single connexin 26 mutation (Putcha et al, 2007). Higher frequencies have been reported in individuals of Spanish, French, and Ashkenazi Jewish descent, and a few cases of SNHL have been associated with two copies of the *GJB6* deletion in the absence of a *GJB2* gene mutation (Schrijver & Gardner, 2006).

DFNB4 Hearing Loss

Mutations in the *SLC26A4* gene (also called *PDS*) are associated with both a syndromic form of hearing loss called Pendred syndrome (discussed later in this chapter) as well as a nonsyndromic form called DFNB4. DFNB4 patients have autosomal recessive, nonsyndromic SNHL with enlarged vestibular aqueducts (EVA) and/or Mondini malformations, but they do not manifest the thyroid abnormalities seen in Pendred syndrome. Hearing loss tends to be congenital, bilateral, severe to profound SNHL, though mild to moderate loss can also be seen; progression and fluctuation are not uncommon (Smith & Van Camp, 2006). On rare occasions, hearing loss onset can occur in childhood. For cases of hearing loss with EVA, ~ 50% of cases from multiplex families (more than one family member affected) and 20% of singleton cases have mutations in the *SLC26A4* (or *PDS*) gene (Smith & Van Camp, 2006).

Mitochondrial Hearing Loss

There are many mitochondrial syndromes in which hearing loss is a component (often associated with neuromuscular disease); however, two forms of mitochondrial hearing loss are usually nonsyndromic. These are caused by mutations in the *MTRNR1* (encoding 12S rRNA) and *MTTS1* (encoding tRNAser[(UCN)]) mitochondrial genes. Due to their location on the mitochondrial chromosome, families with mutations in these genes show maternal inheritance of hearing loss (see **Fig. 3.4** for an explanation of mitochondrial inheritance). However, this pattern of inheritance may not be clear in some families. For instance, some individuals with certain mutations in the *MTRNR1* gene, such as the 1555A>G and 1494C>T mutations, may develop hearing loss only when exposed to aminoglycoside antibiotics (e.g., gentamicin, neomycin, amikacin, tobramycin). The 1555A>G mutation is present in variable percentages of the hearing-impaired population based on geographic and/or ethnic origin: 0.6% Caucasian (Li et al, 2004), 0.7% German (Kupka et al, 2002), 3.5% Asian (Usami et al, 2000), 20% Spanish (del Castillo, Rodríguez-Ballesteros, et al, 2003).

People can lose their hearing because of treatment with high doses of aminoglycoside antibiotics even if they do not have any of these mutations. Also, a person with one of these mutations can develop hearing loss even with no exposure to aminoglycoside antibiotics. Hearing loss from mitochondrial mutations is highly variable; can begin any time from birth to late adulthood; can be flat, sloping, or high–frequency; and can progress, remain stable, or fluctuate (Li et al, 2004; Pandya, 2004). Identifying an *MTRNR1* mutation as the etiology of hearing loss in one individual allows maternally related relatives to prevent exposures that could result in their hearing loss.

Auditory Neuropathy

Auditory neuropathy spectrum disorder (ANSD) is a complex type of hearing loss with multiple etiologies, including environmental (e.g., hyperbilirubinemia, prematurity, and hypoxia) and genetic. More information about ANSD can be found in Chapter 32. Some syndromes, such as Charcot-Marie-Tooth disease and Friedreich ataxia (OMIM, 2012), are associated with ANSD. In addition, two genes—the *OTOF* gene, encoding otoferlin (Yasunaga et al, 1999), and the *DFNB59* gene, encoding pejvakin—are known to be associated with nonsyndromic forms of genetic ANSD (Delmaghani et al, 2006). Individuals with mutations in *OTOF* can present with ANSD or a pure SNHL. The hearing loss is typically prelingual and moderate to profound; a variety of audiometric shapes are observed, including flat, rising, sloping, and bowl-shaped (Varga et al, 2006). Several families have been identified with a unique form of hearing loss that manifests only in the presence of a fever (Varga et al, 2006; Marlin et al, 2010). The genetic basis for this appears to be temperature-sensitive mutations in the *OTOF* gene. Another mutation in *OTOF*, Q829X, is common in the Spanish population and is believed to be responsible for 3% of recessive cases of deafness in this region (Migliosi et al, 2002). In addition, like most patients with ANSD, patients with *OTOF* mutations appear to do well with cochlear implants (Rodríguez-Ballesteros et al, 2003).

Other Genes Related to Nonsyndromic Hearing Loss

Although individually the proportion of nonsyndromic hearing losses due to additional genes may be small, collectively this next tier of genes may account for a significant percentage of hereditary hearing loss. As investigations into the genetics of hearing loss continue, these new and rare genes are being discovered. It is possible that a child for whom a pathogenic variant cannot be identified still has a genetic cause of his or her hearing loss in either mutations in a gene that has yet to be identified or multiple gene interactions that are not yet understood. This is why it is important to create a long-term relationship with a genetics professional to keep up with this ever-growing field.

◆ Syndromic Forms of Genetic Hearing Loss

Approximately 30% of patients with childhood hearing loss also have additional clinical and physical findings that define a particular syndrome. More than 400 such syndromic forms of hearing loss have been characterized; the most complete collection of these disorders is found in Toriello and colleagues' *Hereditary Hearing Loss and Its Syndromes* (Toriello et al, 2004). Some of these syndromes are reviewed in the subsequent sections and are listed in **Table 3.1** with their accompanying phenotypes, responsible genes, and clinical testing information. An excellent source of up-to-date, freely available information on these and other genetic disorders can be found through the GeneTests Web site, where experts in the field contribute comprehensive reviews, called "Gene Reviews," of many genetic disorders (GeneTests, 2012). This Web site can also be queried to determine the availability of gene testing for any genetic disorder.

Alport Syndrome

Alport syndrome (AS) is characterized by renal, cochlear, and ocular involvement and can be inherited in an X-linked (80% XLAS), autosomal recessive (15% ARAS), or autosomal dominant (5% ADAS) manner (Kashtan, 2007). Its prevalence is estimated to be 1 in 50,000 live births (Levy & Feingold, 2000). The characteristic symptom of the disease is microscopic hematuria (blood in the urine), and it can progress to end-stage renal disease. The associated hearing loss is never congenital; initially it affects the high frequencies, with progression to all frequencies over time. Onset occurs by late childhood or early adolescence in individuals with ARAS or males with XLAS, whereas onset is later in individuals with ADAS. Females with XLAS tend to have milder hearing loss and other symptoms, if they have any at all. Although present only in 15 to 20% of patients, the identification of anterior lenticonus, a defect of the lens of the eye, is virtually pathognomonic for Alport syndrome (Kashtan, 2007).

Branchio-Oto-Renal Syndrome

Branchio-oto-renal syndrome (BOR) is a genetic disorder that includes branchial and kidney malformations and hearing loss. The condition is inherited in

Table 3.1 Selected hearing loss syndromes

Syndrome	Features (besides hearing loss)	Inheritance pattern(s)	Gene(s)	Available gene tests*
Alport syndrome	Nephritis, ocular abnormalities	80% XL	XLAS: COL4A5	Yes
		15% AR	ARAS: COL4A3	Yes
		5% AD	ADAS: COL4A4	Yes
Branchio-oto-renal syndrome	Branchial remnants, renal anomalies	AD	EYA1	Yes
			SIX5	Europe only
			SIX1	Yes
CHARGE syndrome	Ocular, ear, and heart defects, delayed growth and development, genital abnormalities	Sporadic or AD	CHD7	Yes
Jervell and Lange-Nielsen syndrome	Cardiac conduction defects	AR	JLN1: KCNQ1	Yes
			JLN2: KCNE1	Yes
Neurofibromatosis type 2	Acoustic neuromas	AD or sporadic	NF2	Yes
Pendred syndrome	Thyroid goiter	AR	SLC26A4 (PDS)	Yes
Usher syndrome	Retinitis pigmentosa, vestibular problems	AR	USH1B: MYO7A	Yes
			USH1C: USH1C	Yes
			USH1D: CDH23	Yes
			USH1E: Unknown	
			USH1F: PCDH15	Yes
			USH1G: USH1G/SANS	Yes
			USH2C: GPR98/VLGR1	Yes
			USH2A: USH2A	Yes
			USH2D: WHRN	Yes
			USH3A: CLRN1	Yes
Waardenburg syndrome	Pigmentary abnormalities of the skin, hair, and eyes	AD or sporadic (AR rare)	WS1: PAX3	Yes
			WS2: MITF, SOX10	Yes
			WS3: PAX3	Yes
			WS4: SOX10, END3, EDNRB	Yes

Abbreviations: AD, autosomal dominant; AR, autosomal recessive; XL, X-linked.

* *Note*: For up-to-date information about test availability go to www.genetests.org.

an autosomal dominant pattern with a prevalence estimated to be 1 in 40,000 to 700,000 individuals (Fraser, 1976; Fraser, Sproule, & Halal, 1980). Expression of the disease is highly variable, even among members of the same family. Malformations of the branchial arches can include cupping of the outer ear; ear pits in front of, or on, the outer ear; tags of skin in front of the ear; and cysts or fistulas on the neck. Renal abnormalities can range from mild renal hypoplasia to bilateral renal agenesis; however, many individuals with BOR either have no renal disease or do not experience symptoms of their renal anomalies. On rare occasions, individuals with BOR may also have blocked tear ducts that interfere with tear flow and require surgical repair. In individuals or families where there is an absence of renal findings, the diagnosis may be branchiootic syndrome (BOS). Most individuals with BOR/BOS (more than 90%) have some degree of hearing loss, and some also have radiologic abnormalities, such as enlarged vestibular aqueducts (Kemperman et al, 2004). The type of loss can be mixed (52%), conductive (33%), or sensorineural (29%); severity ranges from mild to profound; and the loss can be either nonprogressive (~ 70%) or progressive (~ 30%) (Smith, 2006b). Approximately 40% of individuals have a mutation in *EYA1* (Chang et al, 2004), 5% have mutations in the *SIX5* gene (Hoskins et al, 2007), and fewer than 1% have a mutation in *SIX1* (Ruf et al, 2004). The remaining percent of BOR/BOS is likely due to mutations in genes that have yet to be discovered.

CHARGE Syndrome

CHARGE is a mnemonic that stands for the major features of the disease: coloboma, heart defects, choanal atresia, retarded growth and development, genital abnormalities, and ear anomalies (Lalani, Hefner, Belmont, & Davenport 2006). Hearing loss is one of the most common features of CHARGE syndrome and can be sensorineural or conductive because of the presence of Mondini or ossicular malformations, respectively. The sensorineural component of the hearing loss can vary from mild to profound, and the conductive component may fluctuate with middle ear disease, which is common in these patients. The prevalence of CHARGE syndrome is ~ 1 in 8500 (Issekutz, Graham, Prasad, Smith, & Blake, 2005). The majority of individuals with CHARGE syndrome have a mutation in the *CDH7* gene; most cases arise from new mutations, though autosomal dominant inheritance can be observed (Lalani, Safiullah, et al, 2006).

Jervell and Lange-Nielsen Syndrome

Individuals with Jervell and Lange-Nielsen syndrome (JLNS) have congenital deafness and cardiac conduction defects referred to as prolonged QTc intervals (long QT). Long QT is associated with arrhythmias that can result in fainting or sudden death; however, several methods of cardiac management are available. Although the overall prevalence is rare, as many as 1 in 250 deaf children may have JLNS (Schwartz, Periti, & Malliani, 1975). JLNS is inherited in an autosomal recessive pattern and is caused by mutations in *KCNQ1* (JLNS1; 90% of cases) or *KCNE1* (JLNS2; fewer than 10% of cases) (Daley, Tranebjærg, Samson, & Green, 2004). Parents and siblings of a child with JLNS may have an autosomal dominant form of long QT, without hearing loss, called Romano-Ward syndrome.

Neurofibromatosis Type 2

Neurofibromatosis type 2 (NF2) is a rare disease characterized by bilateral acoustic neuromas (benign tumors of the auditory and vestibular nerves), which lead to tinnitus, hearing loss, and balance dysfunction. The average age of onset is typically 18 to 24 years, and the hearing loss is more commonly unilateral (Evans, 2006). Other tumors of the central nervous system can also develop. With comprehensive testing, a mutation can be identified in the *NF2* gene in ~ 60% of patients without a family history and greater than 90% in families with multiple affected family members (Evans 2009). NF2 is inherited in an autosomal dominant pattern; about half of the cases are inherited, and the other half have a new mutation and have no family history for the disorder.

Pendred Syndrome

Pendred syndrome is an autosomal recessive disease that consists of hearing loss associated with temporal bone anomalies and, later, with development of thyroid goiter (which can be hypothyroid or euthyroid). Soon after the discovery that Pendred syndrome is caused by mutations in the *SLC26A4* gene, Usami et al (1999) recognized that many with *SLC26A4* gene mutations are nonsyndromic and do not have thyroid abnormalities (referred to as DFNB4). The temporal bone abnormalities consist of dilation of the vestibular aqueduct (commonly referred to as enlarged vestibular aqueduct, or EVA) with or without cochlear hypoplasia, such as a common cavity or Mondini malformation (Goldfeld et al, 2005). The hearing loss in Pendred syndrome and DFNB4 tends to be congenital, bilateral, and severe to profound SNHL, though mild to moderate severity and unilateral loss can also been seen, and progression and fluctuation are not uncommon (Smith & Van Camp, 2006). On rare occasions, hearing loss onset can occur in childhood. The exact prevalence of Pendred syndrome and DFNB4 hearing loss is not known, but it appears to be a relatively common cause, particularly in patients with temporal bone abnormalities. About 50% of individuals with Pendred syndrome will have a mutation in the *SLC26A4* gene; however, in many individuals only one mutation can be identified (Campbell et al, 2001; Park et al, 2003). Some studies have suggested that the *FOXI1* and the *KCNJ10* genes may account for a small portion of genetic mutations in Pendred syndrome, but to date these genes are being investigated only on a research basis because there is insufficient evidence of a role for them in disease (Yang et al, 2007; Yang et al, 2009).

Usher Syndrome

Usher syndrome is characterized by sensorineural hearing loss and retinitis pigmentosa (RP), with or without vestibular abnormalities. Some studies have suggested that as many as 20% of children with cochlear implants have Usher syndrome (Smith, 2006a).

The disease is divided into three types based on the onset and severity of hearing loss and RP as well as the presence (USH1) or absence (USH2) of vestibular problems (dizziness, loss of balance and coordination, delayed walking) (Keats & Lentz, 2006a; 2006b). RP is a progressive degeneration of the rod and cone functions of the retina. It first causes night blindness and tunnel vision and later results in loss of day vision, although most individuals do not usually become completely blind (Kimberling & Möller, 1995). All three types of Usher syndrome are inherited in an autosomal recessive pattern.

Waardenburg Syndrome

Waardenburg syndrome (WS) is characterized by hearing loss and changes in pigmentation of the hair, skin, and eyes. Eye color can either be pale blue, a combination of two colors in one eye (heterochromia iridis), or a different color in each eye (heterochromia iridum). The eyes appear widely spaced because of the lateral displacement of the inner canthi (dystopia canthorum) in some types of WS. Distinctive hair coloring, such as a patch of white hair or premature graying, is another common sign of the condition. There are four types of Waardenburg syndrome, which are distinguished by their physical characteristics: WS1, WS2, WS3 (Klein-Waardenburg syndrome), and WS4 (Waardenburg-Shah syndrome). Types 1 and 2 are the most common, and individuals with WS1 can have all of the characteristics just described. Close to 60% of WS1 patients have hearing loss, which is usually congenital bilateral profound SNHL, though other types, including unilateral cases, are seen (Milunsky, 2006). Mutations in the *PAX3* gene are responsible for WS1 and WS3 (WS3 also includes upper limb abnormalities). Individuals with WS2 have hearing loss and pigmentation abnormalities but do not have dystopia canthorum. WS2 is caused by mutations in the *SOX10* and *MITF* genes. The *SOX10* gene can also cause WS4, as can mutations in the *EDNRB* and *EDN3* genes. Individuals with WS4 have the pigmentary abnormalities, dystopia canthorum, and Hirschsprung disease (inadequate muscular movement of the bowel, leading to severe constipation and intestinal blockage). The features of Waardenburg syndrome vary among affected individuals, even among members in the same family. The prevalence of Waardenburg syndrome is estimated to be 1 in 20,000 to 40,000 individuals; ~ 3% of people who are deaf have this condition (Milunsky, 2006). The disorder is usually inherited in an autosomal dominant pattern, although autosomal recessive inheritance has been described for WS2, WS3, and WS4.

◆ Genetic Testing for Hearing Loss

As the number of clinical genetic tests for hearing loss grows, the percentage of patients who are able to receive a molecular diagnosis of their hearing loss increases. In almost all cases of childhood SNHL, it is suggested that *GJB2* (connexin 26) testing be ordered because it is substantially more common than any other cause of SNHL and the audiological characteristics can be quite variable, ranging from mild to profound hearing loss. It is even worthwhile to order this test if the patient passed a newborn screen, yet developed hearing loss in early childhood, because an estimated 4% of cases present after birth (Green, Smith, Bent, & Cohn, 2000; Norris et al, 2006). If *GJB2* testing is negative, the most logical next step is to pursuing a comprehensive genetic testing panel for all other causes of hearing loss, given that other causes are all rare. However, there are a few genes or tests that might be considered, given specific presentations.

Special Consideration

- In almost all cases of childhood SNHL, it is suggested that *GJB2* gene (connexin 26 gene) testing be ordered, because it is substantially more common than any other cause of SNHL and the audiologic characteristics can be quite variable, ranging from mild to profound hearing loss.

If a child has a history of exposure to aminoglycoside antibiotics, has a family history of hearing loss consistent with maternal inheritance, or is of Spanish or Chinese ethnicity, testing for mitochondrial mutations in the *MTRNR1* and *MTTS1* genes would be appropriate. Testing for mutations in the *SLC26A4* (*PDS*) gene is indicated if the child has abnormalities of the temporal bone, such as EVA or a Mondini malformation. In a child with a diagnosis of auditory neuropathy/dyssynchrony, testing for *OTOF* and *DFNB59* gene mutations may be appropriate, particularly if there are other affected siblings. Patients with mutations in *OTOF* appear to do well with cochlear implants but not with hearing aids, so diagnosis of this etiology can be useful in management of the hearing loss (Varga et al, 2003).

If a child has any evidence of retinal disease, testing for Usher syndrome may be indicated, given the risk for progressive vision impairment (see the section on Usher syndrome).

Pearl

• An early diagnosis of Usher syndrome would prompt initiation of dietary supplementation, which may slow the progression of vision loss (Berson et al, 1993) as well as aid in managing the hearing loss (i.e., cochlear implants would be preferred over sign language).

Although rare, one additional form of childhood hearing loss for which gene testing is available is DFN3, caused by mutations in the *POU3F4* gene. Unlike most forms of nonsyndromic hearing loss, which are strictly sensorineural, these patients can have conductive, sensorineural, or mixed hearing loss. In addition, the patients often have radiologic abnormalities of the temporal bone and can manifest a perilymphatic gusher during stapedectomy (Chee, Suhailee, & Goh, 2006).

There are very few other presentations that indicate just one or a small number of genes, and therefore, in cases without a unique presentation, a broad hearing loss panel is more useful. The advent of new technologies, such as next-generation sequencing, enables laboratories to look at many genes at once for a lower cost than with traditional methods (Lin et al, 2012).

A summary of all currently available gene tests for nonsyndromic hearing loss is listed in **Table 3.2**

Table 3.2 Clinically available gene tests indicated for types of nonsyndromic hearing loss

Hearing Loss Type	Recommended Gene Tests
Congenital/prelingual SNHL	*GJB2, GJB6*
Congenital/prelingual SNHL with EVA	*SLC26A4*
Congenital auditory neuropathy/ dys-synchrony	*OTOF, DFNB59*
Congenital/prelingual SNHL with retinal disease	Usher syndrome panel
SNHL with aminoglycoside exposure	*MTRNR1*
SNHL with maternal (mitochondrial) inheritance	*MTRNR1, MTTS1*
SNHL ± conductive HL (perilymphatic gusher on stapedectomy)	*POU3F4*
All other forms of hearing loss	Comprehensive panel

Abbreviations: SNHL, sensorineural hearing loss; EVA, enlarged vestibular aqueducts; HL, hearing loss.

along with the most typical type of hearing loss observed. For ongoing updates of available tests, refer to the GeneTests Web site (GeneTests, 2012).

◆ Genetic Counseling for Hearing Loss

As with any condition that may be genetic, it is recommended that families see a genetic counselor. Genetic counseling is the process of providing individuals and families with information on the nature, inheritance, and implications of genetic conditions to help them make informed medical and personal decisions. The process also includes supportive counseling, advocating for the clients and their families, and referring them to community or state support services when needed. Individuals may choose to pursue genetic counseling for various reasons and at different times. Some individuals may choose to seek genetic counseling when the child is first diagnosed to try to understand the cause and make critical decisions about managing the hearing loss. Others may seek genetic counseling when considering family planning or to obtain updated information about genetic testing or research opportunities. Genetic counselors can provide information about recurrence risks, preimplantation genetic diagnosis, or prenatal diagnostic testing.

If genetic testing is pursued, a genetic counselor can discuss the benefits and limitations of genetic testing, including the possible test results, as well as help the family interpret the results of testing when they are received. A potential benefit of genetic testing is that identifying mutations may help to rule out, or predict the development of, additional clinical features, depending on whether a nonsyndromic or syndromic etiology is identified. Identifying the genetic etiology may also help determine whether the hearing loss will progress and may help determine how best to manage the hearing loss. In addition, identification of a genetic cause enables families to know the recurrence risk (chance of having future children with hearing loss). For example, if a hearing couple has a child with hearing loss, the recurrence risk of having a second child with hearing loss is ~ 17.5%, which takes into account the possibility that it may be either genetic or environmental in origin (Green et al, 1999). This risk drops slightly to ~ 14% if connexin 26 testing is negative (Smith & Robin, 2002). In contrast, if genetic testing is positive, more informative risk assessments can be provided.

Pitfall

- Potential limitations of genetic testing are that the test (in the case of a negative result) does not *rule out* a genetic cause for hearing loss.

As described in this chapter, many genes are associated with hearing loss, and currently there is testing for a large number of them. Genetic testing may give unclear results. For instance, if a child with nonsyndromic sensorineural hearing loss is found to have one connexin 26 mutation, as is the case 10 to 50% of the time (Del Castillo, Moreno-Pelayo, et al, 2003), connexin 26 may be in fact responsible for causing the hearing loss, but the second mutation was not detected. However, the child may simply be a carrier for the connexin 26 mutation, and another unidentified cause, genetic or environmental, may be responsible for the hearing loss. In these cases it is not possible to differentiate between the explanations in any given child. Also, genetic testing cannot always predict the characteristics of the hearing loss, such as age of onset, progression, or how severe the loss or associated signs and symptoms will be.

As testing panels grow, the need for thorough pre- and posttest counseling also increases. Patients and families should discuss with a genetic counselor or health care provider what the possible outcomes of genetic testing may be to provide informed consent about genetic testing. For gene panels that include both nonsyndromic and syndromic types of hearing loss, families should be prepared for the possibility that testing may reveal a diagnosis not initially suspected, such as a diagnosis of Usher syndrome in an infant who has presented only with hearing loss. Similarly, it is possible one could find the child is an incidental carrier for a mutation in a hearing loss gene that is unrelated to the child's own hearing loss. This carrier status may have an impact on the patient or other family members in aspects of family planning and risk assessment. In addition, growing numbers of genes queried also increase the chances of finding a variant of unknown significance (VUS). A VUS is a change in which it is unclear whether the change has an impact on the function of the gene or not. Genetic counselors are well trained in patient education and counseling about uncertainty, which can greatly aid in the patient care when discussing genetic testing for hearing loss.

◆ Gene Therapy for Hearing Loss

Much hope has been placed on the concept of gene therapy for genetic disorders. Unfortunately, gene therapy has not been realized to its full potential be-

cause of some very significant practical challenges. These include challenges in the successful development of methods to put the correct gene into the cells that need it, as well as in figuring out ways to maintain the cells with the new genetic material (the body often sees the changed cells as foreign bodies and destroys them). Despite these challenges, there are success stories, some involving immune-related diseases where gene therapy can be performed on blood cells that are taken out of the patient and put back after genetic alteration.

Although gene therapy has not advanced as quickly as hoped, advances have been made, with some of the accomplishments specific to hearing loss. For example, methods have been developed to incorporate genetic material stably into the hair cells of mammals, including mice and guinea pigs. In one study, the addition of the *Atoh1* gene caused the ear to regenerate new hair cells in a guinea pig whose hearing had been destroyed by ototoxic damage. Early studies are now under way to use similar approaches to restore function to mammals with genetically based hearing loss. Such approaches have been successfully used to restore vision to dogs with an early form of genetic blindness (Acland et al, 2005). This holds promise for the ability to prevent blindness in patients diagnosed early with Usher syndrome. Early work on Usher syndrome gene therapy has already begun, and the correction of retinal abnormalities in mice with Usher syndrome has been demonstrated (Hashimoto et al, 2007). Furthermore, recent studies suggest that a future approach to correction of connexin 26–based hearing loss could be to upregulate the neighboring connexin 30 gene in patients (Ahmad et al, 2007). Despite these encouraging advances, it will probably be 10 or more years before such approaches may begin to be used in humans.

◆ Summary

Substantial advancements have been made in understanding, diagnosing, and treating hearing loss. In particular, much has been learned from the discovery of a growing portion of the genes responsible for hearing loss. New technologies are allowing for larger gene panels and more cost-effective testing methods, but many patients still face financial barriers to available genetic testing. The future hopefully holds reduction in cost of genetic testing and increased understanding of the many genes that play a role in hearing. This will enable a genetic evaluation of children with hearing loss to be even better integrated into clinical care than it is now. Such integration will lead to improved diagnoses and more tailored strategies for managing, and eventually curing, hearing loss.

Discussion Questions

1. If your patient is the only individual in his family with hearing loss, can it be genetic?

2. If a couple has a child with congenital SNHL from two mutations in the connexin 26 gene, what is their chance of having a second child with SNHL?

3. If a child tests negative for connexin 26 gene mutations, could his hearing loss still be genetic? What is the chance that the parents will have a second child with hearing loss? Is additional testing available?

4. You have been seeing Michael since he failed his newborn hearing screen and was found to have a bilateral, profound SNHL. He is now 10 years old, and at his last appointment his mother mentioned he was having trouble seeing at night and has always been clumsy. Is there anything to be concerned about? Could these problems be related to his hearing loss? If so, what should you do?

5. A deaf couple shares with you that they are currently pregnant and state that they are interested in knowing the genetic status for deafness in the fetus because they feel they cannot continue a pregnancy that will result in the birth of a hearing child. How would you respond?

References

Acland, G. M., Aguirre, G. D., Bennett, J., Aleman, T. S., Cideciyan, A. V., Bennicelli, J., . . . Jacobson, S. G. (2005). Long-term restoration of rod and cone vision by single dose rAAV-mediated gene transfer to the retina in a canine model of childhood blindness. Molecular Therapy, 12(6), 1072–1082.

Ahmad, S., Tang, W., Chang, Q., Qu, Y., Hibshman, J., Li, Y., . . . Lin, X. (2007). Restoration of connexin26 protein level in the cochlea completely rescues hearing in a mouse model of human connexin30-linked deafness. Proc. Natl. Acad. Sci. USA, 104(4), 1337–1341.

American College of Medical Genetics and Genomics. (2002). Genetics evaluation guidelines for the etiologic diagnosis of congenital hearing loss. Genetic Evaluation of Congenital Hearing Loss Expert Panel. ACMG statement. Genetics in Medicine, 4(3), 162–171.

Angeli, S. (2003). Value of vestibular testing in young children with sensorineural hearing loss. Archives of Otolaryngology–Head & Neck Surgery, 129(4), 478–482.

Berson, E. L., Rosner, B., Sandberg, M. A., Hayes, K. C., Nicholson, B. W., Weigel-DiFranco, C., & Willett, W. (1993). A randomized trial of vitamin A and vitamin E supplementation for retinitis pigmentosa. Archives of Ophthalmology, 111(6), 761–772.

Calvo, J. R. R., Gasparini, P., & Estivill, X. (2007). Connexins and Deafness Homepage, Deafness Research Group (CRG). http://davinici.crg.es/deafness

Campbell, C., Cucci, R. A., Prasad, S., Green, G. E., Edeal, J. B., Galer, C. E., . . . Smith, R. J. (2001). Pendred syndrome, DFNB4, and PDS/SLC26A4 identification of eight novel mutations and possible genotype-phenotype correlations. Human Mutation, 17(5), 403–411.

Centers for Disease Control and Prevention, National Center on Birth Defects and Developmental Disabilities. (2010). 2010 CDC EHDI Hearing Screening & Follow-up Survey (HSFS). Washington, DC: CDC.

Chang, E. H., Menezes, M., Meyer, N. C., Cucci, R. A., Vervoort, V. S., Schwartz, C. E., Smith, R. J. (2004). Branchio-oto-renal syndrome: the mutation spectrum in EYA1 and its phenotypic consequences. Human Mutation, 23(6), 582–589.

Chee, N. W., Suhailee, S., & Goh, J. (2006). Clinics in diagnostic imaging (111): X-linked congenital mixed deafness syndrome. Singapore Medical Journal, 47(9), 822–824, quiz 825.

Daley, S. M., Tranebjærg, L., Samson, R. A., & Green, G. E. (2004). Jervell and Lange-Nielsen syndrome. In GeneReviews at GeneTests: Medical Genetics Information Resource (database online), University of Washington, Seattle. Retrieved from http://www.genetests.org

Del Castillo, F. J., Rodríguez-Ballesteros, M., Martín, Y., Arellano, B., Gallo-Terán, J., Morales-Angulo, C., . . . Del Castillo, I. (2003). Heteroplasmy for the 1555A>G mutation in the mitochondrial 12S rRNA gene in six Spanish families with non-syndromic hearing loss. Journal of Medical Genetics, 40(8), 632–636.

Del Castillo, I., Moreno-Pelayo, M. A., Del Castillo, F. J., Brownstein, Z., Marlin, S., Adina, Q., . . . Moreno, F. (2003). Prevalence and evolutionary origins of the del(GJB6-D13S1830) mutation in the DFNB1 locus in hearing-impaired subjects: a multicenter study. American Journal of Human Genetics, 73(6), 1452–1458.

Delmaghani, S., del Castillo, F. J., Michel, V., Leibovici, M., Aghaie, A., Ron, U., . . . Petit, C. (2006). Mutations in the gene encoding pejvakin, a newly identified protein of the afferent auditory pathway, cause DFNB59 auditory neuropathy. Nature Genetics, 38(7), 770–778.

Evans, D. G. (2006). Neurofibromatosis 2. In GeneReviews at GeneTests: Medical Genetics Information Resource (database online), University of Washington, Seattle. Retrieved from http://www.genetests.org

Evans, D. G. (2009). Neurofibromatosis 2 [Bilateral acoustic neurofibromatosis, central neurofibromatosis, NF2, neurofibromatosis type II]. Genetics in Medicine, 11(9), 599–610.

Fraser, F. C., Sproule, J. R., & Halal, F. (1980). Frequency of the branchio-oto-renal (BOR) syndrome in children with profound hearing loss. American Journal of Medical Genetics, 7(3), 341–349.

Fraser, G. (1976). The causes of profound deafness in childhood. Baltimore, MD: Johns Hopkins University Press.

GeneTests (2012). GeneTests: Medical Genetics Information Resource (database online). University of Washington, Seattle. Retrieved from http://www.genetests.org

Genetic Evaluation of Congenital Hearing Loss Expert Panel (2002). Genetics evaluation guidelines for the etiologic diagnosis of congenital hearing loss. Genetics in Medicine, 4, 162–171.

Goldfeld, M., Glaser, B., Nassir, E., Gomori, J. M., Hazani, E., & Bishara, N. (2005). CT of the ear in Pendred syndrome. Radiology, 235(2), 537–540.

Gorlin, R. J., Toriello, H. V., & Cohen, M. M. (1995). Hereditary hearing loss and its syndromes. New York, NY: Oxford University Press.

Green, G. E., Scott, D. A., McDonald, J. M., Woodworth, G. G., Sheffield, V. C., & Smith, R. J. (1999). Carrier rates in the midwestern United States for *GJB2* mutations causing inherited deafness. Journal of the American Medical Association, 281(23), 2211–2216.

Green, G. E., Smith, R. J., Bent, J. P., & Cohn, E. S. (2000). Genetic testing to identify deaf newborns. Journal of the American Medical Association, 284(10), 1245.

Hashimoto, T., Gibbs, D., Lillo, C., Azarian, S. M., Legacki, E., Zhang, X. M., . . . Jacobson, S. G. (2007). Lentiviral gene replacement therapy of retinas in a mouse model for Usher syndrome type 1B. Gene Therapy, 14(7), 584–594.

Hoskins, B. E., Cramer, C. H., Silvius, D., Zou, D., Raymond, R. M., Orten, D. J., . . . Hildebrandt, F. (2007). Transcription factor *SIX5* is mutated in patients with branchio-oto-renal syndrome. American Journal of Human Genetics, 80(4), 800–804.

Issekutz, K. A., Graham, J. M., Jr, Prasad, C., Smith, I. M., & Blake, K. D. (2005). An epidemiological analysis of CHARGE syndrome: preliminary results from a Canadian study. American Journal of Medical Genetics. Part A, 133A(3), 309–317.

Kashtan, C. E. (2007). Collagen IV-related nephropathies (Alport syndrome and thin basement membrane nephropathy). In GeneReviews at GeneTests: Medical Genetics Information Resource (database online), University of Washington, Seattle. Retrieved from http://www.genetests.org

Keats, B. J., & Lentz, J. (2006a). Usher syndrome type I. In GeneReviews at GeneTests: Medical Genetics Information Resource (database online), University of Washington, Seattle. Retrieved from http://www.genetests.org

Keats, B. J., & Lentz, J. (2006b). Usher syndrome type II. In GeneReviews at GeneTests: Medical Genetics Information Resource (database online), University of Washington, Seattle. Retrieved from http://www.genetests.org

Kemperman, M. H., Koch, S. M., Kumar, S., Huygen, P. L., Joosten, F. B., & Cremers, C. W. (2004). Evidence of progression and fluctuation of hearing impairment in branchio-oto-renal syndrome. International Journal of Audiology, 43(9), 523–532.

Kenna, M. A., Feldman, H. A., Neault, M. W., Frangulov, A., Wu, B. L, Fligor, B., & Rehm, H. L. (2010). Audiologic phenotype and progression in *GJB2* (connexin 26) hearing loss. Archives of Otolaryngology–Head & Neck Surgery, 136(1), 81–87.

Kimberling, W. J., & Möller, C. (1995). Clinical and molecular genetics of Usher syndrome. Journal of the American Academy of Audiology, 6(1), 63–72.

Kupka, S., Braun, S., Aberle, S., Haack, B., Ebauer, M., Zeissler, U., . . . Pfister, M. (2002). Frequencies of *GJB2* mutations in German control individuals and patients showing sporadic non-syndromic hearing impairment. Human Mutation, 20(1), 77–78.

Lalani, S. R., Hefner, M., Belmont, J. W., & Davenport, S. L. (2006). CHARGE syndrome. In GeneReviews at GeneTests: Medical Genetics Information Resource (database online), University of Washington, Seattle. Retrieved from http://www.genetests.org

Lalani, S. R., Safiullah, A. M., Fernbach, S. D., Harutyunyan, K. G., Thaller, C., Peterson, L. E., . . . Belmont, J. W. (2006). Spectrum of CHD7 mutations in 110 individuals with CHARGE syndrome and genotype-phenotype correlation. American Journal of Human Genetics, 78(2), 303–314.

Levy, M., & Feingold, J. (2000). Estimating prevalence in single-gene kidney diseases progressing to renal failure. Kidney International, 58(3), 925–943.

Li, R., Greinwald, J. H., Jr., Yang, L., Choo, D. I., Wenstrup, R. J., & Guan, M. X. (2004). Molecular analysis of the mitochondrial 12S rRNA and tRNASer(UCN) genes in paediatric subjects with non-syndromic hearing loss. Journal of Medical Genetics, 41(8), 615–620.

Lin, X., Tang, W., Ahmad, S., Lu, J., Colby, C. C., Zhu, J., & Yu, Q. (2012). Applications of targeted gene capture and next-generation sequencing technologies in studies of human deafness and other genetic disabilities. Hearing Research, 288(1-2), 67–76.

Marlin, S., Feldmann, D., Nguyen, Y., Rouillon, I., Loundon, N., Jonard, L., . . . Denoyelle, F. (2010). Temperature-sensitive auditory neuropathy associated with an otoferlin mutation: Deafening fever! Biochemical and Biophysical Research Communications, 394(3), 737–742.

Migliosi, V., Modamio-Høybjør, S., Moreno-Pelayo, M. A., Rodríguez-Ballesteros, M., Villamar, M., Tellería, D., . . . Del Castillo, I. (2002, Jul). Q829X, a novel mutation in the gene encoding otoferlin (*OTOF*), is frequently found in Spanish patients with prelingual non-syndromic hearing loss. Journal of Medical Genetics, 39(7), 502–506.

Milunsky, J. M. (2006). Waardenburg syndrome type I. In GeneReviews at GeneTests: Medical Genetics Information Resource (database online), University of Washington, Seattle. Retrieved from http://www.genetests.org

Mitchell, R. E., & Karchmer, M. A. (2004). Chasing the mythical ten percent: Parental hearing status of deaf and hard of hearing students in the United States. Sign Language Studies, 4(2), 138–163.

Morton, N. E. (1991). Genetic epidemiology of hearing impairment. Annals of the New York Academy of Sciences, 630, 16–31.

Morton, C. C., & Nance, W. E. (2006). Newborn hearing screening—a silent revolution. The New England Journal of Medicine, 354(20), 2151–2164.

Norris, V. W., Arnos, K. S., Hanks, W. D., Xia, X., Nance, W. E., & Pandya, A. (2006). Does universal newborn hearing screening identify all children with *GJB2* (connexin 26) deafness? Penetrance of *GJB2* deafness. Ear and Hearing, 27(6), 732–741.

OMIM (2012). Online Mendelian inheritance in man. McKusick-Nathans Institute for Genetic Medicine, Johns Hopkins University (Baltimore, MD) and National Center for Biotechnology Information, National Library of Medicine (Bethesda, MD). Retrieved from http://omim.org/

Pandya, A. (2004). Nonsyndromic hearing loss, mitochondrial. In GeneReviews at GeneTests: Medical Genetics Information Resource (database online), University of Washington, Seattle. Retrieved from http://www. genetests.org

Park, H.J., Shaukat, S., Liu, X.Z., Hahn, S. H., Naz, S., Ghosh, M., . . . Griffith, A. J. (2003). Origins and frequencies of *SLC26A4* (*PDS*) mutations in east and south Asians: global implications for the epidemiology of deafness. Journal of Medical Genetics, 40(4), 242–248.

Putcha, G. V., Bejjani, B. A., Bleoo, S., Booker, J. K., Carey, J. C., Carson, N., . . . Schrijver, I. (2007). A multicenter study of the frequency and distribution of *GJB2* and *GJB6* mutations in a large North American cohort. Genetics in Medicine, 9(7), 413–426.

Rodríguez-Ballesteros, M., del Castillo, F. J., Martín, Y., Moreno-Pelayo, M. A., Morera, C., Prieto, F., . . . del Castillo, I. (2003). Auditory neuropathy in patients carrying mutations in the otoferlin gene (OTOF). Human Mutation, 22(6), 451–456.

Ruf, R. G., Xu, P. X., Silvius, D., Otto, E. A., Beekmann, F., Muerb, U. T., . . . Hildebrandt, F. (2004). *SIX1* mutations cause branchio-oto-renal syndrome by disruption of *EYA1-SIX1*-DNA complexes. Proc. Natl. Acad. Sci. USA, 101(21), 8090–8095.

Schrijver, I., & Gardner, P. (2006). Hereditary sensorineural hearing loss: advances in molecular genetics and mutation analysis. Expert Review of Molecular Diagnostics, 6(3), 375–386.

Schwartz, P. J., Periti, M., & Malliani, A. (1975). The long Q-T syndrome. American Heart Journal, 89(3), 378–390.

Smith, R. J. (2006a). Congenital deafness—*GJB2* and Usher syndrome type 1. First International Symposium on Usher Syndrome and Related Disorders October 3–6, 2006. Omaha, Nebraska.

Smith, R. J. (2006b). Branchiootorenal syndrome. In GeneReviews at GeneTests: Medical Genetics Information Resource (database online), University of Washington, Seattle. Retrieved from http://www. genetests.org

Smith, R. J., & Robin, N. H. (2002). Genetic testing for deafness—*GJB2* and *SLC26A4* as causes of deafness. Journal of Communication Disorders, 35(4), 367–377.

Smith, R. J., & Van Camp, G. (2005). Nonsyndromic hearing loss and deafness, DFNB1. In GeneReviews at GeneTests: Medical Genetics Information Resource (database online), University of Washington, Seattle. Retrieved from http://www.genetests.org

Smith, R. J., & Van Camp, G. (2006). Pendred syndrome/DFNB4. In GeneReviews at GeneTests: Medical Genetics Information Resource (database online), University of Washington, Seattle. Retrieved from http://www.genetests.org

Snoeckx, R. L., Huygen, P. L., Feldmann, D., Marlin, S., Denoyelle, F., Waligora, J., . . . Van Camp, G. (2005). *GJB2* mutations and degree of hearing loss: a multicenter study. American Journal of Human Genetics, 77(6), 945–957.

Toriello, H. V., Reardon, W., & Gorlin, R. J. (2004). Hereditary hearing loss and its syndromes. Oxford, England: Oxford University Press.

Usami, S., Abe, S., Akita, J., Namba, A., Shinkawa, H., Ishii, M., . . . Komune, S. (2000). Prevalence of mitochondrial gene mutations among hearing impaired patients. Journal of Medical Genetics, 37(1), 38–40.

Usami, S., Abe, S., Weston, M. D., Shinkawa, H., Van Camp, G., & Kimberling, W. J. (1999). Non-syndromic hearing loss associated with enlarged vestibular aqueduct is caused by *PDS* mutations. Human Genetics, 104(2), 188–192.

Van Camp, G., & Smith, R. J. H. (2012). Hereditary hearing loss homepage. Retrieved from http://hereditaryhearingloss.org/

Varga, R., Avenarius, M. R., Kelley, P. M., Keats, B. J., Berlin, C. I., Hood, L. J., . . . Kimberling, W. J. (2006). *OTOF* mutations revealed by genetic analysis of hearing loss families including a potential temperature sensitive auditory neuropathy allele. Journal of Medical Genetics, 43(7), 576–581.

Varga, R., Kelley, P. M., Keats, B. J., Starr, A., Leal, S. M., Cohn, E., & Kimberling, W. J. (2003). Non-syndromic recessive auditory neuropathy is the result of mutations in the otoferlin (*OTOF*) gene. Journal of Medical Genetics, 40(1), 45–50.

Yang, T., Gurrola, J. G. II, Wu, H., Chiu, S. M., Wangemann, P., Snyder, P. M., Smith, R. J. (2009). Mutations of *KCNJ10* together with mutations of SLC26A4 cause digenic nonsyndromic hearing loss associated with enlarged vestibular aqueduct syndrome. American Journal of Human Genetics, 84(5), 651–657.

Yang, T., Vidarsson, H., Rodrigo-Blomqvist, S., Rosengren, S. S., Enerback, S., & Smith, R. J. (2007). Transcriptional control of *SLC26A4* is involved in Pendred syndrome and nonsyndromic enlargement of vestibular aqueduct (DFNB4). American Journal of Human Genetics, 80(6), 1055–1063.

Yasunaga, S., Grati, M., Cohen-Salmon, M., El-Amraoui, A., Mustapha, M., Salem, N., . . . Petit, C. (1999). A mutation in OTOF, encoding otoferlin, a FER-1-like protein, causes DFNB9, a nonsyndromic form of deafness. Nature Genetics, 21(4), 363–369.

Chapter 4

Medical Evaluation and Medical Management of Hearing Loss in Children

George Alexiades and Ronald A. Hoffman

Key Points

- Proper medical diagnosis of hearing loss in children is predicated upon a thorough history, good physical examination and proper imaging studies.
- Most congenital hearing losses are hereditary.
- Constant vigilance by parents, pediatricians, and teachers is necessary because many hearing losses develop later in childhood.

Sensorineural hearing loss (SNHL) is the most common birth disorder in the United States (2004 National Consensus Conference on Effective Educational and Health Care Interventions for Infants and Young Children with Hearing Loss). Severe to profound SNHL occurs in one to two children per thousand live births (Brookhouser, 1996), and another two to three per thousand babies are born with partial hearing loss. The cumulative incidence of otitis media with effusion, associated with conductive hearing loss (CHL), is 80% by the age of 4 years (Louis et al, 2005). The proper identification and medical management of these children with hearing loss is a priority if speech and language deficits are to be minimized and progressive otologic disease avoided.

The most important aspect of managing a child with hearing loss is early identification. Universal newborn hearing screening, implemented in most states, allows for the early identification of most children with hearing loss. However, constant vigilance by parents, pediatricians, and teachers is necessary, because many hearing losses develop later in childhood.

Congenital hearing loss is defined as a hearing loss that is present at birth. Congenital hearing loss is not synonymous with hereditary hearing loss, though the two terms are mistakenly used interchangeably. Many hereditary hearing losses manifest themselves later in childhood, and many congenital hearing losses are due to nongenetic causes. Approximately 60% of congenital hearing loss is believed to be heredi-

tary (Morton, 1991). If a child passes newborn hearing screening, but there is a family history of hearing loss, that child must be tested repeatedly over time.

Neonatal hearing loss may be syndromic or nonsyndromic. Syndromic hearing loss occurs in association with other clinical features, though they are not exclusively hereditary in nature (e.g., fetal alcohol syndrome). Approximately 70% of hereditary hearing loss is nonsyndromic (Lalwani & Castelein, 1999), where the hearing loss is the only clinical manifestation. Of these, the inheritance pattern is autosomal recessive in 75%, autosomal dominant in 10–20%, X-linked in 2–3%, and mitochondrial in 1% (Doyle & Ray, 2003). The most common cause of hereditary hearing loss is mutations in connexin 26, which accounts for up to 80% of autosomal recessive nonsyndromic hearing loss (Denoyelle et al, 1997). The hearing loss with connexin 26 mutations can be of any degree, and these children are usually otherwise healthy and normal.

Pearl

- Most hereditary hearing loss is nonsyndromic and autosomal recessive, connexin 26 mutations being the most common cause of disorder.

◆ The Medical Evaluation of the Newly Identified Child

A Thorough History

When a neonate with a newly identified SNHL is seen, the physician begins with a detailed history. That history includes:

- Birth history: Were there any perinatal factors that might predispose to hearing loss, such as prematurity, fetal distress, pregnancy related-illnesses, drug treatments during pregnancy, low birth weight, the need for neonatal intensive care, intravenous ototoxic antibiotics, or kernicterus (high bilirubin)?

- Family history: Is there a family history of hearing loss, suggesting a genetic cause?
- Medical history: Is there any known history of cytomegalovirus (CMV), herpes, or syphilis? Has the child had perinatal meningitis?

Pearl

- The history is the most important piece in identifying the etiology of the hearing loss.

Physical Examination

A physical examination is performed to be sure there are no physical stigmata associated with syndromic hearing loss. For example, widely spaced eyes, heterochromia iridum (eyes of different colors), and a white forelock of hair are typical of Waardenburg syndrome. A hypoplastic malar eminence (flat cheekbones) is a facial deformity that may suggest Treacher-Collins syndrome. The outer and middle ears are carefully examined with an otoscope or operating microscope to ensure there is no atresia of the external ear, or middle ear pathology such as an effusion (fluid). The presence of a middle ear effusion is a major cause of false positives in neonatal hearing screening: the child fails the screen, but in fact there is no SNHL.

Laboratory Testing

The use of laboratory testing to diagnose SNHL at birth is controversial because the yield of useful information is low. Genetic testing may provide a diagnosis for a hearing loss and may help to predict the likelihood of parents' having another child with hearing loss, but it does not influence how the child is managed clinically. Children who are identified as having a severe to profound SNHL should all undergo ophthalmologic examination to rule out Usher syndrome, which is characterized by SNHL and progressive vision loss. Today, earlier identification of these children is possible with an electroretinogram, which can identify these patients before there are any visible retinal changes (Young, Mets, & Hain, 1996). An electrocardiogram is necessary to diag-

nose Jervell and Lange-Nielsen syndrome, which can lead to a potentially fatal cardiac arrhythmia if left untreated. Serologic studies (blood tests) have proven disappointing and, other than for genetic testing, are not recommended. Imaging studies of the inner ear, such as computed tomography (CT) or magnetic resonance imaging (MRI), may provide useful information, particularly regarding the anatomy of the inner ear. However, these are of no pragmatic value during the first 2 years of life, when the only issue is amplification. As the child matures, the identification of large vestibular aqueduct syndrome (LVAS) may influence behavioral modification, since minor head trauma is associated with further hearing loss (Jackler & De La Cruz, 1989). When cochlear implantation becomes an alternative, preoperative imaging is essential.

If a child has had a stable SNHL that then progresses over time or receives limited benefit from amplification, or if there is a fluctuating SNHL, the evaluation algorithm changes and becomes more proactive. Such children should be imaged to identify a cochlear abnormality that may be associated with a perilymphatic fistula, a microscopic leak of fluid from the inner ear. Middle ear exploration and repair of the fistula may be warranted in such cases. There are differing opinions on the utility of surgical exploration in these patients. Several studies have shown improvement mainly in vestibular symptoms, with some improvement or stabilization of hearing (Roman, Bourliere-Najean, & Triglia, 1998). Other recent studies have not shown any benefit in either vestibular or auditory function between surgically repaired patients and those who were only observed (Sim, Jardine, & Beckenham 2009). Blood tests should also be performed to rule out autoimmune disorders, syphilis, or Lyme disease. If the hearing loss is unilateral, a cerebellopontine angle tumor must be ruled out with MRI of the internal auditory canals.

In all cases where a child is identified with SNHL, whether stable or progressive, that child should be followed with at least yearly audiograms and examinations. At the initial stages of identification of the hearing loss, more frequent audiograms, including auditory brainstem response (ABR) and otoacoustic emissions (OAE), are required to document the stability of the hearing loss.

Controversial Point

- Laboratory testing in the work-up of SNHL in children is not productive.

◆ Managing Childhood Hearing Loss: The Role of the Pediatrician

The pediatrician has a critical role in managing the general health and well-being of infants and children. The pediatrician is the "medical home" for all children. The medical home provides health care that is accessible, family centered, continuous, comprehensive, coordinated, compassionate, and culturally competent (Medical Home Initiatives for Children with Special Needs Project Advisory Committee, American Academy of Pediatrics, 2002; American Academy of Pediatrics, 2010). When a child with hearing loss presents in a pediatric practice, the pediatrician has a responsibility to be knowledgeable about the effect of hearing loss on all aspects of the child's development.

Early identification of the hearing loss is essential. When infants fail newborn hearing screening, the pediatrician's role is critical in making certain that families obtain the appropriate evaluations and in providing support and comfort to parents, who likely will be devastated by a diagnosis of hearing loss. If hearing loss is identified, the pediatrician must be certain that appropriate follow-up is obtained so the infant is fitted with technology by 3 months of age and enrolled in an appropriate intervention program by 6 months of age (Joint Commission on Infant Hearing [JCIH], 2007).

Once hearing loss is identified, the otologist and audiologist will be the primary managers of the child's hearing loss; however, other issues will present that will require management by the pediatrician. For example, children with hearing loss often develop otitis media, a medical condition that may exacerbate the child's degree of hearing loss. Because of the significant negative effect of even minor changes in hearing sensitivity on speech and language development, the pediatrician will need to work closely with the audiologist and otologist to manage the medical aspects of the hearing loss and make decisions about the child's overall medical condition. In addition, the pediatrician will work with the otologist to make recommendations for genetic testing and other medical evaluations as needed.

The pediatrician, as the primary care physician, assumes responsibility for coordinating comprehensive health care and working as a team member with the family and all key professionals.

Acquired Hearing Loss

Not all hearing losses are identified at birth. A significant number of children develop hearing loss after the newborn period (Madell & Sculerati, 1991). At each well-baby visit, the pediatrician needs to monitor the child's development; question auditory, speech, and language milestones; and monitor other aspects of growth. When there is any question, the pediatrician needs to refer for appropriate audiologic evaluation.

The Joint Committee on Infant Hearing (JCIH, 2007) has listed risk factors that may result in delayed-onset or progressive hearing loss. These include:

1. Family history of hearing loss and genetic disorders or syndromes associated with hearing loss
2. Caregiver concern regarding hearing, speech, language, or developmental delay
3. Infants admitted to the neonatal intensive care unit (NICU)
4. In-utero infections, such as CMV, herpes, rubella, syphilis, and toxoplasmosis
5. Craniofacial anomalies
6. Physical findings such as a white forelock or atresias
7. Syndromes associated with hearing loss or late-onset or progressive hearing loss
8. Neurodegenerative disorders
9. Culture positive postnatal infections associated with sensorineural hearing loss
10. Serious head trauma
11. Chemotherapy or cancer

Pediatricians should arrange for routine hearing evaluations of children who have these risk factors to ensure that no late-onset hearing loss is missed.

◆ Specific Disease Entities Causing SNHL

Vestibulocochlear Abnormalities

Vestibulocochlear dysplasias cover a wide variety of abnormalities in the inner ear. These may range from isolated semicircular canal abnormalities, with little to no impact on hearing, to a common cavity deformity, where there is one spherical cavity for both the auditory and vestibular systems and a resultant severe to profound SNHL. It is important to identify these abnormalities, as they may have a significant impact on cochlear implantation and postoperative performance. In addition, cochlear dysplasias are associated with a real incidence of perilymphatic fistula, usually through a hole in the footplate of the stapes.

Perilymphatic Fistula

A perilymphatic fistula (PLF) is an abnormal communication between the perilymphatic space and the middle ear cavity. A PLF may occur through the round window, oval window, or both. PLF usually occurs as a result of head trauma or barotrauma. Patients suffer a sudden, progressive, or fluctuating SNHL with or without vestibular symptoms. The key to the diagnosis in an adult is the history. For example, the patient who experiences severe pain on airplane descent with a sudden hearing loss and vertigo must be considered to have a PLF until proven otherwise.

Children, on the other hand, are not likely to be able to provide a history of head trauma, which they experience regularly. Moreover, in the presence of a cochlear malformation, children may suffer from spontaneous PLF, unassociated with head trauma or barotrauma. The key to the diagnosis in a child is the detection of the presence of a cochlear malformation. The diagnosis of a spontaneous PLF in a child without a cochlear malformation is highly controversial. The treatment algorithm for a child with a progressive or fluctuating SNHL with a suspected PLF is outlined in **Fig. 4.1**.

Large Vestibular Aqueduct Syndrome

LVAS is a specific type of inner ear abnormality in which the vestibular aqueduct, the bony channel that houses the endolymphatic duct, is abnormally enlarged. It is the most common inner ear abnormality found on CT scans, with its incidence between 4–10% in children with SNHL (Madden, Halsted, Benton, Greinwald, & Choo, 2003). Genetic testing for Pendred syndrome, which is categorized by abnormal iodine incorporation and resultant enlargement of the thyroid gland, has been found to be associated with LVAS in up to 50% of cases (Berrettini et al, 2005). Conversely, almost all patients with Pendred syndrome have an inner ear abnormality, most of which are LVAS. LVAS is associated with a progressive, fluctuating, or sudden SNHL. Stepwise SNHL is often precipitated by minor head trauma. Therefore, it is recommended that these children abstain from contact sports, as those activities may result in an acute drop in hearing.

Ototoxic Medications

Many medications have been identified as ototoxic in nature, yet are still used due to their efficacy in treating specific medical conditions. The most common class of ototoxic medications used is the aminoglycoside antibiotics, most commonly gentamicin. These are used quite frequently in neonates with suspected sepsis or meningitis. Moreover, they are used commonly in developing nations because of their potency and low cost. Although newer, nonototoxic antibiotics have been developed that cover similar organisms, aminoglycosides are often necessary to treat resistant organisms or serious infections.

Many chemotherapeutic agents are also known to be ototoxic. The most common is cisplatin, used for

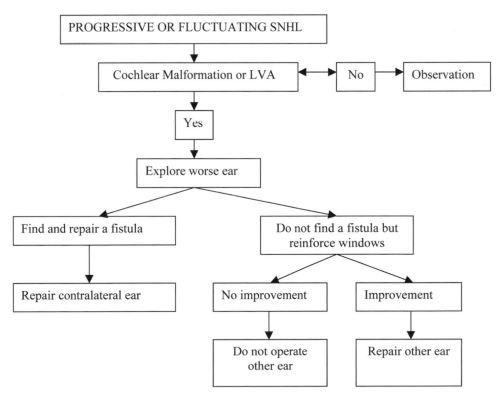

Fig. 4.1 Algorithm for medical management of a child with a progressive or fluctuating SNHL.

a variety of pediatric malignancies. The hearing loss begins with a high-frequency deficit. It is important to obtain a baseline audiogram prior to treatment and to follow up with audiograms throughout the treatment. Evolving hearing loss may necessitate a change to another, less ototoxic agent.

Infections

Meningitis is an inflammation of the lining of the brain, which is often caused by bacteria. Today, *Streptococcus pneumoniae* and *Neisseria meningitidis* are the most common organisms causing meningitis. With the advent of the *Haemophilus influenzae* vaccine, meningitis due to this bacterium has been virtually eliminated. The cochlear aqueduct is a connection between the basal turn of the cochlea and the cerebrospinal fluid space surrounding the brain. On occasion, particularly in young children, the cochlear aqueduct is large and open. The bacteria that cause meningitis can gain access to the inner ear from the infected cerebrospinal fluid via the cochlear aqueduct, resulting in severe to profound hearing loss. Moreover, these bacteria are highly irritative and can cause new bone to form in the cochlea, a condition called labyrinthitis ossificans. This is a dynamic process beginning immediately after the infection and can result in significant blockage of the cochlea in as little as 6 weeks (Tinling, Colton, & Brodie, 2004). It is imperative that these patients be "fast-tracked" through the cochlear implant evaluation process and, if indicated, an implant be inserted as quickly as possible. Should too much time pass, there can be significant ossification of the cochlea, which can result in an incomplete electrode insertion or, in some cases, preclude implantation altogether.

Neoplasms

Neoplasms in the cerebellopontine angle or internal auditory canal are rare in children and comprise only 1% of all intracranial lesions. The most common neoplasms in this area are neurofibromatosis type 2, arachnoid cysts, epidermoid cysts, and meningiomas (Ruggieri et al, 2005). Rarely, an isolated acoustic neuroma will be encountered in a child. Children with such intracranial neoplasms usually present with unilateral SNHL or imbalance and, in the case of neurofibromatosis type 2, frequently have ocular or motor dysfunction due to the multicentricity of the disease. Rarely, malignant neoplasms of the cerebellopontine angle cause unilateral sensorineural hearing loss, as in medulloblastomas and glioblastomas. When a child presents with a new or progressive unilateral sensorineural hearing loss, MRI with gadolinium contrast enhancement is indicated for diagnosis.

◆ Specific Disease Entities Causing Conductive Hearing Loss

Otitis Media with Effusion

Acute suppurative otitis media is the most common infection worldwide and the most common indication for antibiotics in children. Otitis media with effusion (OME) is fluid in the middle ear space without the signs and symptoms of infection (pain, fever, and redness of the tympanic membrane). OME can cause a hearing loss of up to 30 dB. There is a general consensus that OME is overtreated. Decongestants may be indicated if a child suffers with allergies or a sinus condition. Antibiotics are not generally useful. Although oral steroids may resolve OME, the recurrence rate is high, and their use in children is controversial. Current guidelines recommend waiting a minimum of 3 months for OME to clear spontaneously before considering insertion of myringotomy tubes.

Multiple studies have been done on the long-term effect on language development of placing ventilation tubes in children with less than 3 months of OME, as opposed to later. The data clearly show that early insertion of ventilation tubes does not favorably affect speech and language skills long-term (Louis et al, 2005; Paradise et al, 2005). However, no studies have been undertaken in children with underlying SNHL, learning disabilities, or speech and language delay. It is the authors' opinion that in children with additional health or environmental challenges, more aggressive management is appropriate.

The Sequelae of Chronic Otitis Media

Chronic otitis media with effusion and/or recurrent suppurative otitis media, improperly treated over time, can lead to serious pathologic sequelae, including tympanic membrane perforations, adhesive otitis media, cholesteatoma, ossicular destruction, and, in each case, significant conductive hearing loss. Tympanic membrane perforations most often occur in children secondary to prolonged placement of ventilating tubes. Occasionally, perforations result from repeated ruptures of the tympanic membrane due to acute suppurative otitis media. Surgical repair of tympanic membrane perforation should be delayed, if possible, until normal eustachian tube (ET) function has been established. There is no test for adequacy of ET function. If there is a perforation in one ear, the opposite ear can be used as a measure. If the opposite remains free of fluid or infection through a winter, it can be assumed the child has adequate ET function. If perforations are bilateral, one ear should be repaired and observed over a similar period of time. Occasionally, surgery will be mandated by chronic infection. Hearing loss alone is rarely an indication for surgery, as these ears usually can be fitted with hearing aids.

Chronic suppurative otitis media is a chronic infection of the middle ear and mastoid bone and is rare in young children. This condition usually results in a chronic tympanic membrane perforation and intermittent ear drainage. Ossicular erosion can occur and may result in a maximum conductive hearing loss. Chronic suppurative otitis media is usually treated surgically.

Cholesteatoma is a cyst formed from normal skin trapped in the middle ear space. Usually, there is no skin in the middle ear, only in the external auditory canal and on the lateral surface of the tympanic membrane. There are three types of cholesteatoma: congenital, primary acquired, and secondary acquired. Congenital cholesteatoma occurs when a nest of skin becomes trapped in the middle ear space, behind an intact tympanic membrane, during fetal development. The congenital cholesteatoma is usually asymptomatic and is discovered coincidentally on routine physical examination. It presents as white "pearl" anterior to the short process of the malleus. To make this diagnosis, there has to have been no history of tympanic membrane perforation or placement of a myringotomy tube. Primary acquired cholesteatoma is the most common type of cholesteatoma and results when skin shed from the lateral surface of the tympanic membrane collects in a retraction pocket. Retraction pockets usually arise from the weakest part of the tympanic membrane, called the pars flaccida, located above the short process of the malleus. Secondary acquired cholesteatoma occurs when the skin from the lateral surface of the tympanic membrane migrates through a tympanic membrane perforation and grows within the middle ear space. Regardless of the type, cholesteatomas gradually enlarge and can be destructive of surrounding structures. Conductive hearing loss due to ossicular destruction is common (Stapleton, Egloff, & Yellon, 2012). In advanced cases, cholesteatoma can press on the facial nerve, injuring it and causing a facial paralysis. Cholesteatoma becomes particularly aggressive when it gets infected and can lead to meningitis or a brain abscess. The treatment of cholesteatoma is surgical. The abnormal skin must be completely removed from the middle ear and/or mastoid. The tympanic membrane can be repaired and damaged ossicles replaced. There is usually some residual conductive hearing loss.

Pitfall

- Congenital cholesteatoma can be easily missed on exam.

Adhesive otitis media occurs when the tympanic membrane collapses completely and becomes fixed to the ossicles and other middle ear structures. If left untreated, it leads to retraction cholesteatoma. The ossicles can be destroyed by cholesteatoma, as mentioned above, or can be fixed by abnormal scarring and calcification, called tympanosclerosis. The resultant conductive hearing loss can range from mild to moderate.

Congenital Ossicular Abnormalities

Congenital abnormalities of the ossicles can vary in their degree and in which ossicles are involved. Ossicular abnormalities can range from fixation to abnormal shape to absence of the malleus, incus, or stapes. In addition, there can be absence of the oval window, round window, or both. Fixation of the stapes in children can occur due to tympanosclerosis, otosclerosis, or congenital fixation (Welling et al, 2003). Hearing loss due to any of the aforementioned etiologies can be corrected with either surgery or a hearing aid. Appropriate management of these hearing losses is dependent upon the age of the child, the status of the ET, and the etiology of the hearing loss.

Aural Atresia

Aural atresia is a malformation of the external auditory canal and the middle ear. The clinical presentation is very variable, and the extent of abnormality must be defined with CT. In the mildest form, the external auditory canal will be very narrow and threadlike. In more advanced cases, there may be no external auditory canal and the ossicles may be severely deformed or completely absent. There may be no oval window at all, and the facial nerve might take an extremely anomalous course. Aural atresia can be unilateral or bilateral and can be an isolated finding or can occur in association with a syndrome. Aural atresia results in a maximal conductive hearing loss in the affected ear. Occasionally SNHL may coexist. Aural atresia is often found in conjunction with microtia, a malformation of the external ear that can range from a small auricula to total absence of the auricula.

There is controversy in the management of aural atresia because there are considerable complications with its surgical repair. The course of the facial nerve is very variable in these children and is at risk during the atresia repair, especially in inexperienced hands (Jahrsdoerfer & Lambert, 1998). Recurrence of stenosis of the external auditory canal after surgery has been reported in up to 32% of cases (Shih & Crabtree, 1993). Closure of air–bone gaps to within 30 dB occurs in only 60–70% of cases, regardless of the type of ossicular reconstruction (Teufert & De la Cruz, 2004).

Many advocate the use of a bone-anchored implant (BAI), as hearing improvement is more consistent with the device and there are fewer complications.

Controversial Point

- The surgical repair of aural atresia is controversial, especially in unilateral cases.

◆ Bone-Anchored Hearing Technology

In 1980, Anders Tjellström first described the use of a surgically implanted transcutaneous titanium implant for hearing restoration (Tjellström et al, 1980). He transferred technology of penetrating titanium implants, developed for use in dental reconstruction by Dr. Per-Ingvar Brånemark (Brånemark et al, 1969), for creating a better bone conduction hearing aid. This same technology was also used in anchoring auricular reconstruction prostheses. With a device that directly couples to the skull, there was very little loss in power, because skin thickness no longer attenuated the signal. In 1997 the U.S. Food and Drug Administration (FDA) approved the bone-anchored hearing aid Baha (Cochlear Ltd., Sydney, Australia) in patients with conductive or mixed hearing losses who were unable to benefit from traditional hearing aids. (See Chapter 21 for more detailed information about BAIs.) Since that time, there has been an additional indication added: single-sided deafness (SSD).

For patients with SSD, the Baha has been shown to have superior results to the unaided or CROS situations (Bosman, Hol, Snik, Mylanus, & Cremers, 2003; Stewart, Clark, & Niparko, 2011; Wazen, Spitzer, Ghossaini, Kacker, & Zschommler, 2001). The signal is routed transcranially to the functioning cochlea on the contralateral side and eliminates the head shadow effect. Unfortunately, Baha users do not have any improved sound localization (Wazen et al, 2001).

In patients with conductive or mixed hearing losses, the Baha essentially bypasses the conductive component. The gain necessary for the Baha relies solely on the sensorineural loss in the ear. In general, the bone pure tone average of the bone line in the affected ear should be 45 dB or better in order for the patient to have adequate aided benefit.

The surgical procedure is performed in a single stage in adults and older adolescents. In younger children or in adults with thinner skulls, the procedure is usually performed in two stages. The first stage is the placement of the titanium fixture into the skull. The skin is closed and the fixture is allowed to osseointegrate over the next 3 months. Then, a second stage is performed to attach the transcutaneous abutment to the fixture and to thin the surrounding skin and subcutaneous tissue. The two-stage procedure was utilized to decrease the incidence of fixture extrusion and failure to osseointegrate in the thinner, softer bone in children (Davids, Gordon, Clutton, & Papsin, 2007).

Discussion Questions

1. Identify the most common causes of congenital and acquired hearing loss.

2. Discuss the most common causes of conductive hearing loss in children and describe their management.

References

American Academy of Pediatrics. (2010). Task force on improving the effectiveness of newborn hearing screening diagnosis and intervention. Universal newborn hearing screening. Diagnosis and intervention: Guidelines for pediatric medical home providers. Retrieved from http://www.Medical homeinfo.org/how/clinical_care/hearing_screening/

Berrettini, S., Forli, F., Bogazzi, F., Neri, E., Salvatori, L., Casani, A. P., & Franceschini, S. S. (2005). Large vestibular aqueduct syndrome: audiological, radiological, clinical, and genetic features. American Journal of Otolaryngology, 26(6), 363–371.

Bosman, A. J., Hol, M. K., Snik, A. F., Mylanus, E. A., & Cremers, C. W. (2003). Bone-anchored hearing aids in unilateral inner ear deafness. Acta Oto-Laryngologica, 123(2), 258–260.

Brånemark, P. I., Adell, R., Breine, U., Hansson, B. O., Lindström, J., & Ohlsson, A. (1969). Intra-osseous anchorage of dental prostheses. I. Experimental studies. Scandinavian Journal of Plastic and Reconstructive Surgery, 3(2), 81–100.

Brookhouser, P. E. (1996). Sensorineural hearing loss in children. Pediatric Clinics of North America, 43(6), 1195–1216.

Davids, T., Gordon, K. A., Clutton, D., & Papsin, B. C. (2007). Bone-anchored hearing aids in infants and children younger than 5 years. Archives of Otolaryngology—Head & Neck Surgery, 133(1), 51–55.

Denoyelle, F., Weil, D., Maw, M. A., Wilcox, S. A., Lench, N. J., Allen-Powell, D. R., . . . Petit, C. (1997). Prelingual deafness: high prevalence of a 30delG mutation in the connexin 26 gene. Human Molecular Genetics, 6(12), 2173–2177.

Doyle, K. J., & Ray, R. M. (2003). The otolaryngologist's role in management of hearing loss in infancy and childhood. Mental Retardation and Developmental Disabilities Research Reviews, 9(2), 94–102.

Jackler, R. K., & De La Cruz, A. (1989). The large vestibular aqueduct syndrome. The Laryngoscope, 99(12), 1238–1242, discussion 1242–1243.

Jahrsdoerfer, R. A., & Lambert, P. R. (1998). Facial nerve injury in congenital aural atresia surgery. The American Journal of Otology, 19(3), 283–287.

Joint Commission on Infant Hearing [JCIH]. (2007). Retrieved from www.jcih.org

Lalwani, A. K., & Castelein, C. M. (1999). Cracking the auditory genetic code: nonsyndromic hereditary hearing impairment. The American Journal of Otology, 20(1), 115–132.

Louis, J., Burton, M. J., Felding, J. U., Ovesen, T., Rovers, M. M., & Williamson, I. (2005). Grommets (ventilation tubes) for hearing loss associated with otitis media with effusion in children. Cochrane Database of Systematic Reviews, 25(1).

Madden, C., Halsted, M., Benton, C., Greinwald, J., & Choo, D. (2003). Enlarged vestibular aqueduct syndrome in the pediatric population. Otology & Neurotology, 24(4), 625–632.

Madell, J. R., & Sculerati, N. (1991). Non congenital hereditary hearing loss in children. Archives of Otolaryngology, 117, 332–335.

Medical Home Initiatives for Children with Special Needs Project Advisory Committee. American Academy of Pediatrics. (2002). The medical home. Pediatrics, 110(1 Pt 1), 184–186.

Morton, N. E. (1991). Genetic epidemiology of hearing impairment. Annals of the New York Academy of Sciences, 630, 16–31.

Paradise, J. L., Campbell, T. F., Dollaghan, C. A., Feldman, H. M., Bernard, B. S., Colborn, D. K., . . . Smith, C. G. (2005). Developmental outcomes after early or delayed insertion of tympanostomy tubes. The New England Journal of Medicine, 353(6), 576–586.

Roman, S., Bourliere-Najean, B., & Triglia, J. M. (1998). Congenital and acquired perilymph fistula: review of the literature. Acta Otorhinolaryngologica. 18(4, Suppl 59), 28–32.

Ruggieri, M., Iannetti, P., Polizzi, A., La Mantia, I., Spalice, A., Giliberto, O., . . . Pavone, L. (2005). Earliest clinical manifestations and natural history of neurofibromatosis type 2 (NF2) in childhood: a study of 24 patients. Neuropediatrics, 36(1), 21–34.

Shih, L., & Crabtree, J. A. (1993). Long-term surgical results for congenital aural atresia. The Laryngoscope, 103(10), 1097–1102.

Sim, R. J., Jardine, A. H., & Beckenham, E. J. (2009). Long-term outcome of children undergoing surgery for suspected perilymph fistula. The Journal of Laryngology and Otology, 123(3), 298–302.

Stapleton, A. L., Egloff, A. M., & Yellon, R. F. (2012). Congenital cholesteatoma: predictors for residual disease and hearing outcomes. Archives of Otolaryngology–Head & Neck Surgery, 138(3), 280–285.

Stewart, C. M., Clark, J. H., & Niparko, J. K. (2011). Bone-anchored devices in single-sided deafness. Advances in Oto-Rhino-Laryngology, 71(71), 92–102.

Teufert, K. B., & De la Cruz, A. (2004). Advances in congenital aural atresia surgery: effects on outcome. Otolaryngology–Head and Neck Surgery, 131(3), 263–270.

Tinling, S. P., Colton, J., & Brodie, H. A. (2004). Location and timing of initial osteoid deposition in postmeningitic labyrinthitis ossificans determined by multiple fluorescent labels. The Laryngoscope, 114(4), 675–680.

Tjellström, A., Håkansson, B., Lindström, J., Brånemark, P. I., Hallén, O., Rosenhall, U., & Leijon, A. (1980). Analysis of the mechanical impedance of bone-anchored hearing aids. Acta Oto-Laryngologica, 89(1–2), 85–92.

Wazen, J. J., Spitzer, J., Ghossaini, S. N., Kacker, A., & Zschommler, A. (2001). Results of the bone-anchored hearing aid in unilateral hearing loss. The Laryngoscope, 111(6), 955–958.

Welling, D. B., Merrell, J. A., Merz, M., & Dodson, E. E. (2003). Predictive factors in pediatric stapedectomy. The Laryngoscope, 113(9), 1515–1519.

Young, N. M., Mets, M. B., & Hain, T. C. (1996). Early diagnosis of Usher syndrome in infants and children. The American Journal of Otology, 17(1), 30–34.

Part II

Diagnosing Hearing Disorders in Infants and Children

Chapter 5

Newborn Hearing Screening

Karl R. White and Karen Muñoz

Key Points

- The percentage of newborns screened for hearing loss before hospital discharge has increased from fewer than 5% in 1993 to more than 98% in 2010.

- Forty-three states and the District of Columbia have passed legislation requiring newborn hearing screening, and many governmental and professional organizations endorse hearing screening for all newborns.

- Newborn hearing screening is only the first step (and arguably the easiest) in the process of identifying and providing appropriate services to infants and young children who are deaf or hard of hearing (other important steps include at least diagnostic evaluation, early intervention, family support, tracking and data management, and coordination with the child's primary health care provider).

- Equipment, protocols, and procedures used in successful newborn hearing screening programs vary widely depending on the circumstances and preferences of those running the program—there is no one best approach.

- The most successful programs are excellent at involving and communicating with a range of stakeholders (e.g., hospital staff and administrators, primary health care providers, parents, and hearing health professionals).

During the past 20 years (**Fig. 5.1**) the percentage of newborns being screened for hearing loss has increased from 3 to 98% (White & Blaiser, 2011). What has contributed to such a dramatic increase, and what can we learn from these initiatives that will enable us to continue to refine and improve our programs for identifying and serving infants and young children with permanent hearing loss?

◆ Factors Contributing to the Expansion of Newborn Hearing Screening Programs

First, it is important to understand that a variety of factors interacted in a synergistic manner to achieve the growth shown in **Fig. 5.1**: (1) policy initiatives by government, professional associations, and advocacy groups; (2) financial assistance from the federal government; (3) improvements in technology; (4) legislative initiatives; and (5) the demonstrated success of early implementations.

Policy Initiatives

The federal government has been advocating for earlier identification of permanent hearing loss for many years. For example, the Babbidge (1965) Report, issued by the U.S. Department of Health, Education and Welfare, recommended the development and nationwide implementation of "universally applied procedures for early identification and evaluation

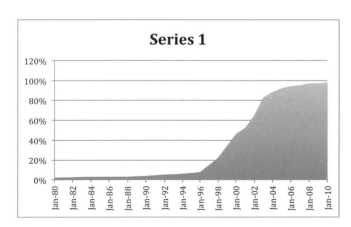

Fig. 5.1 Percentage of newborns screened in the United States for hearing loss from 1980 through 2010.

of hearing impairment" (Babbidge, 1965, p. C-10). A short time later, based on the pioneering work of Marion Downs (Downs & Sterritt, 1964, 1967), the Joint Committee on Infant Hearing (JCIH) was established in 1969 by a group of professional associations (e.g., American Speech Language and Hearing Association, American Academy of Pediatrics [AAP], the American Academy of Otolaryngology—Head and Neck Surgery, among others). Even though the JCIH had little or no budget and no formal authority, the committee has been a powerful force in advocating for earlier identification and better treatment of infants and young children who are deaf or hard of hearing (Olusanya, McPherson, Swanepoel, Shrivastav, & Chapchap, 2006; American Academy of Pediatrics [AAP] & Joint Committee on Infant Hearing [JCIH], 2007).

As new hearing screening technologies became available in the late 1980s, there was increased interest and activity in reducing the age at which hearing loss was identified. These efforts were supported in part by a recommendation from the congressionally mandated Commission on Education of the Deaf that "the Department of Education, in collaboration with the Department of Health and Human Services, should . . . assist states in implementing improved screening procedures for each live birth" (Commission on Education of the Deaf, 1988).

A few years later, *Healthy People 2000* (U. S. Department of Health and Human Services [HHS], 1990) included an objective to "reduce the average age at which children with significant hearing impairment are identified to no more than 12 months." This report went on to state:

> It is difficult, if not impossible, for many [children with congenital hearing loss] to acquire the fundamental language, social, and cognitive skills that provide the foundation for later schooling and success in society. When early identification and intervention occur, hearing impaired children make dramatic progress, are more successful in school, and become more productive members of society. The earlier intervention and habilitation begin, the more dramatic the benefits. (HHS, 1990, p. 460)

Although the concept underlying this objective was similar to what people had been advocating for several decades, the inclusion of a goal related to early identification of hearing loss in *Healthy People 2000* broke new ground, because it required that progress toward each objective be tracked and reported at regular intervals.

In March 1993, the National Institutes of Health (NIH) convened a Consensus Development Panel to review the existing evidence on early identification of hearing loss and make recommendations to improve practice. The panel concluded that "All hearing impaired infants should be identified and treatment initiated by 6 months of age . . . [T]he consensus panel recommends screening of all newborns . . . for hearing impairment prior to discharge" (National Institutes of Health [NIH], 1993).

Some people expected rapid implementation of universal newborn hearing screening programs as a result of the NIH recommendation. Such was not to be the case, however, as it became clear that the research evidence and experience for such broad-scale implementation were lacking. For example, Bess and Paradise (1994) concluded that "the Consensus Panel's recommendation of universal infant screening falls short of being justified on grounds of practicability, effectiveness, cost, and harm-benefit ratio." Two years later the prestigious United States Preventive Services Task Force (USPSTF) (1996) noted that "congenital hearing loss is a serious health problem associated with developmental delay in speech and language function," but concluded that "there is little evidence to support the use of routine, universal screening for all neonates." Similarly, in a 1999 article in *Pediatrics*, Paradise concluded that, "universal newborn hearing screening in our present state of knowledge is not necessarily the only, or the best, or the most cost-effective way to achieve [early identification of hearing loss], and more importantly, . . . the benefits of universal newborn hearing screening may be outweighed by its risks" (Paradise, 1999).

Federal Funding for Early Hearing Detection and Intervention Initiatives

The policy initiatives of the late 1980s and early 1990s led to an increase in projects and initiatives focused on reducing the age at which congenital hearing loss was identified. One of the best known was the Rhode Island Hearing Assessment Project (White & Behrens, 1993), but there were many others (e.g., Barsky-Firkser & Sun, 1997; Finitzo, Albright, & O'Neal, 1998; Mason & Herrmann, 1998; Mehl & Thomson, 1998).

Successful Implementation of Screening Programs

By the mid-1990s the percentage of newborns being screened for hearing loss had increased dramatically (from fewer than 3% in 1993 to 15% in 1996 to 22% in 1998; see **Fig. 5.1**). By 1998 dozens of large-scale universal newborn hearing screening programs had become operational in various states (White, 1997). These projects provided the data and the experience to sustain the momentum that had started during the early 1990s.

Technological Advances

The growth of newborn hearing screening programs was directly linked to the technological advances in hearing screening equipment that occurred during the late 1980s and early 1990s. Without the improvements in automated auditory brainstem response (AABR) (Herrmann, Thornton, & Joseph, 1995) and otoacoustic emissions (OAE) (Kemp, 1978; Lonsbury-Martin & Martin, 1990; Kemp & Ryan, 1993), all of the policy initiatives, federally funded projects, and clinical screening programs that combined to demonstrate the practicality of newborn hearing screening programs would never have happened.

Endorsements by Professional and Advocacy Groups

The demonstrated feasibility of hospital-based screening, coupled with the results of research, led to more endorsements for universal newborn hearing screening by other government, professional, and advocacy organizations. For example, in 1999 the American Academy of Pediatrics "[endorsed] the goal of universal detection of hearing loss in infants before 3 months of age . . . [which] requires universal screening of all infants" (Erenberg, Lemons, Sia, Trunkel, Ziring, AAP, 1999). Other organizations, including the American Speech-Language-Hearing Association, the American Academy of Audiology, March of Dimes, and the American College of Medical Genetics, soon followed suit (National Center for Hearing Assessment and Management [NCHAM], 2012c). Also in 1998, the federal Maternal and Child Health Bureau (MCHB) (2002) began requiring states to report "percent of newborns screened for hearing impairment before hospital discharge" as one of 18 core performance measures that states had to report annually to receive federal MCHB block grant funding. By the end of 2001, every state had established an early hearing detection and intervention (EHDI) program, which was responsible for setting up newborn hearing screening programs and linking babies referred from those programs to diagnostic, early intervention, family support, and other health care services. In 2008 the USPSTF (USPSTF, 2008) revised their earlier statement about newborn hearing screening and concluded that "There is good evidence that newborn hearing screening testing is highly accurate and leads to earlier identification and treatment of infants with hearing loss. . . . Good-quality evidence shows that early detection improves language outcomes. . . . All infants should have hearing screening before 1 month of age."

Legislation Related to Newborn Hearing Screening

The events just described created an atmosphere in which newborn hearing screening programs could be implemented, but legislative action in many states expanded the reach of these programs and increased the probability that they would be continued. The first legislation related to newborn hearing screening was passed in Hawaii in 1990. Spurred on by the demonstrated success of newborn hearing screening programs, 43 states and the District of Columbia now have statutes and/or regulations requiring newborn hearing screening. The increase in legislative activity was probably influenced by the publication of the Position Statement by the AAP in February 1999 and the publication in 1998 of major articles about the feasibility and benefits of implementing large-scale universal newborn hearing screening programs (e.g., Finitzo et al, 1998; Moeller, 2000; Mehl & Thomson, 1998; Yoshinaga-Itano, Sedey, Coulter, & Mehl, 1998). Key provisions of each statute are summarized in **Table 5.1**; the exact wording is made available by NCHAM (2012a).

Pearl

- Many states were screening most of their newborns before passing legislation. Thus, legislation is not essential to have all babies screened but is often most helpful in refining and strengthening the screening program and linking screening results to other services.

◆ Establishing and Operating Successful Newborn Hearing Screening Programs

As a result of work done by JCIH (AAP & JCIH, 2007), MCHB, and the Centers for Disease Control and Prevention (CDC) (2004), most people stopped using the phrase, "universal newborn hearing screening" and began referring to "early hearing detection and intervention" (EHDI) programs. The change in how these programs are described is important, because it underscores that to identify and serve infants and young children with congenital hearing loss, successful screening programs must be coupled with timely audiologic diagnosis; appropriate medical, audiologic, and educational services; coordination with the child's primary health care provider (often referred to as

Table 5.1 Newborn hearing screening legislation in the United States

State	Year passed	Requires screening of:	Advisory committee?	Covered by health insurance?	Report results to state?	Provide educational materials?	Informed consent by parents?
AK	2006	All babies		Yes	Yes	Yes	
AR	1999	Hospitals > 50 births	Yes	Yes	Yes	Yes	
AZ	2007	All babies	Yes		Yes	Yes	
CA	2006	All babies		Medicaid		Yes	Yes
CO	1997	85% of newborns	Yes			Yes	
CT	1997	All babies		Yes		Yes	
DE	2005	All babies		Yes	Yes	Yes	
DC	2001	All babies		Yes			Yes
FL	2000	All babies		Yes		Yes	
GA	1999	95% of newborns	Yes			Yes	
HI	1990	All babies			Yes		
IA	2003	All babies			Yes		
IL	1999	All babies	Yes			Yes	
IN	1999	All babies	Yes	Yes	Yes	Yes	
KS	1999	All babies					Yes
KY	2000	Hospitals > 40 births	Yes		Yes		
LA	1999	All babies	Yes				
ME	1999	> 85%	Yes	Yes	Yes	Yes	
MD	1999	All babies	Yes	Yes	Yes	Yes	
MA	1997	All babies	Yes	Yes	Yes		
MS	1997	All babies	Yes		Yes	Yes	
MI	2006	All babies			Yes		
MN	2007	All babies	Yes		Yes		Yes
MO	1999	All babies	Yes	Yes	Yes	Yes	
MT	2001	All babies	Yes		Yes		
NE	2000	> 95%		Yes	Yes	Yes	
NV	2000	Hospitals > 500 births			Yes	Yes	
NJ	2000	All babies	Yes	Yes	Yes	Yes	Yes
NM	2001	All babies					
NY	1999	Hospitals > 400 births			Yes		
NC	1999	All babies			Yes	Yes	
OH	2002	All babies	Yes	Yes	Yes	Yes	
OK	2000	All babies					
OR	1999	Hospitals > 200 births	Yes		Yes	Yes	
PA	2001	85% of newborns	Yes		Yes	Yes	
RI	1992	All babies		Yes			
SC	2000	Hospitals > 100 births	Yes	Yes	Yes	Yes	
TN	2008	All babies		Yes			
TX	1999	Hospitals > 100 births		Yes	Yes	Yes	Yes
UT	1998	All babies	Yes		Yes	Yes	
VA	1998	All babies	Yes	Yes	Yes	Yes	
WV	1998	All babies	Yes	Yes	Yes		
WI	1999	88% of newborns			Yes		
WY	1999	All babies				Yes	Yes

the child's medical home); and EHDI tracking and data management systems. (Other chapters in this book describe these important aspects of the EHDI system in more detail.)

In the years since the recommendation by NIH that all newborns should be screened before being discharged from the hospital, the techniques, procedures, equipment, and support systems for newborn hearing screening have continued to evolve (White, Forsman, Eichwald, & Muñoz, 2010), and the goal of screening all newborns for hearing loss, which many thought was completely unrealistic in 1993, has been largely attained. The remainder of this chapter summarizes some of the most important considerations and lessons learned about operating a successful newborn hearing screening program.

Creating Stakeholder Support

A successful newborn hearing screening program requires support from dozens of stakeholders, including hospital administrators, primary health care providers, nurses, and parents. All of these people should know that the endorsement of universal newborn hearing screening by so many authoritative groups accompanied by so many successful programs throughout the country and the ready availability of relatively inexpensive equipment and procedures, means that newborn hearing screening has become the de facto "standard of care." Hospitals run a significant liability risk if they do not screen all newborns for hearing loss (White, 2003).

Primary Health Care Providers

Most hospitals have a pediatric committee, a medical policy committee, or other such groups whose members make decisions about what constitutes the standard of care in that hospital. Members of such groups need to understand the benefits associated with newborn hearing screening and how it is done. Physicians, nurse practitioners, and physician assistants in the community who care for babies also need to understand why newborn hearing screening is important and how the process is supposed to work. Ideally, every newborn should have a health care provider who is familiar with the baby and the baby's circumstances and is responsible for ensuring that the baby receives consistent and appropriate health care. Often referred to as the baby's medical home, the baby's primary health care provider is the key to an effective early hearing detection and intervention program (AAP, 2002; Antonelli & Turchi, 2009). Because the baby's primary care physician is responsible for the total health care of the baby, he or she needs to be assured that newborn hearing screening will not interfere with or complicate other health care activities.

Nurses

If the nursing staff in the newborn nursery is not convinced that newborn hearing screening should be happening, it will be almost impossible to have a successful program. If the nurses want newborn hearing screening, they can often convince the physicians and administrators to give it a try. In fact, some of the earliest successful hospital-based newborn hearing screening programs were started and largely operated by nursing staff.

Selecting Equipment and Protocols for the Hospital

One of the first decisions in setting up a newborn hearing screening program is deciding what equipment to use and what type of basic screening protocol to follow. The good news is that there are a lot of options that have been successfully implemented. The bad news is that because there are so many options, some people unnecessarily delay the implementation of a newborn hearing screening program to sort through them all.

The best approach is to talk to people who have tried some of the most frequently used options; devote some brief, but intensive, study time to what type of equipment and protocol is best for the hospital; and then make a choice and move ahead. Waiting to identify the "perfect" solution for every aspect of the program will unnecessarily delay getting started. Adjustments to initial decisions can always be made later. A good starting point is to review the suggestions made by the Joint Committee on Infant Hearing (AAP & JCIH, 2007) regarding screening protocols for both the well-baby and neonatal intensive care nurseries. Additional examples of protocols and procedural guidelines being used by hospitals and state EHDI programs are provided by NCHAM (2012b).

Which Equipment Is Best?

In the past 20 years, a variety of types of equipment have been developed that can be used successfully in universal newborn hearing screening programs. Transient evoked OAE, distortion product OAE, and AABR equipment have all demonstrated their practicality and effectiveness in hospital-based newborn hearing screening programs. Each type of equipment has its proponents, and debates about which technique is best are sometimes quite energetic. It is clear, however, that the particular brand and type of equipment selected is not the most important issue in whether the program will be successful. Equipment continues to be modified and improved, and it is almost certain that better, faster, and easier-to-use equipment will become available. That is no reason, however, to delay implementing a program. Currently available equipment is more than adequate for operating a successful newborn hearing screening program. A brief summary of the issues to be considered in selecting equipment, as well as a listing of names and contact information for different manufacturers, are available from NCHAM (2012b).

How Many Tests Should Be Included in the Screening Protocol?

The purpose of any screening program is to select a subgroup from the general population that is at higher risk of having a particular condition so that a more in-depth diagnostic assessment can be done with members of that group. Therefore, some false positives (that is, infants with normal hearing who do not pass the screening test) and occasional false negatives (infants who pass the screening test but do have a hearing loss) are expected. If only one screening test is done for each baby before hospital discharge, as many as 10–15% of the babies may not pass. Therefore, many hospitals require two or more screening tests if babies do not pass at first. Sometimes this is done with the same type of equipment; sometimes with different types of equipment. Furthermore, some hospitals do a two-stage screening with different types of equipment before the baby is discharged from the hospital; others do a single stage screening before the baby is discharged and then follow with an outpatient screen several days later. Deciding which protocol is best for a given situation is usually based on factors such as the following:

- How long babies typically stay in the hospital before discharge
- How difficult it is in this area to get parents to come back for rescreens
- The availability of different types of equipment
- Who is doing the screening

Pearl

- More important than the type of equipment used or the protocol being followed is having someone in charge of the program who is passionate about the importance of newborn hearing screening and is completely committed to the success of the program.

The fact that successful programs currently use such a variety of protocols suggests that no one protocol is really best for all situations. Regardless of the protocol selected, it is best to have a written document to guide the activities of all people associated with the program. Examples of several such written protocols are provided by NCHAM (2012b).

Dealing with Procedural Issues

Regardless of the technology and protocol used, several procedural issues are important for an efficient, successful program. The World Health Organization (WHO) (2010) recently recommended that all newborn hearing screening programs have:

- Clearly stated goals with well-specified roles and responsibilities for those people who are involved
- A clearly designated person who is responsible for the program
- People doing the screening who have received hands-on training in what they are expected to do
- Regular monitoring to ensure that the protocol is being correctly implemented
- Specific procedures about how to inform parents of results
- Recording and reporting of information about the screening for each child in the health record
- A documented protocol based on local circumstances.

It is often useful to have a written summary describing how the program typically addresses issues such as the following.

Who Is in Charge?

If everyone is responsible for a task, it often remains unfinished. Thousands of hospitals have demonstrated that newborn hearing screening can easily be incorporated into the routine of a hospital. Just like any other procedure, however, it takes attention to detail and someone who is ultimately responsible to make sure that all of the specifics are done. The person responsible for day-to-day operation of the program does not need specific professional certification, but he or she needs to have good connections with the nursery, understand how screening happens, and most of all be committed to the success of the program. Instead of looking for reasons why newborn hearing screening will not work, that person needs to be committed to its success. Depending on how the program is organized, most hospitals find that this person will require 2 to 6 hours per week per 1000 births to coordinate and manage the overall program.

Who Will Do the Screening?

Reports from hundreds of operational programs provide clear evidence that newborn hearing screening can be performed by a wide variety of people, including nurses, audiologists, technicians, health care assistants, volunteers, and students (**Table 5.2**). Some states have laws regarding who can screen for hearing and how they must be supervised; others do not. Regard-

Table 5.2 Who does newborn hearing screening as reported by EHDI program coordinators?

Audiologist	67%
Physician	5%
Nursing staff	95%
Trained volunteer	36%
Trained technician	85%

Percentages sum to more than 100% because many states reported that more than one group of people screened in the same hospital.

less of which individuals do the screening, they must be properly trained and supervised, and data should be kept on each screener's performance to enable timely and appropriate training and assistance when needed.

When Should Screening Be Done?

All other things being equal, newborn hearing screening is faster and easier if babies are quiet and the environment is not too chaotic. Because of this, it is easiest to do screening in the early morning or during the night, when fewer people (such as doctors, visiting relatives, nurses, or parents) want access to the baby. However, depending on who is screening, their other responsibilities, and how the hospital's nursery is organized, screening can be done successfully at other times. Whatever decision is made, dozens of other hospitals are doing it at approximately the same time. The conclusion? There really is no wrong time to do newborn hearing screening.

How Do You Ensure Every Baby Is Screened?

There are many procedures to ensure that no babies are missed. Setting up a system to log the birth and screening of every baby, making sure screeners are available to screen every baby before discharge, and incorporating the hearing screening into the discharge plan should all be considered. Because some hospitals discharge babies after very short stays, seven-day-a-week coverage is usually needed. Many screening program coordinators have found that it is more efficient to incorporate screening duties into the job responsibilities of existing personnel than it is to hire dedicated screening staff.

Should Screening Be Done with Parents Present?

If parents are present for the screening, they will have questions and want to discuss the process. This is wonderful from an educational perspective, but it requires more time and, consequently, increases the cost of the screening program. If it can be afforded, hearing screening provides a great opportunity for educating parents about the importance of hearing and language development. Even if parents are not routinely present for screening, they should certainly be accommodated if they ask to watch. It is important to make sure parents are involved and supported at every opportunity.

Should Parents Be Required to Give Written Permission for Screening?

There are really two different, but related, questions here. First, should there be procedures to ensure that parents understand what happens during newborn hearing screening so they can make an informed decision about whether they want their baby to be screened? Second, should parents be required to sign a written permission before their baby is screened? The answer to the first question is definitely yes; the answer to the second is probably no. With regard to the first question, every effort should be made to educate parents about newborn hearing screening before it happens (what it is, why it is important, how it is done, etc.). Parent education can be accomplished with information in the preadmission materials, prenatal classes, media, or materials placed in the baby's crib. If, based on this information, parents do not want to have their baby screened for hearing loss, they have the right to refuse (it is a good idea to require that they give you a written documentation of that refusal, which is kept on file).

With regard to the second question, it is important to remember that newborn hearing screening is not an experimental research procedure. If it were, written parental permission would probably be required for every baby screened. Although it requires extra time (in some cases, more than the total time required to do screening), a few hospitals still obtain written permission from parents before screening the baby. This does provide an opportunity to explain to parents exactly what the screening is and why it is important, but this could be done more quickly in other ways. Also, some states have laws or regulations regarding such issues.

Communicating with Stakeholders

Many people have a stake in the results of a newborn hearing screening program. It is essential for the success of the program to make sure these people receive timely information. In many cases, it is also important to document that communication has occurred and to have a system to quickly and accurately retrieve information that has been communicated.

Communicating with Parents

Parents are among the most important stakeholders, because they are the ones who have long-term responsibility for ensuring that the baby receives appropriate care. They are also the ones who have the strongest feelings (but usually limited experience) about what it means to have a child with a hearing loss. It is essential that each parent be told the results of their baby's hearing screening test, and this should involve more than just saying that the baby passed or failed. Instead, parents need to know what the result means and what the next steps should be. Even when the baby passes a screening test, it is a great opportunity to help parents understand the importance of monitoring language development and of being aware of the indicators of hearing loss that might occur later. Most successful newborn hearing screening programs use a variety of materials to educate, inform, and follow up with parents. For example, a 6-minute movie that explains how newborn hearing screening is done, why it is important, what the results mean, and what should happen next can be downloaded at no cost (in both English and Spanish) from NCHAM (2012b). Such a video can be used during birthing classes so that mothers know what to expect when the screening is done. Other examples of parent information include information pamphlets about the screening program, parent education materials, letters sent to parents about the results of the test, and cards used to make return appointments for rescreens or diagnostic evaluations; examples of such materials currently being used in other programs are available from NCHAM (2012b).

It is best if parents can be told about the results of the newborn hearing screening test before the baby is discharged. Then, any needed additional screening or testing can be scheduled before the parents leave the hospital, and they can have their questions answered and any misunderstandings clarified. Some health care providers want to be involved in communicating results of screening tests to parents; others do not. Therefore, make sure you have discussed your procedures for informing parents with health care providers in your community.

Some people have worried about creating unnecessary anxiety in parents or disrupting family functioning, because most babies who fail the initial newborn hearing screening test will have normal hearing. There is no evidence that this is really a problem (Tueller, 2006). To avoid creating unnecessary anxiety, make sure parents understand that the screening test is not a diagnostic evaluation and that a referral for further testing does not mean that the baby has a hearing loss.

The activities associated with a newborn hearing screening program also provide an ideal opportunity to help parents understand the importance of language development. Just because a child has passed a newborn hearing screening test does not mean that there will not be future problems with hearing or language development. Materials distributed in conjunction with the newborn hearing screening should emphasize the need to monitor their child's language development and what parents should do if the child does not achieve developmental milestones in a timely manner. It should also be made clear that the newborn hearing screening test provides information about the status of the infant's hearing at the time of discharge. Common childhood diseases can later cause fluctuating or permanent hearing loss that will interfere with language development. Educational materials should emphasize the importance of parents' requesting another hearing evaluation if they have any concerns about their child's language development.

Pitfall

- Some parents mistakenly assume that babies who pass the newborn hearing screening test will always have normal hearing. Babies can have normal hearing at birth and acquire permanent hearing loss later in life.

Communicating with Health Care Providers

From the very beginning, the child's primary health care provider needs to understand how newborn hearing screening contributes to better health care. Distributing written materials to all primary health care providers in the community who see children is a good beginning. It may be useful to do some screening of babies when health care providers typically make their rounds (as long as the screening does not interfere during the time that the physician needs to have access to the baby). A screener's just being there and doing the work will prompt a lot of questions and understanding of what is involved in newborn hearing screening. When a baby with hearing loss is identified, the results must be communicated to that baby's physician. Periodically, reports can be sent to the hospital's pediatric committee or to a newsletter to inform the hospital's medical staff about the success of the program. Anonymous case histories or personal experiences of families whose babies have been helped by the program are particularly useful in such reports and newsletters.

It is also important to have a system to notify each health care provider about the screening results for his or her patients. Although this is particularly important for babies who do not pass the initial screening, it is best to provide information about all babies along with a clear recommendation of what should happen next. Few things will undermine the success of a newborn hearing screening program as much as the baby's health care provider's telling the parent during a well-baby check that it is really not that important to follow up with the outpatient screen or diagnostic evaluation procedures. Instead, it is really important for health care providers to encourage parents to complete recommended testing as quickly as possible. Additionally, if parents have concerns about their baby's hearing or language development, they should be encouraged to see an audiologist who has experience working with infants and young children.

When a baby fails the newborn hearing screening, medical evaluation is an essential part of the diagnostic process, and health care providers need to understand that they are a critical part of that multidisciplinary team. It is also important that everyone involved in the baby's medical management understand how detrimental it is when the diagnostic process requires several months, instead of being completed within a few weeks. For babies without other medical complications, the goal should be to have a definitive diagnosis, to be fitted with hearing aids (if parents choose to do so), and to begin early intervention within a few weeks of birth. For that to happen, however, all members of the team have to recognize the importance of early diagnosis and intervention and then work together to make it happen as quickly as possible.

Communicating with Hospital Administrators and Staff

Hospital administrators, risk managers, nursery supervisors, and community education staff, among others, also need to be kept informed about the newborn hearing screening program. If key people in the hospital are receiving the information they need on a timely basis, the continuation of the newborn hearing screening program is almost guaranteed because the benefits will be well documented and many different groups can work to support and improve the program. It is also important to make sure that hearing screening results are a part of the child's permanent medical record.

Having an effective data management system is important for being able to produce reports on a predetermined schedule or, on request, to show such items of information as the percentage of babies screened, the percentage who passed prior to discharge, the percentage referred from the initial screening who eventually receive diagnostic evaluations, and the number of babies identified with permanent hearing loss. It is also useful to produce a monthly report summarizing the successes of the program, the challenges that still need to be addressed, and the strate-

gies for resolving those challenges. It is particularly valuable to highlight the human side of any success stories so that administrators see that people's lives are better off as a result of this program. Many administrators will also want to know more about program costs. A simple, but complete, cost analysis of the program after the first year, and then at periodic intervals thereafter, is very useful.

Pearl

- Accurate reporting about key variables related to the newborn hearing screening program is valuable in identifying weaknesses and in improving the program as well as in building support among various stakeholders.

Training Newborn Hearing Screeners

Regardless of which screening equipment or protocol is used, screeners will become proficient much faster if there is hands-on, competency-based training. Sales representatives can demonstrate how to operate the equipment, but the best training is done by people who are experienced screeners. Ideally, such training should include ample time for the people being trained to do supervised screening. Once a person acquires skill with the screening equipment, it is easily remembered. An excellent online training module (the interactive Newborn Hearing Screening Training Curriculum or NHSTC) is available at no cost from NCHAM (2012b).

The number of screeners needed to operate a universal newborn hearing screening program depends on the annual number of births and how the program is organized. Because some babies are discharged just a few hours after being born, seven-day-a-week coverage will be needed. However, the total amount of screening time is relatively small. Many hospitals make the mistake of training too many people (e.g., all of the nursing staff). Not only does this require extra time for training and supervision, but it often results in a less efficient program, because responsibility for screening babies is diffused and the quality of screening suffers.

Although it is often said that practice makes perfect, it is more accurate to say that practice makes permanent. Consequently, it is important to provide timely feedback to people who are just learning to screen so that errors can be corrected before they become ingrained. Subsequently, there should be regular one-on-one observation and feedback. A regular report that shows each screener's performance with regard to variables such as the number of babies screened, babies passed, invalid tests, and screens completed per hour of work can be useful in identifying screeners who are having difficulty and need assistance. Such supervision should be organized so that it is viewed as assistance instead of punishment.

Operating an Efficient Program

Regardless of the type of technology or protocol used, the goal of newborn hearing screening is to create the smallest reasonable subset of the general population that still contains all of the infants with hearing loss. In other words, without missing any babies, it is generally best to minimize the number of infants who fail the screening test and are referred for a diagnostic evaluation. The following strategies should be considered to ensure that most of the babies who have normal hearing will pass the screening test.

Do Screening When Babies Are Quiet

Even though it is possible to screen babies who are awake and restless, screening is easier and quicker when the baby is quiet (or even asleep), well fed, and comfortable. Therefore, if possible, most screening should be done when babies are most likely to be in this optimal state. When and where screening is done will depend on other activities, routines, and available space at the hospital.

Test a Second Time before Discharge for Babies Who Do Not Pass at First

Typically, the first attempt to screen the baby is made shortly after birth. It is best not to spend too much time with the baby during this initial attempt. If the baby passes (as the majority will do), screening is finished. If not, wait several hours and try again. Regardless of the equipment or protocol being used, these second efforts before discharge can substantially reduce the number of babies who need to come in for outpatient screens or diagnostic procedures. Instead of spending 30 minutes with the baby during an initial attempt, it is much more efficient to make a quick first attempt, followed by a second or even third attempt a few hours later. It is not appropriate (and not an efficient use of time) to screen a particular baby more than three times in each ear before discharge.

Minimize Noise and Confusion in the Screening Area

It is not necessary to take extraordinary measures to make the screening area quiet. As an example, newborn hearing screening is routinely done in crowded and noisy neonatal intensive care units. However, other things being equal, screening will be faster and more effective if the screening area is relatively quiet. In other words, where possible, do the screening when physicians are not making their rounds; do not screen directly under a ventilator fan; and screen in an area that is not adjacent to a bathroom, where running water creates unnecessary noise. Where sensible and inexpensive modifications can be done to reduce noise (e.g., carpeting on the floor, curtains on windows), they can make screening more efficient.

Have Backup Equipment and Supplies Readily Available

Because some babies are discharged after just a few hours in the nursery, arrangements should be made to have backup equipment in case there is a breakdown. Most newborn hearing screening equipment is extremely reliable. However, if the equipment unexpectedly stops operating and it takes 3 days to get a replacement, 10% of the babies born at the hospital that month will be missed. Although such babies can come back for screening, it is extra work for everyone and unlikely to be completely successful. Thus, it is best to have made arrangements to obtain replacement or loan equipment within a very short time from the salesperson, a neighboring hospital, or a nearby university. It is also important to have sufficient supplies.

Pitfall

- It is possible to become so fixated on achieving very low "fail" rates that the quality of the program suffers. Remember, the object of a newborn hearing screening program is to find babies with permanent hearing loss, not to have every baby pass the screening test.

Managing Data and Patient Information

Ensuring that babies with hearing loss are enrolled as quickly as possible in appropriate intervention programs requires coordination with the baby's medical home, one or more audiologists, and various state and local agencies who are responsible for providing services to infants and young children with hearing loss. The screening that happens before hospital discharge is only the first step. Most screening program managers report that keeping track of what happens in the screening program and managing babies through the referral and diagnostic process are the most challenging part of an EHDI program. Data and patient information management includes keeping track of which babies have been screened, what screening or diagnostic procedures should happen next, and which babies have missed appointments and need to be located. It also involves generating reports for program management, accountability, and program continuation, and generating letters to parents and physicians concerning the outcome of various screening and evaluation procedures. If such data and patient information management is not handled appropriately, it can be much more time-consuming than the actual screening.

Arranging for a data and patient information management system is the kind of task on which it is easy to procrastinate. The amount of information that needs to be managed continues to multiply as more and more babies are born. If a system is not in place when the screening program starts, screening personnel will soon find that they are overwhelmed, and the whole system begins to collapse in piles of paper and yellow sticky notes.

Summarizing data from individuals into understandable reports, generating letters to parents and health care providers at different times based on the most recent outcomes, and sending reminders about upcoming and overdue screening and diagnostic activities are all easily done with a computer-based program. Information about several data and patient information packages that can be used for newborn hearing screening programs is available from NCHAM (2012b).

Program Coordination

The person in charge of the newborn hearing screening program needs a continual flow of information, including:

- The number of babies born at the hospital
- The percentage of babies successfully screened
- The percentage of babies who fail the screening test
- The percentage of babies rescreened and/or diagnosed
- The number of babies identified with hearing loss
- How well each of the screeners is functioning

Regular and timely summaries of such information are critical if the program is to be successful. There should be regular coordination meetings (at least monthly) to review such information. This meeting should be attended by the program coordinator, a representative of the screening staff, the nursery coordinator, an audiologist who is involved with the program, and a health care provider who cares for newborns at that hospital. The purpose of the meeting is to review the functioning of the program during the previous time period to make sure that its goals are being accomplished. Results from a computer-based data and patient information management program will provide all of the necessary data, but the meeting must still be convened and follow-up done.

Over the long term, an efficient newborn hearing screening program will identify ~ 3 babies per 1000 with permanent hearing loss (White et al, 2010). However, because hearing loss is a low-incidence condition, it may take 10,000 or more babies to achieve that average. In other words, it is not unusual for a hospital to screen 1000 babies and not find a single infant with permanent hearing loss. That same hospital, however, may find 5 or 6 infants in the next 1000.

Pearl

- Don't be discouraged if it takes a while to identify the first baby with a hearing loss.

Discussion Questions

1. What factors have contributed to the dramatic increase in percentage of newborns screened for hearing loss during the past 15 years?

2. What other components of an EHDI system are important to have in place to make newborn hearing screening effective?

3. Why is it important for stakeholders to know that newborn hearing screening is now considered to be a medical "standard of care"?

4. In what ways does an effective data management and tracking system contribute to a successful newborn hearing screening program?

5. Assume you are consulting with a hospital that has an unusually high percentage of newborns who fail the newborn hearing screening test. What factors should be considered to achieve a more reasonable percentage of newborns who fail the test?

6. Why is it important to have screeners available to do newborn hearing screening seven days per week?

7. What information do parents need to know about their baby's newborn hearing screening test and when do they need to know it?

References

American Academy of Pediatrics. (2002). The Medical Home Policy Statement. Pediatrics, 110(1). Retrieved from http://www.aap.org/policy/s060016.html

American Academy of Pediatrics & Joint Committee on Infant Hearing. (2007). Year 2007 position statement: Principles and guidelines for early hearing detection and intervention programs. Pediatrics, 120(4), 898–921.

Antonelli, R., & Turchi, R. M. (2009). This issue: the family-centered medical home in pediatrics. Pediatric Annals, 38(9), 472–476.

Babbidge, H. (1965). Education of the deaf in the United States: report of the Advisory Committee on Education of the Deaf. Washington, DC: U.S. Government Printing Office.

Barsky-Firkser, L., & Sun, S. (1997). Universal newborn hearing screenings: a three-year experience. Pediatrics, 99(6), E4.

Bess, F. H., & Paradise, J. L. (1994). Universal screening for infant hearing impairment: not simple, not risk-free, not necessarily beneficial, and not presently justified. Pediatrics, 93(2), 330–334.

Centers for Disease Control and Prevention. (2004). National EHDI goals. Retrieved from http://www.cdc.gov/ncbddd/ehdi/nationalgoals.htm

Commission on Education of the Deaf. (1988). A report to the Congress of the United States: toward equality. Washington, DC: U.S. Government Printing Office.

Downs, M. P., & Sterritt, G. M. (1964). Identification audiometry for infants: a preliminary report. The Journal of Auditory Research, 4, 69–80.

Downs, M. P., & Sterritt, G. M. (1967). A guide to newborn and infant hearing screening programs. Archives of Otolaryngology, 85(1), 15–22.

Erenberg, A., Lemons, J., Sia, C., Trunkel, D., & Ziring, P.; American Academy of Pediatrics (AAP). (1999). Newborn and infant hearing loss: detection and intervention. American Academy of Pediatrics. Task Force on Newborn and Infant Hearing, 1998-1999. Pediatrics, 103(2), 527–530.

Finitzo, T., Albright, K., & O'Neal, J. (1998). The newborn with hearing loss: detection in the nursery. Pediatrics, 102(6), 1452–1460.

Herrmann, B. S., Thornton, A. R., & Joseph, J. M. (1995). Automated infant hearing screening using the ABR: development and validation. American Journal of Audiology, 4, 6–14.

Kemp, D. T. (1978). Stimulated acoustic emissions from within the human auditory system. The Journal of the Acoustical Society of America, 64(5), 1386–1391.

Kemp, D. T., & Ryan, S. (1993). The use of transient evoked otoacoustic emissions in neonatal hearing screening programs. Seminars in Hearing, 14, 30–44.

Lonsbury-Martin, B. L., & Martin, G. K. (1990). The clinical utility of distortion-product otoacoustic emissions. Ear and Hearing, 11(2), 144–154.

Mason, J. A., & Herrmann, K. R. (1998). Universal infant hearing screening by automated auditory brainstem response measurement. Pediatrics, 101(2), 221–228.

Maternal and Child Health Bureau. (2002). National core and performance outcome measures. Retrieved from http://205.153.240.79/search/core/cormenu.asp

Mehl, A. L., & Thomson, V. (1998). Newborn hearing screening: the great omission. Pediatrics, 101(1), E4.

Moeller, M. P. (2000). Early intervention and language development in children who are deaf and hard of hearing. Pediatrics, 106(3), E43.

National Center for Hearing Assessment and Management. (2012a). EHDI Legislation: overview. Retrieved from http://www.infanthearing.org/legislation

National Center for Hearing Assessment and Management. (2012b). NCHAM. Retrieved from http://www.infanthearing.org

National Center for Hearing Assessment and Management (2012c). Policy statements regarding newborn hearing screening. Retrieved from http://www.infanthearing.org/resources_home/positionstatements

National Institutes of Health (1993). Early identification of hearing impairment in infants and younger children. Rockville, MD: National Institutes of Health.

Olusanya, B., McPherson, B., Swanepoel, W., Shrivastav, R., & Chapchap, M. (2006). Globalization of infant hearing screening: the next challenge before JCIH? Journal of the American Academy of Audiology, 17(4), 293–295, discussion 295–296.

Paradise, J. L. (1999). Universal newborn hearing screening: Should we leap before we look? Pediatrics, 103(3), 670–672.

Tueller, S. J. (2006). Maternal worry about infant health, maternal anxiety, and maternal perceptions of child vulnerability associated with newborn hearing screen results. Master's thesis, Utah State University, Logan.

U.S. Department of Health and Human Services. (1990). Healthy people 2000: national health promotion and disease prevention objectives. Washington, DC: Public Health Service.

U.S. Preventive Services Task Force. (1996). Screening for hearing impairment. In U.S. Preventive Services Task Force guide to clinical preventive services (2nd ed., pp. 393–405). Baltimore, MD: Williams & Wilkins.

U.S. Preventive Services Task Force. (2008). Universal screening for hearing loss in newborns: U.S. Preventive Services Task Force recommendation statement. Pediatrics, 122(1), 143–148.

White, K. R. (1997). Universal newborn hearing screening: issues and evidence. Retrieved from www.infanthearing.org/summary/prevalence.html

White, K. R. (2003). The current status of EHDI programs in the United States. Mental Retardation and Developmental Disabilities Research Reviews, 9(2), 79–88.

White, K. R., & Behrens, T. R. (1993). The Rhode Island Hearing Assessment Project: implications for universal newborn hearing screening. Seminars in Hearing, 14, 1–22.

White, K. R., & Blaiser, K. M. (2011). Strategic planning to improve EHDI programs. The Volta Review, 111, 83–108.

White, K. R., Forsman, I., Eichwald, J., & Muñoz, K. (2010). The evolution of early hearing detection and intervention programs in the United States. Seminars in Perinatology, 34(2), 170–179.

World Health Organization. (2010). Newborn and infant hearing screening: Current issues and guiding principles for action. Outcome of a WHO informal consultation held at WHO Headquarters, Geneva, Switzerland, 09–10 November 2009.

Yoshinaga-Itano, C., Sedey, A. L., Coulter, D. K., & Mehl, A. L. (1998). Language of early- and later-identified children with hearing loss. Pediatrics, 102(5), 1161–1171.

Chapter 6

Hearing Test Protocols for Children

Jane R. Madell and Carol Flexer

Key Points

- Pediatric audiologic assessments involve the selection of developmentally appropriate protocols that include the cross-check principle.

- Before testing, the child's cognitive age and physical status must be determined.

- A case history contributes valuable diagnostic information, provides an opportunity to observe the child, and allows a rapport to be established between the audiologist and the family.

- Functional auditory assessments, in the form of paper-and-pencil surveys, can assist in monitoring the baby's or child's auditory progress over time.

◆ The Cross-Check Principle for Test Batteries

There are four main purposes for a pediatric audiologic assessment: (1) to obtain a measure of peripheral hearing sensitivity that rules out or confirms hearing loss as a cause of the baby's or child's problem; (2) to confirm the status of the baby's or child's middle ear; (3) to assess auditory functioning using speech perception measures when possible; and (4) to observe and interpret the baby's or child's auditory behaviors.

To this end, a test battery approach employing the "cross-check" principle is standard (American Academy of Audiology [AAA], 2012). The cross-check principle, originally described by Jerger and Hayes (1976), posits that several appropriate behavioral and electrophysiologic tests must be used to determine the extent of a child's auditory function (Stach, 1998). A test battery approach furnishes detailed information, avoids drawing conclusions from a single test, allows for the identification of multiple pathologies, and provides a comprehensive foundation for observing a child's auditory behaviors. **Table 6.1** summarizes each test in the pediatric threshold test battery and discusses when each is appropriate.

The purpose of this chapter is to discuss the audiologic tests in the various pediatric test protocols, to emphasize the need for behavioral audiologic assessments for all infants and children, to detail the steps in administering a test protocol (including selecting the appropriate protocol), to describe obtaining pediatric case histories, and, finally, to summarize functional auditory assessments.

◆ Pediatric Audiologic Test Protocols

The American Speech-Language-Hearing Association (ASHA) (2004) and the AAA (2012) recommend the following test protocols according to the chronological/developmental age of the child:

1. Birth through 6 months of age (age is adjusted for prematurity): When infants are very young or experiencing severe developmental disabilities, ASHA and AAA recommend that the testing of infants or children should rely primarily on physiologic measures of auditory function, such as auditory brainstem response (ABR) and auditory steady state responses (ASSR) using frequency-specific stimuli to estimate the audiogram. In addition, otoacoustic emissions (OAE) and acoustic immittance measures should be used to supplement ABR and ASSR results. Case history, parent/caregiver report, behavioral observation of the infant's responses to a variety of sounds, developmental screening, and functional auditory assessments should also be performed.

Table 6.1 A summary of tests used in pediatric assessments

Test	Expected infant/ child response	Cognitive age range	Benefit	Challenges
Behavioral Observation Audiometry (BOA)	Change in sucking in response to auditory stimulus; other behavioral changes are not accepted because they usually indicate supra-threshold response.	Birth–6 months	• Enables the audiologist to obtain valuable behavioral responses in infants; part of the cross-check principle. • Testing can be conducted in sound-fields, with earphones or with bone oscillator, hearing aids, or cochlear implants. • Enables accurate fitting of technology because minimal response levels (MRLS) can be obtained.	• Requires careful observation of infant sucking by the audiologist. • Cannot be used with infants who do not suck (e.g., infants who use feeding tubes). • Testing can be performed only when the infant is in a calm awake or light sleep state. • BOA has not been generally accepted in the audiology community because audiologists typically have not been trained to use a sucking response paradigm.
Visual Reinforcement Audiometry (VRA)	Conditioned head turn to a visual reinforcer; usually a lighted animated toy.	5–36 months	• Enables the audiologist to obtain valuable behavioral responses in infants and young children; part of the cross-check principle. • Because responses are conditioned, more responses can be obtained in one test session. • Testing can be conducted in soundfield, with earphones or with bone oscillator, hearing aids, or cochlear implants. • Enables accurate fitting of technology because MRL can be obtained. • The state of the infant or child is less problematic than in BOA because the child can be more easily involved in the task.	• Some children will not accept earphones, so obtaining individual ear information can be challenging.
Conditioned Play Audiometry (CPA)	Child performs a motor act in response to hearing a sound (e.g., the listen and drop task)	30 months to 5 years	• Accurate responses can be obtained at threshold level. • Testing can be conducted in sound field or with earphones, with bone oscillator, hearing aids, or cochlear implants.	• Keeping the child entertained and involved long enough to obtain all the necessary information can be challenging.
Immittance	None	All	• Provides information about middle ear functioning and about intactness of the auditory system reflex arc.	• The child must sit still, not speaking or moving during the test battery.
Transient Otoacoustic Emissions (TOAE)	None	All	• Measures out hair cell function. • Presence of emissions indicates no greater than a mild hearing loss. • Contributes to evaluation of the overall function of the auditory system.	• Cannot rule out mild hearing loss.
Distortion Product Otoacoustic Emissions (DPOAE)	None	All	• Measures out hair cell function. • Presence of emissions indicates no greater than moderate hearing loss. • Contributes to evaluation of the overall function of the auditory system.	• Cannot rule out moderate hearing loss.
Auditory Brainstem Response Testing (ABR)	None	All	• Tonal ABR provides frequency-specific threshold information. • Click ABR provides information about the intactness of the auditory pathways, including measures contributing to the diagnosis of auditory neuropathy.	• The infant or child must be asleep, sedated, or very still for the duration of testing. • ABR testing is not a direct measure of hearing and is not a substitute for behavioral audiologic testing.

- The authors of this book propose a primary role for behavioral audiologic assessment, even for this very young population. See Chapter 7 and the DVD.

2. Five months through 24 months of age: At these ages, ASHA (2004) and AAA (2012) suggest that behavioral assessments should be performed first, with VRA (visual reinforcement audiometry) being the behavioral test of choice. OAEs and ABRs should be assessed only when behavioral audiometric tests are unreliable, ear-specific thresholds cannot be obtained, behavioral results are inconclusive, or auditory neuropathy is suspected. Developmental screening and functional auditory assessments also should be performed; please refer to **Table 6.4** at the end of the chapter for a summary of functional auditory assessments. See Chapter 8 for detailed information about VRA.
3. Twenty-five months through 60 months of age: ASHA (2004) and AAA (2012) suggest that behavioral tests (VRA or CPA [conditioned play audiometry]) and acoustic immittance tests are usually sufficient. Speech perception tests should also be performed in combination with developmental screening and functional auditory assessments.

The expected outcomes of pediatric audiologic protocols are extensive and include: (1) identification of hearing loss; (2) identification of auditory neuropathy, if present, or of a potential central auditory processing/language disorder; (3) quantification of hearing status based on behavioral and electrophysiologic tests; (4) development of a comprehensive report of historical, physical, and audiologic findings, and recommendations for treatment and management; (5) implementation of a plan for monitoring, surveillance, and habilitation of hearing loss; and (6) provision of family-centered counseling and education.

◆ Why Behavioral Audiologic Tests Need to Be Included in the Evaluation of All Infants and Children

The *Guidelines for the Audiologic Assessment of Children from Birth to 5 Years of Age* (ASHA, 2004) and the *Audiologic Guidelines for the Assessment of Hearing in Infants and Young Children* (AAA, 2012) both suggest that behavioral testing is not the preferred

method for evaluating hearing in infants from birth to 4 months of age for identifying hearing loss and selecting hearing aids because of (1) the prolonged cooperation required from the child, (2) excessive test time needed, (3) poor frequency resolution, and (4) poor test–retest reliability. There is no doubt that evaluating hearing in infants and young children is time consuming and can require prolonged cooperation. However, these challenges should not lead to the conclusion that behavioral testing should not be conducted. If we believe that the information obtained from behavioral testing is valuable, if not critical, our goal should be to develop procedures that will permit us to obtain reliable behavioral test results. It would not occur to any of us to make a determination about auditory function or to fit amplification on a normally developing 5-year-old without a good behavioral audiogram, and for good reason. The behavioral audiogram provides valuable information not available from electrophysiological testing, and within certain limits, it should be possible to obtain good-quality behavioral evaluations on infants and children of any age or developmental status.

Chapters 7 to 11 describe in detail the techniques for the behavioral evaluation of infants and children. In addition, the DVD that accompanies this book will demonstrate these behavioral test techniques. We hope that the text and DVD together will assist the audiologist in learning the necessary skills to optimize behavioral test results. The DVD may also be helpful to the experienced clinician who wishes to update skills.

◆ Steps to Take Before Initiating Behavioral Audiologic Testing of Infants and Children

Selecting the Appropriate Test Protocol

A pivotal factor in obtaining reliable test results is the selection of the appropriate test protocol. To do so, it is essential to know the child's cognitive level and physical abilities. Knowledge of what tasks the child is capable of performing *before* initiating testing is critical.

Cognitive Age

There are three behavioral techniques, each of which is appropriate for children at different developmental levels, allowing for some flexibility at upper and lower age limits. Behavioral observation audiometry (BOA) is the appropriate behavioral technique for infants from birth to 6 months cognitive age; VRA is appropriate for infants from 5 months to 36 months cognitive age; and conditioned play audiometry (CPA) is the appropriate technique for children whose cognitive age is 30 to 36 months and older. Knowing the child's cognitive age allows the audiologist to select the appropriate test method, which is essential. For example, it would not be a good idea to ask a 2-month-old to raise her hand when she heard a sound. Doing so would lead to the conclusion that every 2-month-old child is deaf.

Pitfall

- It is critical to know the cognitive age of the child to select the appropriate test protocol. Although many children have compatible cognitive and chronological ages, some do not. Without knowing the correct cognitive age, the audiologist runs the risk of selecting the wrong test protocol and thus obtaining unreliable test results.

Unfortunately, it is not always possible to rely solely on chronological age to determine cognitive level. Although many children function at the same levels cognitively and chronologically, not all do. Much of the information obtained from the case history will be helpful in determining cognitive level. If speech and language skills are at or close to age level, one can assume that chronological and cognitive ages are the same or relatively close. Unfortunately, many children undergo audiologic evaluations because they are not developing speech and language skills, so other information is needed to determine cognitive level. Motor development can be a useful marker. If a child's motor skills are at age level, the child is usually cognitively close to chronological level, at least for the purpose of the tasks that are necessary for testing hearing.

Reports from other clinicians, including speech-language pathologists and pediatricians, can provide very useful information about developmental level. A variety of scales used by pediatricians can give the audiologist an idea about developmental level. Experience spending time with young children also will assist the audiology student in developing an "intuition" that will support the selection of the appropriate test protocol.

It is not a good idea to use the trial-and-error method to choose a test protocol; this method may work some, but not all, of the time. If a child's cognitive and chronological levels are too far apart, using an inappropriate test may give the false appearance of hearing loss or yield inaccurate thresholds because the child will not respond appropriately to the test stimulus.

Physical Status

Once a child's cognitive level has been established, her physical condition needs to be evaluated to be certain that the child is capable of performing the test tasks. For BOA, we are primarily looking for changes in sucking, which is relatively easy to discern. Does the child suck? If yes, the audiologist can implement the BOA procedure (see Chapter 7, Behavioral Observation Audiometry for detailed test techniques). An infant may have an eating problem and receive food through feeding tubes, but if she uses a pacifier, sucking still can be observed. However, if the infant does not suck, it is probably not possible to obtain reliable observation audiometry responses. (See Chapter 10 for alternative test techniques for evaluating hearing in children with special needs.)

VRA uses a conditioned head turn in response to presentation of a sound stimulus, which requires the child to have vision good enough to see the reinforcing toy, and neck control sufficient to turn and look for the reinforcing toy. This task is most often performed with the child sitting either in a highchair or on someone's lap. A child who cannot sit can be placed in an adaptive supported position, such as an infant seat, that will still allow a conditioned head turn to be made. If the child cannot make a head turn, it will not be possible to use VRA. If the child is blind or, for some other reason, cannot see the reinforcer, it will not be possible to use standard VRA protocols. A creative audiologist may be able to generate some adaptive protocols (see Chapter 10).

Play audiometry requires that the child perform a motor task in response to the presentation of a sound. The ability to accomplish this task is limited only by the creativity of the audiologist. If the child cannot hold a toy and drop it in a bucket, she may be able to blink, move a finger, or push a button, for example. Specific test information about the various behavior protocols is discussed in the following chapters.

Setting Up the Test Room

Using a Two-Room Setup

There are several ways to set up a test room for evaluation of hearing in infants and young children. The most common is a two-room setup with an audiologist and audiometer in one room and the child, parent, and test assistant in the other. When using this setup, the audiologist and the test assistant must have a full view of the child. The audiologist, who is presenting the test stimuli, needs to be able to observe the child's behavioral state to know when and when not to present stimuli (e.g., do not present a stimulus if the child is fidgeting or trying to get out of the chair), and both testers need to be able to judge the presence or absence of a response.

It is also important that the two testers are able to communicate. If possible, the test assistant should have an earphone to hear directions or suggestions from the audiologist in the control room. A wireless system also can work well for clinician-to-clinician communication. It is important that the test assistant knows when the stimulus is being presented in order to determine whether or not to reinforce a child's response. For example, if a child looks toward the VRA toy when a sound has been presented, the test assistant must be enthusiastic, clapping and laughing. If the child looks toward the toy when there has been no test stimulus, the test assistant must not reinforce the response. If the test assistant does not have earphones or a wireless system, the tester and test assistant must develop visual cues to ensure that they are communicating.

Pearl

- A communication system needs to be set up so that the audiologist and the test assistant can communicate about test protocols and so that the test assistant knows when a sound is being presented to the child.

Using a One-Room Setup

Some audiologists use a one-room test setup, either for all testing or for selected testing. The advantage of a one-room test setup is that testing can be accomplished with only one audiologist, who now performs both the tester and test assistant roles, thus having more control of the test situation. To accomplish this type of testing, the audiologist places the audiometer in the test room where the child will be. The setup should be arranged so that the child cannot see the audiometer controls and does not know when the interrupter switch is being pressed. The controls for the reinforcer toy for VRA also need to be located in a place not visible to the child. The audiologist can sit in front of the child and provide the stimulus, test assistance as needed (such as handing the child toys for play audiometry or distracting the child for VRA), and reinforcement as needed (either social or VRA). Even in centers where a two-room test setup is the norm, there are times when it is convenient to have the tester and child in the same room.

Experimenting with a variety of test setups will assist the audiologist in finding the one that is most comfortable for each test situation. See **Table 6.2** for a summary of steps that need to be taken before the actual pediatric assessment is initiated.

Obtaining a Case History

A good case history is a valuable tool and an often overlooked part of an audiologic evaluation (Ehrlich, 1983). All diagnosticians recognize the need to obtain some information before beginning testing, and the amount needed will vary according to the reason for the evaluation. If the evaluation is a presurgical or postsurgical evaluation because a child is scheduled for insertion of pressure equalization tubes, it

Table 6.2 Necessary steps before beginning the pediatric assessment

1. Determine the child's cognitive age from:
   – Case history
   – Reports from other evaluations
   – Infant developmental screening scales

2. Evaluate the child's physical status in terms of:
   – Upper-torso control
   – Head and neck control
   – Vision
   – Ability to manipulate toys

3. Choose the test room setup:
   – One room with one audiologist
   – Two rooms with two audiologists, or one audiologist and one test assistant
   – Two rooms with one audiologist and one parent who also functions as a test assistant

may not be necessary to obtain an extensive history. If, however, the child is being seen for evaluation because of concern about hearing, speech and language development, developmental delay, or problems in school, an extensive history is needed. Failure to obtain sufficient history information may reduce the quantity and quality of data obtained from the evaluation and diminishes the role of both the assessment and the audiologist to a technical one rather than a professional and diagnostic one.

Taking a case history obviously provides information necessary to learn about a child's development and health. A case history also provides an opportunity to observe the child and to become acquainted with the family and caregivers to understand their concerns and needs and to assess their objectivity. If different family members have dissimilar viewpoints, this difference of opinion frequently emerges during the interview process. The time spent obtaining a history also provides an opportunity to observe the child and his interactions with family members and others, and it may uncover differences of opinion or interpretation between the audiologist's observations and those of the family members. Finally, taking a case history provides an excellent opportunity to develop rapport with and insights into the family, which may increase their willingness to accept the audiologist's assessment results and subsequent recommendations for management.

By the end of the interview, the audiologist should have a good picture of the child's cognitive and developmental status as well as an initial estimate of the child's auditory skills.

Collecting Case History Information

Some clinics mail out questionnaires in advance of the appointment and have families complete them before coming in for the evaluation. This method allows the family to think about answers, to check with other family members or clinicians if needed, and to find addresses of health care providers and schools, for example. Advance information is especially helpful if the child is brought to the evaluation by someone other than the parents (e.g., older sibling, grandparents, or foster parents). If the child is a foster child, mailing out the questionnaires in advance enables the responsible social service agency to provide the necessary information. However, not all families will complete forms even if they are received in advance.

Pearl

- Obtaining a case history permits the audiologist to learn about the child and to understand the parents' concerns and assessment expectations. History taking also facilitates the development of a rapport between the audiologist and the family that will be invaluable when counseling about test results.

Some programs give families questionnaires to complete when they arrive at the center just before being seen for evaluation. Although this method limits the time for completing the form and for thinking about the answers and does not permit obtaining information that is not easily recalled, it ensures that some information will be obtained.

Even when history forms are completed in advance by the family, the audiologist still needs to ask questions and spend time reviewing the information before initiating testing. This review will frequently reveal incomplete answers that will need to be finished before testing can begin. Some audiologists prefer to collect history information by asking all the questions themselves. Although this method allows the audiologist to direct specific questions as needed and expand or delete questions in certain areas, it extends the time scheduled for an evaluation, because all information must be obtained at the time of the audiologic assessment.

Some basic areas should be reviewed in any history. Other questions will present themselves as the interviewer learns more about the child and the concerns of the parents or caregivers. A printed history form is frequently useful because it provides basic information; however, it is important not to let the form limit the questions.

Caution

- The case history form should be viewed simply as a guide to the interview process.

Topics to Cover in a Case History

A complete history covers several content areas, and depending on the reason for the evaluation, emphasizes different segments of information. For example, if this evaluation is an initial one or if the child has not been seen recently, the obvious first question is, "Why have you brought your child here today?" By determining the reason for the visit, the audiologist can find out what the parent's or caregiver's concerns are and begin to get a picture of the goals of the evaluation. (Asking an older child why he is here today helps the audiologist understand what the child thinks is happening.) The next step is obtaining specific information. See **Table 6.3** for a list of case history topics.

◆ Summary

Obtaining a history takes time but provides valuable information. At the very least, by the end of obtaining a history, the audiologist should have a very good sense of:

- The child's cognitive status and motor abilities, which are critical for selecting the appropriate behavioral test protocol (BOA, VRA, or CPA)
- The child's speech, language, and developmental levels, which are important in selecting test materials for speech perception testing

During the audiologic evaluation, the audiologist determines whether the initial impressions were accurate or not. It may be helpful to try to estimate the audiogram from history information and from observation of the child before beginning the test. Doing so over a period of time will improve the audiologist's ability to take a history and make accurate observations of a child's auditory status.

◆ Functional Auditory Assessments

An important part of a basic test battery for an infant or child of any age is an evaluation of auditory function. Numerous tests and surveys have been developed for this purpose. Functional auditory assessments are typically accomplished by having the teacher, student, or parent complete a questionnaire before and after the use of a hearing aid, cochlear implant, personal FM, or sound field system or the delivery of therapy or educational services. Most important, functional auditory assessments can monitor the child's auditory progress over time by repeating assessments periodically. **Table 6.4** displays a summary of functional auditory assessment tools.

Table 6.3 Information to obtain in important case history content areas

Birth and prenatal history	Communication history: Hearing

– Previous pregnancies
– Illnesses during the pregnancy, including the week of pregnancy an illness occurred
– RH incompatibility, ABO blood incompatibility
– Medications, drugs (legal and illegal) taken during the pregnancy
– Complications during the pregnancy
– Length of the pregnancy
– Delivery: caesarean section or vaginal
– Birth weight
– Complications at birth: anoxia, jaundice, Apgar scores, breech, other
– Length of hospitalization
	– Parents' thoughts of child's hearing
	– Sounds to which child responds
	– Does the child distinguish between sounds (phone, doorbell)?
	– Does the child want TV/CD/DVD/computer loud?
	– Does hearing fluctuate? Under what conditions?
	– Are sounds comfortable? What sound? Under what conditions?
	– Amplification history:
	  – Does the child wear a hearing aid and/or a cochlear implant?
	  – Name and model number of the instruments(s)? Which ears?
	  – Does the child wear an FM system? Name and model number of the instrument? Which ears?
	  – Who recommended the devices?
	  – When were they acquired?
	  – When does the child wear them? (e.g., all day? only at school?)

Health history	Communication history: Speech and language
– Colds, allergy, ear infections – High fevers – Immunizations – Meningitis – Other viruses (mumps, cytomegalovirus) – Immunization history; reaction to immunizations – Drugs taken regularly and drug reactions – Feeding or swallowing problems – Seizures – Head injury	– Age of babbling, first word, phrases, sentences – Does the child understand verbal requests with, without visual cues? – How does the child communicate his/her needs? Voice? Gesture? Sign? – Has there been a change in the child's speech and language? – Did the child speak and then stop?

Developmental history	Social history
– Motor milestones: sitting, crawling, walking – Age of visual response to parents – Is walking clumsy? Does the child fall a lot? – Feeding and eating history – Age of toilet training	– When did the child feed himself? Dress himself? – Does she play with other children? – What toys or objects does the child like to play with? – Does the child have any behavior problems? – How does the child get along with other children? Adults? Family? – Have there been any changes in the child's behavior? – Does the child respond to others? Make eye contact?

Educational history	Special services
– Current school – Type of educational program – Previous school placements – Reasons for change in school placement – Special services received in school – Describe educational problems or concerns	– What special services does the child receive in school? Outside of school? – Speech-language therapy – Hearing (auditory) therapy – Occupational therapy – Physical therapy – Psychological services – Educational tutoring – Other

Other evaluations	
– What other evaluations has the child had (evaluator, dates, and results)? – Audiologic – Speech-language – Hearing (auditory) therapy – Occupational therapy – Physical therapy – Psychological – Educational – Pediatric – Otolaryngologic – Neurologic – Psychiatric	

Table 6.4 Functional auditory assessment tools for infants and young children

Measurement tool	Authors	Age range	Purpose
Auditory Behavior in Everyday Life (ABEL) (2002)	Purdy, Farrington, Moran, Chard, & Hodgson, 2002	Children 2–12 years	Twenty-four-item questionnaire with three subscales (aural-oral, auditory awareness, social/conversation skills) which evaluates auditory behavior in everyday life
Children's Home Inventory for Listening Difficulties (CHILD) (2000)	Anderson & Smaldino, 1998, 2000	Children 3–12 years	Parent and self-report versions that assess listening skills in 15 natural situations
Children's Outcome Worksheet (COW) (2003)	Williams, 2003	Children 4–12 years	Teacher, parent, and child rating scales of classroom and home listening situations with amplification device; to specify five situations where improved hearing is desired
Early Listening Function (ELF) (2000)	Anderson, 1989, 2000	Infants and toddlers; 5 months–3 years	Parent observational rating scale of structured listening activities conducted over time to record distance learning
Functional Auditory Performance Indicators (F.A.P.I) (2003)	Stredler-Brown & Johnson, 2003	Infants through school-age	Parent or interventionist assessment of functional auditory skills over time
Infant-Toddler Meaningful Auditory Integration Scale (IT-MAIS) (1991)	Robbins, Renshaw, & Berry, 1991	Infant-toddler and older child versions	Structured parent interview scale designed to assess spontaneous auditory behaviors in everyday listening situations
Listening Inventories for Educations (L.I.F.E.) (1998)	Anderson & Smaldino, 1998, 2000	6 years and above	Student and teacher rating scales designed to assess listening difficulty in the classroom
LittleEARS (2003)	Kuhn-Inacker, Weichbold, Tsiakpini, Coninx, & D'Haese, 2003	Birth and up	Questionnaire for the parent with 35 age-dependent questions that assess auditory development
Meaningful Auditory Integration Scale (MAIS) (1991)	Robbins, Renshaw, & Berry, 1991	Children 3 to 4 years and up	Parental interview with 10 questions that evaluates meaningful use of sound in everyday situations; attachment with hearing instrument, ability to alert to sound, ability to attach meaning to sound
Parent's Evaluation of Aural/Oral Performance of Children (PEACH) (2000)	Ching, Hill, & Psarros, 2000	Preschool to 7 years	Interview with parent with 15 questions targeting the child's everyday environment. Includes scoring for five subscales (use, quiet, noise, telephone, environment)
Preschool Screening Instrument for Targeting Educational Risk (Preschool SIFTER) (1996)	Anderson & Matkin, 1996	3 to 6 years	Questionnaire with 15 items completed by the teacher that identifies children at risk for educational failure; has five subscales (academics, attention, communication, class participation, behavior)
Screening Inventory for Targeting Educational Risk (SIFTER) (1989)	Anderson, 1989, 2000	6 years through secondary school	Teacher questionnaire designed to target academic risk behaviors in children with hearing problems; has five subscales (academics, attention, communication, class participation, behavior)
Teacher's Evaluation of Aural/Oral Performance of Children (TEACH) (2000)	Ching, Hill, & Psarros, 2000	Preschool to 7 years	Interview with teacher having 13 questions targeting the child's everyday environment. Includes scoring for five subscales (use, quiet, noise, telephone, environment)

Discussion Questions

1. Discuss the factors that need to be taken into consideration before beginning the actual pediatric assessment.

2. Identify five reasons for taking a case history.

3. Detail some of the reasons for performing functional auditory assessments, and summarize four tools.

4. Discuss the tests that are included in a pediatric test battery for a typical 12-month-old baby; include the concept of the cross-check principle.

References

American Academy of Audiology. (2012). Guidelines for the assessment of hearing in infants and young children. Retrieved from http://www.audiology.org/resources/documentlibrary/Pages/PediatricDiagnostics.aspx

American Speech-Language-Hearing Association. (2004). Guidelines for the audiologic assessment of children from birth to 5 years of age. Retrieved from http://www.asha.org/members/deskref-journals/deskref/default

Anderson, K. (1989). Screening Instrument for Targeting Educational Risk (SIFTER). Tampa, FL: Educational Audiology Association. Retrieved from http://www.hear2learn.com

Anderson, K. (2000). Early Listening Function (ELF). Retrieved from http://www.hear2learn.com

Anderson, K., & Matkin, N. (1996). Screening Instrument for Targeting Educational Risk in Preschool Children (age 3–kindergarten) (Preschool SIFTER). Retrieved from http://www.hear2learn.com

Anderson, K., & Smaldino, J. (1998). The Listening Inventory for Education: an efficacy tool (LIFE). Retrieved from http://www.hear2learn.com

Anderson, K., & Smaldino, J. (2000). Children's Home Inventory for Listening Difficulties (CHILD). Retrieved from http://www.hear2learn.com

Ching, T. C., Hill, M., & Psarros, C. (2000). Strategies for evaluation of hearing aid fitting for children (PEACH and TEACH). Paper presented at the International Hearing Aid Research Conference, August 23, Lake Tahoe, NV. Retrieved from http://www.nal.gov.au

Ehrlich, C. (1983). A case history for children. In Handbook of clinical audiology (3rd ed., pp. 607–620). J. Katz (Ed.). Baltimore, MD: Williams and Wilkins.

Jerger, J. F., & Hayes, D. (1976). The cross-check principle in pediatric audiometry. Archives of Otolaryngology (Chicago, Ill.), 102(10), 614–620. PubMed

Kuhn-Inacker, H., Weichbold, V., Tsiakpini, L., Coninx, S., & D'Haese, P. (2003). Little ears: Auditory questionnaire. Innsbruck, Austria: MED-EL.

Purdy, S. C., Farrington, D. R., Moran, C. A., Chard, L. L., & Hodgson, S. A. (2002). ABEL: Auditory behavior in everyday life. American Journal of Audiology, 11, 72–82.

Robbins, A. M., Renshaw, J. J., & Berry, S. W. (1991). Evaluating meaningful integration in profoundly hearing impaired children (MAIS). American Journal of Otolaryngology, 12, 144–150.

Stach, B. A. (1998). Clinical audiology: an introduction. San Diego, CA: Singular Publishing Group.

Stredler-Brown, A., & Johnson, D. C. (2003). Functional Auditory Performance Indicators: an integrated approach to auditory development. Retrieved from http://www.arlenestredlerbrown.com

Williams, C. (2003). The Children's Outcome Worksheets (COW): an outcome measure focusing on children's needs (ages 4–12). News from Oticon, January 2005. Retrieved from http://www.oticon.com

Chapter 7

Using Behavioral Observation Audiometry to Evaluate Hearing in Infants from Birth to 6 Months

Jane R. Madell

Key Points

- Auditory brainstem response (ABR), auditory steady state response (ASSR), and otoacoustic emission (OAE) testing provide critical information about the status of the auditory pathways, but are not direct measures of hearing.

- Only behavioral testing can provide a direct measure of hearing.

- When carefully performed, using appropriate criteria (including changes in sucking as an indication of a response), behavioral observation audiometry (BOA) can accurately measure thresholds in infants younger than 6 months.

- ABR, ASSR, and OAE cannot be used to monitor auditory performance and benefit from technology, whereas behavioral testing can be used to monitor performance and benefit from technology.

Nonbehavioral tests, such as ABR testing, ASSR testing, and OAEs, are frequently used to assist in estimating peripheral hearing in infants (American Speech-Language-Hearing Association [ASHA], 2004; American Academy of Audiology [AAA], 2012). Although these tests are an important part of the audiology practice, they are, in fact, not tests of hearing. The only true test of hearing is behavioral assessment. ABR, ASSR, and OAE measures provide information about the integrity of specific sites within the auditory system (Delaroche, Thiebaut, & Dauman, 2004; Gravel, 2000; Hicks, Tharpe, & Ashmead, 2000; Sininger, 1993). Only behavioral testing truly tests hearing, since it measures the response of the entire auditory system from the outer ear through the cerebral cortex. Behavioral tests permit measurement of what an infant actually perceives, so they are measures of functional hearing abilities.

Numerous authors have posited the necessity for cross-checking physiological results with behavioral data by using a battery of tests to determine hearing sensitivity (Bess & Humes, 2003; Gravel, 2000; Hicks et al, 2000; Jerger & Hayes, 1976; Madell, 1998, 2008; Northern & Downs, 2002). Behavioral testing of infants 6 months and older is a well-documented part of the clinical practice of audiology (ASHA, 2004; AAA, 2012). Behavioral evaluation of infants younger than 6 months is more difficult to achieve and less well documented. This chapter will describe a behavioral technique that can be used to successfully evaluate hearing in infants younger than 6 months.

◆ The History of Behavioral Testing of Infants

As early as the 1940s, attempts were made to develop behavioral techniques to assess hearing in infants (Ewing & Ewing, 1940, 1944; Froeschels & Beebe, 1946). Sir Alexander and Lady Ewing used percussion sounds and pitch pipes to elicit aural reflex responses (eye blinks). Wedenberg began infant screening in Sweden in 1956 using pure tones to elicit the auro-palpebral reflex (Wedenberg, 1956). Froding continued Wedenberg's work using a small gong and mallet. Some clinicians used the infant's ability to turn toward the sound to assess hearing. Frisina (1963) reported that, between 2 and 4 months of age, infants could turn toward a sound. However, Northern & Downs (2002) reported that head turning does not occur before the age of 6 months, and Gerber (1977) reported the average age of head turn to be at 7½ months.

Noisemakers

Noisemakers were the most common sound source employed for early hearing tests. They were selected for testing because they were readily available, simple, and inexpensive and could be used in any setting (a sound room was not required) and it was believed that infants would respond more reliably to noisemakers than to pure tone stimuli. The difficulty with noisemakers is that they usually have very broad frequency responses. Furthermore, their intensity is not easy to control even with practice exerting the pressure necessary to make the sound and stabilizing the distance from the infant's ear. Bove and Flugrath (1973) and Poblano, Chayo, Ibarra, and Rueda (2000) analyzed different noisemakers to determine their frequency responses so that response to noisemakers could provide more useful information. Even if noisemakers cannot provide sufficient information to be used to assess hearing, they can provide some gross information about how an infant responds to sound. Specifically, noisemakers can provide some evidence of an infant's ability to alert to sound and to localize the source (Northern & Downs, 2002).

Noisemakers should be used, primarily, to gain an understanding of how a baby will respond to sound—not as a measure of hearing. Before using any noisemakers, information should be obtained about the auditory signals they emit, including their frequency response and intensity. Results of noisemaker tests must be viewed with caution. For example, a noisemaker may have the bulk of its energy in the 2000–4000 Hz range but also have energy at 500 Hz at 30 to 40 dB less intensity than the high frequencies. What can be surmised about the infant's response to this stimulus? It is possible that the infant hears the high-frequency component of the stimulus, but it is also possible that the infant has a high-frequency hearing loss, does not hear the high-frequency part of the signal, and is responding to the low-frequency component.

Early Infant Hearing Screening Programs

The first large-scale infant hearing screening program in the United States was a citywide hearing screening project in Denver, conducted by Marion Downs and Graham Sterritt in 1964. They used a handheld noise generator that emitted a 90-dB sound pressure level (SPL) noise centered at 3000 Hz. Downs and Sterritt (1964, 1967), Northern and Downs (1991), and Werner and Gillenwater (1990) attempted to develop a standardized procedure to assess an infant's behavioral arousal, but a significant number of false positive test results made the testing unreliable. Several authors have described techniques for assessing behavioral responses in infants, including observa-tion of eye widening, quieting, eye shifting, grimacing, head orienting, limb movement, and changes in respiration. Attempts have been made to calibrate the observer (Mencher, McCulloch, Derbyshire, & Dethlefs, 1977; Weber, 1969), to assess the state of the infant (Eisenberg, 1969), and to calibrate the signal precisely (Thompson & Thompson, 1972). A major problem with using the auro-palpebral reflex, the Moro reflex, or changes in limb movement or respiration is that these behaviors are not elicited by threshold stimuli but rather are responses to suprathreshold stimuli. Although some infants with hearing loss were identified using these methods, many with less than severe to profound hearing losses were missed. In spite of all attempts to improve test protocols, BOA continued to be considered "unreliable."

Infant Thresholds

Because behavioral test protocols frequently did not reveal threshold responses, some audiologists proposed that responses at 60 to 70 dB SPL be interpreted as normal hearing for very young infants (McConnell & Ward, 1967, Northern & Downs, 1974). However, others demonstrated that infants hear at essentially adult levels (Berg & Smith, 1983; Eisele, Berry, & Shriner, 1975; Madell, 1995a, 1998, 2008; Olsho, 1984; Olsho, Koch, Carter, Halpin, & Spetner, 1988; Werner & Gillenwater, 1990). Olsho (1984), Olsho, Koch, and Halpin (1987), Olsho et al (1988), and Nozza (2006) reported that average behavioral thresholds of 3-month-olds were worse than thresholds for young adults by 15 to 20 dB between 250 and 4000 Hz and by ~ 30 dB at 8000 Hz. By 6 months of age, hearing sensitivity in the high frequencies improves, but thresholds at 250 Hz remain elevated by ~ 15 dB. Thresholds improved by 20 dB between 3 and 6 months. Olsho et al (1988) discussed how the audibility curve of younger infants may differ in shape compared with the curve of older infants and adults. It was assumed that this audibility curve difference was, at least in part, due to the characteristics of the external and middle ears in infants. Olsho et al (1988) postulated that some of the threshold differences may be related to sensory immaturity.

Gravel (2000), Hicks et al (2000), Olsho, Koch, Halpin, and Carter (1987), Olsho, Koch, and Halpin (1987), and Olsho et al (1988) use an observer-based procedure developed by Olsho to reduce tester bias in evaluating hearing in infants as young as 2 to 5 weeks. In this method, a trial consists of a sound or a no-sound interval. One or two trained observers watch the infant and make a determination as to whether the interval contained a sound, or no sound, based on the infant's response. The observer receives feedback as to whether a sound is present. Once the observer demonstrates a false-positive rate of less than 25% reliable, testing begins. Hicks et al (2000) used this technique with two observers testing 2- and 4-month-old infants. They successfully obtained thresholds for 4-month-olds, but were not successful in obtaining thresholds for 2-month-olds. Werner (2011) reports that BOA can be used when operant conditioning audiometry is not successful. Several authors evaluating hearing in infants report that results could be optimized by enhancing the test conditions. This enhancement included reducing visual distractions (Muir, Clifton, & Clarkson, 1989), using a salient auditory stimulus (Thompson & Thompson, 1972), reinforcing desired behaviors (Olsho, Koch, Halpin, & Carter, 1987; Olsho et al, 1988), and using changes in sucking as the response criteria (Delaroche et al, 2004; Madell, 1995a, 1998, 2008). Because of the critical need to obtain reliable test results on infants, research in this area will need to continue.

The Need for Behavioral Testing of Infants

Over time, the demand for infant hearing screening has increased significantly, so most states have mandated newborn hearing screening requirements. (See Chapter 5 for a complete discussion of newborn hearing screening.) As more infants survive and as hearing screening becomes more universal, audiologists are being asked to assess hearing in very young infants who have failed newborn screening and to manage hearing loss when it is identified. One of the first steps in hearing loss management is the selection and fitting of appropriate amplification. Hearing aid fitting requires an accurate assessment of the degree and type of hearing loss, with both ear- and frequency-specific information obtained by air and bone conduction.

Many audiologists feel comfortable testing hearing in infants older than 6 months using visual reinforcement audiometry (VRA) but do not feel comfortable testing younger infants, developmentally delayed infants, or critically ill infants. If an infant fails a hearing screening at birth, hearing aids should be fitted within a few weeks. Work by Apuzzo and Yoshinaga-Itana (1995), Yoshinaga-Itano, Coulter, and Thomson (2001), Dettman et al (2007), and others have demonstrated that infants who are fitted with appropriate technology before they are 6 months old can develop speech and language skills commensurate with their normal-hearing peers and that infants fitted with technology when they are older than 6 months do not catch up to those fit earlier. Sharma, Dorman, and Spahr (2002) and Sharma et al (2009) have demonstrated that infants who receive auditory stimulation at a sufficiently early age have evoked potential latencies similar to those of normal-hearing peers, but infants who do not have sufficiently early access do not. While information obtained through electrophysiological testing provides critical information,

it cannot be used to assess benefit from technology. Without assessing technology benefit, we cannot know whether a child is receiving sufficient auditory access to develop speech and language. Without this information, we are not appropriately monitoring auditory performance.

Behavioral testing allows the parents to participate in testing by allowing them to assist in determining when the infant is responding to a sound. If parents are provided with information about what to observe, they can be active participants in testing, facilitating acceptance and understanding of hearing loss and motivating families to proceed with treatment (Gravel & McCaughey, 2004). Electrophysiologic testing, on the other hand, provides little for a family to observe.

It is clear that we must develop test techniques for evaluating very young infants that will provide the ear- and frequency-specific information necessary for the evaluation, selection, and fitting of amplification. Real-ear measures provide good information about how much sound is reaching the eardrum, but this information is difficult to interpret without good information about the status of the infant's unaided hearing. Tonal ABR and ASSR measures provide some of this information, but thresholds obtained may vary by ±15 dB. BOA techniques can assist in obtaining ear- and frequency-specific information and can provide confirmation of information obtained from electrophysiologic tests.

◆ Diagnostic Audiologic Evaluation of Neonates

The goal of an audiologic evaluation of an infant is usually to determine whether the child has sufficient hearing to develop speech and language. A complete diagnostic evaluation of infants should include immittance testing (to assess middle ear status) and a test technique that will provide frequency- and ear-specific information, ideally for both air and bone conduction. The most common test protocols for evaluating neonates include immittance testing with a high-frequency probe tone, auditory brainstem response testing (ABR), auditory steady-state evoked potential (ASSEP), and OAE.

Immittance testing assesses middle ear status but does not provide information about hearing. ABR and ASSEP provide information about the auditory system's ability to receive sound but are not direct measures of hearing. OAEs assess function of the outer hair cells of the cochlea but, again, are not a direct measure of hearing. Information about an infant's ability to hear and attend to auditory stimuli can be obtained only with behavioral testing. For that reason, no at-risk infant or child should be released from audiologic follow-up until behavioral test results are obtained. (See Chapter 12 for a discussion of immittance testing, Chapter 13 for a discussion of OAE testing, and Chapter 15 for a discussion of ABR and ASSEP testing.)

Pearl

- Although ABR, ASSR, and OAE testing provides important information about the status of the auditory system, only behavioral testing directly tests hearing. For this reason, it is critical that audiologists have a behavioral technique that is accurate for assessing hearing in infants younger than 6 months.

The Basics of Behavioral Observation Audiometry

Who Is a Candidate for Behavioral Observation Audiometry?

Behavioral observation testing, using the protocol discussed in this chapter, is intended as a threshold technique. It is not a protocol for general observation of responses to noise. This protocol uses observation of sucking responses and is appropriate only for infants who are cognitively at birth to 6 months of age and who are capable of sucking. The technique may be useful for older infants who, because of developmental delay, are cognitively less than 6 months of age. Infants older than 6 months' cognitive age will likely not suck consistently, so the responses may be less reliable. In addition, at 6–7 months of age, infants can be reliably tested using visual reinforcement audiometry (see Chapter 8).

What Is Being Observed?

Historically, many behaviors have been used to assess hearing in infants (arousal, limb movement, respiration changes, facial grimace, eye blink), but these behaviors have not proven to be sufficiently repeatable, and, more importantly, they have not been good indicators of threshold. The behavior most likely to provide threshold responses is a change in sucking (Delaroche et al, 2004; Madell, 1988, 1995a, 1998, 2008; Widen & Keener, 2003). Arousal responses, limb movements, and eye blinks frequently reveal suprathreshold-level responses but rarely threshold, since these behaviors typically are elicited by louder stimuli. Sucking responses, however, although present at suprathreshold levels, are frequently observed at, or close to, threshold. Either initiation or cessation

of sucking is an acceptable response. Some infants will start sucking when a sound is presented, others will cease sucking, and some will do both.

Pearl

- Cessation or initiation of sucking is the only reliable response for obtaining behavioral thresholds in infants younger than 6 months.

Maximizing Observation of the Sucking Response

Sucking can be observed with a bottle, nursing at the breast, or a pacifier. The family should be instructed to bring the infant to the evaluation session hungry so that he will be ready to suck. The infant needs to be as comfortable as possible during testing, so, if the infant normally drinks from a bottle, the family should bring one. If the infant normally nurses, it would be best if the infant is nursed during testing. For this test procedure to succeed, the mother has to be comfortable being observed nursing, and some women are not. If the mother understands the reason for the intrusion on her privacy, she usually acquiesces. If the infant uses a pacifier, the family should bring one along. After the infant is finished eating, testing can frequently continue by observing sucking with a pacifier. If an infant is very hungry, it is best to allow him a little time to eat to enable him to get over that initial extreme hunger before beginning testing.

As soon as the baby settles down, testing can begin. The best way to observe the sucking response is to be able to see the infant's mouth close-up. A good view of the mouth can easily be obtained by having a video camera in the test room that can be adjusted from the control room. By using the zoom on the camera, it is possible to focus directly on the infant's mouth, which will enable the audiologist to have an excellent view of sucking. If a camera is not available, the audiologist needs to be certain that she can clearly see changes in sucking to use this technique.

How Does One Know That the Sucking Is a Response to a Sound Stimulus?

As with all other behavioral responses, timing is the key factor. When using play audiometry with a child, we question the validity of the child's response if it comes a long time after presentation of the stimulus. With any test protocol, behavioral or electrophysiologic, responses can be accepted only if they fall within a reasonable time window after presentation of the stimulus. Infants are fairly consistent, internally. Some respond to the "on" of the stimulus, and others respond to the "off." The timing of the response is also usually consistent. Infants respond at about the same number of seconds after presentation of the stimulus each time, with the response time slightly shorter for louder stimuli (Madell, 1998, 2008; Northern & Downs, 2002; Widen & Keener, 2003).

Positioning the Infant

The necessity of appropriately positioning the infant cannot be overstated. Positioning may, in fact, be the most important factor in obtaining accurate test results with behavioral observation audiometry. To obtain reliable test results, the infant needs to be resting in a comfortable position with full support of the head and torso and must be visible to the testers. If the child is nursing, the mother will be holding the child in her arms. If the child is using a bottle or a pacifier, the child may be held in someone's arms or placed in an infant seat (**Fig. 7.1a–c**). The advantage of an infant seat is that the infant will not be receiving any "signals" from the mother when he hears the sound. Involuntary movements, such as stiffening by the mother in response to sound or movement of the breast or bottle, can be transmitted to the infant; therefore, changes in sucking may occur that are not related to the auditory stimuli. If the infant is being held, the mother or other person holding the infant should be very carefully instructed about the need to remain silent and still throughout testing to eliminate interfering with test results. It is sometimes useful to have the mother wear earphones to prevent her from hearing and being influenced by the sound; however, many mothers prefer not to wear earphones because they want to hear what their baby is hearing.

The Role of the Test Assistant

BOA is best accomplished by using two or more observers. One is the audiologist controlling the test equipment, usually outside the room where the infant is placed. The second observer typically is sitting next to the infant. Positioning of all players needs to be carefully orchestrated to be certain that both testers can easily see the infant.

The test assistant has several responsibilities. He must constantly be monitoring the infant to be certain that the baby's head and torso are comfortably balanced to minimize or preclude fussing and straining. If the infant becomes fussy, testing will need to stop until the infant can be made comfortable (Madell, 1998, 2008). For older infants, or infants using a bottle or a pacifier, the test assistant must keep the infant focused at the midline, again so that the infant is comfortable and not distracted. It is sometimes helpful to hold a colorful toy (Madell, 1998, 2008) or a light emitting diode (LED), usually a small red light (Hicks et al, 2000; Olsho, Koch, Halpin, & Carter, 1987), in front of the infant in a position that allows the infant's head to be centered. The toy should not be held above the infant's head so he needs to move his neck to see it. Visual distractions need to be kept to a minimum (Muir et al, 1989) to be certain that extraneous stimuli are not interfering with observation of responses. It is important that the person holding the toy or LED make no change in the movement of the toy when the sound is presented. Any change in movement can confound the interpretation of whether the infant is responding to the sound or to the change in the distracter. If the infant is in an infant seat, the test assistant may be the one holding the bottle or pacifier and holding the visual distracters. Finally, the test assistant will be one of the observers who judges whether or not the infant responded to the sound presentation by changing his or her sucking behavior.

The Role of the Parents

The parents cannot be relied on as observers, and certainly not as the primary observers. Their stakes are too high, they are not experienced in the task, and they may not understand exactly what constitutes an acceptable response. Parents are, however, very valuable in helping the testers to understand the baby and in assisting in making the baby com-

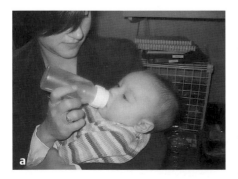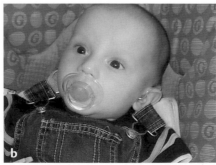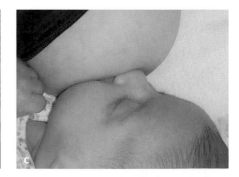

Fig. 7.1a–c   Positioning the infant for testing: **(a)** using a bottle, **(b)** using a pacifier, and **(c)** nursing at the breast.

fortable. At least one parent needs to be in the test room to assist in understanding the test protocols and test results. If both parents are present, the other parent can observe from the control room. The audiologist in the control room can point out responses during testing to assist in the parents' understanding of the tests. Their observation of how the baby does or does not respond will be helpful when interpreting the final test results and presenting subsequent follow-up recommendations (Flasher & Fogel, 2004).

Testing Protocol of Behavioral Observation Audiometry

Soundfield versus Earphone Testing

A complete audiogram includes air and bone conduction thresholds in each ear at frequencies of 250 to 8000 Hz. However, infants will provide only a limited number of responses in one test session, so testing protocols need to be designed to obtain the most information with the fewest responses. The goal of the initial audiologic evaluation of an infant is usually to be certain that the infant has sufficient hearing to develop speech and language. It may not be necessary to obtain ear-specific information at the first visit. (Occasionally, a child is referred to a pediatric audiologist because of a medical condition that requires ear-specific information immediately, but this is more frequently the exception rather than the rule. When detailed information is required during the first test session, the test protocol will obviously have to change.) Ear specific information is important and must be obtained prior to releasing an infant from audiologic follow-up, but the more important question at the time of the initial evaluation is whether the infant hears enough to learn language. Should the initial audiologic evaluation indicate that hearing is normal in at least one ear utilizing soundfield testing, it may not be critical to obtain information about each ear separately at that visit. However, if the initial testing indicates that hearing is not within normal limits in the soundfield, then ear-specific information is critical so that management can proceed. No infant should be released from audiologic follow-up until ear-specific information is obtained.

Under most conditions, testing should begin in soundfield. Soundfield testing is less stressful for the infant and allows two ears to be stimulated at the same time. This ensures testing of the best-hearing ear. It also permits parents to hear the sounds; this can be very useful in their understanding of the test results. Earphone testing can follow later in the initial test session or in a subsequent test session. When earphone testing is being attempted, insert earphones are the earphones of choice for infants. Insert earphones (**Fig. 7.2**) will remain appropriately seated in the ear canal and will provide the most accurate

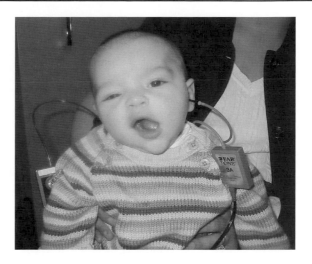

Fig. 7.2 Infant with insert earphones.

results in tiny ears. Circumaural earphones are frequently too large and are very difficult to keep well positioned.

If testing indicates thresholds at lower than normal hearing levels, bone conduction testing is essential. The bone vibrator should be held in place with either a pediatric-sized headband or a fabric one that goes around the head and across the forehead using Velcro to secure it in place. If a metal headband is used, soft material such as foam or other padding should be used for comfort and to keep the headband from moving. If a hearing loss is confirmed, the same test protocols can be used to assess functional gain with amplification in soundfield.

Test Stimuli

When planning the test session, it is important to keep in mind that infants will provide only a limited number of responses, so each stimulus presentation must be considered carefully. The goal of the testing is to obtain frequency-specific test results. Warble tones or narrow bands of noise will provide this information. Broadband stimuli, such as music, conversational speech, or white noise, will not. Narrow bands of noise are frequently easier for an infant to respond to (Gravel, 2000; Madell, 1998, 2008) and may provide thresholds that are 5 to 10 dB softer than those obtained with warble tones.

Speech awareness thresholds to low- (ba), mid-high- (sh), and high- (s) frequency speech stimuli can be used to confirm warble tone/noise band thresholds. The threshold for "ba" should be close to the threshold obtained at 500 Hz, "sh" should be close to the threshold obtained at 2000 Hz, and "s" should be close to the threshold obtained at 3000 to 4000 Hz (Ling, 2002; Madell, 1995b, 1998, 2008). A broadband speech stimulus, such as running speech or music, is not a good test stimulus, since it is not frequency-specific and cannot provide information that could be useful in fitting technology or in developing a management protocol.

Presentation of Test Stimuli

Many normal-hearing infants respond better to high-frequency stimuli, so it is reasonable to begin at a high frequency, usually 2000 Hz. To explain, if there is concern about middle ear pathology, low-frequency hearing could be compromised, so it may be better to begin with a high-frequency stimulus (2000 Hz). On the other hand, if a significant sensorineural hearing loss is suspected, hearing may be better at low frequencies, so testing should begin with 500 Hz. After obtaining thresholds at 500 and 2000 Hz, make a determination about what is the next most important piece of information to have. For example, if thresholds at both 500 and 2000 Hz are normal, it would be more important to obtain a threshold at 4000 Hz than at 1000 Hz, since hearing is likely also to be normal at 1000 Hz. However, if hearing at 500 Hz is at 30 dB HL and hearing at 2000 Hz is at 70 dB HL, it would be very important to know what hearing is at 1000 Hz.

Several indications can clue the audiologist about which frequencies and intensities should be used to begin testing:

- Observe the infant's responses to noisemakers.
- Observe the infant's responses to voice and environmental sounds.
- Question the parents about the infant's response to sound before testing.

Presentation of stimuli should begin at a soft level slightly above where you expect the infant to respond, and then should be increased in 10-dB steps until a response is observed. The initial stimulus should not be so loud as to startle the infant. If the initial stimulus is much louder than threshold, it may be difficult to regain the infant's attention to threshold-level stimuli. When the infant responds, decrease intensity in 10-dB steps, decreasing stimuli in 5-dB steps when close to estimated threshold, and then increase intensity in 5- or 10-dB steps as would be done with any other population. *Especially with infants, no response should be recorded until it is observed at the same level three times.*

Timing is critical. If stimuli are presented too quickly, the infant will ignore them. A sound that comes out of silence is more likely to elicit a response. To obtain reliable responses, it is important to observe the infant carefully. If an infant startles to a sound, it is probably significantly above threshold. The way the baby responds when the stimulus is loud will provide clues about the type of response and latency that can be expected. This information can be used to interpret responses when the stimulus intensity decreases (**Table 7.1**).

Other Factors That Influence Behavioral Observation Audiometry Test Results with Infants

The audiologist must know something about the infant to obtain reliable test results. Spending a little time with the infant before beginning testing will increase the likelihood of obtaining reliable test results. It is important to have a good estimate of the infant's developmental, neurologic, and behavioral status. Can the infant do whatever is required for testing? If we are looking for sucking changes, we need to know that the infant sucks steadily. Some infants take a few sucks and stop, then start again. When an infant has an irregular sucking pattern, it becomes very difficult to use sucking to assess hearing. Some infants, because of serious medical conditions, will be fed with a gastrointestinal tube. If the infant uses a pacifier, it may still be possible to test hearing by measuring nonnutritive sucking responses. However, if the infant does not use a pacifier, it will not be possible to measure hearing using a sucking technique.

Are there concerns about the infant's neurologic status that could affect testing? For example, is the

Table 7.1 Behavioral observation audiometry test protocol

1. Bring infant into test room in hungry state.
2. Seat infant so torso is supported and infant is not fidgety, and so tester(s) can easily see mouth.
3. Monitor infant state during testing and stop if infant becomes fidgety.
4. Instruct parents not to respond to test stimuli or responses from the child.
5. Test assistant will keep infant centered, observe responses, and monitor parents' behavior.
6. Begin testing in soundfield.
7. Begin testing with a stimulus that is slightly above estimated threshold.
8. Test one low (500 Hz) and one high (2000 Hz) frequency initially and select additional frequencies to test depending on initial responses.
9. Reduce thresholds in 10-dB steps and increase in 5- to 10-dB steps to bracket threshold. Record a response after three reversals.
10. Take breaks as needed to calm the infant and increase usable test time.
11. If soundfield testing indicates a hearing loss, test bone conduction.
12. If infant is still responding, or at the next test session, test with insert earphones.
13. Test with technology as needed.

child alert to the environment? A baby may indicate visual and tactile awareness by making postural changes and meaningful eye-gaze to people and environmental events. In a visually alert baby, lack of response to sound is strongly suggestive of a true hearing loss. However, if the infant is not alert to visual or tactile stimuli, an inability to respond to auditory stimuli may not be an indication of hearing loss.

Adding Objectivity to Behavioral Observation Audiometry

The Test Setting

Infant State and Positioning

Monitor the infant's state to increase the likelihood that it will be possible to observe responses accurately. "State" refers to the infant's level of arousal, from deep sleep to hysterical crying (**Fig. 7.3**).

Movement of Test Assistant and Parent/Caregiver

Everyone in the test room with the child must:

- Be still and nonresponsive to the test stimuli
- Keep the infant focused at midline
- Be reminded not to respond to the stimulus by altering the movement of the toy or facial expressions

Test Stimuli and Response

The most critical element in obtaining reliable responses is to predetermine what will constitute a response (Flexer & Gans, 1986; Madell, 1998, 2008; Widen, 1993). If it has been decided that sucking is the acceptable response, the audiologist should not then also accept eye widening or a head turn as a response. Changing response criteria during testing runs the risk of accepting behaviors as responses

that are not actually responses. The response must be time-locked to the presentation of the stimulus. All of the infant's responses must be repeatable. The use of multiple observers to determine whether a response is present also will increase reliability, as will the use of silent controls (Gravel & McCaughey, 2004; Madell, 2008).

Comparison of Behavioral Observation Audiometry Thresholds to VRA, CPA, and ABR

By carefully following the sucking test protocols detailed in this chapter and observed on the accompanying DVD, observation responses can be used to obtain reliable thresholds. **Figs. 7.4a-d** are typical of many multiple audiograms that demonstrate that thresholds can be obtained accurately by using BOA. These audiograms make the best possible case for the reliability of the BOA sucking technique by comparing thresholds obtained with BOA, VRA, and play audiometry over several years on four children. Results of clinical work with many children, and by many clinicians, over many years indicates that BOA, appropriately conducted, using the sucking paradigm discussed in this chapter and demonstrated on the accompanying DVD, can more accurately identify hearing levels in infants than ABR thresholds can.

Developing Comfort Using Behavioral Observation Audiometry

Clinicians who are comfortable using ABR to assess infants may want to add BOA to their protocol to gain experience with the technique before making behavioral testing a regular part of clinical practice. As with most other skills, it takes experience to become a competent tester when using the BOA sucking paradigm detailed in this chapter. It is important to be certain that the test situation is appropriately organized so as to maximize the ability to observe changes in sucking. The clinicians should have good communication with each other to enable them to share information during testing. All infant responses should be repeatable. Viewing the DVD that accompanies this book will be helpful in developing the necessary BOA skills.

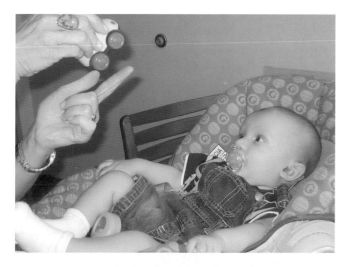

Fig.7.3   Position of infant for observation audiometry.

Discussion Topics

1. Discuss why behavioral observation audiometry has not been considered a good clinical tool in the past.
2. Discuss why sucking is a more reliable threshold response when testing infants.
3. Discuss ways to maximize objectivity in BOA.

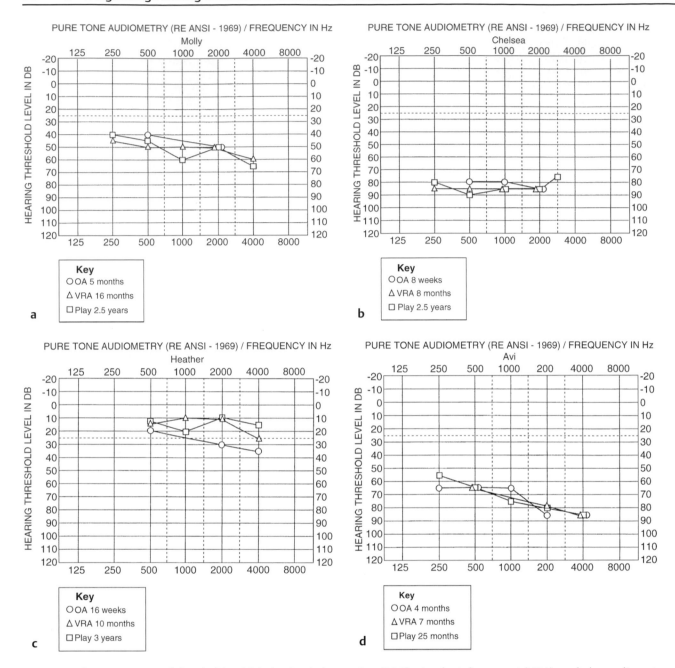

Fig. 7.4a–d   Comparison of thresholds with behavioral observation (BOA), visual reinforcement (VRA), and play audiometry.

References

American Academy of Audiology. (2012) Guidelines for the assessment of hearing in infants and young children. Retrieved from http://www.audiology.org/resources/documentlibrary/Pages/PediatricDiagnostics.aspx

American Speech-Language-Hearing Association. (2004). Guidelines for the Audiologic Assessment of Children from Birth to 5 Years of Age. Retrieved from http://www.asha.org/members/deskref-journals/deskref/default

Apuzzo, M. L., & Yoshinaga-Itana, C. (1995). Early identification of infants with significant hearing loss and the Min-

nesota Child Development Inventory. Seminars in Hearing, 16, 124–139.

Berg, K. M., & Smith, M. C. (1983). Behavioral thresholds for tones during infancy. Journal of Experimental Child Psychology, 35(3), 409–425.

Bess, F. H., & Humes, L. E. (2003). Audiology: the fundamentals (3rd ed.). Philadelphia, PA: Lippincott Williams & Wilkins.

Bove, C., & Flugrath, J. M. (1973). Frequency components of noisemakers for use in pediatric audiological evaluations. The Volta Review, 75, 551–556.

Delaroche, M., Thiebaut, R., & Dauman, R. (2004). Behavioral audiometry: protocols for measuring hearing thresholds in babies aged 4–18 months. International Journal of Pediatric Otorhinolaryngology, 68(10), 1233–1243.

Detteman, S. J., Pinder, D., Briggs, R. J., Dowell, R.C., & Leigh, J.R. (2007). Communication development in children who receive the cochlear implant younger than twelve months: risks vs benefits. Ear Hear, Apr 28 (2 Suppl), 11S-18S.

Downs, M. P., & Sterritt, G. M. (1964). Identification audiometry for neonates: a preliminary report. The Journal of Auditory Research, 4, 69–80.

Downs, M. P., & Sterritt, G. M. (1967). A guide to newborn and infant hearing screening programs. Archives of Otolaryngology, 85(1), 15–22.

Eisele, W. A., Berry, R. C., & Shriner, T. H. (1975). Infant sucking response patterns as a conjugate function of change in the sound pressure level of auditory stimuli. Journal of Speech and Hearing Research, 18, 296–307.

Eisenberg, R. B. (1969). Auditory behavior in the human neonate: functional properties of sound and their ontogenetic implications. International Audiology, 8, 34–45.

Ewing, J. R., & Ewing, A. W. G. (1940). Discussion on audiometric tests and the capacity to hear speech. The Journal of Laryngology and Otology, 55, 339–355.

Ewing, J. R., & Ewing, A. W. G. (1944). The ascertainment of deafness in infancy and early childhood. The Journal of Laryngology and Otology, 54, 309–333.

Flasher, L. V., & Fogel, P. T. (2004). Counseling skills for speech-language pathologists and audiologists. Clifton Park, NY: Delmar Learning.

Flexer, C., & Gans, D. P. (1986). Distribution of auditory response behaviors in normal infants and profoundly multihandicapped children. Journal of Speech and Hearing Research, 29(3), 425 429.

Frisina, R. (1963). Measurement of hearing in children. In J. F. Jerger (Ed.), Modern developments in audiology. New York, NY: Academic.

Froeschels, E., & Beebe, H. (1946). Testing the hearing of newborn infants. Archives of Otolaryngology, 44(6), 710–714.

Gerber, S. E. (1977). Audiometry in infancy. New York, NY: Grune and Stratton.

Gravel, J. (2000) Audiologic assessment for the fitting of hearing instruments: big challenges from tiny ears. In R. Seewald (Ed.), A sound foundation through early amplification. Proceedings of an international conference (pp. 33–46). Nashville, TN: Vanderbilt–Bill Wilkerson Press, Phonak, AG, 2000.

Gravel, J. S., & McCaughey, C. C. (2004). Family-centered audiologic assessment for infants and young children with hearing loss. Seminars in Hearing, 25, 309–317.

Hicks, C. B., Tharpe, A. M., & Ashmead, D. H. (2000). Behavioral auditory assessment of young infants: methodological limitations or natural lack of auditory responsiveness? American Journal of Audiology, 9(2), 124–130.

Jerger, J. F., & Hayes, D. (1976). The cross-check principle in pediatric audiometry. Archives of Otolaryngology, 102(10), 614–620.

Ling, D. (2002). Speech and the hearing impaired child (2nd ed.). Washington, DC: Alexander Graham Bell Association of the Deaf and Hard of Hearing.

Madell, J. R. (1988). Identification and treatment of very young children with hearing loss. Infants and Young Children, 1, 20–30.

Madell, J. R. (1995a). Behavioral evaluation of infants after hearing screening: Can it be done? Hearing Instruments, 12, 4–8.

Madell, J. R. (1995b). Speech audiometry for children. In S. E. Gerber (Ed.), Pediatric audiology (pp. 84–103). Washington, DC: Gallaudet University Press.

Madell, J. R. (1998). Behavioral evaluation of hearing in infants and young children. New York, NY: Thieme.

Madell, J. R. (2008). Using behavioral observation audiometry to evaluate hearing in infants from birth to 6 months. In J. R. Madell & C. Flexer (Eds.), Pediatric audiology: diagnosis, technology, and management (pp. 54–64). New York, NY: Thieme.

McConnell, F., & Ward, P. (1967). Deafness in childhood. Nashville, TN: Vanderbilt University Press.

Mencher, G. T., McCulloch, B., Derbyshire, A. J., & Dethlefs, R. (1977). Observer bias as a factor in neonatal hearing screening. Journal of Speech and Hearing Research, 20(1), 27–34.

Muir, D. W., Clifton, R. K., & Clarkson, M. G. (1989). The development of a human auditory localization response: a U-shaped function. Canadian Journal of Psychology, 43(2), 199–216.

Northern, J., & Downs, M. (1974). Hearing in children. Baltimore, MD: Williams and Wilkins.

Northern, J., & Downs, M. (1991). Hearing in children (4th ed.), Baltimore, MD: Williams and Wilkins.

Northern, J. L., & Downs, M. P. (2002). Hearing in children (5th ed.). Baltimore, MD: Lippincott Williams & Wilkins.

Nozza, R. (2006). Developmental psychoacoustics: auditory function in infants and children. Paper presented at the 4th Widex Congress of Paediatric Audiology, Ottawa, Canada, May 19–21, 2006.

Olsho, L. W. (1984). Infant frequency discrimination. Infant Behavior and Development, 7, 27–35.

Olsho, L. W., Koch, E. G., Halpin, C. F., & Carter, E. A. (1987a). An observer-based psychoacoustic procedure for use with young infants. Developmental Psychology, 23, 627–640.

Olsho, L. W., Koch, E. G., & Halpin, C. F. (1987b, Aug). Level and age effects in infant frequency discrimination. The Journal of the Acoustical Society of America, 82(2), 454–464.

Olsho, L. W., Koch, E. G., Carter, E. A., Halpin, C. F., & Spetner, N. B. (1988). Pure-tone sensitivity of human infants. The Journal of the Acoustical Society of America, 84(4), 1316–1324.

Poblano, A., Chayo, I., Ibarra, J., & Rueda, E. (2000). Electrophysiological and behavioral methods in early detection of hearing impairment. Archives of Medical Research, 31(1), 75–80.

Sharma, A., Dorman, M. F., & Spahr, A. J. (2002). A sensitive period for the development of the central auditory system in children with cochlear implants: implications for age of implantation. Ear and Hearing, 23(6), 532–539.

Sharma, A., Nash, A. A., & Dorman, M. (2009). Cortical development, plasticity and re-organization in children with cochlear implants. Journal of Communication Disorders, 42(4), 272–279.

Sininger, Y. S. (1993). Evaluation of hearing in the neonate using the auditory brainstem response. In Consensus development conference on early identification of hearing impairment in infants and young children (pp. 95–97). Bethesda, MD: National Institutes of Health.

Thompson, M., & Thompson, G. (1972). Response of infants and young children as a function of auditory stimuli and test methods. Journal of Speech and Hearing Research, 15(4), 699–707.

Weber, B. A. (1969). Validation of observer judgments in behavioral observation audiometry. Journal of Speech and Hearing Research, 34(4), 350–355.

Wedenberg, E. (1956). Auditory tests on newborn infants. Acta Oto-Laryngologica, 46(5), 446–461.

Werner, L., & Gillenwater, J. (1990). Pure tone sensitivity of 2–5 week old infants. Infant Behavior and Development, 13, 355–375.

Werner, L. (2011) Behavioral audiometry with infants. In R. Seewald & A. M. Tharpe (Eds.), Comprehensive handbook of pediatric audiology. San Diego, CA: Plural.

Widen, J. E. (1993). Adding objectivity to infant behavioral audiometry. Ear and Hearing, 14(1), 49–57.

Widen, J. E., & Keener, S. K. (2003). Diagnostic testing for hearing loss in infants and young children. Mental Retardation and Developmental Disabilities Research Reviews, 9(4), 220–224.

Yoshinaga-Itano, C., Coulter, D., & Thomson, V. (2001). Developmental outcomes of children with hearing loss born in Colorado hospitals with and without universal newborn hearing screening programs. Seminars in Neonatology, 6(6), 521–529.

Chapter 8

Using Visual Reinforcement Audiometry to Evaluate Hearing in Infants from 5 to 36 Months

Jane R. Madell

Key Points

- Once infants reach 5 to 6 months of age, most can be conditioned to make a head turn response to the presence of an auditory stimulus.

- Positioning is critical. The infant should be seated to maximize torso control. If the child is having a problem sitting upright and balancing, it will be difficult to make a head turn.

- Reinforcement should be provided only when it is certain that the child is responding to the stimulus. Turning on the reinforcing toy when the child has not heard the sound will decrease the reliability of conditioning.

- Visual reinforcement audiometry (VRA) can be used to test children using earphones, the bone conduction transducer, hearing aids, cochlear implants, and FM systems.

Behavioral methods are the first choice for diagnostic testing of auditory function because they provide the most information about an infant's ability to use hearing. Once infants reach 5 to 6 months of age, behavioral testing becomes much easier to accomplish because infants can be conditioned to respond to sound (American Speech-Language-Hearing Association [ASHA], 2004; American Academy of Audiology [AAA], 2012). The most common test techniques involve training the infant to make a conditioned head turn in response to a test stimulus. Infants only a few months of age will naturally turn toward a sound source. Most infants will turn toward the sound source a few times, but the head-turning behavior will habituate to repeated stimuli. Fortunately, this head-turning behavior can be shaped using an operant discrimination procedure that permits obtaining numerous responses to auditory stimuli. The sound stimulus is used to cue the child to seek the visual reinforcement. Use of a positive reinforcement, such as a lighted toy or short video clip, will increase the number of responses before the responses are extinguished. Conditioned responses have the advantage of being more repeatable than unconditioned responses, and more responses usually can be obtained during one sitting.

Several visual conditioning techniques have been used. VRA (Lidén & Kankkunen, 1969) and conditioned orienting response (COR) (Suzuki & Ogiba, 1960) are the most commonly used protocols. VRA uses a conditioned head turn reinforced by a lighted toy. COR requires that the infant localize the sound source before reinforcement with a lighted toy, and reinforcement is provided only if the child turns toward the correct side.

◆ Test Protocols

Visual Reinforcement Audiometry

VRA is the most commonly used reinforcement procedure. It is used to evaluate hearing in children who are cognitively between 5–6 and 36 months of age. Operant conditioning is a process by which the frequency of occurrence of a behavior (in this case, a conditioned head turn) is modified by what happens when the behavior occurs. VRA uses a conditioned head-turning response that is shaped by the examiner's control of a stimulus–reinforcement paradigm. The foundation for VRA was laid by Suzuki and Ogiba (1960), and the term itself was first used by Lidén and Kankkunen (1969). The technique was refined by Wilson and Thompson (1984), by Wilson, Moore, and Thompson (1976) and Moore, Wilson, and

Thompson (1977), and in numerous other publications between 1977 and 1984. The audiologist presents a stimulus. If the child detects the stimulus, she will turn toward it. The audiologist then activates a reinforcer. After a few repetitions, the child learns to seek the reinforcer when she hears the sound (Primus & Thompson, 1985; Primus, 1987).

Conditioning Orienting Response Audiometry

COR testing, originally described by Suzuki and Ogiba (1960), uses the same conditioning techniques as VRA. Sound may be presented from either the right or left loudspeaker, but the child will be reinforced only when turning to the correct side. Standard hearing testing requires only the ability to identify whether a sound is present. It does not require that the listener identify where the sound is coming from. Young babies may have a difficult time determining which way to turn, but older babies and children will be able to perform the task. The ability to localize a sound close to threshold can be difficult for anybody.

◆ Visual Reinforcers

A variety of toys are available for use as reinforcers. Moore, Thompson, and Thompson (1975) investigated use of different reinforcers and their effect on responses. They compared no reinforcement, social reinforcement, blinking lights, and complex visual reinforcement and concluded that the complex reinforcement resulted in significantly more localizations than simple reinforcers did. The best reinforcers are novel and interesting. Mechanical toys that are brightly illuminated, such as clowns that play drums, dogs that bark, or elephants that eat ice cream cones, are excellent.

The reinforcer should be enclosed in a translucent plastic box so that it is not easily observable until it is turned on. Stacking two or three toys on top of each other in individual plastic boxes permits the audiologist to vary the reinforcer and increase the novelty, thereby increasing the length of time a child will attend to the task (**Fig. 8.1**). Most VRA systems permit turning on the sound and lights separately or together. This on-off switch is particularly useful when a child is frightened by the noise made by the reinforcing toy. Occasionally, children react negatively to the reinforcers. Some children are frightened by the sound or the movement. If the sound is the problem, it can be turned off and the lights can be used alone. If the movement is a problem, the toy can be held still and a light can be flashed on and off as a reinforcer. If the child is disturbed by the toys regardless of whether or not they are making noise, there are two alternatives. One is to use video clips as the re-

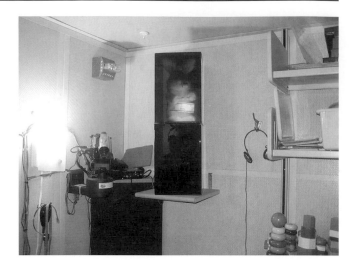

Fig. 8.1   VRA toys.

inforcer using a small TV and a DVD player, and the second is to darken the test room and shine a flashlight through the test room window as a reinforcer. The light can either flash on and off or can be waved around in circles. A head turn toward the tester's window will be used to determine a response. (If this protocol is going to be used, the test room will usually need to be reorganized so that the child is seated facing away from the test room window.)

For older children, or children who are no longer interested in the VRA toys, a cartoon video works particularly well as a reinforcer (**Fig. 8.2**). The TV sound should be off so as not to interfere with test stimuli. Because the video is constantly changing, it will be of ongoing interest. A small TV monitor can be placed above the loudspeaker with the DVD player on the tester's side of the booth. The audiologist can activate the video in the same way as a mechanical toy.

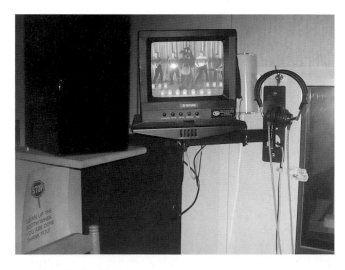

Fig. 8.2   Video VRA.

◆ Positioning the Infant or Child

A critical factor for obtaining reliable VRA thresholds is the ability to keep the infant's or child's attention focused at midline in a position that easily permits a head turn. Proper positioning is critical. The child needs to be seated comfortably so that the upper body is steady and allows the infant or child to turn easily to look at the toy. The child should not be leaning over trying to get something from the floor, trying to maintain balance, or looking for something or someone seated behind. Older children with very good body control may be able to make a head turn of 180 degrees to look for the reinforcer, but a young or neurologically impaired child will not. For these children, a head turn of more than 90 degrees is very difficult and may significantly reduce their ability to respond, and so it is critical that the children be carefully focused at midline (**Fig. 8.3**).

An infant who does not yet have good upper body control because of young age or neurologic or developmental concerns, and does not sit comfortably, will have difficulty making a head-turning response. Positioning for these children will be especially critical. A child without good upper body control should be seated leaning back in a reclining seat or leaning against a parent so that she does not need to struggle to maintain position. This position will leave the infant with enough energy to make a head turn toward the reinforcer.

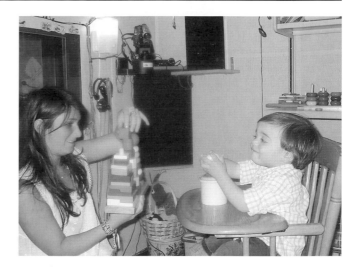

Fig. 8.3   Positioning for VRA.

quently very useful, provided they are not too noisy. (Crunchy food will interfere with listening, and food that takes too long to swallow can significantly extend test time and interfere with the flow of testing.)

Pearl

- Positioning is critical. The infant needs to be seated so that she can easily make a conditioned head turn. If the child does not sit up easily, she should be positioned in a reclining position, leaning back against someone or in a reclining chair, so she does not need energy to control her torso.

◆ The Test Assistant

Accurate VRA depends on the ability of the examiner or test assistant to keep the child attentive. An audiologist, test assistant, or parent needs to be responsible for keeping the infant facing forward. The test room should not be cluttered. Toys that are not being used should be out of view so that the infant will not be distracted by anything except the adult who is keeping the child focused. (See Chapter 14 for more information about the test assistant's responsibilities.)

The test assistant may be an audiologist, an audiology student, or an audiology assistant. An experienced test assistant will make testing most efficient. When a test assistant is not available, parents or caregivers can often be very good at this task. With limited instruction they can frequently do this job very well, especially with typically developing children. They know their children well and know how to entertain them. If a parent is going to have the responsibility of distracting the child, she needs to be told to be relatively quiet so as not to interfere with presentation of test stimuli. Even more critical, she must understand that she must not react to the sound in any way that might cue the child. Instructions for the parent or the test assistant should include the following:

- Don't respond to the sound.
- Don't look at the reinforcement toy until after the child does.

◆ Distractors

A variety of toys can be useful as distractors. They should be quiet, simple, and interesting but not engrossing. Colorful toys, puppets, finger games, stacking toys, toys with pieces that connect, magnets on a magnet board or on the test room wall, or the test assistant making funny faces will keep the infant focused straight ahead so that a clear head turn can be observed. Young children should view the toys being manipulated by the test assistant but should not manipulate them, since this will likely be too distracting. Older children may be able to manipulate some toys as long as they are not too interesting or require too much concentration. Edible distractions are fre-

- Don't change your body language when the sound is presented.
- Don't alter the way you are playing with the toys when the sound is presented.
- Act "deaf" to the sound.

◆ Training and Conditioning the Response

The operant conditioning paradigm begins with a discriminative stimulus; the subject then makes a response and receives reinforcement. In VRA, the stimulus will be tones, noise bands, or speech stimuli. The infant's response will be a head turn, and the reinforcer will be either a moving toy or a video and may include cheering from the test assistant. The VRA procedure involves two distinct phases. The first is the training/conditioning phase, where the baby or toddler is conditioned to respond to the visual reinforcer. The second is the testing phase, during which thresholds are obtained once the baby is conditioned.

Operant behavior is willful behavior elicited by a stimulus and controlled by the behavior that is increased or decreased by changes in the environment (Diefendorf & Gravel, 1996; Gravel, 2000; Widen, 2011). In VRA or COR, the head-turning response is increased by the positive reinforcement of the reinforcing toy. There are two approaches to training the response. The first approach is to pair the stimulus with the reinforcer, turning both on at the same time. The child will frequently turn to the reinforcing toy and learn the task. If the child looks up but does not turn, the audiologist can attract the child's attention to the reinforcer. The second approach is to begin by observing the child's response and then providing a reinforcer when the child naturally turns to the sound. During the training/conditioning phase, the stimulus should always be presented at an intensity that the audiologist is sure the child can hear, and every correct head turn should be reinforced. If the reinforcer is activated when there is no stimulus or when the child cannot hear the stimulus, the infant will not be able to make the association between the sound and the reinforcer and will only be confused. If there is any question at all about whether or not the child heard the stimulus, the reinforcer should not be activated. Training/conditioning is considered complete when the infant consistently turns when a stimulus is presented and when there are very few random head turns.

The stimulus used for conditioning can be the same stimuli used for testing: noise bands, warble tones, or speech stimuli. Research by Thompson and Folsom (1984) and others has demonstrated that the particular stimulus used for training will not affect test results.

◆ Testing

Once the infant or child is conditioned to the visual reinforcer, the testing phase can begin.

Test Room Setup

It is usually best to begin testing in soundfield. Inserting earphones may be stressful to the child and reduce cooperation. Beginning testing in soundfield will provide basic information about hearing, and once that is obtained, testing can proceed with insert earphones or with the bone vibrator. By then the child will be more comfortable in the test situation and may be more willing to accept insert earphones.

To perform soundfield testing, the test room needs to be large enough to be able to have loudspeakers set up at a sufficient angle and distance from the infant to permit an obvious head turn. If the room is too small, the loudspeakers and reinforcing toy may be within the child's line of sight, making it difficult to see a change in head position. Since the response we are seeking is a conditioned head turn, the child should be seated at no less than a 45-degree angle from the loudspeakers and reinforcer, and preferably at 90 degrees (**Fig. 8.3**, **Fig. 8.4**). The reinforcing toy should not be in the child's line of sight when she is facing forward. The test setup needs to be such that there is no doubt whether the infant made a head turn, rather than a casual gaze toward the toy. When performing VRA, the sound is usually presented from one loudspeaker, and the reinforcing toys are on the same side of the test room as the loudspeaker. No matter whether the child hears the sound in the right or left ear, she will turn toward the same toy.

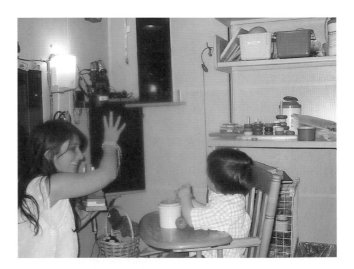

Fig. 8.4   Turning toward reinforcer.

Positioning

Ideally the child should be seated in a highchair and not on a parent's lap. If the child is on someone's lap, the adult may respond to the sound and inadvertently give a cue to the child. If the child must sit on an adult's lap because she will not sit alone or does not have sufficient torso control to sit alone, the adult needs to be instructed not to respond in any way to the presentation of the sound stimulus. Noise-canceling earphones can be used to keep the adult from responding to the sound stimulus. However, the use of earphones may make it very difficult for the adult to interact with the infant, which may make both the infant and the adult uncomfortable. Most parents are capable of sitting still and not responding when the reason is made clear to them. In addition, parents usually prefer to hear what their child is hearing so that they can better understand the test results.

Beginning Testing

If a child has anything less than severe or profound hearing loss, it should be relatively easy to get an initial response. The child should be seated in the high chair or on a parent's lap and facing forward. The room does not need to be silent, but it should be relatively quiet. The audiologist begins by presenting stimuli at a level at which the child is expected to respond. If the child hears the sound, she will likely look up from the toy and search for the sound source. If there is no response, the audiologist increases the intensity until there is a response. Once a response is obtained, the reinforcer is turned on. If the infant looks up but does not turn to the reinforcer, the test assistant should attract the child's attention to the reinforcer. When this has been done a few times, the infant will usually have learned the task and testing can begin. Before attracting the child's attention to the reinforcer, it is *essential* that the audiologist be absolutely certain that the child heard the sound. **Fig. 8.4** shows a child making a conditioned head turn to the VRA toy. Control trials, in which no sound is presented, should be included during training to be certain that responses are truly being obtained to the test stimuli and are not random.

Conditioning Children with Very Profound Hearing Loss

Children with severe to profound hearing loss, or with auditory attention or auditory processing problems, may not have the ability to localize to sound. For these children in particular, it will be necessary to pair the stimulus with the sound and teach the child to seek the reinforcer. If the child does not re-

spond to even very loud sounds, it may be useful to train the child to respond to a low-frequency tactile stimulus, since even a child with no usable hearing will be able to feel the bone vibrator. Place a bone vibrator in the child's hand or on the knee and have the test assistant or parent hold it in place. The sound or vibration is then paired with the reinforcer and the child is conditioned to that stimulus. After the child responds consistently to a tactile stimulus, return to an air-conducted stimulus in soundfield or under earphones and try again. Sometimes pairing the tactile stimulus with an auditory stimulus will assist in training the response. If the reason for lack of response is severity of hearing loss, it is essential that the infant accept earphones, because earphone signals can almost always be presented at a louder intensity than those from loudspeakers (**Fig. 8.5**).

The intensity of the initial test stimuli is important. Ideally the stimulus should be presented slightly above threshold but not too much above threshold. Several researchers (Eilers, Miskiel, Ozdamar, Urbano, & Widen, 1991; Gravel, 2000; Tharpe & Ashmead, 1993) have demonstrated that the starting level influences false responses: the louder the starting intensity, the greater the false response rate. Wilson and Moore (1978) and Wilson, Moore, and Thompson (1976) demonstrated that once a child is conditioned for VRA, responses do not vary as a function of age. Data from 6- to 7-month-olds and 11- to 13-month-olds indicated that thresholds did not vary by age.

Frequency of Reinforcing the Response

The tendency of most testers is to reinforce every response the child makes in the effort to be sure to condition the response. The anxiety to be sure to re-

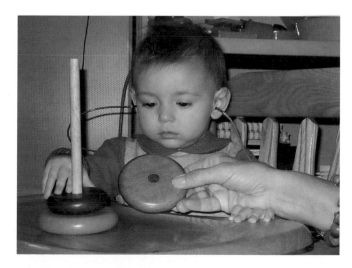

Fig. 8.5   Infant with insert earphones.

inforce every appropriate response can occasionally result in the audiologist's providing reinforcement when, in fact, the infant has not really provided a head turn and may not have heard the stimulus. This will confuse the child and reduce response reliability. In addition, frequent reinforcement will cause more rapid habituation of the response. Research on behavioral conditioning has demonstrated that intermittent reinforcement is more reliable than constant reinforcement and provides more responses. The best reinforcement schedule begins with 100% reinforcement and decreases to less frequent reinforcement. Occasionally failing to reinforce the response will increase the total number of responses the infant is likely to provide in any individual test session. If there is any question about whether or not the child heard the stimulus, the reinforcer should not be activated. The rule is "If in doubt, don't." Nothing is lost by failing to reinforce when a stimulus is present, but a great deal may be lost by reinforcing when the infant does not hear a stimulus.

Pitfall

- If in doubt—don't. It is critical that the reinforcer be turned on only when the child has made an appropriate head turn. If the reinforcer is turned on when the child has not heard a sound, the child becomes confused and response reliability is decreased.

Test Stimuli

Any test stimulus used in behavioral testing can be used with VRA or COR. Speech stimuli are frequently used as the initial test stimulus with children because they are familiar and are likely to get their attention. Any speech stimulus can be used to obtain a speech awareness threshold. To obtain frequency-specific speech information, it will be necessary to use low-, mid-high-, and high-frequency stimuli (such as *ba*, *sh*, and *s*, respectively), which will be in agreement with pure tone thresholds at low, mid-high, and high frequencies. Using a broadband stimulus, such as music or running speech (e.g., "Hello Jody, how are you today?"), will provide a threshold that is in agreement with the softest pure tone threshold. (See Chapter 11 for more information about speech audiometry with children.)

To obtain a complete audiogram, thresholds are needed at several if not all frequencies. Although pure tones are usually the stimulus of choice, other stimuli are also very useful and may be helpful in obtaining a complete audiogram. Narrowband noise may be more interesting to infants and young chil-

dren and may hold their attention longer than pure tones. Alternating between pure tones, warble tones, and narrow noise bands may also increase interest and the number of repeatable responses. Narrowband noise stimuli are easier for young infants to respond to than warble tone or pure tone stimuli (Gravel, 2000). Noise band thresholds may be 5 to 10 dB softer than those obtained with pure tones; this needs to be taken into consideration when evaluating the responses. For soundfield testing, noise bands or warbled pure tones are the stimuli of choice.

Test Conditions

Visual reinforcement audiometry can be reliably used in all test conditions required for the evaluation of hearing in infants and young children. Testing can be accomplished in soundfield, with insert earphones, with circumaural earphones, with a bone vibrator, and with technology (hearing aids, cochlear implants, or FM systems). These conditions will permit us to obtain almost all required audiologic information.

Test Order

Some audiologists begin every evaluation with immittance testing. Although there is no doubt about the usefulness of this procedure, it is important to take the child into consideration when selecting tests and test order. An infant who is frightened of the test facility or the tester may be very distressed by having a stranger come up to him to place an immittance probe in the ear at the beginning of the evaluation. If you proceed to do the test and the child becomes very distressed, the rest of the testing may be difficult or impossible to accomplish. If the child seems distressed or even wary, it may be better to wait until the end of the session for immittance testing.

The same can be said for the decision to begin testing using earphones or in soundfield. Day, Bamford, Parry, Shepherd, and Quigley (2000) tested typically developing infants both in soundfield and with insert earphones and demonstrated that significantly more responses were obtained for soundfield testing than for insert earphone testing. No doubt earphone testing is the goal, but it may be better to get some information in soundfield before presenting earphones. When testing very young children, it is useful to assume that each response may be the last one obtained. Therefore, it is very important to think carefully about the order of testing. If earphones are tried first and the child becomes upset and gives only one reliable response, very little information is obtained. However, if the child is kept happy by starting in soundfield and thresholds are obtained at 500 and 2000 Hz, something is known about her hearing even if testing has to stop at that point.

Frequency-Specific Stimuli

Using the theory that each threshold obtained may be the last requires good planning when testing children. After beginning at 500 Hz or 2000 Hz, depending on whether there is concern about conductive hearing loss (CHL) or sensorineural hearing loss (SNHL), a decision must be made about how to proceed. If the concern is for CHL, begin testing at 2000 Hz in each ear and then go to 500 Hz, because for most patients with CHL, hearing will be better at high frequencies, facilitating conditioning. If the concern is that the infant or child may have SNHL, begin at 500 Hz, then proceed directly to 2000 Hz, because for most patients with SNHL, hearing is better in the low frequencies. Depending on the contour of the partial audiogram and the cooperativeness of the child, decide whether it would be better to proceed with 4000 Hz, 1000 Hz, 250 Hz, bone conduction, or earphones. If there is a significant difference between the thresholds at 500 and 2000 Hz, it will be critical to test 1000 Hz before proceeding to other frequencies to obtain a good picture of the audiometric contour. If the audiogram is fairly flat, the 1000 Hz threshold may be left to last and can frequently be estimated from the rest of the thresholds if time is limited or the child stops cooperating. If sound-field testing indicates hearing loss, bone conduction testing might be selected as the next test procedure to determine whether hearing loss is conductive or sensorineural. If it is not possible to obtain bone conduction thresholds, either because the child can no longer attend or because it is not possible to get the child to accept the bone oscillator, immittance may provide sufficient information to begin a plan of treatment. If the child is still cooperative, earphone testing should be attempted. No child should be dismissed from audiologic follow-up until earphone testing has been accomplished (**Table 8.1**).

Enticing a Child to Wear Earphones

Enticing a young child to wear earphones can be a little tricky but is usually possible. Start by having the test assistant wear the earphones, then the parents, and then offer them to the child. If the child refuses at first, let everyone have another turn, and then offer the earphones to the child once more. If she still refuses, it is important to make a judgment about how serious the refusal is. If the protest is minimal, try pushing the matter. Someone needs to keep the child occupied with a toy while someone else puts the earphones on. Frequently, once the child hears a sound or music and can observe the reinforcer, the resistance will stop or at least be reduced to a low enough level to permit testing to proceed. If it doesn't, and the child starts to become very upset, it may be

Table 8.1 Protocol for visual reinforcement audiometry

1. Seat child in high chair, in a child's chair, or on a parent's lap.

2. The test assistant or parent keeps child's attention focused to the front using quiet toys.

3. The auditory stimulus is presented at a comfortably loud level above expected threshold. The conditioning/reinforcing toy is turned on, and if the child does not turn, the test assistant calls attention to the toy. The auditory stimulus and the conditioning toy are kept on together for 3–4 seconds.

4. Step 3 is repeated until the child consistently turns to the auditory stimulus.

5. When the child is conditioned to respond, the auditory stimulus is presented without turning on the conditioning/reinforcing toy. If the child turns toward the sound, the reinforcing toy is turned on and conditioning is complete.

6. Testing proceeds obtaining thresholds for one low- (500 Hz) and one high- (2000 Hz) frequency stimulus. The stimulus intensity is decreased until the child stops responding, and is then increased to bracket threshold. Three responses at the same intensity are sufficient.

7. Additional frequencies to be tested will be determined by the responses to the initial frequencies tested.

8. Testing proceeds using insert earphones, bone vibrator, and technology (hearing aids, cochlear implants, and FM systems).

9. The reinforcing toy is turned on only when the child makes a conditioned head turn in response to a sound. When in doubt, do not turn on the reinforcer.

better to hold off and try again at a later date, or try different earphones (inserts versus circumaural), or try a handheld circumaural earphone at the child's ear. Circumaural earphones are easy to put on and can frequently be put in place in a couple of seconds. However, they can be heavy for a little head, making it difficult for the baby or toddler to turn toward the reinforcer, and they can fall off with movement. In addition, positioning of the headphones is critical for obtaining accurate thresholds, especially in high frequencies. Insert earphones are more comfortable to wear because they are very lightweight and, because they are always well positioned, may provide more accurate thresholds, but they take more effort to insert. If after really trying, the child will not accept earphones, ask the parents to try to persuade the child to accept earphones at home. It is sometimes easy to persuade a child to accept earphones by having the parents plug earphones into the TV at home, and not allowing the child to watch videos or TV without wearing the earphones. In a few days the child will be wearing them consistently at home, and once he wears them at home there should be no problem persuading him to wear them in the clinic.

If testing can be performed using a combination of loudspeakers, earphones, and bone conduction transducers, consider testing different frequencies with each transducer. The combination of information can provide a fairly complete picture of the child's hearing (**Fig. 8.6**).

Stimuli Presentation

When testing children, audiologists frequently feel the need to obtain many responses at one intensity before recording thresholds. This is understandable, but it may significantly reduce the total number of thresholds obtained. Infants and young children will respond for only a limited time. Each presentation needs to be carefully considered. Eilers et al (1991) and Gravel (2000) used computer simulation to test infants and determined that more than three reversals were not useful in obtaining thresholds. There was less than a 3-dB difference when more than three reversals were obtained. So, bite the bullet and trust the responses that are observed.

A mistake that is frequently made when testing young children is related to timing of presentation of the stimulus. When testing infants, test time is limited, so there is a tendency to present stimuli too quickly. If a child is asked to make a conditioned head turn frequently, both the stimulus and the reinforcer will become uninteresting and the child will stop responding. Taking time and presenting stimuli after a longer period of silence will increase the likelihood that the stimulus is interesting, causing the child to look up. On the other hand, having a very extended "off" period can also have a negative effect. The correct timing will vary from child to child.

In the attempt to eliminate tester bias in recording responses, a computer-controlled test protocol was developed by Widen (1984, 1990, 2011). The technique uses only one examiner, who is in the test room with the child. When the examiner determines that the child is centered, a button is pushed, which calls for a trial. The examiner votes whether the child makes a head turn during the predetermined response interval. The software determines whether a sound is present during the interval. If a sound is present and the examiner records a response, the software provides the reinforcement. The signal level and type are determined by the software (**Fig. 8.7**).

What Is Normal Hearing?

There has been much discussion about what is considered normal hearing in infants. Early data (Primus, 1991) indicated that normally hearing infants did not respond to sound until it was at ~ 60 decibels hearing level (dB HL). Several other studies (Berg &

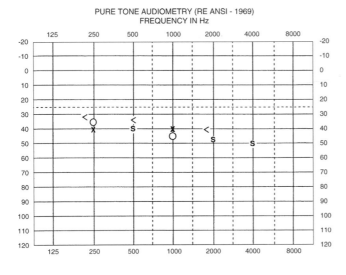

Key
X Left ear
O Right ear
S Soundfield
< Bone

Fig. 8.6 Audiogram with different information from different transducers.

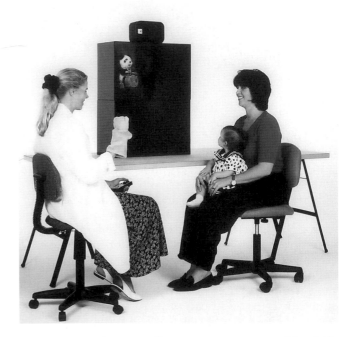

Fig. 8.7 IVRA (From Intelligent Hearing Systems, Miami, FL. Reprinted with permission.)

Smith, 1983; Diefendorf & Gravel, 1996; Gravel, 2000, Madell, 1995, 1998, 2008; Sinnott, Pisoni, & Aslin, 1983; Widen et al, 2000; Wilson et al, 1976; Wilson & Moore, 1978; Nozza & Wilson, 1984; Olsho, Koch, Carter, Halpin, & Spetner, 1988) demonstrated that infants with normal hearing respond to sound at only slightly higher than adult levels. Infant responses should be no more than 15 to 20 dB HL, and by 1 year of age, children should be responding at adult levels. Widen et al (2000) demonstrated that 94% of high-risk infants have essentially normal hearing sensitivity (20 dB HL) at 1000, 2000, and 4000 Hz in both ears.

The concept of minimal response level (MRL) is useful when evaluating children. The responses we obtain may not be threshold in the way we think of thresholds for adults, but they are repeatable and reliable and may be close to true threshold.

◆ Summary of Factors That Affect Test Results

Many factors affect the reliability of test results.

- Developmental age is critical. As mentioned before, it is essential to know the child's developmental age to select the appropriate test protocol.
- Neurologic status is also critical. The child must be capable of attending and of making the appropriate physical response (in this case, a conditioned head turn). If the child's neurologic status will not permit a head turn, the test will not be valid.
- Behavioral status is also important. If a child is very fussy or uncomfortable, it may not be possible to elicit the best results. It may be worth it to take the time to make the child comfortable (change diapers, provide food and comfort) before proceeding with the test.

- Positioning is very important. If the child is seated in such a way as to reduce upper body control, there is very little chance that he will be able to make reliable conditioned head turns. If the neurologic status is a concern, the range of the required head turn may be limited. Requiring a head turn of more than 90 degrees will likely not be successful with many children with neurologic concerns (see Chapter 10 for a discussion of evaluating children with special needs).
- Distractors must be interesting but not too engrossing.
- Reinforcers must be interesting and attractive.
- Parents and other adults in the test room must be careful not to be distracting and not to clue the infant as to the presence of an auditory stimulus.
- The test stimuli should be varied to keep the child's attention.
- Presentation timing of stimuli should be varied so as to be unpredictable.

For a new tester this sounds like a great deal to keep in mind, and initially it is. But with experience, controlling these factors becomes second nature. However, during any evaluation, even the most experienced testers should stop when test problems arise, review what they are doing, and try to think about what might be changed to improve test results. Behavioral testing is both a science and an art.

Discussion Topics

1. Describe the conditioning paradigm.
2. Discuss factors to consider in keeping a child's attention and increasing test time.
3. Discuss the reliability of VRA for obtaining audiometric thresholds.

References

American Academy of Audiology. (2012). Guidelines for the assessment of hearing in infants and young children. Retrieved from http://www.audiology.org/resources/documentlibrary/Pages/PediatricDiagnostics.aspx

American Speech-Language-Hearing Association. (2004). Guidelines for the audiologic assessment of children from birth to 5 years of age. Retrieved from http://www.asha.org/members/deskref-journals/deskref/default

Berg, K. M., & Smith, M. C. (1983). Behavioral thresholds for tones during infancy. Journal of Experimental Child Psychology, 35(3), 409–425.

Day, J., Bamford, J., Parry, G., Shepherd, M., & Quigley, A. (2000). Evidence on the efficacy of insert earphone and sound field VRA with young infants. British Journal of Audiology, 34(6), 329–334.

Diefendorf, A. O., & Gravel, J. S. (1996). Behavioral observation and visual reinforcement audiometry. In S. Gerber (Ed.), Pediatric audiology (pp. xxx–xxx). Washington, D.C.: Gallaudet University Press.

Eilers, R. E., Miskiel, E., Ozdamar, O., Urbano, R., & Widen, J. E. (1991). Optimization of automated hearing test algorithms: simulations using an infant response model. Ear and Hearing, 12(3), 191–198.

Gravel, J. S. (2000). Behavioral audiologic assessment for hearing aid fitting: big challenges from tiny ears. In R. Seewald (Ed.), A sound foundation through early amplification. Proceedings of an international conference (pp. 33–46). Nashville, TN: Vanderbilt–Bill Wilkerson Press; Phonak, AG.

Lidén, G., & Kankkunen, A. (1969). Visual reinforcement audiometry. Acta Oto-Laryngologica, 67(2), 281–292.

Madell, J. R. (1995). Behavioral evaluation of infants after hearing screening: Can it be done? Hearing Instruments, December, 4–8.

Madell, J. R. (1998). Behavioral evaluation of hearing in infants and young children. New York, NY: Thieme.

Madell, J. R. (2008) Using behavioural observation audiometry to evaluate hearing in infants from birth to 6 months. In J. R. Madell & C. Flexer (Eds.), Pediatric audiology: diagnosis, technology, and management (pp. 54–64). New York, NY: Thieme.

Moore, J. M., Thompson, G., & Thompson, M. (1975). Auditory localization of infants as a function of reinforcement conditions. The Journal of Speech and Hearing Disorders, 40(1), 29–34.

Moore, J. M., Wilson, W. R., & Thompson, G. (1977). Visual reinforcement of head-turn responses in infants under 12 months of age. The Journal of Speech and Hearing Disorders, 42(3), 328–334.

Nozza, R. J., & Wilson, W. R. (1984). Masked and unmasked pure-tone thresholds of infants and adults: development of auditory frequency selectivity and sensitivity. Journal of Speech and Hearing Research, 27(4), 613–622.

Olsho, L. W., Koch, E. G., Carter, E. A., Halpin, C. F., & Spetner, N. B. (1988). Pure-tone sensitivity of human infants. The Journal of the Acoustical Society of America, 84(4), 1316–1324.

Primus, M. A. (1987). Response and reinforcement in operant audiometry. The Journal of Speech and Hearing Disorders, 52(3), 294–299. PubMed

Primus, M. A. (1991). Repeated infant thresholds in operant and nonoperant audiometric procedures. Ear and Hearing, 12(2), 119–122.

Primus, M. A., & Thompson, G. (1985). Response strength of young children in operant audiometry. Journal of Speech and Hearing Research, 28(4), 539–547.

Sinnott, J. M., Pisoni, D. B., & Aslin, R. N. (1983). A comparison of pure tone auditory thresholds in human infants and adults. Infant Behavior and Development, 6, 3–17.

Suzuki, T., & Ogiba, Y. (1960). A technique of pure-tone audiometry for children under three years of age: conditioned orientation reflex (COR) audiometry. Revue de Laryngologie—Otologie—Rhinologie, 8, 33–45.

Thompson, G., & Folsom, R. C. (1984). A comparison of two conditioning procedures in the use of visual reinforcement audiometry (VRA). The Journal of Speech and Hearing Disorders, 49(3), 241–245.

Tharpe, A. M., & Ashmead, D. H. (1993). Computer simulation technique for assessing pediatric auditory test protocols. Journal of the American Academy of Audiology, 4(2), 80–90.

Widen, J. E. (1984). Application of visual reinforcement audiometry (VRA) to high risk infants. Paper presented to Audiology Update. Pediatric Audiology, Newport, RI.

Widen, J. E. (1990). Behavioral screening of high risk infants using visual reinforcement audiometry. Seminars in Hearing, 11, 342–356.

Widen, J. (2011). Behavioral audiometry with infants. In R. Seewald & A. M. Tharpe (Eds.), Comprehensive handbook of pediatric audiology (pp. 483–495). San Diego, CA: Plural.

Widen, J. E., Folsom, R. C., Cone-Wesson, B., Carty, L., Dunnell, J. J., Koebsell, K., . . . Norton, S. J. (2000). Identification of neonatal hearing impairment: hearing status at 8 to 12 months corrected age using a visual reinforcement audiometry protocol. Ear and Hearing, 21(5), 471–487.

Wilson, W. R., & Moore, J. M. (1978). Pure-tone earphone thresholds of infants utilizing visual reinforcement audiometry (VRA). Paper presented at American Speech and Hearing Association Convention, San Francisco, CA.

Wilson, W. R., Moore, J. M., & Thompson, G. (1976). Sound-field auditory thresholds of infants utilizing visual reinforcement audiometry (VRA). Paper presented at American Speech and Hearing Association Convention, Houston, TX, 1976.

Wilson, W. R., & Thompson, G. (1984). Behavioral audiometry. In J. Jerger (Ed.), Pediatric audiology (pp. 47–63). San Diego, CA: College Hill Press.

Chapter 9

Using Conditioned Play Audiometry to Test Hearing in Children Older Than 2½ Years

Jane R. Madell

Key Points

- Play audiometry can be successfully accomplished with children once they reach a cognitive age of ~ 30 months.
- By being creative, the pediatric audiologist can find tasks that keep the young child interested and sufficiently cooperative to obtain necessary testing information.
- The audiologist needs to own the responsibility for obtaining test results. If testing is not completed, the audiologist must take responsibility and say "On this day, I cannot test this child."

Play audiometry, or conditioned play audiometry (CPA), was first described by Hoversten, Lowell, Rushford, and Stoner (1956). Their technique provided valuable guidance for the audiologic evaluation of very young children. Audiologists have been following their protocol, with slight modifications, since that time.

As has been known for decades, once children reach a cognitive age of ~ 30 months, they can begin to cooperate voluntarily in hearing testing. By this age, children can be taught to drop a toy in a bucket or put a ring on a ring stand when they hear a sound. If the child can be enticed to cooperate, a great deal can be learned about his hearing. The challenging task for the pediatric audiologist is to find ways to keep the young child entertained for a long enough time to complete the hearing test.

◆ Assessing the Child's Cognitive Age

As with all other behavioral test techniques, the first task is to determine the child's cognitive age. Regardless of the child's chronologic age, behavioral testing requires that the child's cognitive age be determined. Play audiometry will be easily accomplished with children who are cognitively older than 3 years and will not be easily accomplished for children younger than 2½ years. Some children around 2 years of age will be able to perform play tasks, but many will not, and those who can may not be able to perform the task for a sufficiently long time to complete an audiogram. Selecting the wrong test procedure means that one may be unable to obtain any thresholds, may obtain very few thresholds, or may obtain inaccurate thresholds (American Academy of Audiology [AAA], 2012; Diefendorf, 2002; Madell, 1998; Martin & Clark, 1996; Thompson, Thompson, & Vethivelu, 1989).

Cognitive information can be obtained in several ways. A good case history will provide some information. If the child's motor development is within normal limits and the child has no other significant developmental issues, such as autism or pervasive development disorder (PDD), she should be able to perform the play task. If speech and language development are grossly within normal limits, as determined by observation and discussion with parents (Lidén & Harford, 1985), cognitive levels can be assumed to be close to normal as well. If a child has other developmental disabilities, cognitive levels will be harder to ascertain and results of specific developmental tests may be required. Once it is determined that a child is cognitively older than 30 months, play audiometry can be attempted. Children who have frequent hearing tests, such as those with hearing loss or recurrent otitis media, are likely to learn the listen-and-drop task earlier. Visual reinforcement audiometry (VRA) often becomes boring after repeated test sessions, so when a child becomes familiar with the audiologist and the test environment, the child may be willing to try the play task at a younger age.

◆ Training a Child for Play Audiometry

When conditioning a child to play audiometry, it is critical that the child actually hears the stimulus used to train the response. If the child does not hear the sound, the audiologist will be conditioning the child to silence, resulting in a great deal of confusion and inaccurate test results. After obtaining a case history and interacting with the child during the interview, the audiologist should have some idea about the loudness level at which to begin presenting stimuli. If the child responds to speech at a normal conversational level, testing can probably begin by presenting test stimuli at 40 to 50 dB hearing level (HL). If the child does not respond to speech at a normal conversational level but seems to be developing normally in other ways (motor development and play activities), it is possible that the child has significant hearing loss and a loud stimulus will be needed.

Training the Task

The play audiometry task requires the child to hold a toy up to his ear and perform a motor task (drop the toy in the bucket, etc.) when the sound is presented (AAA, 2012). The toy is held up to the ear for two reasons: (1) as a specific signal that the child is ready to listen and (2) as a clear indication of the motor act of dropping the toy in the bucket. To explain, if the child is playing with the toy or holding it right above the bucket, it is not clear, when the toy goes into the bucket, whether the drop was truly a response to the sound or whether the child just decided to drop the toy at that moment. When training the listen-and-drop task, begin with an easy play activity, such as dropping a block in a bucket. Do not start with a task that requires good dexterity, such as slipping a chip into a slot or fitting a small peg into a hole (**Fig. 9.1**).

Pearl

- Having a variety of interesting toys will increase the probability of keeping the child's attention long enough to get the information needed for testing.

There are several ways to begin the training. The audiology assistant can begin by demonstrating the task. She holds the toy to her ear and, when the sound is presented, says "I hear that" and drops the toy in the bucket. If the child seems hesitant, allow the parent to try for one or two sound presentations. Then hand the child the toy, hold his hand up to his ear, and, when the sound is presented, say "We heard that" and, hand over hand, with the tester's hand over the child's hand, move the child's hand to drop the

---

toy in the bucket. After a few tries, the tester should feel the child's hand start to move when the sound is presented. That is the clue to let the child carry out the task alone. If the child seems hesitant and you are certain that he hears the sound, give his hand a little nudge to help him get going. If he still needs assistance, try demonstrating the task again saying "Okay, it's my turn." Doing the task together, with both the tester and the child holding a toy and dropping it in the bucket when the sound is presented, may help. It is important to be careful that the child is not simply imitating the motor task or dropping the block when the audiology assistant does, but is, in fact, responding to a sound stimulus. After several attempts, the child will need to do the listen-and-drop task himself. Say "It's your turn" and let the child do the task. If the child looks up when the sound is presented but is hesitant about putting the toy in the bucket, it is all right to say, "You heard that, put it in." If the child continues to look to the audiology assistant for approval before putting the toy in the bucket, the audiology assistant should look at the floor or at the bucket to signal to the child that he is on his own. If the child is still unable to execute the task, start over again and retrain the task.

If there is uncertainty as to whether the child has heard the sound even at loud levels, try conditioning the child with the bone vibrator from the audiometer. Even a child with no hearing will feel the tactile stimulation of the bone vibrator at 250 Hz at maximum output. Place the vibrator on the mastoid with a headband, or in the child's hand or on the knee and hold his hand closed with your own. Use your other hand to help the child hold the toy up to his ear, and then place it in the bucket when the vibrator is turned on (**Table 9.1**). Once the child learns the task with the vibrator, return to an air-conducted stimulus and try again.

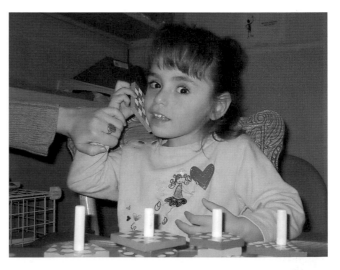

Fig. 9.1   Helping a child get ready to listen for play audiometry.

Table 9.1 Test protocol for conditioned play audiometry

1. Set the child in a highchair or at a children's table so the child is comfortably seated.

2. Select a toy that will be enjoyable for the child and within the child's skill range.

3. Begin using a test stimulus that you expect the child to be able to hear.

4. Begin by demonstrating the task. The audiology assistant holds the toy to her ear. When she hears the sound she says "I hear that" and drops the toy into the bucket.

5. After a few presentations, the child is given the toy and the audiology assistant holds the toy to the child's ear. When the sound is heard, the audiology assistant helps the child drop the toy into the bucket.

6. Care must be taken to encourage the child to drop the toy in the bucket *only* when you are certain the child heard the sound.

7. This is repeated until the child is able to perform the task without assistance.

8. Once the child is conditioned and performing reliably, testing can begin.

9. If the child appears to be bored, change toys to increase interest.

10. Testing can be accomplished by air and bone conduction, with hearing aids, cochlear implants, Baha, and FM systems.

◆ Test Protocol

Choosing the Test Stimulus

If a child responds to speech (e.g., if the child answers when called), it may be best to begin with a speech stimulus. The easiest speech utterance may be the command "Put it in." The child will understand the verbal command and learn the task easily. Use of a speech stimulus will provide a speech awareness threshold but will not give any frequency-specific information. Once the child is conditioned to the listen-and-drop task, change the stimulus to tones or narrowband noise to obtain an audiogram.

If the child displays some developmental concerns, such as autism, PDD, or multisystem developmental delay, the child may not respond to speech stimuli. In that case, testing should begin with tones, noise bands, or music. (See Chapter 10, Evaluation of Hearing in Children with Special Needs.)

Test Order

Test protocol needs to take into consideration the fact that 2-, 3-, and 4-year-olds are not always very cooperative. Testing should begin with the tasks that

require the least cooperation and move on to more difficult tasks as the child becomes more comfortable. It is easiest to begin testing in soundfield, since many children initially object to earphones. If a child has anything less than severe-profound hearing loss, there should be no problem hearing a stimulus in soundfield. If conductive hearing loss (CHL) is the concern, begin with a high-frequency stimulus, which should be more easily heard. If the concern is that the child might have a sensorineural hearing loss (SNHL), begin with a low-frequency stimulus, since hearing is likely to be better in the low frequencies.

After obtaining at least one low- and one high-frequency threshold, the audiologist has to make a decision about which test information is most crucial and about how likely the child is to accept earphones. If CHL is the concern and a decision needs to be made about insertion of pressure equalization (PE) tubes, discrete ear information and bone conduction thresholds can be critical. If the concern is SNHL, separate ear information is still important, but it may be more important to obtain an idea of the contour of the audiogram before trying earphones on the child. Remember, once earphones are used, twice as many thresholds are required. That is, twice as many responses from the child are necessary to obtain an audiogram because each frequency needs to be tested for both ears.

When the audiologist is ready to try earphone testing, a decision needs to be made about whether to begin with circumaural headphones or with insert earphones. Circumaural headphones are easy to put in place quickly. However, they can be heavy for a small head, and even little children are amazingly quick at removing them or pushing them out of position. Circumaural headphones need to be positioned directly over the ear canal to provide accurate thresholds. Insert earphones will definitely be in the right place (directly in the ear canal), but they require more effort to insert, and poking at the child's ears may be distressful to the child. Nevertheless, whenever possible, it is best to attempt to persuade the child to accept insert earphones because they will provide the best test results (AAA, 2012).

Regardless of the type of hearing loss suspected, an attempt should be made to obtain bone conduction thresholds. Once the child accepts the bone vibrator, thresholds are usually easy to obtain. If time or attention is a problem, two to three thresholds should be sufficient. For CHL, the most critical thresholds to obtain by bone conduction are probably 250, 500, and 2000 Hz. If hearing loss is sensorineural, 500, 2000, and 4000 Hz are probably the most critical frequencies to test by bone conduction. It is not unusual with SNHL to have bone conduction thresholds at levels that are better than air conduction thresholds in the low frequencies, probably as a result of a tactile (not auditory) response. If a standard bone conduction headband of metal is used, a piece of foam should be used to make it more comfortable and to improve fit. A Velcro headband can also be used; this is often more comfortable for little heads. (See **Fig. 9.2** for different bone conduction headbands.)

Test Room Setup

For many children, testing is most easily accomplished using two testers in a two-room test setup. One audiologist will present test stimuli from the control room, and the audiology assistant will work with the child in the test room. This two-room test procedure is especially important for soundfield testing.

When earphone testing is being performed, it is possible to have one tester sit next to the child in the sound room and act as both tester and test assistant. In a one-tester situation, it is difficult to test hearing in soundfield. If there is only one tester, and if there is concern that the child will not accept earphones immediately, it is possible to train the child to perform the listen-and-drop task before the earphones are placed on her head. Put the earphones on the test table near the child and set the signal to a loud level that the child can be expected to hear based on previous observations. Then train the child to perform the play audiometry task. Once the child is responding reliably, place the earphones on her head and proceed in the usual way. Some test setups allow for the audiometer in the test room to be attached to loudspeakers so that all testing can be performed in a one-room setup. This has its benefits in that it does not require two audiologists to test a child, but the audiologist may sometimes feel the need for more than two hands to accomplish everything smoothly, especially with a difficult-to-test child.

Testing Children with Hearing Loss

Children with mild or moderate hearing loss or with CHL do not require any special test adaptation, except that the audiologist may need to be creative in keeping the child entertained and cooperative through repeat testing. However, children with severe and profound hearing loss may need some test adaptations. If the child does not respond to soundfield stimuli at the audiometric limits, it may be possible to obtain a response using a bone vibrator either held in the child's hand, on the knee, or on the mastoid. No matter how severe a child's hearing loss, he will feel the vibrator at 250 Hz, since this is a tactile stimulus, not an auditory one. Once the child responds consistently to the tactile stimulus, begin testing with earphones at 250 or 500 Hz. Insert earphones are usually preferable if the child will accept them. (For more information, see Chapter 10, Evaluation of Hearing in Children with Special Needs.)

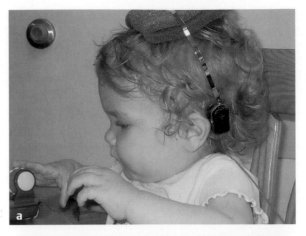

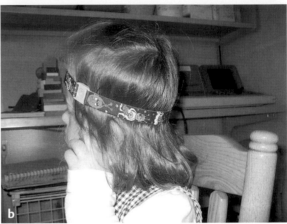

Fig. 9.2   (a) Bone conduction headband with foam to improve comfort. **(b)** Bone conduction headband held in place with Velcro.

◆ Special Test Techniques

Tangible Reinforced Operant Conditioning Audiometry

Tangible reinforced operant conditioning audiometry (TROCA) was developed for use with special populations (Lloyd, 1966; Lloyd, Spradlin, & Reid, 1968; Martin & Coombes, 1976; Northern & Downs, 2002). TROCA uses food or tokens as reinforcers instead of a movable toy. A clown or other toy is frequently used to dispense the reinforcer when the child pulls its arm, head, or other lever.

TROCA can be useful for children with developmental disabilities, for children who are not interested in the visual reinforcer, or for children with visual disabilities who cannot see a reinforcer that is a few feet away. Very small pieces of food are used to prolong the length of time the child will respond. The food selected needs to be something that will be quickly swallowed so that the test can proceed in a timely fashion. Cheerios are a useful reinforcer. Candy has been used and is reinforcing for children, but many parents are not happy about having their children fed sugar. Once the child is no longer interested in the food, testing will need to end.

◆ Computer-Assisted Reinforcement

A computer-assisted reinforcement procedure uses a laptop computer that is placed in the sound room with the child, parent, and audiology assistant. On the computer screen is an interesting PowerPoint program that is controlled by a remote mouse operated by the audiologist in the control room. Every click of the mouse adds a feature to a picture on the screen so as to complete a clown face, for example. The child has a mouse or other apparatus that is not actually connected to the computer. The child is conditioned to click his mouse every time he hears a sound. Of course, his mouse does not do anything, but the child does not know that. If the child clicks his mouse when a sound is presented, the audiologist uses her remote mouse to add a feature to the picture on the screen. If the child clicks his mouse when a sound is not presented, no feature is added to the picture. Computer pictures or games can be changed as needed to maintain the child's interest.

◆ What to Do If the Child Will Not Cooperate

A child is a child. Especially with a very young child, the audiologist, not the child, should be in control. If testing cannot be accomplished, the audiologist needs to accept responsibility and say, "I was not able to test this child," rather than "This child is not testable." Owning responsibility for a test failure encourages the audiologist to try many procedures before giving up. There are some children from whom it is not possible to obtain good cooperation. However, there should be very few children for whom little or no information is available at the end of a test session.

The answer to the question of what to do if the child will not cooperate really starts with what *not* to do. First, do not offer choices that are not bona fide choices. For example, do not ask the child if he wants to have a hearing test or if he wants to put on earphones when there actually is no choice about the matter. Genuine choices can be offered about which of two games the child wants to play, or whether he wants to start testing with words or beeps. Those are realistic choices that can permit the child to feel he has some control over the situation. Next, do not give

up. If cooperation is difficult to obtain, try taking a short rest. Have the child go for a walk or take a drink from the water fountain and then try again. Try some new toys. Try a new audiology assistant. Perhaps a parent would be a better test assistant for a particular child. Try using different test stimuli to make the game more interesting; children need to be entertained. Try a different test room, a different chair, or allow the child to sit on a parent's lap.

Do *not* try to use a different test technique if that technique is not appropriate. For example, if a child is cognitively at 3 to 4 years of age, do not try to use visual reinforcement audiometry. Although the child may make a few responses using VRA, the older child will quickly become bored. Moreover, it will not be possible to obtain more than a few responses, and it will be difficult to determine whether the responses were really at threshold. However, VRA reinforcers may be used to support the play task. Tell the uncooperative child that if he cooperates, the toy will be turned on.

Pitfall

- When a child is not cooperating, it is tempting to try a different test protocol, such as moving from play audiometry to VRA. This is almost always a bad choice. If the child is cognitively old enough to do play, testing with VRA will give inaccurate test results, and may suggest hearing loss that is not present.

Other "bribes" may also be useful. Promises such as "after we are finished you can have . . ." work very well. Possible rewards include stickers, stamps, food, and candy. Sometimes it is useful to offer the treat during testing. Providing occasional reinforcement during the test session if the child seems to be fading (such as a piece of a cookie, fruit, raisins, Cheerios, or candy) may prolong the child's cooperation. As with all other promises, when a child is told that something will or will not occur, the promise should be fulfilled. For example, if a sticker is promised after putting five blocks in the box, be sure to provide the sticker after exactly five blocks. If the child is told he cannot leave until the game is finished, that promise too, needs to be kept. In other words, think about what is promised to children before the words are spoken, and be prepared to carry out any promises that are made.

Giving some indication about how long the task will take is very useful. The audiologist can say something like "When all of these marbles are put in the jar, we will be finished." Children have no idea how long an audiometric test will take unless a concrete referent is provided for them.

◆ Parents in the Test Room

Under most circumstances, parents should be involved in test situations. Their role will be limited, but they are a source of comfort for the child. In addition, seeing how the child performs and hearing what the child can and cannot hear are very helpful when counseling about test results. When two parents accompany a child, one can sit with the child and the other can observe from the control room. Having a parent on the control room side permits the audiologist to point out events and behaviors that are happening during testing that will assist in later counseling. For example, pointing out that a child is having increased difficulty hearing the soft speech signal may help the parent understand the effect of hearing loss.

On the other hand, for some children, having a parent in the test room reduces cooperation. Some parents have a parenting style that does not require the child to carry out tasks he does not want to complete. For some parents, if the child becomes distressed or frustrated, the parent will remove the child from the situation rather than have the child be distressed. If that is the case, it may be best to have the parent leave the room and watch from the control room. As a last resort, and one that should be used only very, very rarely, it is sometimes necessary to tell children that if they do not cooperate, the parent will have to wait outside. Sending the parent out for a short time may increase the child's cooperation. Removing parents is not a procedure that should be tried on a first visit, but it may be considered at a reevaluation if testing cannot be accomplished because of the child's uncooperative behavior.

◆ Summary

With a little creativity, play audiometry is easy to accomplish with children. The following tips are useful to consider:

- Keep the test room orderly to avoid distracting the child.
- Be prepared to change toys frequently to maintain the child's attention.
- Offer only choices that are authentic; for example, do not ask a child whether he wants a hearing test when that is not a genuine choice.
- Include parents in the testing process to assist them in understanding audiologic results.
- CPA can be performed in all necessary conditions including using earphones or technology (hearing aids, cochlear implants, Baha, and frequency modulation [FM] systems).

Discussion Questions

1. What are some techniques for persuading a child to cooperate when he is not interested in doing so?

2. What are the steps in deciding what frequencies to test in what order for a child with suspected SNHL; for a child with suspected CHL?

References

American Academy of Audiology. (2012). Audiologic guidelines for the assessment of hearing in infants and young children. Retrieved from http://www.audiology.org/resources/documentlibrary/Documents/201208_AudGuideAssessHear_youth.pdf

Diefendorf, A. O. (2002). Detection and assessment of hearing loss in infants and children. In J. Katz (Ed.), Handbook of clinical audiology (5th ed.). Baltimore, MD: Lippincott Williams & Wilkins.

Hoversten, G., Lowell, E. L., Rushford, G., & Stoner, M. (1956). Evaluation of pure tone audiometry with preschool age children. The Journal of Speech and Hearing Disorders, 21(3), 292–302.

Lidén, G., & Harford, E. R. (1985). The pediatric audiologist: from magician to clinician. Ear and Hearing, 6(1), 6–9.

Lloyd, L. L. (1966). Behavioral audiometry viewed as an operant procedure. The Journal of Speech and Hearing Disorders, 31(2), 128–136.

Lloyd, L. L., Spradlin, J. E., & Reid, M. J. (1968). An operant audiometric procedure for difficult-to-test patients. The Journal of Speech and Hearing Disorders, 33(3), 236–245.

Madell, J. R. (1998). Behavioral evaluation of hearing in infants and young children. New York, NY: Thieme.

Martin, F. N., & Clark, J. G. (1996). Behavioral hearing tests with children. In F. N. Martin & J. G. Clark (Eds.), Hearing care for children. Needham Heights, MA: Allyn & Bacon.

Martin, F. N., & Coombes, S. (1976). A tangibly reinforced speech reception threshold procedure for use with small children. The Journal of Speech and Hearing Disorders, 41(3), 333–338.

Northern, J. L., & Downs, M. P. (2002). Hearing in children (5th ed.). Baltimore, MD: Lippincott Williams & Wilkins.

Thompson, M., Thompson, G., & Vethivelu, S. (1989). A comparison of audiometric test methods for 2-year-old children. The Journal of Speech and Hearing Disorders, 54(2), 174–179.

Chapter 10

Evaluation of Hearing in Children with Special Needs

Jane R. Madell

Key Points

- By appropriately controlling the test environment and using the appropriate test protocols, almost any child can be tested using behavioral techniques.

- If a child cannot be tested, the audiologist needs to take ownership for the inability to test and say "I was unable to test this child" rather than "This child is untestable."

Testing an infant or child with special needs demands unique skills from the audiologist in all areas, from taking a case history to modifying test protocols and tasks. Frequently, parents bring a child for evaluation because they have concerns about her development. If a child is not speaking, the first question is "Does she hear?" The audiologist is often the first person to evaluate a child, especially if the disability has not been identified in the newborn nursery. To begin with, when taking a case history, a parent may report that the child has been diagnosed with autism, pervasive developmental disorder (PDD), Down syndrome, or some other condition. It is the audiologist's responsibility to find out about the particular disorder so that he can more effectively test and be an effective participant on the team.

The audiologist must be familiar with multiple disorders that can either cause hearing loss or interfere with a child's using hearing to learn. These disorders include autism, PDD, Down syndrome, CHARGE (coloboma of the eye, heart anomaly, choanal atresia, retardation, and genital and ear anomalies) syndrome, and other developmental disorders. Although the audiologist is not the professional who diagnoses these disorders, he should be able to recognize them and understand their effect on hearing. Doing so will enable him to select

test protocols, make referrals for additional evaluations, and arrange for management.

Many developmental disabilities do not result in hearing loss—that is, when appropriately tested, the children have normal audiograms. However, because of other contributing factors, they may have problems learning language and responding to sound. It is frequently a difficult task to make the appropriate diagnosis, but doing so will improve the likelihood that the child will be directed toward appropriate follow-up.

A very old textbook (Myklebust, 1954) provides wonderful descriptions of various auditory disorders. Although the terminology is outdated and the book is now out of print, it has a lot of useful information, and for clinicians interested in becoming pediatric audiologists, it is well worth the effort to search out and read the book. It can be found in many audiology libraries as well as on the Internet.

◆ Testing Hearing in Infants and Children with Severe and Profound Hearing Loss

Children with severe and profound hearing loss who are developing normally should be able to be taught auditory test tasks in the same way as their normally hearing peers, except that the sound will need to be much louder. Since children with severe and profound hearing loss frequently do not hear sounds, they may not know how to attend to auditory signals. Therefore, it may take more than the usual number of presentations for the child to learn to respond to the conditioning task. It is critical that the audiologist be absolutely certain that the child hears the sound before either turning on the visual reinforcer when using visual reinforcement audiometry (VRA) or signaling to the child to "listen and drop" for conditioned play audiometry (CPA).

For very young children, testing usually begins in soundfield. If the room is quiet and activities are kept to a minimum, it should be fairly easy to see whether the child responds to a loud stimulus. Begin with low-frequency stimuli, because children with hearing loss commonly hear low-frequency signals better than high frequencies. If the child does not respond, it will be useful to encourage her to accept earphones, since most audiometers can present an earphone signal at a greater intensity than can be obtained in sound-field. Centers that see large numbers of children with severe and profound hearing loss may want to consider installing power amplifiers and loudspeakers to permit soundfield testing of more intense signals.

If the child is not responding to an auditory stimulus, it may be possible to obtain a response using a tactile stimulus. Condition the child to a tactile stimulus by placing a bone vibrator in her hand, on the knee, or on the mastoid. Even if the child cannot hear the stimulus, she will feel it and should easily become conditioned to the task. Once the child is conditioned, it is useful to pair the tactile and auditory stimuli, then fade the tactile stimulus and see whether the child continues to respond. It may take several attempts, but unless the child has no measurable hearing, it should be possible to teach her to respond to an auditory signal using this tactile technique.

Because children with hearing loss are evaluated frequently, they are likely to grow tired of hearing testing. A great deal of creativity will be demanded of the audiologist to keep the child interested. Using multiple VRA toys could maintain the child's interest for a little while longer, but creative toys alone may be insufficient. Using video VRA (a TV with cartoons) as a reinforcer may be more interesting for a 2-year-old child than standard VRA toys are. Children with hearing loss frequently learn the listen-and-drop task of play audiometry earlier than their normal hearing peers because they are tested so often. An interesting and enthusiastic audiologist with many good toys may be able to keep a child's attention long enough to obtain a sufficient number of thresholds using either VRA or CPA (Madell, 1998).

It is not reasonable to expect that any young child will be able to attend long enough to obtain air conduction thresholds in each ear, bone conduction thresholds, speech audiometry measures, and assessment of performance with technology (monaurally and binaurally) in one test session. Parents need to be advised in advance that it is not likely that all the necessary information will be obtained in one test session and that, depending on the child, it may take two or three test sessions to complete each evaluation. When parents understand that the audiologist is trying to maximize the child's functioning, they are usually understanding about the need for repeat visits.

◆ Testing Hearing in Infants and Children with Developmental Delay

Unfortunately, having one disability does not prevent a child from having another. Many children with developmental disabilities have also been identified with hearing loss. Some of the syndromes and disorders associated with developmental disabilities (e.g., Down syndrome, CHARGE syndrome, cytomegalovirus, premature birth) are also associated with impaired hearing. Abilities of these children vary greatly. Some have mild delays, and others have significant ones. Some of these children have structural deformities of the ear, and many have significant middle ear disease (Shoup & Roeser, 2007). As a result, every child identified with any developmental disability or delay should be followed audiologically until ear- and frequency-specific information is obtained. If no hearing loss is identified, and if the disorder is not a progressive one, the infant can be discharged from follow-up. However, if the disorder has the potential for being progressive (e.g., cytomegalovirus, central nervous system dysfunction) or fluctuating (e.g., conductive hearing loss in Down syndrome), children should be monitored on a regular basis. It is very helpful for the audiologist to learn as much as possible about the disorders that frequently present in the audiology clinic and the specific disorder that any one child may express. Understanding a disorder will help the clinician understand what kind of behavior may be expected from the child, what types of auditory disorders are expected, and the prognosis for development of speech, language, and hearing. However, it is important to remember that every disorder presents in variable ways. The developmental delay may be mild or severe, and the auditory disorder may be mild or severe. Information about the disorder is a starting place for effective audiologic assessment, but only a start.

When evaluating normally developing children, the audiologist makes assumptions about developmental age that he cannot make when evaluating children with developmental disabilities. With all children, and especially with infants and children with special needs, it is critical to know the cognitive age in order to select the appropriate test protocol. Flexer and Gans (1985) demonstrated that by carefully assessing the developmental age of children with profound multiple disabilities, they could obtain thresholds at the same levels as with normally developing children of the same developmental age. This confirms that children with developmental delay can be accurately evaluated for hearing loss if their developmental age is correctly determined. If the child is in an early intervention or educational program, the staff at the program should be able to provide information about developmental age. The pediatrician may also be able to provide this information. With experience evaluating children, most pediatric audiologists will develop the necessary intuition to determine enough about cognitive level to select the appropriate test protocol. It is most important to look at motor and play skills. Language, especially for a child with hearing loss who has not had sufficient auditory input, is not likely to be a good indicator of cognitive age. Once the child's cognitive age is known, it is possible to select the appropriate test protocol: behavioral observation audiometry (BOA), VRA, or CPA (Kile, 1996; Madell, 1998).

Positioning

The specific test protocols described in Chapters 7, 8, and 9 (BOA, VRA, and CPA) emphasize that positioning of the child is critical. The infant needs to be situated so that she is comfortable, is not straining, and can attend to auditory stimuli. A great deal of care needs to be taken to keep a child with any neurologic disorder centered. A child with a neurologic disorder and for whom motor activity is difficult will have trouble making a significant head turn. The child must be focused straight forward with the visual reinforcer at 45 degrees and no more than 90 degrees from midline. If the child does not have good trunk control, she needs to be seated in a chair that will provide trunk stabilization. Infants will be able to use standard infant seats or will lean against a parent. Older children will need adaptive chairs or strollers that can offer the necessary support to facilitate head, trunk, and neck control. Many children will be able to turn toward a reinforcement toy if seated in a chair that affords trunk and neck stabilization.

For children who are engaged in play audiometry, positioning needs to permit optimum range of motion of arms and hands. Some children may need to be held upright to provide the upper body support that enables them to use their arms and hands for the play activity. Play tasks should be carefully selected to be within the child's skill range. Putting pegs into a pegboard may be too difficult, but throwing pegs into a basket may be a motor skill the child can accomplish (Madell, 1998). Tangible reinforced operant conditioning audiometry (TROCA) (Lloyd, Spradlin, & Reid, 1968) is a play audiometry task that was designed to assist in testing children with developmental disabilities. For more information about TROCA, see Chapter 9.

Timing of Test Stimulus Presentation

Delivery of the test signal may require a little more consideration with this population. Because motor control is an issue for many children with neurologic disorders, the audiologist needs to observe the child carefully to be certain she is stabilized and comfortable before the audiologist presents a stimulus. If the child is squirming and trying to attain a stabilized position, she may not be able to respond to a stimulus. In that case, absence of response is not an indication of inability to hear the stimulus.

Difficulties in Obtaining Responses

There are several issues to be considered in obtaining and interpreting reliable responses from children with developmental disabilities. First, the response the child makes may be qualitatively different from that obtained from normally developing children. For example, it may take the child longer to focus on a reinforcer and to refocus on the distraction toy. There may be a longer latency between presentation of the test stimulus and the response. In some cases, the child may demonstrate a very short latency, turning almost as soon as the stimulus is presented. An extremely rapid response may be an indication of sound sensitivities. More commonly, however, motor responses may be slower than with normally developing children. The audiologist will need to be sensitive to this latency differential and change the timing of stimulus presentation accordingly.

Children with developmental delays may fatigue more quickly and may habituate more rapidly to test stimuli and reinforcers. The child may fixate on the visual reinforcer and thus require a great deal of effort from the audiology assistant to refocus the child's attention after each stimulus presentation. To maximize test results, the audiology assistant needs to be very alert to the child's mood and change distractors, reinforcers, and play toys quickly to keep her interested and alert. Social reinforcers are frequently very helpful.

Some children with neurologic disorders may react negatively to the visual reinforcer toys; they may become fearful and anxious. When this happens, the audiologist needs to react quickly. Most VRA systems allow the audiologist to set the reinforcement toy so that it can be presented with only a light or with

◆ Testing Hearing in Children with Attention Deficit/Hyperactivity Disorder

A child with attention deficit/hyperactivity disorder (ADHD) comes into the clinic with a great deal of energy. He has a difficult time attending and sitting still; as a result, testing may take longer than expected. If he enters the test room before the audiologist, he may start opening drawers and cabinets and disassembling headphones. When he selects a toy, he may leave it and go to another, and even with direction, he has difficulty stopping and putting away toys he is no longer using. Such a child is frequently talking; he interrupts others and has difficulty listening to the audiologist and following directions (Shoup & Roeser, 2007; Madell, 1998). To accomplish the audiologic evaluation successfully, the test room must be carefully organized. A structured test environment includes seating the child in a highchair or at a table with the chair pulled in close to encourage him to stay seated, and so that his feet are firmly placed on the floor or on a stool. If his feet are hanging loosely, the child is likely to fidget. The audiologist needs to remind the child constantly to attend and should change toys frequently to keep interest. Stimuli should be presented only when the child is attending. If the child becomes bored, it may be possible to gain more test time by taking a small break, by doing jumping jacks in the test room, or by taking a walk to the water fountain.

◆ Testing Hearing in Infants and Children with Visual Impairment

Testing children with visual impairment using VRA is obviously difficult. If the child cannot see the reinforcer, she cannot respond to it. If the child has limited vision, she can be moved closer to the reinforcer or the reinforcer can be moved closer to the child to make it easier for the child to see. If this modification is not sufficient, an alternative is to darken the test room and use a bright flashlight close to the child's face. If the child does not have sufficient vision to see the bright light, a tactile stimulus such as a bone vibrator may be successful. The bone vibrator can be used as the reinforcer by moving the child's hand to the vibrator when the sound is presented. If the child likes the vibrator, she will make the association and reach for it when she hears the sound. The air-puff technique previously described for children with developmental delay may be useful (Friedlander et al, 1973; Lancioni et al, 1989; Lancioni & Coninx, 1995; Verpoorten & Emmen, 1995). Children who are blind and who function at the 3-year-old level and higher should be able to perform play audiometry tasks by selecting toys that do not require difficult manipulation.

◆ Testing Hearing in Graduates of the Neonatal Intensive Care Unit

Neonatal intensive care unit (NICU) graduates need to be evaluated in the same way as other infants. Research by Smith, Zimmerman, Connolly, Jerger, and Yelich (1992) indicates that as many as 35% of NICU graduates may have hearing loss, which makes it clear that hearing testing of this population is critical. Testing should be delayed until the infant is stable, and it is frequently delayed until a few days before hospital discharge. However, if the infant is to be hospitalized for several months, it is necessary to test earlier than discharge so that if there is hearing loss, she will not be functioning without auditory stimulation during critical developmental months. It is very important that every attempt be made to identify hearing loss if present and to fit the infant with appropriate amplification so that she is not left without auditory stimulation for an extended period of time. ABR and OAE will be the first tests for this population, but behavioral testing should also be considered.

Although NICU graduates are evaluated in the same way as other infants, there may be some additional testing difficulties. As with other infants, it is critical to obtain an accurate developmental age and use the appropriate test protocol. Some NICU graduates function like children with developmental delays, even after age is corrected for prematurity, and will need the same considerations as are suggested for that population. Many have feeding problems and may not suck. If that is the case, it will be very difficult to accomplish BOA, but air-puff audiometry may be possible (Friedlander et al, 1973; Lancioni et al, 1989; Lancioni & Coninx, 1995; Verpoorten & Emmen, 1995). NICU babies live in a very noisy environment and, as a result, may not attend to sound. The audiologist who works with NICU patients may be able to assist in monitoring the auditory environment and in helping to control noise levels.

◆ Testing Hearing in Children with Functional Hearing Loss

It is not unusual for children between the ages of 8 and 12 years to occasionally demonstrate functional hearing loss (Berk & Feldman, 1958; Shoup & Roeser, 2007). Functional hearing loss, sometimes called malingering or faking, occurs when a child knowingly exaggerates hearing thresholds. The typical scenario is that a child fails a hearing screening either in school or in the pediatrician's office and is referred to an audiologist for a complete evaluation. The audiologist may suspect that hearing loss is functional if the following occur: (1) Test results do not agree with the child's ability to communicate (i.e., the child seems to understand with no difficulty although thresholds indicate moderately severe hearing loss, or she has a great deal of difficulty communicating when thresholds are near normal); (2) speech recognition thresholds are much better or worse than pure tone thresholds; (3) responses to speech stimuli are unusual (e.g., consistently saying only half the spondee word); (4) test results are not repeatable; or (5) unmasked bone conduction thresholds are much poorer in one ear than in the other.

If functional hearing loss is suspected, try first to reinstruct the child. It may be helpful to suggest to the child, "Maybe you did not understand the directions. This is hard to do. You need to raise your hand even if the sound is very, very soft." Alternatively, the audiologist can suggest that there may be something wrong with the equipment, which is causing the problem. "There must be something wrong with this equipment. It is making it seem that you have much worse hearing than I know you have. Let's go into a different test room and try again." You are not exactly telling the child that you think she is faking hearing loss, but you are making it clear that you know the results are not accurate.

If cooperative test results are not obtained on the second try, it will be necessary to rely on alternative techniques to get results. It is very helpful to use a portable audiometer and have the child seated next to you so that you can make eye contact. It is much more difficult for a child to say she does not hear a sound when looking you in your eye.

If the child's responses still are not providing accurate results, have him "count the beeps." Tell the child that he will hear one, two, or three beeps and to tell you how many he hears. Start at a level that the child admits to hearing. For example, if the child admits to hearing at 40 dB HL, present two beeps at 40 dB HL and when the child says "two," present two beeps at 40 dB HL and one beep at 35 dB HL. If the child responds, "three," you know that the child heard three beeps at both 35 dB HL and 40 dB HL. Continue in this fashion until consistent thresholds are obtained.

Obtaining the audiogram is actually the easy part. Now the audiologist needs to explain test results to both the child and the parent. One could simply say that the child has normal hearing and send him home, but that may be begging the issue. Why did the child feel the need to simulate hearing loss?

If the audiologic evaluation takes this "crutch" away, will the child substitute something else? It is probably useful to tell the child that she has normal hearing. However, it is important to discuss with the parents or caregivers that the child may have difficulties that are causing stress and suggest that they find out whether anything is bothering the child. It is possible that simply being aware that the child is under stress will help the parents provide the necessary support. If not, telling them about the child's behavior during testing can alert them to seek help.

◆ Conclusion

Children with all types of developmental, behavioral, and auditory disorders are testable using behavioral procedures. A review of the literature and the experience of many pediatric audiologists clearly indicate that reliable test results can be obtained from almost any child. The audiologist has to believe he can test the child and be creative in finding ways to accomplish the task. If test results cannot be obtained, the audiologist needs to take ownership of the problem and assume responsibility for the unfavorable outcome. It is not the child's fault testing could not be completed. The audiologist needs to say (at least to himself) "I was unable to test this child." On another day, testing may be more successful, especially if the audiologist can identify the problems that were apparent during the failed testing and make changes to improve results. The reward of accurately assessing the hearing of a child who is difficult to evaluate is well worth the effort.

Discussion Questions

1. How is testing different when evaluating a child with autism compared with a typically developing child?

2. What special protocols could be used to test children with significant motor impairments?

3. What kind of evaluation protocol should be used to test children who are diagnosed with ADHD?

References

Berk, R. L., & Feldman, A. S. (1958). Functional hearing loss in children. The New England Journal of Medicine, 259(5), 214–216.

Davis, R., & Stiegler, L. N. (2005). Toward more effective audiologic assessment of children with autism spectrum disorders. Seminars in Hearing, 26, 241–252.

Downs, D., Schmidt, B., & Stephens, T. J. (2005). Auditory behaviors of children and adolescents with pervasive developmental disorders. Seminars in Hearing, 26, 226–240.

Egelhoff, K., Whitelaw, G., & Rabidoux, P. (2005). What audiologists need to know about autism spectrum disorders. Seminars in Hearing, 26(4), 202–209.

Flexer, C., & Gans, D. P. (1985). Comparative evaluation of the auditory responsiveness of normal infants and profoundly multihandicapped children. Journal of Speech and Hearing Research, 28(2), 163–168.

Friedlander, B. Z., Silva, D. A., & Knight, M. S. (1973). Selective responses to auditory and auditory-vibratory stimuli by severely retarded deaf-blind children. The Journal of Auditory Research, 13, 105–111.

Gomot, M., Giard, M. H., Adrien, J. L., Barthelemy, C., & Bruneau, N. (2002). Hypersensitivity to acoustic change in children with autism: electrophysiological evidence of left frontal cortex dysfunctioning. Psychophysiology, 39(5), 577–584.

Gravel, J. S., Dunn, M., Lee, W. W., & Ellis, M. A. (2006). Peripheral audition of children on the autistic spectrum. Ear and Hearing, 27(3), 299–312.

Greenspan, S. (1995). The challenging child. Reading, MA: Addison-Wesley.

Greenspan, S., & Weider, S. (1998) The child with special needs. Reading, MA: Perseus.

Kile, J. E. (1996). Audiologic assessment of children with Down syndrome. American Journal of Audiology, 5, 44–52.

Lancioni, G. E., Coninx, F., & Smeets, P. M. (1989). A classical conditioning procedure for the hearing assessment of multihandicapped persons. Journal of Speech and Hearing Research, 54, 88–93.

Lancioni, G. E., & Coninx, F. (1995). A classical condition procedure for auditory testing: air puff audiometry. Scandinavian Audiology, 24, 43–48.

Lloyd, L. L., Spradlin, J. E., & Reid, M. J. (1968). An operant audiometric procedure for difficult-to-test patients. The Journal of Speech and Hearing Disorders, 33(3), 236–245.

Madell, J. R. (1998). Behavioral evaluation of hearing in infants and young children. New York, NY: Thieme.

Myklebust, H. (1954). Auditory disorders in children, a manual for differential diagnosis. New York, NY: Grune and Stratton.

Shoup, A. G., & Roeser, R. (2007). Audiologic evaluation of special populations in audiology. In R. J. Roeser, M. Valente, & H. Hosford-Dunn (Eds.), Audiology diagnosis (pp. 314–334). New York, NY: Thieme.

Smith, R. J. H., Zimmerman, B., Connolly, P. K., Jerger, S. W., & Yelich, A. (1992, Dec). Screening audiometry using the high-risk register in a level III nursery. Archives of Otolaryngology–Head & Neck Surgery, 118(12), 1306–1311.

Verpoorten, R. A., & Emmen, J. G. (1995). A tactile-auditory conditioning procedure for the hearing assessment of persons with autism and mental retardation. Scandinavian Audiology, 41, 49–50.

Chapter 11

Evaluation of Speech Perception in Infants and Children

Jane R. Madell

Key Points

- Speech perception testing is a critical part of the audiologic test battery. It provides information about how a child can be expected to function in daily listening situations.

- Selecting a test at the appropriate language level is critical.

- Testing should be conducted with and without technology (hearing aids, cochlear implants, and FM systems).

- Testing should be conducted at normal and soft conversational levels in quiet and with competing noise.

Pearl

- Speech perception testing is the only part of the audiology test battery that functionally assesses auditory performance. Speech perception information can be used to determine how a child is functioning with and without technology, in quiet, and with competing noise. Speech perception information should be used to plan remediation, including suggesting modifications in technology and in selecting and managing educational placement.

◆ Speech Perception Testing

Purpose of Speech Perception Testing

Speech audiometry, appropriately used, can be an extremely valuable part of the clinical audiology test battery, particularly for evaluating and monitoring auditory function in children. Pure tone testing provides information about degree and type of hearing loss, but it does not provide information about auditory function. How a person is able to use hearing for the perception of speech is critical for the development of language and accurate speech production. Speech perception testing is the only part of the audiologic test battery that assesses how a child hears speech (Madell, 2007, 2008; Van Vliet, 2006).

Evaluating speech perception skills can be very helpful in determining the kind of auditory difficulties a child may be having and in planning remediation. For example, word recognition scores that are poorer than expected compared with pure tone thresholds at normal and soft conversational levels can be strong indicators for aggressive treatment—medical, audiologic, or educational—and for the need to assess auditory processing skills. Testing at soft conversational levels and in the presence of competing noise can effectively demonstrate the need for technology, the need to change technology, the need for a frequency modulation (FM) system in the classroom, or the need for auditory therapy.

Information available from the evaluation of large numbers of adults and children (Boothroyd, Hanin, & Hnath, 1985; Boothroyd, 2004) indicates that word recognition ability decreases as the degree of hearing loss increases. However, the effect of hearing loss is much more significant for children than for adults because of the impact that even mild hearing loss can have on the development of speech and language (Clopton & Silverman, 1977; McKay, 2008; Ross & Giolas, 1978; Wallace, Gravel, McCarton, & Ruben, 1988). Word recognition testing evaluates the extent to which a child's hearing loss has adversely affected speech perception and put development of speech and language at risk.

For children who have identified hearing losses or auditory processing disorders, word recognition testing is useful in monitoring progress during treatment. Almost everyone agrees that, regardless of the mode of communication families choose for educating their children who experience hearing loss, all children should be given the opportunity to maximize their auditory skills. Providing appropriate technology is a necessary but incomplete step toward this goal. Children must be taught to use residual hearing for perception of speech and language. Even young children with profound hearing losses, when fitted with the proper technology, can learn to use audition for the reception of speech and language. The use of audition will positively affect language growth and improve speech production (Boons et al, 2012; Geers, Strube, Tobey, Pisoni, & Moog, 2011).

The audiologist who evaluates a child annually, semiannually, or quarterly may be in a better position to evaluate auditory progress than the therapist or teacher who sees the child several times a week. If a therapy program is successful, the child's word recognition should continue to improve and, over time, the child should be able to perform more difficult auditory tasks. During routine evaluations the audiologist can monitor the child's progress and assist teachers and therapists in modifying treatment goals to improve the child's auditory functioning.

Pearl

- The audiologist who sees a child less frequently is in a better position to monitor changes in performance than teachers and other clinicians who see the child daily or weekly.

How Speech Perception Is Evaluated

The goal of speech audiometry is to obtain as much information as possible about a child's speech perception abilities. There are several ways to evaluate speech perception, and each procedure provides different information. Erber's classic work (Erber & Alencewicz, 1976; Erber, 1979) describes an auditory skills matrix that is a useful way to think about the different components of speech perception testing and auditory listening tasks. Four response tasks can be used to assess performance:

1. *Detection* is the ability to tell when a stimulus is present. Detection is assessed using threshold tests (speech awareness threshold).
2. *Discrimination* is the ability to determine whether two stimuli are the same or different. Discrimination is tested in such tasks as the Visually Reinforced Infant Speech Discrimination (VRISD) procedure, in which an infant is tested on signaling when the stimulus changes (e.g., in [ba] [ba] [ba] [ba] [ba] [s] [s]).
3. *Identification* is the ability to recognize the stimulus being presented and to identify it by repeating, pointing, or writing. Identification is assessed during word recognition testing. Repeating back without understanding the word is an identification task.
4. *Comprehension* is the ability to understand what the stimulus means. The child may point to a picture and indicate that he also comprehends the stimulus, or may simply repeat back the words without understanding, which indicates identification.

The most common task for assessing speech perception skills in English uses a monosyllabic word as the stimulus. Results can be scored by recording the number of *words* identified correctly or by scoring the number of *phonemes* repeated correctly. Phoneme testing is the most difficult task in the stimulus hierarchy because it is the least redundant and provides the fewest cues; however, phoneme scoring provides valuable information about exactly what is perceived. Connected discourse, on the other hand, is easiest to understand, since the listener may acceptably extrapolate words he does not correctly perceive from contextual cues. Unfortunately, connected discourse provides very little information about which specific phonemes are being misperceived and are causing perception difficulties. As a result, connected discourse testing is not usually performed during audiologic testing but is more frequently used during therapy to improve auditory skills.

Word recognition can be influenced by multiple factors: *acoustic* variables (including intensity and duration of the signal), *phonetic* variables (manner, place, and voicing), and *lexical* variables (word familiarity, word frequency, neighborhood frequency, and density). Wilson, McArdle, and Roberts (2008) studied word recognition performance in young adults with normal hearing and reported that acoustic variables accounted for 5%, lexical variables accounted for 3%, and phonetic variables accounted for 40% of the total variance, with manner accounting for 24% and final consonants 14%. What does this mean for children with hearing loss? If a child with hearing loss cannot hear phonetic variables, speech perception will be significantly decreased, resulting in a decrease in language exposure and language development.

What Speech Perception Testing Measures

Speech perception testing can help determine how a child is functioning in everyday listening situations with and without technology and can assist in making decisions about management. Children who are hearing well at normal and soft conversational levels in quiet and in noise should be able to hear well in the classroom, although they may still benefit from an FM system to reduce the strain of listening. Children who can hear well at normal conversational levels in quiet, but who do not hear soft speech well or cannot hear well in noise, will have a difficult time hearing in a typical classroom. They may be able to hear the teacher with the FM, but they will not hear other children, resulting in a decrease in incidental learning. Research demonstrates that incidental learning accounts for ~ 90% of what young children learn about the world (Akhtar, Jipson, & Callanan, 2001), so difficulty perceiving soft speech will have significant negative effects. Children who cannot understand speech, even at normal conversational levels, will not be able to rely on audition to learn in the classroom. Knowing what a child can hear, with and without technology, will help the educational team determine whether a technology is appropriate or needs to be modified, and it will assist in identifying appropriate classroom placement and the need for ancillary services.

Speech perception testing can:

- Demonstrate benefit with technology (hearing aids, cochlear implants, and FM systems)
- Demonstrate improvement in auditory functioning over time
- Identify problems that develop over time, including:
  - Reduction in auditory functioning
  - Equipment deterioration or failure
- Identify specific speech perception errors that require remediation
- Demonstrate habilitation and rehabilitation needs
- Demonstrate whether therapy is providing improvement in the child's auditory performance
- Assist in selecting the appropriate educational environment

Goal of the Audiologic Evaluation

In addition to the basic audiologic assessment of degree and type of hearing loss, a critical part of the evaluation of children is the measurement of the actual use of hearing in daily listening situations (in quiet and with competing noise), including assessment with technology if it is used. Although audi-

ologists routinely evaluate speech perception under earphones during basic hearing testing, speech perception testing is not routinely measured in sound-field (unaided) to assess functional auditory skills and is not routinely assessed with technology.

Asking a child, parents, or, for that matter, an adult with hearing loss whether he is "doing well" with technology will not provide enough information about auditory function. Some users have low expectations about what is possible with technology and do not expect to understand speech in difficult listening situations; others may expect to hear better than normal-hearing peers when using technology. Observing the child's communication skills during casual conversation will provide some information but cannot lead to an accurate evaluation of auditory functioning, because the listener will be using general knowledge to "fill in the blanks" for what is not heard. Without speech perception testing, it is not possible to predict:

- What the child hears
- What the child does not hear
- Whether there has been a change in auditory perception
- Whether something can be done to improve auditory functioning

When Speech Perception Should Be Measured

Speech perception should be measured when hearing loss is identified, at every reevaluation, when selecting or changing technology, when changing technology settings, or at any time that concern develops about auditory functioning. For young children with hearing loss, speech perception should be reevaluated about four times per year. Older children should be evaluated twice yearly, and adults, who ought to be better able to monitor their own functioning, should be evaluated annually (Madell, 2002, 2008).

◆ Speech Threshold Tests

Speech threshold information is very useful in:

- Providing basic information about auditory status
- Confirming pure tone thresholds
- Determining the level to begin speech perception testing

Speech Awareness or Speech Detection Thresholds

The speech awareness threshold (SAT) or speech detection threshold (SDT) is a test that uses speech stimuli to determine threshold—the lowest level at which a person can detect the presence of the stimulus 50% of the time. SATs are usually used only when more complex speech stimuli cannot be used, such as when testing a very young child who does not have the vocabulary for other speech testing, or when testing a person with extremely poor or no word recognition ability—as may be seen in some children with profound hearing loss who have not been fitted with appropriate technology or who have not had the benefit of good auditory therapy.

Using voice (running conversation) or music will provide general information that sound is being heard. However, because both are very broadband stimuli, a threshold obtained with conversational speech or music does not offer frequency-specific information. A threshold to music at 40 dB HL tells us that at some frequency the person is hearing at 40 dB HL; it does not tell us whether that is a low or a high frequency or whether the person is hearing throughout the frequency range required for speech.

More useful information is obtained by using individual phonemes, such as in the Ling Six-Sound Test (Ling, 2002). The test items are selected to provide frequency-specific information to low, midhigh-, and high-frequency stimuli and include [a], [i], [u], [ʃ], [m], and [s]. The vowels [a] and [u] and the consonant [m] assess perception of low-frequency stimuli, [i] includes both low- and mid- to high-frequency information, [sh] assesses perception of mid- to high-frequency information, and [s] assesses perception of high-frequency information.

A shorter version of the Ling Six-Sound Test (Madell, 1998, 2007, 2008) uses three sounds: [ba] for assessing low-frequency information, [sh] for assessing mid- to high-frequency information, and [s] for assessing high-frequency information. Although it takes slightly longer to obtain these three thresholds than to obtain one, the information is much more valuable than that obtained using a single broad-frequency stimulus. The information is frequency-specific and provides information about how a person can be expected to perceive stimuli across the frequency range needed for speech. In addition, since the test is frequency-specific, it can be more directly compared with pure tone thresholds.

However, for children to develop language, they need to be able to hear all 44 phonemes in English or the phonemes in their native language, not simply the Ling six sounds. The Ling test should be considered a screening test; it should not be used to evaluate speech perception skills.

Speech Reception Threshold

The speech reception threshold (SRT) determines the lowest level at which a person can identify speech stimuli 50% of the time. It differs from detection tasks, which require only that the person be aware of the presence of

speech, not identify the stimulus. The test materials selected will depend on the individual being tested. When possible, it is desirable to use test materials and procedures that are standardized on adults so that results are comparable across patients. Older children with good language skills will be able to perform well on the standard tests that were developed for adults. Young children may not have the vocabulary or may be too shy to repeat back what the tester has said. For these children, a task that requires pointing to pictures, objects, or body parts will be easier and will produce useful results (Madell, 1998, 2007, 2008; Ramkissoon, 2001).

The test procedure for SRTs requires that the person be familiar with the material being presented. Familiarity will make testing easier and result in a threshold at a softer level than that obtained from a test in which any vocabulary word might be used. Standard testing uses spondee words (two syllable words with equal stress on both syllables). With children who can perform this task, the audiologist reads the list of words at a comfortably loud level, permitting speech reading if necessary, with the child repeating the word to verify that the word is correctly identified. Once the child is familiar with the words, the audiologist begins testing using audition alone, reducing the intensity until the child begins making errors. The audiologist then ascends and descends, establishing the level at which the child can correctly repeat the words 50% of the time. The guidelines of the American Speech-Language-Hearing Association (ASHA) (2004) and the American Academy of Audiology (AAA) (2012) for SRT testing describe a complex procedure that, while resulting in an accurate threshold, may be too time-consuming for use with some children. Cramer and Erber (1974) found that best results were obtained by asking the child to say the word and point at the same time. This combined task may increase the child's attention to the task and results in improved scores. Litovsky (2003, 2005; Litovsky, Johnston, Parkinson, Peters, & Lake, 2004; Litovsky, Parkinson, et al, 2004) has developed the CRISP and CRISP, Jr. (Children's Realistic Index for Speech Perception) closed-set spondee tests, which can be performed with a picture book or on a computer. The tests are designed to be used with or without competing noise. When used without competing noise, they are threshold tests.

◆ Infant Speech Discrimination Tests

Bertoncini and Berger (2004) describe a protocol based on the VRISD procedure that can be used to test discrimination of speech contrasts and to categorize various speech stimuli. The original VRISD protocol was developed by Eilers, Wilson, and Moore (1977) and is described by Werker, Shi, and Desjardins (1998); it uses a task in which an infant is asked to identify a change in the speech stimulus. For example, the phoneme [a] may be presented and contrasted with [ʃ] as follows: [a] [a] [a] [a] [a] [a] [ʃ] [ʃ] [ʃ] [a] [a] [a]. Infants are trained to make a conditioned head turn at the change in stimulus, and the standard VRA procedure can be used as reinforcement. Older children can use other tasks to indicate that they have heard the change in stimulus.

Martinez, Eisenberg, Boothroyd, and Visser-Dumont (2008) have developed a speech patterns contrast test for young children ages 6 months to 5 years, based on the Speech Patterns Contrast Test developed by Boothroyd (1984). It is a progressive test beginning with a Visual Reinforcement Assessment of the Perception of Speech Pattern Contrasts (VRASPAC), then progressing to Play Assessment of the Perception of Speech Pattern Contrasts (PLAYSPAC), then to Online Imitative Test of Speech Feature Perception (OLIMSPAC) and Video Speech Pattern Contrast Test (VIDSPAC). All measures use the same six phonetic contrasts: vowel height (e.g., [aː] versus [uː]), vowel place (e.g., [iː] versus [uː]), consonant voicing (e.g., [d] versus [t]), consonant continuance or manner (e.g., [t] versus [s]), consonant place in the front (alveolar versus bilabial position, e.g., [d] versus [b]), and consonant place in the rear position (alveolar versus velar, e.g., [d] versus [g]). This type of complex testing can provide detailed information about speech perception that can be used to determine benefit from technology and to provide information about possible changes in technology settings that might improve perception.

◆ Children's Speech Perception Testing

Speech perception tests are designed to evaluate a child's ability to understand speech under different listening conditions. Unlike threshold testing, word recognition testing is performed at suprathreshold levels. Testing may be conducted at different intensities and under varying conditions of competing noise. The selection of test materials and test conditions will depend on the child's vocabulary level and the child's ability to cooperate. Scoring requires accurate perception of all the phonemes in any word to obtain a correct score. By modifying the response task and types of reinforcement, it is possible to learn a great deal about a child's speech perception skills. Several factors affect speech perception test results.

Selecting the Appropriate Test

Vocabulary Level

It is essential that the audiologist know the child's vocabulary level to select the appropriate test. The child's vocabulary age may be determined by using a stan-

dardized vocabulary test, by obtaining information from testing at another evaluation, or from the reports of parents, speech-language pathologists, or teachers. When the previous alternatives are not available, it will be necessary for the audiologist to make a determination about vocabulary level through conversation with the child. Selecting test materials that contain vocabulary words that are not in the child's lexicon will result in a score that does not accurately reflect the child's speech perception abilities. If the information cannot be obtained in another way, the audiologist can perform a receptive language test to obtain an estimate of the child's receptive language level.

Degree of Hearing Loss

Degree of hearing loss should not be a factor in selecting tests of speech perception. Tests should be selected based on the individual child's abilities. It is unfair to the child to make assumptions about how he will be able to perform based on the pure tone audiogram alone. Many children with profound hearing losses are capable of using residual hearing for reception of auditory information (especially with the availability of cochlear implants). However, it is undoubtedly true that profound hearing loss makes it more difficult to receive information using the auditory channel for children using hearing aids, not cochlear implants. For children who have not had the advantage of early intervention, who have not been trained in a program that emphasizes the use of audition, or who do not have the ability to use audition, special tests have been developed that make speech perception testing possible. (See the discussion of Tests for Severe and Profound Hearing Loss in this chapter.)

Closed-Set versus Open-Set Testing

Word recognition tests can be divided into two categories: closed-set tests and open-set tests. In closed-set testing, the number of possible items is restricted. Items might be numbers, body parts, pictures, or alphabet letters to which the child will point. The child being tested understands what all the possible test stimuli are and will select his response from that limited number of potential items. By simply guessing and pointing to a picture, a child has some chance of attaining a correct score.

Open-set testing, on the other hand, offers no clues. The child is asked to repeat what he hears without any indicators. Any word in the child's vocabulary is a possibility. In some cases, the child may be asked to repeat what he hears even if it is not a word (e.g., nonsense syllables). Open-set testing is much more difficult than closed-set testing, and it will frequently result in lower scores. However, open-set paradigms will provide a more realistic picture of speech perception capabilities in conversation. As soon a child is capable of the task, open-set testing should be used, since it will provide a more accurate representation of how the child is performing when compared with children of the same age. By the time a child reaches kindergarten, open-set testing should be attempted.

Recorded versus Monitored Live Voice Testing

Recorded testing has the advantage of being more easily comparable from test session to test session and from one audiologist to another (Roeser & Clark, 2008). It avoids the possibility of the tester modifying his voice, either intentionally or unintentionally, to assist the child in obtaining a higher score. On the other hand, recorded testing is more time consuming and prevents the audiologist from making the adaptations that are sometimes needed when testing young children. A child may require:

- More off-time between stimuli than the recording permits to be able to attend
- Repetition of an item if the child becomes distracted or begins to talk to a parent or the test assistant
- Time out for encouragement

It is certainly possible to stop a compact disc (CD) player and reset, but this is often difficult to accomplish efficiently. Experienced pediatric audiologists who are aware of the pitfalls can obtain accurate results using monitored live voice (MLV) testing, but MLV testing should be used only when it is not possible to perform recorded testing (AAA, 2012; ASHA, 2004; Madell, 2008).

Table 11.1 shows speech perception scores for an 8-year-old with normal hearing who was tested with MLV and then tested with recorded stimuli. It is clear that the monitored live voice testing can overestimate the child's auditory functioning. The recorded testing was in agreement with the parent's and school's description of the child's functioning and made a case for referring the child for an auditory processing evaluation.

Table 11.1 Word recognition testing for an 8-year-old using monitored live voice and recorded testing demonstrating different results

Conditions	MLV	Recorded
50 dB	100%	100%
35 dB	100%	95%
50 dB +5 SNR	100%	50%
50 dB 0 SNR	100%	50%
35 dB 0 SNR	88%	32%

Abbreviations: dB, decibels; SNR, signal-to-noise ratio.

Pearl

- MLV testing, because it is easier for children than recorded testing, and because it may be easier for the audiologist as well, will frequently show higher scores than recorded testing and thus overestimate the child's actual auditory abilities. Therefore, it is important to use recorded tests whenever the child is capable of doing the task. Recorded testing will provide a more accurate representation of auditory performance.

Phoneme Scoring versus Whole-Word Scoring

Most of the tests that we use to evaluate speech perception are scored according to whether or not the person correctly identifies the whole word. If the person makes an error on one phoneme, the entire word is scored as wrong. The whole-word method of scoring may be depriving us of useful information.

Boothroyd has written extensively about phoneme scoring and its advantages; he has developed tests that rely on phoneme scoring (Boothroyd, 1968, 1984, 2004; Boothroyd, Springer, Smith, & Schulman, 1988). Actually, phoneme scoring can be used with any test. By recording the phoneme errors that a child makes during any speech perception test, we can learn what parts of the auditory spectrum are not being appropriately perceived. For example, vowel errors indicate insufficient low-frequency information. Inability to perceive sibilants correctly indicates insufficient high-frequency information or possible upward spread of masking caused by too much low-frequency amplification. Knowing the exact spectral bands of the phonemes that are misperceived will provide even more specific information. Such information may permit us to make changes in the frequency response of the child's hearing aids or cochlear implants, to make earmold modifications, and to make suggestions about auditory training goals.

Half List versus Full List

The issue of using only a half list of words in a test versus using the entire or full list has been debated in the field of audiology for years. Obviously, using a full 50-word list reduces the chance of scoring error. However, when working with young children, several additional factors need to be considered. With young children, time is of the essence. It is necessary to acquire a great deal of information in a short period of time, and it may not be possible to obtain test results in all the necessary test conditions if too much time is spent on any one test. However, the necessity for speed does not justify using fewer than the required number of stimuli to obtain reliable results. Short lists should be used only when a short-list protocol has been validated. The number of words used must be sufficient to obtain all the information necessary to assess the child's speech perception abilities. This assessment can usually be achieved with 25 words on most tests, but not with only 10 words. Except in rare cases, such as the Isophonemic Word Lists (Boothroyd, 1968), which have been standardized as 10-word (30-phoneme) lists, 10 words will not provide a sufficient number or variety of stimuli to obtain an accurate score.

Use of a Carrier Phrase

Most word recognition tasks were designed to be used with a carrier phrase. The carrier phrase alerts the child to attend and places the word in a sentence context that more accurately represents its use in normal conversation. The carrier phrase usually ends with a vowel so that the carrier phrase does not influence the word. Common carrier phrases are "you will say," "show me the," "where is the," or "tell me."

◆ Description of Children's Speech Perception Tests

Closed-Set Tests

The most frequently used closed-set tests for very young children are Northwestern University Children's Hearing in Pictures (NU-CHIPS) (Elliot & Katz, 1980), and the Word Intelligibility by Picture Identification (WIPI) (Ross & Lerman, 1970). The NU-CHIPS is a four-item test with vocabulary appropriate for children aged 3 to 5 years, and the WIPI is a six-item test with vocabulary appropriate for children aged 4 to 6 years. The foils in the WIPI are more similar to each other, requiring finer auditory skills, which, along with the larger number of items, make the test more difficult.

The Alphabet Test (Ross & Randolph, 1990) asks the child to point to one or two alphabet letters. The errors are scored according to how phonemically close to correct the answer is. For example, if the stimulus is [p] and the child points to [b], the answer is wrong by only one distinctive feature (voicing). If the child had pointed to [z], the response would have been off by three distinctive features (voicing, manner, and place), indicating a much more significant problem in auditory perception, and the child would have received a lower score.

The Auditory Numbers Test (ANT) (Erber, 1980), is a fun way to test number perception. There are pictures of one, two, three, or more ants on cards. The tester says a number and the child selects the appropriate card. The same information can be obtained by having the child repeat the number spoken by the tester. Number identification requires only vowel perception, so scores obtained with numbers are measuring only low-frequency perception.

The Children's Realistic Inventory of Speech Perception (CRISP) and CRISP Jr. (Litovsky, 2003, 2005; Litovsky, Johnston, et al, 2004; Litovsky, Parkinson, et al, 2004) are closed-set, four-item forced-choice tests that use spondee words and different levels of competing noise. The noise level at which a child can identify spondees accurately is determined. The test can be performed using either a computer or a book format, with the child pointing to the selected picture.

When standardized tests cannot be used, body parts or names of familiar objects can be substituted as test stimuli. However, if a very small set of stimuli is used, the results must be interpreted with caution.

Open-Set Tests

Word Tests

Open-set testing, because it does not have a limited set from which the listener selects an answer, is more difficult than closed-set testing. The response is limited only by the vocabulary of the person being tested.

The NU-CHIPS and WIPI word lists can be used without the pictures, making the task open-set rather than closed-set. These tests are useful because vocabulary level can be easily identified.

The Phonetically Balanced Kindergarten (PBK) test (Haskins, 1949) is an open-set test with kindergarten-level vocabulary.

The Isophonemic Word Lists (Mackersie, Boothroyd, & Minniear, 2001) use 10-item consonant–nucleus–consonant (CNC) word lists with school-age vocabulary and are scored for phonemes and whole words correct.

The Minimal Pairs Test (Robbins, Renshaw, Miyamoto, Osberger, & Pope, 1988) was designed for use with cochlear implant patients. The listener is shown two pictures with words that differ by only one phoneme (e.g., *bear* and *pear*). For each pair, the difference is one phonologic contrast (e.g., place, manner, or voicing). During the course of the test, manner, place and voicing are tested for consonant discrimination, and vowel place and height are tested for vowel discrimination.

The Lexical Neighborhood Test (LNT) and Modified Lexical Neighborhood Test (MLNT) (Kirk, Pisoni, & Osberger, 1995) were designed for cochlear implant evaluations and use words that do not have similar words or confusions. This makes these tests easier than some of the other open-set tests. There are a limited number of test lists of comparable difficulty, reducing the number of conditions that can be tested.

Older children and adults can be tested using the more familiar Consonant Nucleus Consonant Test (CNC) (Peterson & Lehiste, 1962) or NU 6 (Tillman & Carhart, 1966) word lists. As a child's vocabulary increases and skills improve, the more difficult tests should be used, since they provide a measure of performance that can better be compared with scores obtained for typically hearing peers.

The University of Western Ontario Plurals Test (Scollie et al, 2012; Glista & Scollie, 2012) is a test of high-frequency perception skills. It consists of five randomized lists of 30 words that have simple plural forms with the addition of a final /s/ or /z/. Children are asked to repeat what they hear. The test is useful in determining whether the child hears high-frequency sounds, which is critical, since research (Pittman, 2008) has demonstrated that children with normal hearing and hearing loss learned new words faster with a 9-kHz bandwidth than with a 4-kHz bandwidth.

Sentence Tests

Sentence tests provide beneficial information about how a person communicates in general conversation; they provide clues about the ability of the child to "fill in the blanks" when he or she receives only part of the message. Even though sentence tests are useful, they may not be a substitute for monosyllabic word tests, which often provide more specific information and are more helpful in planning remediation. However, some new sentence tests have been developed that are demonstrating comparable results to those obtained with monosyllabic word tests.

The Hearing in Noise Test (HINT) (Nilsson, Soli, & Sullivan, 1994) and the Hearing in Noise Test for Children [HINT-C] (Nilsson, Soli, & Gelnett, 1996) were developed for evaluating cochlear implant candidates who had very profound hearing losses and who, prior to receiving a cochlear implant, would not have had good auditory access. The results with these tests are considerably better than those for monosyllabic words and thus overestimate everyday performance.

The CUNY (City University of New York) sentences (Boothroyd et al, 1985) is a more difficult test and useful for older children and adults.

The Matrix Test (Tyler & Holstad, 1987) is intended for children 4 to 6 years of age. It uses a closed-set format and has two levels of difficulty of materials. The child has a test plate with several pictures. The child is presented with a sentence containing one word from each column. The child can either repeat the sentence or point to two correct pictures.

The AzBio tests (Spahr et al, 2012) and the Baby Bio (Spahr, Dorman, Loiselle, & Oakes, 2011) are more difficult sentence tests that provide results comparable to monosyllabic word tests. The sentence testing likely will elicit more cooperation from children, and the results will be useful in determining candidacy for cochlear implantation.

The North American Listening in Spatialized Noise-Sentences Test (NA LiSN-S) (Cameron et al, 2009) is a speech-in-noise test designed to evaluate children with suspected central auditory processing disorder. It is a computerized test that presents sentences from 0° azimuth in competing speech that varies in respect to location. The test is standardized for use in the United States, Canada, and Australia.

Tests for Special Populations

Tests for Very Young Children

Because young children have limited vocabularies, tests need to be selected with care to be certain that testing is assessing auditory perception and not vocabulary knowledge. Possible test stimuli for very young children include body parts and familiar toys or objects.

Standardized tests include Early Speech Perception Test (ESP) (Moog & Geers, 1990), which has a low-verbal version that uses objects, for very young children, and a standard version that uses pictures. Subtest 1 assess syllabification (monosyllabic [shoe], bisyllabic [two syllables with unequal stress—baby], spondee [equal stress on both syllables—airplane], or trochee [three syllables—ice cream cone]). Subtest 2 is a spondee test. Subtest 3 assesses perception of monosyllabic words using primarily vowel perception.

The Mr. Potato Head Task (Robbins, 1994) uses the familiar Mr. Potato Head game (Hasbro, Pawtucket, RI) to assess perception by asking the child, for example, to "give Potato Head the blue shoes." With the increasing number of Potato Head pieces currently available, this test can be used in a complex way to assess speech perception and language.

Tests for Children with Profound Hearing Loss

Tests for children with profound hearing loss are based on the assumption that such a child will not be able to perform on the more common standardized tests. With newborn hearing screening identifying affected infants within weeks of birth, and with technology available to provide good acoustic access to almost every child, most children can use standard tests. Limited speech perception ability may be true for some patients, but with cochlear implants, expectations are changing. Tests for children with profound hearing loss should be used only when the child cannot perform on standard tests.

The tests most commonly used for children with profound hearing loss are closed-set tests. These include the ANT (Erber, 1980), the ESP (Moog & Geers, 1990), the Mr. Potato Head Task (Robbins, 1994), and the Alphabet Test (Ross & Randolph, 1990). Other tests are the Minimal Auditory Capabilities (MAC) Test (Owens, Kessler, Telleen, & Schubert, 1981), and the Test of Auditory Comprehension (TAC) (Los

Angeles County, Office of the Los Angeles County Superintendent of Schools, Audiology Services, and Southwest School for the Hearing Impaired, 1980).

◆ Selecting the Appropriate Test Protocol

It is clearly important to select the appropriate test protocol. The first step in selecting the appropriate test is to know the child's auditory language age—the language the child has developed through listening.

> **Caution**
>
> - A child may have a sign language vocabulary or a lipreading vocabulary at a 9-year-old level but have only a preschool-age vocabulary when using listening alone without visual cues.

Because audiologic speech perception tests are performed using listening alone, it is important that the test we select be based on auditory skill level. **Fig. 11.1** describes the protocol for beginning testing. If a child's auditory language level is lower than 2 years, the ESP is a good initial test, and if the auditory language age is 9 years, testing will begin with a test at the level of the NU 6 or CNC.

Fig. 11.2 describes the general concept of proceeding through the tests. If the child does extremely well, it is possible that a test has been selected that is too easy. The subsequent step should be to proceed to the next more difficult test and repeat testing. For example, if a child obtains a score of 90% on the

NU-CHIPS, that test is too easy. The test can be made more difficult by:

- Testing in more difficult conditions, such as moving to open-set testing at 50 dB HL
- Continuing using closed set-testing at soft conversational speech levels (at 35 dB HL)
- Presenting speech in noise (50 dB HL +5 dB signal-to-noise ratio [SNR])
- If vocabulary permits, moving to a more difficult test

In this example, testing could proceed to the WIPI, the PBK, the CNC, or NU 6 test, depending on the child's vocabulary level.

Figs. 11.3, 11.4, 11.5, 11.6 and **11.7** describe the protocol to use when starting with specific tests.

Testing in soundfield should always begin at a normal conversational level of 50 dB HL. If the child does well at that level, testing continues at a soft speech level of 35 dB HL and then in noise, at a normal conversational level of 50 dB +5 SNR. If a child does well at this noise level, additional testing should be performed at 50 dB at 0 SNR and at 35 dB at 0 SNR.

◆ Evaluating Functional Listening

Testing speech perception skills under earphones reveals important information about the functioning of individual ears, but it does not provide information about performance in daily listening. Standard audiologic test protocol suggests testing speech perception at 40 dB louder than the speech threshold (40 dB SL). A significant body of research has indicated that testing at this level is likely to provide the best word recognition scores for people with normal hearing. If the child has normal hearing, this level may be

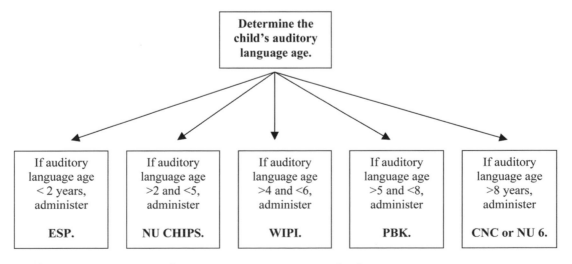

Fig. 11.1   Speech perception test protocol. Determining appropriate start level.

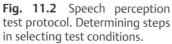

Fig. 11.2 Speech perception test protocol. Determining steps in selecting test conditions.

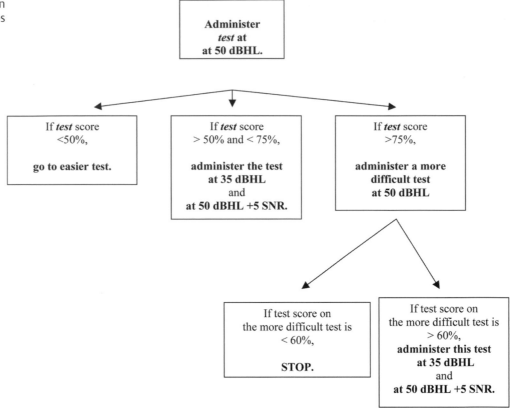

Fig. 11.3 Speech perception test protocol. Test sequence when using the ESP for children with an auditory language age younger than 2 years.

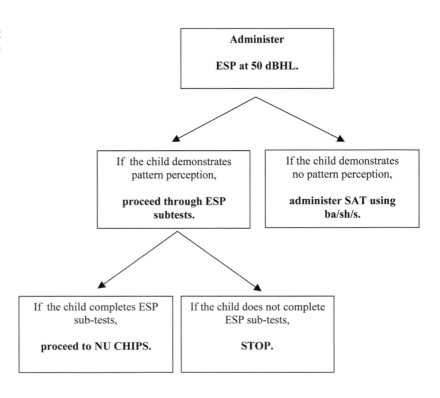

Fig. 11.4 Speech perception test protocol. Test sequence when using the NU-CHIPS for children with an auditory language age between 2 and 5 years.

Fig. 11.5 Speech perception test protocol: Test sequence when using the WIPI for children with an auditory language age between 4 and 6 years.

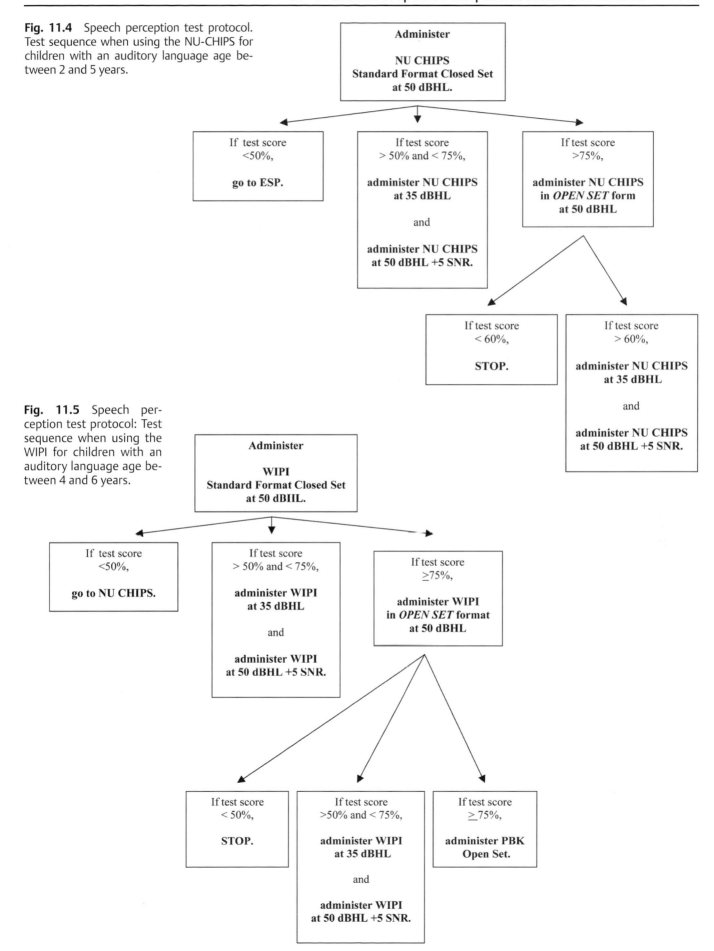

Fig. 11.6 Speech perception test protocol. Test sequence when using the PBK for children with an auditory language age between 5 and 8 years.

Fig. 11.7 Speech perception test protocol. Test sequence when using the NU 6 or CNC test for children with an auditory language age older than 8 years.

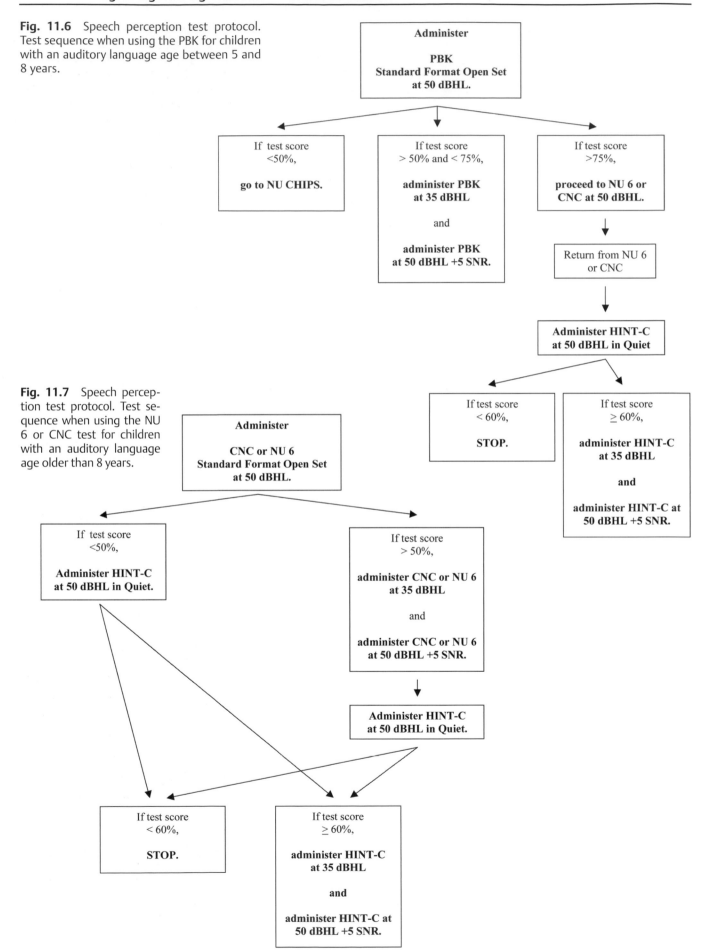

close to the typical conversational level of 50 dB HL. However, if the child's speech threshold is 30 dB HL and speech perception is tested at 70 dB HL, we are not seeing a realistic picture of how the child hears normal conversation in daily listening situations. To obtain a more realistic picture of how a child is performing in day-to-day situations, it is useful to assess speech perception at normal (50 dB HL) and soft (35 dB HL) conversational levels in quiet.

It is also necessary to assess hearing in the presence of competing noise, since the child must hear in noisy environments at school and at home. It is useful to test normal conversational levels at +5 and 0 dB SNR, and soft speech at 0 dB SNR. Speech noise or white noise will provide the easiest competing noise condition, since it is not confused with speech and is relatively easy to ignore. Single-talker babble poses a very difficult listening task, because it is easy to understand what the distracting person is saying and therefore it will be difficult to tune-out. Multitalker babble with numerous talkers (10 to 12 talkers) is easier to tune out than four-talker babble because the number of talkers makes it difficult to identify individual words. Four-talker babble is a relatively difficult stimulus, since it is possible to understand some of what is said, so the babble adds to the confusion when listening to the primary signal. For this reason, four-talker babble is a good stimulus to use, since it is difficult but realistic. Bodkin, Madell, and Rosenfeld (1999) reported on testing of 126 children with normal hearing age 3–17. Testing in multiple noise conditions revealed a mean score of 91–99% in different conditions for different age groups. These results demonstrate that speech-in-noise testing is possible in children and should be part of the standard test battery.

By testing in more difficult conditions, the audiologist will be able to identify children who may have auditory processing problems and who require additional testing. Children with otitis media who are experiencing problems that indicate difficulty hearing in a classroom may also be identified (Rosenfeld, Madell, & McMahon, 1997).

◆ Evaluating the Use of Technology

When evaluating the benefit that the child receives from technology, and to be certain the technology is providing the expected benefit, it is important to assess:

- Each piece of equipment, individually
- Each ear, separately
- Both ears, together, with the FM system

Without doing this precise testing, it will not be possible to identify problems with individual pieces of equipment. If, for example, one hearing aid is providing insufficient gain, or if speech perception with one hearing aid is significantly poorer than with the other hearing aid, binaural testing will not identify the problem, and the audiologist will not know there is a discrepancy that requires attention (**Fig. 11.8**).

Fig. 11.8 shows test results for a child who has poorer word recognition in the left ear that is resulting in poor binaural word recognition. If testing had been performed binaurally only, the audiologist would not know that the child has good speech perception in the right ear. Since aided gain is the same for both ears, speech perception discrepancies may indicate that there is some distortion in the left hearing aid or that the child has poor auditory skills in the left ear and needs auditory training work on the left ear alone.

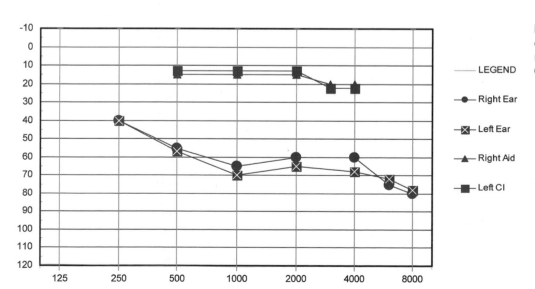

Fig. 11.8 Binaural speech perception is poorer than the best monaural speech perception. CI, cochlear implant.

LEGEND

—●— Right Ear

—⊠— Left Ear

—▲— Right Aid

—■— Left CI

◆ Developing a Speech Perception Test Protocol

The first thing to consider when developing a test protocol is the purpose of the test. Is the test being performed to obtain the best possible score? If that is the case, it would be best to select very easy test materials on which the person can be expected to do very well. On the other hand, if the purpose is to see how the person compares to normal-hearing peers, testing must be conducted with tests that would be used to test normal-hearing peers. If the purpose is to monitor technology or technology settings, testing should be performed with each piece of equipment alone, and also in whatever combinations the equipment is used on a daily basis. If the purpose is to assess areas needing habilitation/rehabilitation and to plan for educational placement, it will be important to monitor performance in difficult listening situations and to score appropriate vocabulary-level tests using both whole word and phoneme scoring.

Test Materials

Test materials must be linguistically appropriate, neither too easy nor too difficult.

It may be necessary to select different tests for each ear if the two ears function differently (**Fig. 11.9**). The evaluation report must be clear about what tests were used in which condition so that they can be appropriately interpreted. The level of complexity of the test material must be considered. To obtain a complete picture of a person's auditory abilities, it may be useful to test monosyllabic words, nonsense syllables, and sentences, all of which can be scored for number of words and phonemes correctly identified.

Test Conditions

When testing speech perception using earphones, it is standard practice to test at 40 dB SL (louder than the pure tone average), or 40 dB above the SRT. When testing with technology, test at levels that will provide a good indication of how the person functions in a variety of daily listening situations (**Table 11.2**). With technology, test monaurally, binaurally, and with FM system.

Test Modality

Testing in the auditory-only mode will provide information about how the child is using auditory information. Auditory-only testing is critical for monitoring technology to determine whether adjustments need to be made to the technology, and to understand how the person functions when visual cues

Table 11.2 Suggested test conditions for speech perception testing in soundfield, with and without technology

Testing in quiet
Normal conversation 50 dB HL
Soft conversation 35 dB HL
Testing in competing noise (4-talker babble)
Normal conversation 50 dB HL at +5 SNR
Normal conversation 50 dB HL at 0 SNR
Soft conversation 35 dB HL at 0 SNR

Abbreviations: dB, decibels; HL, hearing level; SNR, signal-to-noise ratio.

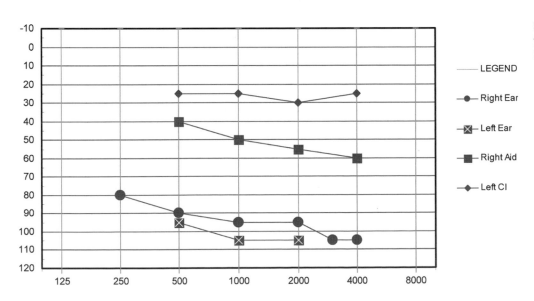

Fig. 11.9 Using different tests for different ears. CI, cochlear implant.

LEGEND

—●— Right Ear

—☒— Left Ear

—■— Right Aid

—◆— Left CI

are not available. Testing in the visual-only mode will provide information about how the child is using visual information, primarily speech reading. Testing in the auditory–visual mode will provide information about a combination of auditory and visual skills.

Audiological emphasis on testing in the auditory-only mode does not imply that a child will be asked to ignore visual cues in daily communication. Auditory-only testing is simply the best way to obtain information about auditory skills and necessary audiological modifications to improve communication. Information about auditory perceptual skills is critical no matter what communication approach the child uses.

Stimulus Presentation

Recorded testing is the preferred test method because it is most repeatable. This makes it easy to compare test results over time. Some young children who cannot sit still and attend consistently may require that testing be adaptable. For these children, MLV testing is easier to use. When MLV testing is used, the audiologist must monitor the voice level using a volume unit (VU) meter to be certain that the level is well controlled. When using MLV testing, rate of presentation should be close to that of the recorded test. If an adaptive test protocol is used (if test stimuli are eliminated or words are repeated), this must be noted and taken into account when describing test results. As children age and skills improve, testing should advance to using recorded stimuli.

Scoring Speech Perception Tests

What is a good score on a speech perception test? Does it matter how speech perception tests are scored? Yes, it does! If the audiologist believes that a child is performing well on a speech perception test there is no reason to work on improving auditory access. If however, test results are perceived as being poor the audiologist has a responsibility to improve auditory performance. Madell et al (2011) surveyed audiologists and auditory therapists to determine what was considered good speech perception. They were distressed to learn that what was viewed as "good" speech perception varied significantly—from 40 to 90%. The authors also asked recipients if children with hearing loss needed to hear as well as children with normal hearing and respondents agreed that they did. If that is the case, tests need to be scored in the same way as tests are scored for children with normal hearing.

The following scoring is recommended:

Excellent	90-100%
Good	80-89%
Fair	70-79%
Poor	< 70%

Reports should accurately report speech perception performance. Children who are performing at 68% cannot be described as having good or excellent speech perception. They do not. By honestly reporting performance, all professionals working with the children know that they have to work to improve performance. Audiologists may need to change technology, and teachers, speech-language pathologists, and auditory therapists need to work on improving auditory skills.

Test Format

Closed-set tests are easier for the child to perform because the possible choices are limited, and all targets are present for the child to select. Open-set format is the preferred method because it is a more realistic estimate of everyday performance.

◆ Items to Consider When Reviewing the Report of an Audiologic Evaluation

When reviewing a report of an audiologic evaluation, it is important to know how testing was accomplished. Was testing accomplished in open- or closed-set? Was testing performed recorded or MLV? How loud was the test signal? Was each ear tested separately with technology? Closed-set, MLV testing may be appropriate for a 3-year-old, but it is not the appropriate test protocol for a 10-year-old in a mainstream setting. The NU-CHIPS (Elliot & Katz, 1980) is an appropriate test for a preschool child or a child with a preschool vocabulary, but it is no longer appropriate for a mainstreamed third-grader, who should have a vocabulary significantly above the preschool level.

> **Pitfall**
>
> • Assessing a child's speech perception capabilities with a test that is too easy will result in an inflated test score that will not provide an accurate estimate of the child's daily functioning.

If a child performs well binaurally at a normal conversional level but does not do well at a soft speech level or with competing noise, the child will have problems hearing at school and at home. The audiologist will then need to try to improve the child's ability to hear soft speech and to hear in noise. With a hearing aid, it may be possible to increase gain. With a cochlear implant, it may be possible to increase the sensitivity. If the technology cannot be adjusted, it indicates the need for a change in technology (a different hearing aid or moving from a hearing aid to a cochlear implant), or for the use of an FM system in many listening situations for auditory access.

By recording and evaluating phoneme scoring, it is feasible to determine which phonemes are not being heard. It is then possible to extrapolate the frequencies that the child cannot access. For example, if a child is not hearing [s], it is likely that there is insufficient gain between 4000 Hz and 8000 Hz. Knowing this specific frequency information will assist the audiologist in determining how to change technology settings and in suggesting to the auditory therapist what needs to be emphasized during auditory therapy.

Pearl

- Recording phoneme errors can assist in identifying specific areas of the frequency spectrum that may be possible to access by changing hearing aid or cochlear implant settings to improve auditory performance.

◆ Conclusion

It is critical that everyone working with a child who has hearing loss have high expectations for what the child is capable of achieving and what the technology is capable of providing. If the child cannot hear some sounds, audiologists need to modify the technology settings. If the child is using the best possible hearing aid and cannot hear a portion of the speech signal, it may be time to consider moving to cochlear implants. The goal of audiologic management is to have the child hear as much as possible to maximize auditory learning. By fully evaluating auditory skills, the audiologist can go a long way to improving auditory functioning.

When a child performs well at normal conversational levels (50 dB HL) but poorly for soft speech (35 dB HL) and in competing noise (50 dB HL +5 SNR), it is very easy to demonstrate the need for an FM system in school and in other difficult listening situations (e.g., ballet class, sports, the car, restaurants). By comparing test results under several conditions with and without the FM system, the child, parents and school district will be convinced of the need for

Table 11.3 Speech perception evaluation form

Word tests	Right unaided	Left unaided	Soundfield, no technology	Right technology	Left technology	Binaural technology	FM + technology
50dB HL							
Word score							
Phonemes							
35 dB HL							
Word score							
Phonemes							
50 dB HL + 5 SNR							
Word score							
Phonemes							
50 dB HL 0 SNR							
Word score							
Phonemes							
35 dB HL 0 SNR							
Word score							
Phonemes							
Sentences							
50 dB HL							
35 dB HL							
50 dB HL + 5 SNR							

consistent FM use. Children who perform well at loud levels but poorly at normal and soft levels will have difficulty hearing everyday speech at home and in school. This difficulty may indicate the need for a change in technology or technology settings, the need to use an FM on a full-time basis, or that it may be time to consider a move from hearing aids to cochlear implants.

Table 11.3 is an example of a test form that can be used to record test scores. At first look it appears to be daunting, but the more boxes that are filled in, the more information the audiologist has by which to make treatment decisions. Although not all boxes will be completed at each evaluation, the more boxes that are filled in, the more information the audiologist has at her fingertips.

Speech perception testing offers the best opportunity for the audiologist to learn about a child's audi-tory performance and to make critical modifications in technology and recommendations for management. Although it may be time consuming, its value is well worth the effort. In the long run, it may be one of the most important services we can offer the children we have the privilege to work with.

Discussion Questions

1. Which factors need to be considered in developing a test battery for a 3-year-old with a severe hearing loss?
2. Which factors need to be considered in developing a test battery for a 15-year-old with a mild hearing loss?
3. What are the considerations in selecting test levels?

References

Akhtar, N., Jipson, J., & Callanan, M. A. (2001). Learning words through overhearing. Child Development, 72(2), 416–430.

American Academy of Audiology. (2012). Guidelines for the assessment of hearing in infants and young children. Retrieved from http://www.audiology.org/resources/documentlibrary/Pages/PediatricDiagnostics.aspx

American Speech-Language-Hearing Association. (2004). Guidelines for the audiologic assessment of children from birth to 5 years of age. Retrieved from http://www.asha.org/members/deskref-journals/deskref/default

Bertoncini, J., & Berger, B. (2004). Assess speech perception capacities in young children with cochlear implants: a psycholinguistic approach. International Congress Series, 1273, 296–299.

Boons, T., Brokx, J. P., Dhooge, I., Frijns, J. H., Peeraer, L., Vermeulen, A., . . . van Wieringen, A. (2012). Predictors of spoken language development following pediatric cochlear implantation. Ear and Hearing, 33(5), 617–639.

Bodkin, K., Madell, J., & Rosenfeld, R. (1999). Word recognition in quiet and noise for normally developing children. Miami, FL: American Academy of Audiology.

Boothroyd, A. (1968). Developments in speech audiometry. Sound, 2, 3–10.

Boothroyd, A. (1984). Auditory perception of speech contrasts by subjects with sensorineural hearing loss. Journal of Speech and Hearing Research, 27(1), 134–144.

Boothroyd, A. (2004). Measuring auditory speech perception capacity in very young children. International Congress Series, 1273, 292–295.

Boothroyd, A., Hanin, L., & Hnath, T. (1985). A sentence test of speech perception: reliability, set equivalence, and short term learning (internal report RCI 10). New York: City University of New York.

Boothroyd, A., Springer, N., Smith, L., & Schulman, J. (1988). Amplitude compression and profound hearing loss. Journal of Speech and Hearing Research, 31(3), 362–376.

Cameron, S., Brown, D., Keith, R., Martin, J., Watson, C., & Dillon, H. (2009). Development of the North American Listening in Spatialized Noise-Sentences Test (NA LiSN-S): sentence equivalence, normative data, and test-retest reliability studies. Journal of the American Academy of Audiology, 20(2), 128–146.

Clopton, B. M., & Silverman, M. S. (1977). Plasticity of binaural interaction. II. Critical period and changes in midline response. Journal of Neurophysiology, 40(6), 1275–1280.

Cramer, K. D., & Erber, N. P. (1974). A spondee recognition test for young hearing-impaired children. The Journal of Speech and Hearing Disorders, 39(3), 304–311.

Eilers, R. E., Wilson, W. R., & Moore, J. M. (1977). Developmental changes in speech discrimination in infants. The Journal of Speech and Hearing Research, 20(4), 766–780.

Elliot, L., & Katz, D. (1980). Development of a new children's test of speech discrimination. St Louis, MO: Auditec.

Erber, N. P. (1979). An approach to evaluating auditory speech perception ability. The Volta Review, 81, 16–24.

Erber, N. P. (1980). Use of the Auditory Numbers Test to evaluate speech perception abilities of hearing-impaired children. The Journal of Speech and Hearing Disorders, 45(4), 527–532.

Erber, N. P., & Alencewicz, C. M. (1976). Audiologic evaluation of deaf children. The Journal of Speech and Hearing Disorders, 41(2), 256–267.

Geers, A. E., Strube, M. J., Tobey, E. A., Pisoni, D. B., & Moog, J. S. (2011). Epilogue: factors contributing to long-term outcomes of cochlear implantation in early childhood. Ear and Hearing, 32(1, Suppl), 84S–92S. PubMed

Glista, D., & Scollie, S. (2012). Development and evaluation of an English language measure of detection of word-final plurality markers: the University of Western Ontario Plurals Test. American Journal of Audiology, 21(1), 76–81.

Haskins, H. (1949). A phonetically balanced test of speech discrimination for children. Master's thesis, Northwestern University, Evanston, IL.

Kirk, K. I., Pisoni, D. B., & Osberger, M. J. (1995). Lexical effects on spoken word recognition by pediatric cochlear implant users. Ear and Hearing, 16(5), 470–481.

Ling, D. (2002). Speech and the hearing impaired child (2nd ed.). Washington, DC: Alexander Graham Bell Association of the Deaf and Hard of Hearing.

Litovsky, R. Y. (2003). Method and system for rapid and reliable testing of speech intelligibility in children. U.S. Patent No. 6,584,440.

Litovsky, R. Y. (2005). Speech intelligibility and spatial release from masking in young children. The Journal of the Acoustical Society of America, 117(5), 3091–3099.

Litovsky, R. Y., Johnston, P., Parkinson, A., Peters, R., & Lake, J. (2004). Bilateral cochlear implants in children: effect of experience. International Congress Series, 1273, 451–454.

Litovsky, R. Y., Parkinson, A., Arcaroli, J., Peters, R., Lake, J., Johnstone, P., & Yu, G. (2004). Bilateral cochlear implants in adults and children. Archives of Otolaryngogy—Head & Neck Surgery, 130(5), 648–655.

Los Angeles County, Office of the Los Angeles County Superintendent of Schools, Audiology Services, and Southwest School for the Hearing Impaired. (1980). Test of Auditory Comprehension. North Hollywood, CA: Forworks.

Mackersie, C. L., Boothroyd, A., & Minniear, D. (2001). Evaluation of the Computer-Assisted Speech Perception Assessment Test (CASPA). Journal of the American Academy of Audiology, 12(8), 390–396. PubMed

Madell, J. (1998). Behavioral evaluation of hearing in infants and young children. New York, NY: Thieme.

Madell, J. (2002). Speech audiometry for children. In S. Gerber (Ed.), The handbook of pediatric audiology (pp. xxx–xxx). Washington, DC: Gallaudet University Press.

Madell, J. (2007). Using speech perception testing to maximize auditory performance. Volta Voices, 14(2), 16–20.

Madell, J. (2008). Evaluation of speech perception in infants and children. In J. Madell & C. Flexer (Eds.), Pediatric audiology: diagnosis, technology and management (pp. 89–105). New York, NY: Thieme.

Madell, J., Batheja, R., Klemp, E., & Hoffman, R. (2011). Evaluating speech perception performance. Audiology Today, September–October, 52–56.

McKay, S. (2008). Managing children with mild and unilateral hearing loss. In J. Madell & C. Flexer (Eds.), Pediatric audiology: diagnosis, technology and management (pp. 291–298). New York, NY: Thieme.

Martinez, A., Eisenberg, L., Boothroyd, A, & Visser-Dumont, L. (2008). Assessing speech pattern contrast perception in infants: early results on VRASPAC. Otology and Neurotology, 29(2):183–188.

Moog, J., & Geers, A. (1990). Early Speech Perception Test for profoundly hearing-impaired children. St Louis, MO: Central Institute for the Deaf.

Nilsson, M., Soli, S. D., & Sullivan, J. A. (1994). Development of the Hearing in Noise Test for the measurement of speech reception thresholds in quiet and in noise. The Journal of the Acoustical Society of America, 95(2), 1085–1099.

Nilsson, M., Soli, S. D., & Gelnett, D. J. (1996). Development of the Hearing in Noise Test for Children (HINT-C). Los Angeles, CA: House Ear Institute.

Owens, E., Kessler, D. K., Telleen, C. C., & Schubert, E. D. (1981). The Minimal Auditory Capabilities (MAC) battery. Hearing Aid Journal, 34, 9–34.

Peterson, G. E., & Lehiste, I. (1962). Revised CNC lists for auditory tests. The Journal of Speech and Hearing Disorders, 27, 62–70.

Pittman, A. L. (2008). Short-term word-learning rate in children with normal hearing and children with hearing loss in limited and extended high-frequency bandwidths. Journal of Speech, Language, and Hearing Research: JSLHR, 51(3), 785–797.

Ramkissoon, I. (2001). Speech recognition thresholds for multilingual populations. Communication Disorders Quarterly, 22, 158–162.

Robbins, A. M. (1994). The Mr. Potato Head Task. Indianapolis, IN: Indiana University School of Medicine.

Robbins, A. M., Renshaw, J. J., Miyamoto, R. T., Osberger, M. J., & Pope, M. L. (1988). Minimal Pairs Test. Indianapolis, IN: Indiana University School of Medicine.

Roeser, R., & Clark, J. L. (2008). Live voice speech recognition audiometry—stop the madness! Audiology Today, 20(1), 32–33.

Rosenfeld, R. M., Madell, J. R., & McMahon, A. (1997). Auditory function in normal hearing children with middle ear effusion. In D. J. Lim, et al. (Eds.), Proceedings of the Sixth International Symposium on Recent Advances in Otitis Media (pp. 354–356). Ontario, BC: Decker Periodicals.

Ross, M., & Giolas, T. G. (1978). Auditory management of hearing impaired children: principles and prerequisites for intervention. Baltimore, MD: University Park.

Ross, M., & Lerman, J. (1970). A picture identification test for hearing-impaired children. Journal of Speech and Hearing Research, 13(1), 44–53.

Ross, M., & Randolph, K. (1990). A test of the auditory perception of alphabet letters for hearing impaired children: the APAL test. The Volta Review, 92, 237–244.

Scollie, S., Gilista, D., Tenhaaf, J., Dunn, A., Malandrino, A., Keen, K., & Folkeard, P. (2012). Stimuli and normative data for detection of Ling-6 sounds in hearing level. American Journal of Audiology, 21(2), 232–241.

Spahr, A. J., Dorman, M. F., Loiselle, L., & Oakes, T. (2011) A new sentence test for children. 10th European Symposium on Pediatric Cochlear Implantation. Athens, Greece, May 12–15.

Spahr, A. J., Dorman, M. F., Litvak, L. M., Van Wie, S., Gifford, R. H., Loizou, P. C., . . . & Cook, S. (2012). Development and validation of the AzBio sentence lists. Ear and Hearing, 33(1), 112–117.

Tillman, T. W., & Carhart, R. (1966). An expanded test for speech discrimination utilizing CNC monosyllabic words (N.U. Auditory Test No 6). Technical Report SAM-TR-66–55. Brooks Air Force Base, TX, USAF School of Aerospace Medicine.

Tyler, R. S., & Holstad, B. (1987) A closed set speech perception test for hearing-impaired children. Iowa City, IA: University of Iowa.

Van Vliet, D. (2006). When it comes to audibility, don't assume, measure. Hearing Journal, 59(1), 89.

Wallace, I. F., Gravel, J. S., McCarton, C. M., & Ruben, R. J. (1988). Otitis media and language development at 1 year of age. The Journal of Speech and Hearing Disorders, 53(3), 245–251.

Werker, J. F., Shi, R., & Desjardins, R. (1998). Three methods for testing infants' speech perception. In A. Slater (Ed.), Perceptual development: visual, auditory, and speech perception in infancy. East Sussex, UK: Psychology Press.

Wilson, R. H., McArdle, R., & Roberts, H. (2008). A comparison of recognition performances in speech-spectrum noise by listeners with normal hearing on PB-50, CID W-22, NU-6, W-1 spondaic words, and monosyllabic digits spoken by the same speaker. Journal of the American Academy of Audiology, 19(6), 496–506.

Chapter 12

Middle Ear Measurement in Infants and Children

M. Patrick Feeney and Chris A. Sanford

Key Points

- Development of the external and middle ear over the first 6–8 months of life results in tympanometric data that may not reflect middle ear function when using a 226 Hz probe tone.

- Evidence is mounting to suggest that 1000 Hz tympanometry and wideband assessment techniques may provide greater sensitivity to middle ear disorders in neonates and young infants.

- Otoscopy should be conducted prior to the admittance evaluation to ensure that the test can be conducted safely, and to gather information for test interpretation.

- If published normative data are used for middle ear assessment, ensure that measurements are obtained using the same test parameters (e.g., probe frequency, pump speed) as the published studies, or collect local norms.

- The results of the middle ear test battery should be cross-checked with other behavioral and physiologic test results.

- A quantitative description of the tympanogram is desirable in addition to a description of its shape.

- The measurement of infant acoustic stapedius reflexes should be conducted with a high-frequency probe tone. Power measures of middle ear function using a wideband *probe* signal may also prove useful as this becomes available.

- Acoustic reflex activator stimuli for insert phones are calibrated in a 2 cm³ cavity and may be reported in dB HL. This calibration is not appropriate for infant ears and likely underestimates the level of the reflex activator in the infant ear canal.

Middle ear measurement is a fundamental component of the audiologic test battery, and its importance is nowhere more evident than in pediatric assessment. Tympanometry and acoustic reflex testing are the basic components of the middle ear test battery, which provides information about the middle ear, cochlea, auditory nerve, auditory brainstem, and cranial nerve VII. Therefore, the middle ear test battery is useful as a cross-check with other physiological and behavioral tests (see Chapter 6 for information about hearing test protocols for infants and children). However, because of the anatomical development of the conductive mechanism of the peripheral ear over the first 6–8 months of life, tests that we can readily use to detect middle ear status in older infants and children with a 226 Hz probe tone provide little useful information in young infants. An approach to this problem using 1000 Hz tympanometry and wideband immittance (e.g., reflectance or absorbance) measurements will be discussed. This chapter will also focus on when and how to conduct middle ear testing in children including the interpretation of test results. Although a brief overview will be provided here, it is assumed that the reader has a basic knowledge of the principles of acoustics and aural acoustic immittance, which form the foundation for current middle ear measurement (see Feeney & Keefe, 2012; Keefe & Feeney, 2009; Margolis & Hunter, 1999; Wiley & Fowler, 1997).

◆ The Role of the Middle Ear and Developmental Aspects

The middle ear contains the tympanic membrane, ossicles, ligaments, muscles, and an air space. This system serves to transfer acoustic vibrations in air to the fluid-filled cochlea. If the middle ear were removed from this process, a 60 dB hearing loss would result. Sounds at more intense levels would reach the cochlea through skull vibration. The gain in sound transfer to the cochlea is provided in part by two simple machines. The area difference between the tympanic membrane and the oval window of the stapes increases the force per unit area on the stapes footplate, much as a thumbtack allows us to puncture wood with our thumb. The second simple machine is a lever provided by the size and orientation of the malleus and incus, which also boosts sound energy at the stapes footplate. These two factors combine for as much as a 30 dB gain in sound transfer to the cochlea. If the middle ear were missing entirely, sound would strike the oval and round windows of the cochlea approximately in phase, causing an additional reduction in the efficiency of sound transfer to the cochlea, leading to the maximal conductive hearing loss of 60 dB.

The acoustic stapedius reflex (ASR) is a response of the auditory system to high levels of sound. It is detected clinically by noting a small change in acoustic middle ear function as the stapedius muscle contracts to pull on the stapes and stiffen the annular ligament in the oval window. The ASR, a bilateral effect, involves activation of fibers in the auditory nerve and brainstem, which trigger a response from the motor nucleus of the seventh (facial) nerve to activate the facial nerve and contract the stapedius muscle. For this cascade of events to occur, each station along the way must be functional. Thus, the reflex may be absent because of a lesion anywhere along the pathway. By examining the pattern of ASR responses for ipsilateral and contralateral stimulation, the audiologist derives a wealth of knowledge about the function of the peripheral auditory system from the middle ear to the brainstem. It has been demonstrated that infants with auditory dyssynchrony may pass a newborn hearing screening with otoacoustic emissions (OAEs), a preneural phenomenon, while the auditory brainstem response (ABR) and ASR are absent (Berlin et al, 2005). This suggests a role for the ASR as a tool for newborn hearing screening when paired with OAE screening. Both tests could be conducted with the same probe without the need for more costly ABR screening.

There are significant changes in the human external and middle ear over the first postnatal months of life that likely affect its sound conduction properties (Ruah, Schachern, Zelterman, Paparella, & Yoon, 1991; Saunders, Kaltenbach, & Relkin, 1983). These changes include: (1) growth of the bony portion of the ear canal wall and resulting decrease in the length of the cartilaginous portion of the canal; (2) an increase in the overall size of the ear canal; (3) a decrease in the density of the ossicles over the first 6 months of life due to ossification and absorption of residual mesenchyme (Eby & Nadol, 1986); (4) changes in the orientation of the tympanic membrane to be more vertical (Ikui, Sando, Sudo, & Fujita, 1997); and (5) progressive stiffening of the ossicular joints (Saunders et al, 1983). Studies by Keefe, Bulen, Arehart, and Burns (1993) and by Sanford and Feeney (2008) using wideband energy reflectance,

an emerging tool for middle ear assessment, suggest that the acoustic properties of the infant ear change markedly over the first 6 months of life.

◆ Some Basic Principles of Middle Ear Measurement

An acoustic transfer function (ATF) can be thought of as the ratio of the response of an acoustic system to the acoustic input. During traditional tympanometry, a tone is presented to the hermetically sealed ear canal, and its level is monitored using a microphone. The level of the tone is held constant using an automatic gain control circuit while the static pressure in the ear canal is varied using an air pump (**Fig. 12.1**). The frequency of the probe tone is specified as 226 Hz at a level ≤ 90 dB sound pressure level (SPL) (American National Standards Institute [ANSI], 2012). The ease of energy flow through the ear, its acoustic admittance as a function of frequency, Y_a, is an ATF equal to the ratio of total acoustic volume velocity of the source, u, to the total sound pressure, p,

$$Y_a = \frac{u}{p} \qquad \text{(Eq. 12.1)}$$

The u is the rate at which the acoustic displacement over a surface, such as a speaker cone, varies with time. Assuming a constant u source in clinical admittance systems, the voltage to the probe-tone amplifier required to keep the tone at a fixed SPL is directly proportional to the Y_a.

The term *acoustic immittance* refers to a family of ATFs, including acoustic admittance and its inverse, acoustic impedance ($Y_a = \frac{1}{Z_a}$). Y_a can be represented in the complex plane as a vector composed of two components (acoustic conductance, G_a, and acoustic susceptance, B_a), which can be plotted in Cartesian coordinates (**Fig. 12.2**). We can solve for the

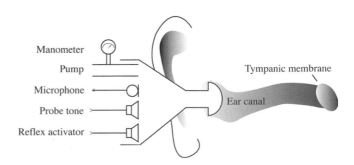

Fig. 12.1 The basic components of a tympanometer. One receiver is used for the presentation of the probe tone, which is monitored by the microphone. The second receiver is used for the presentation of an ipsilateral acoustic stapedius reflex activator. The pump varies the air pressure in the ear canal.

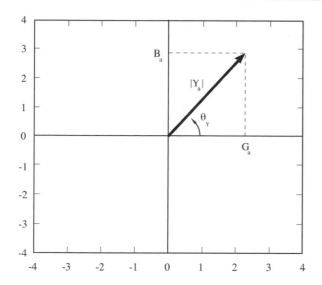

Fig. 12.2 Cartesian plot of the acoustic admittance vector. $|Y_a|$ represents the magnitude of the admittance vector. The acoustic susceptance B_a has both compliant (+) and mass (–) components. The acoustic conductance, G_a, is in phase with flow of energy through the system. The symbol θ_Y represents the admittance phase angle.

admittance magnitude $|Y_a|$ by using the Pythagorean theorem:

$$|Y_a| = \sqrt{G_a^2 + B_a^2} \qquad \text{(Eq. 12.2)}$$

G_a on the horizontal axis is the portion of Y_a directly related to energy transfer through the ear and ranges from zero (no energy transfer) to positive values to the right. The conductance is positive for the middle ear, in which frictional forces are responsible for dissipating energy. This causes the admittance vector to lie in the right half of the complex plane (**Fig. 12.2**). A condition of G_a near zero might occur in the measurement of a fluid-filled middle ear with little or no acoustic energy transfer to the middle ear. B_a is the portion of Y_a related to energy storage in the system, which is composed of two opposing forces: compliant susceptance (positive) and mass susceptance (negative).

The value B_a for a 1 cm³ volume of air at 226 Hz at sea level is approximately equal to 1 mmho, the unit of admittance, making it straightforward to calibrate admittance instruments using this probe frequency. In a calibration cavity there would be no energy transfer, so that $G_a = 0$. When a system like the ear is at its resonance frequency, around 1000 Hz for adults, the positive and negative values of B_a cancel, leaving G_a to dominate energy flow through the system. In this case the phase angle, θ_Y, between the admittance vector and the conductance would be 0°. The opposite situation occurs in the case of measurement in a calibration cavity where $G_a = 0$, and

$\theta_Y = +90°$, a pure compliant susceptance. If the system were mass dominated, θ_Y would be negative and the admittance vector would be pointed down in the bottom right quadrant (**Fig. 12.2**).

To circumvent the problem of trying to measure the middle ear admittance with the added admittance of the ear canal as measured at the plane of the probe tip, we can use vector tympanometry, a measurement of Y_a as a function of ear canal pressure (**Fig. 12.3**). In theory, the middle ear admittance is reduced to near zero with high positive or negative air pressure in the ear canal. What is left is the admittance of ear canal space, Y_{ec}. We can then subtract Y_{ec} from the total admittance measured at the tympanometric peak to arrive at the admittance of the middle ear Y_{me}, also referred to as peak-compensated static acoustic admittance, *peak* Y_{tm} (ANSI, 2012). Another clinically useful measurement of the vector tympanogram is its width (*TW*) in daPa measured at half the height of *peak* Y_{tm} calculated from the positive tail (**Fig. 12.3**).

Another useful quantity, the equivalent volume (V_{ea}), may be calculated in terms of the susceptance as:

$$V_{ea} = \frac{\rho c^2 B_a}{2\pi f} \qquad \text{(Eq. 12.3)}$$

where ρ (rho) represents the density of air, and c equals the speed of sound. V_{ea} varies with frequency and, when measured in adult ear canals, is positive at low frequencies and becomes negative at high frequencies. V_{ea} for a low-frequency probe tone is useful for determining such things as the patency of pressure-equalization (PE) tubes or the possibility of a tympanic membrane perforation.

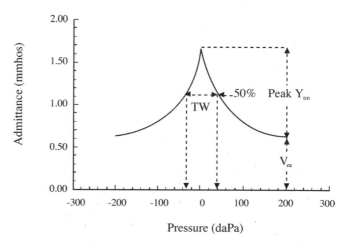

Fig. 12.3 Measurements made with a tympanogram include V_{ea}, which is the equivalent volume in cm³; *peak* Y_{tm}, which is the peak-compensated static acoustic admittance in millimhos (mmho); and *TW*, the tympanometric width, which is the width of the tympanogram in daPa measured at one half its height.

Several studies have recently shown that wideband measurement of the acoustic power transfer to the middle ear may be a family of ATFs useful in pediatric assessment (Allen, Jeng, & Levitt, 2005; Feeney & Sanford, 2005; Hunter, Feeney, Lapsley-Miller, Jeng, & Bohning, 2010; Keefe et al, 2000; Keefe & Simmons, 2003; Merchant, Horton, & Voss, 2010; Sanford et al, 2009; Werner, Levi, & Keefe, 2010). The acoustic pressure reflectance is the ratio of the reflected pressure to the incident pressure. Middle ears with low admittance tend to reflect more sound pressure than they absorb. The energy reflectance is the square of the magnitude of the pressure reflectance. The absorbance equals 1 − energy reflectance and represents the ratio of the energy absorbed by the middle ear to the incident energy. Energy reflectance (and absorbance) is approximately the same no matter where along the ear canal they are measured, and thus these ATFs have an advantage over admittance, which is affected by the ear canal volume. Results comparing these ATFs with 1 kHz tympanometry in newborns will be presented in subsequent sections.

◆ Conducting Middle Ear Measurements

Otoscopic Examination

An otoscopic examination is essential prior to undertaking the admittance evaluation. For young children and infants it is often helpful if the child sits on the parent's lap during otoscopy and subsequent admittance testing. The parent should be advised that if little hands make a grab for the ear, the parent should intercept. Prior to otoscopic examination, children are often comforted to be shown that the clinician is holding a "flashlight" and they can see the light shining on them. A cursory look into the parent's ears by the audiologist may also be reassuring for the child. It is best not to ask permission of the child to look in his ear; rather, just go about your business in a confident and comforting manner, letting the child know what you are doing. If the child is reluctant to let you perform otoscopy, you may be able to complete the task with the help of an assistant who can distract the child momentarily with an interesting toy, similar to the role of a toy waver in behavioral testing. This toy distraction technique may also be useful during tympanometry and ASR testing.

The appropriately sized speculum should be selected based on an observation of the child's external ear. The best view will be obtained with a speculum tip slightly smaller than the ear canal diameter, allowing it to be inserted into the canal while providing the maximum lumen for viewing purposes. It is important to create a bridge between the scope and the patient's head with the pinky and/or ring fingers of the hand holding the scope. This bridge will allow your hand to move with sudden movements of the patient's head rather than dislodging the speculum or pushing it uncomfortably against the canal wall. The other hand may be used to straighten the ear canal by gently pulling horizontally backward on the pinna. This last step should be undertaken with great care, especially if there is a history of ear pain.

Once the speculum is positioned in the canal, you may move your eye close to the scope to view the canal. As you may have only a quick look with some pediatric patients, it is important to see whether the ear canal is: (1) clear enough to allow the insertion of an admittance probe tip; (2) free from excessive cerumen; (3) free from other obstructions such as PE tubes that have been extruded from the tympanic membrane; and (4) not draining excessively so that the probe would be plugged. It is also important in this quick look to see whether: (1) the normal landmarks of the tympanic membrane can be seen (light reflex, umbo, and short process of malleus); (2) the tympanic membrane appears normal or is inflamed or perforated; (3) a PE tube appears to be in place or not; and (4) there is any scarring or tympanosclerosis of the tympanic membrane, which could lead to abnormal tympanometry.

Tympanometry

Preparing to Test

Daily calibration of the tympanometer with the included calibration cavities ensures valid test data. It is also helpful to check that instrument defaults are to your liking when you work with other audiologists. A self-administered tympanogram is also useful in that it provides a biological check and ensures that the system has not developed an internal pressure leak. For pediatric assessment, one should have an admittance instrument capable of multiple probe frequencies, and the calibration of each should be checked per the manufacturer's recommendations. The standard 226 Hz probe tone specified by ANSI (2012) S3.39 may be used from age 7 months to adulthood, but higher-frequency probe tones are required to test young infants, as discussed subsequently.

Many tympanometers allow the examiner to adjust other test parameters in addition to probe frequency. A rapid pressure sweep rate, often available in a screening-test mode, may be useful in obtaining data quickly in children. Some systems offer a rapid sweep rate, such as 600 daPa/s, except near the tympanogram peak, where the rate slows to 200 daPa/s. Care must be taken to duplicate the probe frequency and sweep rate if test results are compared with published normative data. For example, *peak* Y_{tm} increases with pressure sweep rate (Shanks & Wilson, 1986). Otherwise, locally collected age-specific normative data are preferable. Many commercial systems offer a standard ear canal pressure range (e.g., +200 to –300 daPa) and an extended pressure range (e.g., +300 to –600 daPa). The extended range is useful in detecting a tympanogram peak in cases of extreme negative middle ear pressure, where rising admittance is often noted with increasing negative pressure in the standard pressure range, but the pressure limit is reached before the tympanogram peak is observed. Extreme negative middle ear pressure could help to explain the presence of normal hearing in an ear with a flat tympanogram obtained within the standard pressure range. However, the extended pressure range should be used judiciously, as the standard range is sufficient for most ears and is more comfortable for the patient, which increases the likelihood that both ears will be tested.

Obtaining a Seal

The otoscopic examination provides an opportunity to judge the size of the probe tip appropriate for the patient. A standard admittance probe tip will be inserted in the ear canal to obtain a hermetic seal and thus should be large enough to afford a snug fit. If using a screening tip, this will be held against the canal during the test and should be larger than the canal opening, but smaller than the concha bowl for a good fit. With some devices, the tympanometer itself is a hand-held device, which is used with a screening probe tip held against the opening of the ear canal. As with otoscopy, gently pulling horizontally back on the pinna straightens the ear canal and makes it less likely that it will be collapsed when the probe tip is inserted. Although beginning clinicians often have difficulty obtaining a hermetic seal to complete the test and may be notified repeatedly that there is a "leak," the art of consistently obtaining an appropriate seal comes with practice. However, on occasion, even the most seasoned clinician will have difficulty obtaining a seal for tympanometry. If selecting a different probe tip does not solve the problem, reexamine the ear with the otoscope to make sure you have the correct angle on the ear canal when inserting the probe tip. Note that an ear with a patent PE tube or a perforation may register a very large equivalent volume including the ear canal, middle ear, and mastoid air spaces. This volume may exceed the measurable limit on some equipment, causing the instrument to register a leak. Similarly, some equipment may register a blocked probe in the presence of a normal but very small ear canal volume, such as in an infant ear. It is impor-

tant to know these limitations for your equipment and what the upper and lower limits of measurable equivalent volume are.

Most systems default to a starting pressure of +200 daPa and then sweep pressure from a positive to negative direction. However, the difficulty in obtaining a seal may be increased by starting the sweep with positive air pressure, as this may act to push the probe out of the ear canal. When having difficulty maintaining a seal, changing to a negative starting pressure may allow a tympanogram to be obtained, because in this case the starting pressure is not acting to push the probe out of the ear. However, it should be noted that negative-to-positive pressure sweeps may result in increased complexity of tympanogram shape (Shanks & Wilson, 1986).

Considerations When Testing Infants

Based on results from several studies, low-frequency tympanometry measurements are generally considered valid and reliable predictors of middle ear function by about 7 months of age (Cantekin et al, 1980; Hunter & Margolis, 1992; Keefe & Levi, 1996; Roush, Bryant, Mundy, Zeisel, & Roberts, 1995). Several studies have investigated the developmental changes in traditional immittance measurements in infants to elucidate this issue (De Chicchis, Todd & Nozza, 2000; Holte, Margolis, & Cavanaugh, 1991; Meyer & Jardine, 1997; Roush et al, 1995).

Two studies of infants and children, with participants ranging in age from 6 months to 4 years, reported a small but statistically significant increase in static acoustic admittance and a decrease in tympanometric width as a function of age (De Chicchis et al, 2000; Roush et al, 1995). Holte et al (1991) conducted a longitudinal study of multifrequency tympanometry in newborn infants through 4 months of age. They reported that admittance magnitude stayed approximately the same across age for a 226 Hz probe tone but increased with age at higher frequencies (400 to 900 Hz). However, at all frequencies above 226 Hz, irregular tympanometric patterns were observed that were inconsistent with the Vanhuyse model, which demonstrates the progression of tympanogram shapes with increasing probe frequency in multifrequency tympanometry (Hunter & Margolis, 1992). Holte et al showed that, by 4 months of age, tympanograms followed the Vanhuyse model fairly consistently up to 900 Hz. They also reported that, while general changes in development of Y_{tm} and θ_Y were observed, these responses were characterized by substantial intersubject variability.

> **Pearl**
>
> • Unsure about the Vanhuyse model? A good reading of Hunter and Margolis (1992) will go a long way toward improving your understanding of this model and demonstrate just how important it is in interpreting tympanometry results.

To investigate suggestions that pressure-induced changes in the external ear canal influenced middle ear measurements, Holte et al (1991) introduced positive and negative pressure pulses in the ear canal and used video monitoring to determine a percent change in ear canal diameter relative to resting diameter. They found that the pressure-induced change in ear canal diameter steadily decreased as a function of age, dropping from an 18% change at 1–7 days to no change at 4 months of age. They reported that in some cases, where no ear canal wall motion was observed, there were still multiple peaks in the 226 Hz tympanograms. Correlations that were computed to assess the relationship between complexity of tympanometric patterns and amount of wall distention failed to reach significance. Based on this result, the authors suggested that ear canal wall mobility and tympanometric patterns were not related.

Meyer et al (1997) documented changes in Y_a tympanograms for a single infant using 226 and 1000 Hz probe frequencies. They reported results similar to those of Holte et al (1991), in that change in resonant frequency progressed from low to high frequency with age. This was evidenced by more complex tympanometric shapes observed with a 226 Hz probe tone at younger ages. Results when using a 226 Hz probe tone showed gradual change from complex to simple tympanometric shapes with age, indicating a shift from a mass- to a stiffness-dominated middle ear system with age. The opposite effect was observed for tympanometric results for the 1000 Hz probe tone, with tympanograms gradually changing from simple to more complex with age. In addition, Meyer et al reported a flat 1000 Hz tympanogram in conjunction with a normal 226 Hz tympanogram during a period of time when the infant presented with middle ear pathology.

Tympanogram Interpretation

Children Older Than 7 Months of Age

Single-frequency 226 Hz admittance-vector tympanometry is universally used in clinical assessment for adults and children. Tympanograms were initially interpreted qualitatively in terms of pressure continua (Jerger, 1970; Lidén, 1969). A tympanogram with normal single-peaked shape, normal amplitude, and normal peak pressure is a Type A. Type B is flat, indicative of ears with effusion or tympanic membrane perforation; Type C displays a peak with excessive

negative pressure (usually exceeding –150 to –200 daPa). Other subtypes were used to describe various conditions, such as Type A_S, normal pressure peak but abnormally shallow amplitude, often seen in otosclerosis. Many audiologists and physicians continue to refer to tympanograms using this system. However, in addition to describing the shape of the tympanogram, most audiologists provide a quantitative assessment made possible with the advent of calibrated admittance instruments and ANSI (2012) S3.39. This allows for a quantitative assessment of *peak Y_{tm}*, *TW*, V_{ea}, and tympanometric peak pressure (TPP).

The next step is to determine whether the tympanogram is within normal limits. Some general guidelines will be provided, but normative data collected with your preferred instrumentation settings is ideal. For all ages, flat tympanograms, where Y_{tm} is 0 mmho, are abnormal, with the caveat that a flat tympanogram with a standard pressure range may be masking an ear with extreme negative pressure. Flat tympanograms with large equivalent volumes ($V_{ea} \geq 1$ cm^3) are suggestive of a patent PE tube or a perforation, and if pre- and post-PE-tube insertion measurement are available, a change in $V_{ea} \geq 0.4$ cm^3 suggests that the tube is patent (Shanks, Stelmachowicz, Beauchaine, & Schulte, 1992). These criteria were obtained with insert-type probe tips with a 226 Hz probe tone as measured at +200 daPa in children ranging from infancy to 7 years. A large V_{ea} in an ear without a tube is suggestive of a tympanic membrane perforation, and thus a medical referral is indicated.

A flat tympanogram with normal ear canal volume and a tympanogram with an abnormally low *peak Y_{tm}* or abnormally wide *TW* are suggestive of middle ear effusion (MEE). Specifically, Nozza, Bluestone, Kardatzke, and Bachman (1994) found that a *TW* criterion of > 275 daPa had the best test performance for detecting MEE in children 1 to 12 years of age. For ages 6 to 30 months, a value of *peak Y_{tm}* < 0.2 mmho is suggestive of MEE. This is also the case for ears with *peak Y_{tm}* ≥ 0.3 mmho, but *TW* > 235 daPa (Roush et al, 1995). These criteria were obtained with an automatic tympanometer with a 226 Hz probe tone and a +200 daPa compensation. American Speech-Language-Hearing Association (ASHA) (1997) screening criteria suggest that children 1 year to school age should be referred for retest if *peak Y_{tm}* < 0.3 mmho with a +200 daPa compensation or with *TW* > 200 daPa (see also American Academy of Audiology [AAA], 2011; Margolis & Hunter, 1999). TPP is an indicator of middle ear pressure and should be reported. However, efforts to use TPP as a screening tool and basis for referral have not been successful (see Margolis & Hunter, 1999, for a review).

Children Younger Than 7 Months of Age

As noted previously, the young-infant middle ear is dominated more by mass contributions than by stiffness. While the exact developmental time course is not known, 226 Hz tympanometry measurements are, for the most part, adult-like by about 6 to 8 months of age and are generally considered valid predictors of middle ear function (Hunter & Margolis, 1992; Keefe et al, 1993; Roush et al, 1995). Although research suggests that 1000 Hz tympanometry is more sensitive to changes in middle ear status in infants, compared with 226 Hz tympanometry (Alaerts, Luts, & Wouters, 2007; Calandruccio, Fitzgerald, & Prieve, 2006), there is no consensus regarding a single method for interpreting 1000 Hz tympanometric data. Similar to strategies for interpreting 226 Hz tympanometry, both quantitative and qualitative methods have been proposed.

Margolis, Bass-Ringdahl, Hanks, Holte, and Zapala (2003) and Kei et al (2003) evaluated 1000 Hz tympanometry results and reported normative data, including compensated admittance *magnitude* values. Margolis et al suggested a low cutoff value (5th percentile for peak-to-*negative*-tail compensated admittance) of 0.60 mmho, while Kei et al (2003) suggested a low cutoff value (5th percentile for peak-to-*positive*-tail compensated admittance) of 0.39 mmho. Margolis et al used their suggested pass/fail criterion of 0.60 mmho and assessed 1000 Hz tympanometric test performance in predicting whether a newborn infant passed or failed a distortion product otoacoustic emission (DPOAE) test. Using the DPOAE test outcome as the reference standard, the 1000 Hz test had a specificity of 91% but a sensitivity of only 50%.

The 1000 Hz Y_a tympanograms of a neonate who was referred for failing a newborn hearing screening (DPOAE) for the right ear as well as a secondary ABR screening with a click stimulus at 30 dBnHL are shown in **Fig. 12.4**. The infant passed both screening tests for the left ear. Note that the right tympanogram is essentially flat, while the left tympanogram shows a relatively normal shape. The infant is being followed for right ear conductive hearing loss, which is expected to be transient. Application of normative data from Kei et al (2003) and Margolis et al (2003) to these results would result in a similar classification for the right ear, but peak Y_{tm} for the left ear falls in between the two suggested criterion of 0.39 and 0.60 mmho, respectively.

A different quantitative analysis method proposed by Margolis and Hunter (2000) utilizes the individual admittance components (conductance, G, and susceptance, B) to generate compensated admittance *component* values. Instead of simply subtracting the admittance magnitude at the positive tympanogram tail from the admittance magnitude at the tympanogram peak, the individual component (G and B) peak-to-tail values are calculated, and then the component compensated admittance (Y_{cc}) is calculated as:

$$|Y_{cc}| = \sqrt{G_{pt}^2 + B_{pt}^2}$$

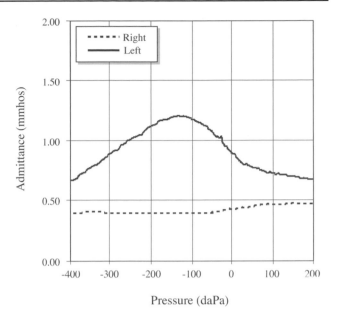

Fig. 12.4 The Y_a 1000 Hz tympanograms for a neonate who failed his newborn hearing screening for the right ear (*dashed line*) and passed on the left ear (*solid line*). The *peak* Y_{tm} on the right was 0.53 mmho with either +200 or −200 daPa compensation.

where G_{pt}^2 and B_{pt}^2 are the squared peak-to-tail values for conductance and susceptance, respectively. The rationale for using the individual components lies in the fact that for adults, when a 226 Hz probe tone is used, the uncompensated peak admittance and admittance at the positive tail have a similar phase angle. However, when a 1000 Hz probe tone is used in an infant ear, the phase angles may not be the same. To estimate the admittance of the middle ear most accurately, it is necessary to calculate admittance using individual admittance components. Several studies have reported data obtained using this analysis method (Calandruccio et al, 2006; Kei, Mazlan, Hickson, Gavranich, & Linning, 2007; Mazlan, Kei, & Hickson, 2009) and suggested that the larger mean admittance values produced with the compensation method (versus admittance magnitude) may allow greater separation between data obtained from normal and abnormal middle ears. This method requires the "extraction" of B and G component data; however, some immittance systems calculate and display component-compensated tympanograms for the user.

Baldwin (2006) used a qualitative analysis method similar to one first proposed by Marchant et al (1986) and a traditional visual classification system (Type A, B, etc.) (Lidén, 1969; Jerger, 1970) to assess middle ear function in 2 to 21-week-old infants. For the Marchant et al (1986) method, a line was drawn between the *susceptance* (B) tympanogram tails at +300 and −400 daPa and a peak susceptance was measured from the baseline to the susceptance peak.

Baldwin (2006) modified this method and, instead, drew a line between the *admittance* tympanogram tails at +200 and –400 daPa (**Fig. 12.5**). A middle ear generating either positive- or negative-going admittance tracings (e.g., "peaks") relative to the drawn line between pressure extremes was classified as having either normal or abnormal middle ear function, respectively; "indeterminate" tracings (with both positive and negative peaks) were put in the negative peak category and were classified as having abnormal middle ear function. Tympanometry results obtained with 226, 678, and 1000 Hz probe tones from 107 infants were organized using the Lidén/Jerger types and the alternative ("Baldwin") method. The infants were grouped as having either normal or disordered middle ear function based on results from a combination of air and bone conduction ABR results and behavioral assessments. The Baldwin method for classifying 1000 Hz tympanograms provided the best results, with sensitivity of 0.99 and specificity of 0.89. This qualitative approach to classifying 1000 Hz tympanograms showed excellent test performance for differentiating between normal and abnormal middle ears for infants 2 to 21 weeks of age and is simple to perform.

Both 226 and 1000 Hz tympanograms from the left ear of a 15-day-old infant who passed a DPOAE screening are shown in **Fig. 12.5**. In this case, the presence of the positive peak would suggest that this ear has normal middle ear function; the 226 Hz tympanogram appears normal too. Tympanograms from the right ear of a 39-day-old infant are shown in **Fig. 12.6**. In this case, the 226 Hz tympanogram appears normal, but the presence of a negative-going admittance tracing with the 1000 Hz tympanogram (right panel) would suggest middle ear dysfunction; this result is consistent with a failed DPOAE screening for the right ear.

While the need to use 1000 Hz-probe-tone tympanometry for young infants is clear and some normative data and interpretation strategies have been published, to date there is no consensus on which specific strategy is best. For a more in-depth review of these interpretation strategies and a summary of normative data, see the individual cited studies above and Kei and Zhao (2012).

> **Pitfall**
>
> - Be careful interpreting equivalent ear canal volume (V_{ea}) data when conducting 1000 Hz tympanometry tests. The straightforward relationship between physical volume and admittance when using a 226 Hz probe tone (e.g., 1 cm³ volume of air has an admittance of 1 mmho) does not hold true when using other frequencies. Clinicians can use 226 Hz probe-tone tympanometry to obtain V_{ea} data and 1000 Hz probe-tone tympanometry to interpret the admittance characteristics of the middle ear. Alternatively, some equipment uses a calculation method to estimate V_{ea}, when using probe tones other than 226 Hz; know what your equipment capabilities are and how to interpret the data.

Sanford et al (2009) examined the test performance of 1000 Hz tympanometry and wideband absorbance in predicting the conductive status (e.g., ear canal and/or middle ear) of ears that passed or referred in newborn hearing screening tests based on DPOAEs. The tests of conductive status in newborn ears included measurements of 1000 Hz tympanograms and wideband absorbance at ambient pressure, as well as wideband tympanograms (e.g., wideband absorbance measured in the presence of

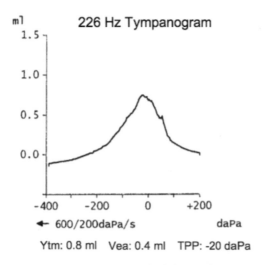
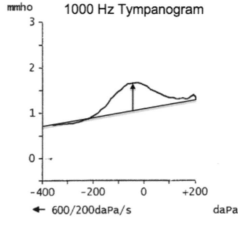

Fig. 12.5 Tympanograms obtained from the left ear of a 15-day-old infant using both 226 and 1000 Hz probe tones. The 1000 Hz tympanogram on the right illustrates a qualitative method of interpreting 1000 Hz tympanograms in young infants; in this case, a positive-going admittance tracing (relative to the horizontal line) would suggest a normal middle ear.

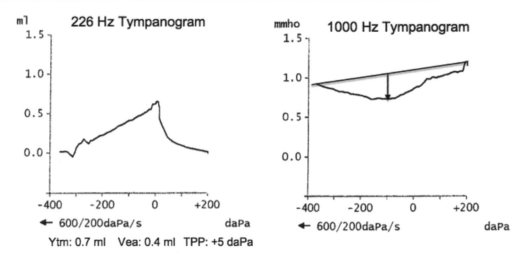

Fig. 12.6 Tympanograms obtained from the right ear of a 39-day-old infant using both 226 and 1000 Hz probe tones. The 1000 Hz tympanogram (*right panel*) illustrates a qualitative method of interpreting 1000 Hz tympanograms in young infants; in this case, a negative-going admittance tracing (relative to the horizontal line) would suggest an ear with middle ear dysfunction.

pressure changes in the ear canal). The Pass group of one-day-old infants included 375 ears, and the Refer group included 80 ears. The Pass ears had higher absorbance on the ambient pressure test than Refer ears in the frequency range of 1000–8000 Hz. The median and interquartile range of the absorbance at ambient pressure from Sanford et al (2009) are plotted in **Fig. 12.7** for both the Pass and Refer groups. Ears that passed the DPOAE screening tended to have higher absorbance than Refer ears in the frequency range of DPOAE testing.

A receiver operating characteristic (ROC)-curve analysis by Sanford et al (2009) revealed that wideband absorbance was more accurate than 1000 Hz tympanometry in predicting DPOAE test outcomes in a newborn hearing screening program. Similar results showing that wideband energy reflectance at ambient pressure had better test performance than 1000 Hz tympanometry in predicting which newborn infants passed or referred on a DPOAE test were reported by Hunter et al (2010). Although these wideband tests show promise as potentially useful diagnostic tools, more evidence is needed across wider age ranges and from ears with a variety of middle ear disorders.

Acoustic Stapedius Reflex Testing

ASR testing typically follows tympanometry, using the same equipment and probe placement, with ear canal pressure adjusted to peak tympanometric pressure for maximum sensitivity. For screening purposes, many systems offer an automated search for the presence of a reflex at several levels, stopping when a criterion admittance shift is obtained (typically 0.02 or 0.03 mmho for a 226 Hz probe tone). Two important caveats are related to ASR testing in young infants. A 226 Hz probe tone results in absent

reflexes in the majority of neonates, whereas with a 1000 Hz probe tone, nearly all neonates have a measurable reflex. Second, ipsilateral ASR activator signals are typically calibrated in a 2 cm³ coupler to establish a dB HL value. This calibration is not appropriate for infant ears and underestimates the level of the reflex activator in the infant ear canal. Otherwise, it has been shown that ASR thresholds for children are similar to those for adults. For more in-depth discussions and case study presentations of ASR testing in infant populations, see Mazlan et al (2009), Kei (2012), and Kei and Zhao (2012), respectively.

> **Pitfall**
>
> - To avoid confusion, when reporting contralateral ASR results, it is helpful to specify which ear received the activator stimulus (e.g., with the probe in the left ear and activator in the right ear, ASR results were within normal limits).

When an ASR occurs, there is a frequency-dependent shift in admittance. In adults, the reflex causes a decrease in admittance at frequencies below ~ 700 Hz and an increase in admittance above this frequency, with a positive peak admittance shift around 1000 Hz (Feeney et al, 2003) (**Fig. 12.8**). This shift as a function of frequency is age dependent, although the time course for the development of an adult-like ASR shift is not known. Feeney and Sanford (2005) showed that, for 6-week-old infants, there was a maximal negative shift in admittance at 1000 Hz during a contralateral ASR reflex, compared with the maximal positive shift for adults (**Fig. 12.8**). Although the time course is not known, the zero-

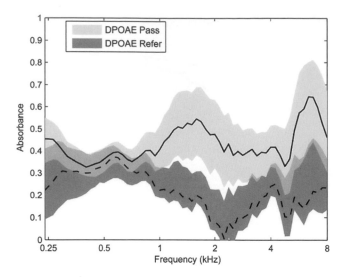

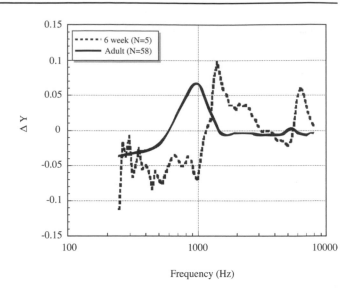

Fig. 12.7 Ambient energy absorbance from newborn ears that passed or referred on a DPOAE screening test. Shaded areas represent the 25th to 75th percentile ranges, with the light gray shading representative of the Pass group and the dark gray shading representative of the Refer group. Dashed and solid lines represent the 50th percentile for the refer and pass groups, respectively. From "Physiologyical Mechanisms Assessed by Aural Acoustic Transfer Functions" by M.P. Feeney and D.H. Keefe in Translational Perspectives in Auditory Neuroscience: Hearing Across the Lifespan—Assesssment and Disorders (p. 116) by K.L. Tremblay and R.F. Burkard (Eds.). Copyright © 2012 Plural Publishing Inc. All rights reserved. Used with Permission.

Fig. 12.8 The average shift in admittance as a function of frequency during the contralateral ASR for five infants from Feeney and Sanford (2005) and 58 ears for 34 adults from Feeney et al (2003). The reflex shifts were normalized by dividing the shift by the baseline admittance ($\Delta Y = [|Y|$ activator $- |Y|$ baseline] $/ |Y|$ baseline). Note that at 1000 Hz there was a maximal positive shift in admittance for the adults and a maximal negative shift in admittance for the infants.

crossing point will shift down in frequency with development and at some point would occur near 1000 Hz, presumably making the reflex difficult to detect with a 1000 Hz probe tone. It is suggested that a wideband probe signal such as a chirp or click would be more successful in detecting a reflex across development in infants than a single frequency.

Keefe, Fitzpatrick, Liu, Sanford, and Gorga (2010) investigated the usefulness of including a wideband ASR test as part of a wideband ATF test battery aimed at classifying ears that passed or referred on an OAE newborn hearing screening test. ASR thresholds were obtained in 97% and 90% of infants who passed or referred on an OAE screening test, respectively. A wideband test battery, which included ASR tests, showed improved test performance in predicting a NHS outcome, relative to 1000 Hz tympanometry and a wideband test battery without ASR tests. However, the wideband test battery with ASR was not significantly better at classifying ears than were wideband tests without ASR included. Additional data on acoustic reflexes in infants across the first 6 months of life, when the middle ear is undergoing significant change, will help further our understanding of infant auditory development and reveal potential uses of ASR in audiological evaluation of infants (Keefe et al, 1993; Sanford & Feeney, 2008).

Discussion Questions

1. What components are included in a vector tympanogram, and how do they relate to the function of the middle ear?

2. What quantitative and qualitative descriptors should be used to report on the results of vector tympanometry?

3. Is there a reason to obtain special middle ear measurement equipment for pediatric assessment? Why or why not?

4. You are seeing a 5-year-old child who recently had PE tubes inserted. His hearing has improved in one ear, but he continues to have a conductive hearing loss in the other ear. The otoscopic examination reveals that the tubes appear to be in place in both ears. What can admittance measurement contribute to the assessment of this child?

5. An 18-month-old is referred to you for a hearing evaluation by her pediatrician because of parental concern that she hasn't started to talk. You are unable to condition the child for VRA, but you obtain normal 226 Hz tympanograms and normal OAEs. In addition to scheduling the child for repeat behavioral assessment, what additional test(s) should be conducted or scheduled?

◆ Acknowledgments

The authors thank Monica Feeney for the preparation of figures. The content of this chapter does not represent the views of the Department of Veterans Affairs or of the United States Government.

References

Alaerts, J., Luts, H., & Wouters, J. (2007). Evaluation of middle ear function in young children: clinical guidelines for the use of 226- and 1,000-Hz tympanometry. Otology & Neurotology, 28(6), 727–732.

Allen, J. B., Jeng, P. S., & Levitt, H. J. (2005). Evaluation of human middle ear function via an acoustic power assessment. Journal of Rehabilitation Research and Development, 42(4, Suppl 2), 63–78.

American Academy of Audiology. (2011). Clinical practice guidelines for childhood hearing screening. Retrieved from http://www.audiology.org/resources/documentlibrary/Documents/ChildhoodScreeningGuidelines.pdf

American National Standards Institute. (2012). Specifications for instruments to measure aural acoustic impedance and admittance (aural acoustic immittance) (ANSI S3.39–1987–R2012). New York, NY: ANSI.

American Speech-Language-Hearing Association. (1997). Guidelines for audiologic screening. Rockville, MD: ASHA.

Baldwin, M. (2006). Choice of probe tone and classification of trace patterns in tympanometry undertaken in early infancy. International Journal of Audiology, 45(7), 417–427.

Berlin, C. I., Hood, L. J., Morlet, T., Wilensky, D., St John, P., Montgomery, E., & Thibodaux, M. (2005). Absent or elevated middle ear muscle reflexes in the presence of normal otoacoustic emissions: a universal finding in 136 cases of auditory neuropathy/dys-synchrony. Journal of the American Academy of Audiology, 16(8), 546–553.

Calandruccio, L., Fitzgerald, T. S., & Prieve, B. A. (2006). Normative multifrequency tympanometry in infants and toddlers. Journal of the American Academy of Audiology, 17(7), 470–480.

Cantekin, E. I., Bluestone, C. D., Fria, T. J., Stool, S. E., Beery, Q. C., & Sabo, D. L. (1980). Identification of otitis media with effusion in children. The Annals of Otology, Rhinology & Laryngology. Supplement, 89(3 Pt 2), 190–195.

De Chicchis, A. R., Todd, N. W., & Nozza, R. J. (2000). Developmental changes in aural acoustic admittance measurements. Journal of the American Academy of Audiology, 11(2), 97–102.

Eby, T. L., & Nadol, J. B., Jr. (1986). Postnatal growth of the human temporal bone. Implications for cochlear implants in children. The Annals of Otology, Rhinology, and Laryngology, 95(4 Pt 1), 356–364.

Feeney, M. P., & Keefe, D. H. (2012). Physiological mechanisms assessed by aural acoustic transfer functions. In K. Tremblay & R. Burkard (Eds.), Translational perspectives in auditory neuroscience: hearing across the life span—assessment and disorders (pp. 85–122). San Diego, CA: Plural.

Feeney, M. P., & Sanford, C. A. (2005). Detection of the acoustic stapedius reflex in infants using wideband energy reflectance and admittance. Journal of the American Academy of Audiology, 16(5), 278–290.

Feeney, M. P., Keefe, D. H., & Marryott, L. P. (2003). Contralateral acoustic reflex thresholds for tonal activators using wideband reflectance and admittance measurements. Journal of Speech, Language, and Hearing Research: JSLHR, 46, 128–136.

Holte, L., Margolis, R. H., & Cavanaugh, R. M., Jr. (1991). Developmental changes in multifrequency tympanograms. Audiology, 30(1), 1–24.

Hunter, L. L., & Margolis, R. H. (1992). Multifrequency tympanometry: Current clinical application. American Journal of Audiology, 1, 33–43.

Hunter, L. L., Feeney, M. P., Lapsley-Miller, J. A., Jeng, P. S., & Bohning, S. (2010). Wideband reflectance in newborns: normative regions and relationship to hearing-screening results. Ear and Hearing, 31(5), 599–610.

Ikui, A., Sando, I., Sudo, M., & Fujita, S. (1997). Postnatal change in angle between the tympanic annulus and surrounding structures. Computer-aided three-dimensional reconstruction study. The Annals of Otology, Rhinology, and Laryngology, 106(1), 33–36.

Jerger, J. (1970). Clinical experience with impedance audiometry. Archives of Otolaryngology, 92(4), 311–324.

Keefe, D. H., & Feeney, M. P. (2009). Principles of acoustic immittance and acoustic transfer functions. In J. Katz (Ed.), Handbook of clinical audiology (6th ed., pp. 125–156). Baltimore, MD: Lippincott Williams and Wilkins.

Keefe, D. H., & Levi, E. (1996). Maturation of the middle and external ears: acoustic power-based responses and reflectance tympanometry. Ear and Hearing, 17(5), 361–373.

Keefe, D. H., & Simmons, J. L. (2003). Energy transmittance predicts conductive hearing loss in older children and adults. The Journal of the Acoustical Society of America, 114(6 Pt 1), 3217–3238.

Keefe, D. H., Bulen, J. C., Arehart, K. H., & Burns, E. M. (1993). Ear-canal impedance and reflection coefficient in human infants and adults. The Journal of the Acoustical Society of America, 94(5), 2617–2638.

Keefe, D. H., Fitzpatrick, D., Liu, Y. W., Sanford, C. A., & Gorga, M. P. (2010). Wideband acoustic-reflex test in a test battery to predict middle-ear dysfunction. Hearing Research, 263(1-2), 52–65.

Keefe, D. H., Folsom, R. C., Gorga, M. P., Vohr, B. R., Bulen, J. C., & Norton, S. J. (2000). Identification of neonatal hearing impairment: ear-canal measurements of acoustic admittance and reflectance in neonates. Ear and Hearing, 21(5), 443–461.

Kei, J. (2012). Acoustic stapedial reflexes in healthy neonates: normative data and test-retest reliability. Journal of the American Academy of Audiology, 23(1), 46–56.

Kei, J., & Zhao, F. (2012). Assessing middle ear function in infants. San Diego, CA: Plural.

Kei, J., Allison-Levick, J., Dockray, J., Harrys, R., Kirkegard, C., Wong, J., & Tudehope, D. (2003). High-frequency (1000 Hz) tympanometry in normal neonates. Journal of the American Academy of Audiology, 14(1), 20–28.

Kei, J., Mazlan, R., Hickson, L., Gavranich, J., & Linning, R. (2007). Measuring middle ear admittance in newborns using 1000 Hz tympanometry: a comparison of methodologies. Journal of the American Academy of Audiology, 18(9), 739–748.

Lidén, G. (1969). The scope and application of current audiometric tests. The Journal of Laryngology and Otology, 83(6), 507–520.

Marchant, C. D., McMillan, P. M., Shurin, P. A., Johnson, C. E., Turczyk, V. A., Feinstein, J. C., & Panek, D. M. (1986). Objective diagnosis of otitis media in early infancy by tympanometry and ipsilateral acoustic reflex thresholds. The Journal of Pediatrics, 109(4), 590–595.

Margolis, R. H., & Hunter, L. L. (1999). Tympanometry: Basic principles and clinical applications. In F. E. Musiek & W. F. Rintelmann (Eds.), Contemporary perspectives in hearing assessment (pp. 89–130). Boston, MA: Allyn and Bacon.

Margolis, R. H., & Hunter, L. L. (2000). Acoustic immittance measurements. In R. Roeser, M. Valente, & H. Hosford-Dunn (Eds.), Audiology diagnosis (pp. 381–423). New York, NY: Thieme.

Margolis, R. H., Bass-Ringdahl, S., Hanks, W. D., Holte, L., & Zapala, D. A. (2003). Tympanometry in newborn infants—1 kHz norms. Journal of the American Academy of Audiology, 14(7), 383–392.

Mazlan, R., Kei, J., & Hickson, L. (2009). Test-retest reliability of the acoustic stapedial reflex test in healthy neonates. Ear and Hearing, 30(3), 295–301.

Merchant, G. R., Horton, N. J., & Voss, S. E. (2010). Normative reflectance and transmittance measurements on healthy newborn and 1-month-old infants. Ear and Hearing, 31(6), 746–754.

Meyer, S. E., Jardine, C. A., & Deverson, W. (1997). Developmental changes in tympanometry: a case study. British Journal of Audiology, 31(3), 189–195.

Nozza, R. J., Bluestone, C. D., Kardatzke, D., & Bachman, R. (1994, Aug). Identification of middle ear effusion by aural acoustic admittance and otoscopy. Ear and Hearing, 15(4), 310–323.

Roush, J., Bryant, K., Mundy, M., Zeisel, S., & Roberts, J. (1995). Developmental changes in static admittance and tympanometric width in infants and toddlers. Journal of the American Academy of Audiology, 6(4), 334–338.

Ruah, C. B., Schachern, P. A., Zelterman, D., Paparella, M. M., & Yoon, T. H. (1991). Age-related morphologic changes in the human tympanic membrane. A light and electron microscopic study. Archives of Otolaryngology–Head & Neck Surgery, 117(6), 627–634.

Sanford, C. A., & Feeney, M. P. (2008). Effects of maturation on tympanometric wideband acoustic transfer functions in human infants. The Journal of the Acoustical Society of America, 124(4), 2106–2122.

Sanford, C. A., Keefe, D. H., Liu, Y.-W., Fitzpatrick, D. F., McCreery, R. W., Lewis, D. E., & Gorga, M. P. (2009). Sound-conduction effects on distortion-product otoacoustic emission screening outcomes in newborn infants: test performance of wideband acoustic transfer functions and 1-kHz tympanometry. Ear and Hearing, 30(6), 635–652.

Saunders, J. C., Kaltenbach, J. A., & Relkin, E. M. (1983). The structural and functional development of the outer and middle ear. In R. Romand (Ed.), Development of auditory and vestibular systems. New York, NY: Academic Press.

Shanks, J. E., & Wilson, R. H. (1986). Effects of direction and rate of ear-canal pressure changes on tympanometric measures. Journal of Speech, Language, and Hearing Research: JSLHR, 29(1), 11–19.

Shanks, J. E., Stelmachowicz, P. G., Beauchaine, K. L., & Schulte, L. (1992). Equivalent ear canal volumes in children pre- and post-tympanostomy tube insertion. Journal of Speech, Language, and Hearing Research: JSLHR, 35(4), 936–941.

Werner, L. A., Levi, E. C., & Keefe, D. H. (2010). Ear-canal wideband acoustic transfer functions of adults and two- to nine-month-old infants. Ear and Hearing, 31(5), 587–598.

Wiley, T. L., & Fowler, C. G. (1997). Acoustic immittance measures in clinical audiology. San Diego, CA: Singular.

Chapter 13

Otoacoustic Emissions in Infants and Children

Beth A. Prieve and Lisa M. Lamson

Key Points

- Otoacoustic emissions (OAEs) are excellent screening tools for detection of hearing loss in newborns.
- OAEs are an integral part of the pediatric diagnostic test battery. They can help determine site-of-lesion and can be used as cross-checks against other results from the test battery.
- Published literature is available to guide us in using OAEs in screening and diagnostic test batteries.

Kemp's (1978) description of otoacoustic emissions (OAEs) has significantly changed our understanding of cochlear processing and has impacted clinical audiology. OAE measurements are now a standard part of the pediatric test battery, helping us in the identification and diagnosis of hearing loss and assisting in choosing appropriate (re)habilitation. OAE measurements are noninvasive and quick to perform, essential attributes for pediatric patients. Audiologists can obtain ear-specific information when it cannot be obtained through pure tone audiometry.

The focus of this chapter is to provide basic information about how clinicians can use measures of OAEs in infants and children for identification and diagnosis of hearing loss. Toward this goal, supporting articles have been chosen that illustrate certain points and offer current, relevant literature pertaining to infants and children. This chapter is not meant to be an exhaustive source describing OAEs and their clinical use. There are hundreds of excellent publications about basic properties of OAEs and their clinical use, but reviewing such an extensive bibliography is beyond the scope of this chapter.

Pearl

- Do you want more in-depth knowledge about OAEs? Good sources are books by Dhar and Hall III (2012) and Robinette and Glattke (2007).

◆ Important Background Information

Three essential areas of background information are needed for clinicians to use OAEs effectively in the clinic. First, it is critical to have a basic understanding of the generation of OAEs so that hearing loss can be properly diagnosed. OAEs are linked to the normal functioning of the outer hair cells (OHCs) and are believed to be a byproduct of cochlear amplifier processing. They reflect mechanical, rather than neural, cochlear responses. OAEs are considered "preneural." Two observations supporting this thinking are that (1) they can be generated even when the eighth nerve has been severed (Siegel & Kim, 1982) and (2) OAEs reverse polarity along with the stimulus. Moreover, OAEs are reduced or absent in persons with cochlear loss. While the majority of hearing loss involves OHC loss and can be detected by OAE testing, some etiologies of hearing loss, such as auditory neuropathy spectrum disorders (ANSD), involve dysfunction of neural pathways and not the cochlea (see Chapter 32 for more information about ANSD). Consequently, OAEs are particularly useful for diagnosing the location of auditory lesions.

The mechanical source for the cochlear amplifier and OAEs is under investigation. Currently, there are two main hypotheses being considered. One hy-

133

pothesis is that somatic motility, which is the rapid changes in outer hair cell length and shape with electrical stimulation, is linked with OAEs (Liberman et al, 2002). The second hypothesis is that the source of the cochlear amplifier and OAEs is in the nonlinearity of the outer hair cell stereocilia bundle (for overview, see Ricci, 2003). It is possible that both OHC somatic motility and stereocilia contribute to the production of OAEs in mammals and that the contributions of these mechanisms change depending on the stimulus level (Liberman, Zuo, & Guinan, 2004).

Second, although OAEs can be evoked with virtually any auditory stimuli, OAEs evoked by clicks (referred to as transient-evoked OAEs, or TEOAE) and two sinusoids (distortion product OAEs) are used clinically. In measuring a TEOAE, a click is presented to the ear at a fixed rate. The OAE occurs in the time period following the click. Responses are averaged to reduce the noise. A typical click level is 75–80 dB peak sound pressure level (pSPL), and often a specialized stimulus presentation paradigm and subtraction process is used to eliminate possible artifacts due to the transducers and middle ear. Two separate waveforms are collected in tandem, which allows determination of whether an OAE is present by analyzing how similar the two responses are to each other. **Fig. 13.1** illustrates the time waveform of a TEOAE in the large panel and the corresponding frequency response in the inset panel.

When using TEAOEs to identify or diagnose hearing loss, the broadband TEAOE in the frequency domain is analyzed into smaller bands, such as half-octave bands. Three response attributes in each band can be used to assess whether the response is an OAE: (1) the absolute level; (2) the emission level compared with the noise level (emission-to-noise ratio, or ENR); and (3) the reproducibility between the two waveforms.

Distortion product OAEs (DPOAEs) are the other type of OAE used clinically. To record DPOAEs, two sinusoids (called primaries) are presented to the ear at the same time. The lower-frequency primary is referred to as f_1, and the higher-frequency primary is f_2. When two primaries are presented to a healthy ear, it will produce intermodulation distortion products that are mathematically related to the frequencies of the primaries. The distortion product at the frequency $2f_1 - f_2$ is the one used clinically. A typical frequency ratio (f_2:f_1) to evoke the DPOAE is 1.22. Common primary levels for f_2 and f_1 are 55 dB SPL and 65 dB SPL, respectively, because research has shown that the mid-level stimuli are better at identifying hearing loss than high-level stimuli (e.g., Stover et al, 1996). Usually, pairs of primaries with a fixed ratio and level difference between f_1 and f_2 are presented sequentially at frequencies matched to those used on the audiogram. Stimuli are presented and DPOAEs averaged for a pair of stimuli before presentation of the next pair of stimuli. DPOAE level at $2f_1 - f_2$ is plotted as a function of f_2 frequency by the solid line, and the corresponding noise is represented by a dashed line, in **Fig. 13.2**.

This type of recording and display of DPOAEs is often referred to as a "DP-gram." To decide whether a DPOAE is present, absolute DPOAE level is used or the DPOAE level compared with the noise (ENR). In most clinical equipment, the noise is the average level in a few frequency bands lower and higher in frequency than the DPOAE frequency.

Finally, it is essential for clinicians to understand that OAEs change level and frequency content as the infant/child develops. TEOAE and DPOAE levels are higher in newborns than they are in adults (for re-

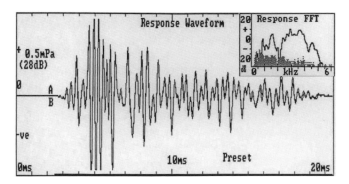

Fig. 13.1 The large panel illustrates a TEOAE plotted as a function of time for an infant aged 2 months. The inset shows TEOAE level (*open area*) and noise level (*shaded areas*) as a function of frequency. The TEOAE was evoked by an 80 dB pSPL click.

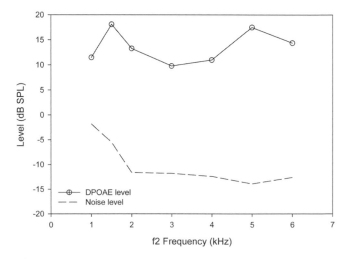

Fig. 13.2 "DP-gram" from an infant aged 6 months. The solid line illustrates DPOAE level as a function of frequency, and the dashed line is the corresponding noise.

view, see Prieve, 2007). Moreover, TEAOE and DPOAE levels in infants are higher than they are in older children and young adults, and children aged 1–5 years have higher OAE levels than older children and adults. The changes in OAE levels across age are frequency-dependent, with no significant decrease for frequencies 1500 Hz and higher (Prieve, Fitzgerald, & Schulte, 1997; Prieve, Fitzgerald, Schulte, & Kemp, 1997). Among preterm infants, DPOAE and TEOAE levels increase with postconception age (Smurzynski, 1994). In addition, TEOAE levels increase between birth and 4 weeks of age (Prieve, Hancur-Bucci, & Preston, 2009; Welch et al, 1996).

Pitfall

- Although there are differences in TEOAE and DPOAE levels with age, there are few age-dependent norms for clinical use.

◆ Screening

Newborns

DPOAEs and TEOAEs, as well as screening auditory brainstem response (SABR), are recommended by the Joint Committee on Infant Hearing (JCIH) as screening tools in universal newborn hearing screening programs (Joint Committee on Infant Hearing [JCIH], 2007). The JCIH recommended that SABR, not OAEs, be used as the screening tool in the NICU because of the possibility that infants may have normal OHC function but neural hearing loss. In the well-infant nursery, OAEs or SABR may be utilized, with both screening and rescreening using the same technology.

Numerous articles have been published about screening programs that have used OAEs, either alone or in combination with SABR. Data from screening programs with large numbers of babies demonstrate that OAE is a feasible screening tool; 90 to 96% of babies pass screening criteria. Factors affecting the percentages of babies passing include the use of different pass criteria, length of training of personnel, ambient noise, and age of babies at time of test (Prieve, 2007). Most important to consider, however, is how well TEOAEs and DPOAEs actually identify hearing loss.

To determine how well a test identifies hearing loss, all infants, whether they pass or do not pass a hearing screening, must have their screening outcome compared with their hearing status (normal hearing or hearing loss) using a "gold standard." There are many gold standards that can be used to evaluate screening accuracy, such as TB-ABR thresh-

olds or behavioral, audiometric thresholds obtained when the infant is older. One large-scale, multicenter study in which behavioral thresholds were used as the gold standard was funded by the National Institutes of Health (NIH). It was designed to determine which screening tool (TEOAEs, DPOAEs, or SABRs), identified hearing loss with the greatest accuracy. A total of 7170 infants were enrolled in the study, which included 4478 infants who were cared for in the NICU. The remaining babies were cared for in the well-baby nursery and included 353 well babies with risk indicators for hearing loss (JCIH, 1994). TEOAEs were evoked by 80 dB pSPL clicks, DPOAEs were evoked using two pairs of primaries at different levels (f_2 level = 50 dB SPL; f_1 level = 65 dB SPL; f_1 and f_2 levels both 75 dB SPL), and SABRs were evoked by click levels of 30 dB nHL. A computerized test program was used that randomized the order of tests in both ears. Details for passing criteria, stopping rules, noise/artifact rejection, and response filtering can be found in Gorga et al (2000), Norton, Gorga, Widen, Vohr, et al (2000), and Sininger et al (2000).

Of the total number of infants, ~ 3100 had their hearing tested behaviorally using visual reinforcement audiometry (VRA) with insert earphones when they were 8–10 months of age. Minimal response levels (MRLs) were measured to pulsed, frequency-modulated tones presented at 1000 Hz, 2000 Hz, and 4000 Hz and to speech presented monitored-live voice (MLV) to obtain a speech awareness threshold (SAT). The lowest level at which stimuli were presented was 20 dB HL, and the intensity step size was 10 dB (Widen et al, 2000). Minimal response levels less than 30 dB HL were considered to be consistent with normal hearing sensitivity. Minimal response levels equal to or higher than 30 dB HL were considered to be indicative of hearing loss. The MRLs were used as the "gold standard" against which screening results were compared. Receiver operating characteristic (ROC) curves were constructed for TEOAEs and DPOAEs by comparing different OAE ENRs at 1, 2, or 4 kHz to the MRL of the corresponding frequency. The "best" ENR at any of the three frequencies was compared against the SAT MRL. For construction of SABR ROC curves, different F_{sp} values, which are an ABR equivalent of signal-to-noise ratio, were compared with MRLs obtained using each of the four stimuli (for a description of F_{sp}, refer to Sininger et al, 2000). The area under the ROC curve is an indication of how well the screening test identified normally hearing and hearing-impaired ears, with 1.0 indicating that hearing status was identified perfectly. The areas under the ROC curves for the screening tools ranged from 0.70 to 0.92 when infants suspected of having progressive hearing loss and middle ear pathology were excluded.

Based on these ROC areas, several important conclusions can be made. First of all, no area was 1.0, indicating that no screening test identified hearing loss with 100% accuracy. Second, TEOAEs, DPOAEs and SABR all identified hearing loss with approximately the same accuracy, although some small differences were noted. DPOAEs evoked by mid-level primaries (f_1 level = 65 dB SPL and f_2 level = 50 dB SPL) identified hearing loss better those evoked by primaries presented at 75 dB SPL. TEOAEs and DPOAEs evoked by mid-level stimuli outperformed SABR slightly at identification of hearing loss at 2000 Hz and 4000 Hz, SAT, and pure tone average (PTA) based on hearing loss at 2000 Hz and 4000 Hz. Screening ABR outperformed TEOAEs and DPOAEs at identification of hearing loss at 1000 Hz and was slightly better at identifying hearing loss using a PTA that included 1000 Hz. All of the screening tools identified almost 100% of moderate, severe and profound hearing losses, but mild hearing loss was identified only at a rate of ~ 50%. Another important finding from the NIH study was that the percentage of infant passes was similar for SABRs, TEOAEs, and DPOAEs using the mid-level primaries (Norton et al, 2000b).

Based on the NIH study, the question arises: "Are there recommended criteria to use for identification of hearing loss?" **Table 13.1** lists the calculated top and bottom of the range of OAE ENRs, as well as the 25th, 50th, and 75th percentiles of the best DPOAE and TEOAE ENRs at 2000 Hz and 4000 Hz from infants having normal hearing and hearing loss based on PTAs including 2000 Hz and 4000 Hz.

The table indicates that the range of ENRs is different for both types of OAEs in infants with normal hearing and in those with hearing loss; however, there is no one criterion that screening programs can use that will identify hearing loss but "pass" infants with normal hearing. For example, some infants who had normal PTAs did not have measurable DPOAEs or TEOAEs, given that the bottom of the range has ENRs of negative numbers. While the 75th percentile of ENRs for infants with hearing loss indicates that no OAE was present, some infants with hearing loss had DPOAEs and TEOAEs that were between the 50th and 75th percentile of ENRs for infants with normal hearing.

Table 13.1 Calculated lower and upper range and percentiles of TEOAE and DPOAE ENR collected using a newborn screening procedure

	DPOAE, ENR (dB)		TEOAE, ENR (dB)	
	NH	HL	NH	HL
Bottom of range	–8	–28	–5	–30
25%-ile	3	–18	7	–18
50%-ile	5	–10	10	–9
75%-ile	10	–7	15	–5
Top of range	22	8	28	11

Values were calculated from Figure 5 in Norton et al (2000b).

Pearl

- In spite of the fact that there is no criterion that identifies hearing loss perfectly, clinicians should keep in mind that OAEs do detect the majority of moderate, severe, and profound hearing loss.

Knowledge of the results from screening programs using particular pass criteria will allow clinicians to make informed judgments about the characteristics of their own universal newborn hearing screening program. The stimuli and pass criteria for TEOAEs and the DPOAE measures that were used by the NIH study are provided in **Table 13.2**. Other programs have used different "pass" criteria; however, in these studies the results of screening were not compared with behavioral hearing in all children. One large-scale study has used 75% reproducibility in frequency bands at 2000, 3000, and 4000 Hz, rather than ENR (Vohr, Carty, Moore, & Letourneau, 1998) and many other programs use OAEs in combination with SABR (e.g., Prieve & Stevens, 2000; Wessex Universal Neonatal Hearing Screening Trial Group, 1998) to identify hearing loss.

Pearl

- The description and results of the entire NIH newborn hearing screening study can be found in the October 2000 issue of the journal *Ear and Hearing*.

Children

Because of the success of using OAEs in newborn hearing screening programs, OAE screening has also been explored for screening in toddlers (Eiserman et al, 2008) and preschool children (Yin, Bottrell, Clarke, Shacks, & Poulsen, 2009). Eiserman et al (2008) performed TEOAE screening on 4519 children 3 years of age or younger. TEOAEs were screened by laypeople who worked regularly with the children. Of the children who completed the entire screening process, 5.9% were referred for further evaluation. Of those that were referred, 42% had medically identified problems, including middle ear dysfunction, wax in the external ear, and permanent hearing loss. An earlier study compared TEOAE and pure tone screening results in children aged 2.5–3.5 years. The authors concluded that TEOAEs were useful for screening in this population if an audiologist was not available (Beppu, Hattori, & Yanagita, 1997). The use of laypeople as screeners is novel, as the American-Speech-Language-Hearing Association (ASHA) (1997)

Table 13.2 Pass criteria for TEAOEs and DPOAEs used in the NIH study

| | Stimulus | | |
	Type	Levels	Pass Criteria
TEOAE[a]	Customized click	80 dB pSPL	SNR in 4 out of 5, ½-octave bands 3 dB SNR at 1.0 and 1.5 kHz 6 dB SNR at 2, 3, and 4.1 kHz
DPOAE[b]	f_2= 1.0, 1.5, 2.0, 3.0, 4.0 kHz f_2/f_1 ratio = 1.22	f_1 = 65 dB SPL f_2 = 50 dB SPL	SNR at ⅘, f_2 frequencies 3 dB higher than 2 SDs above the mean noise

[a] Norton et al, 2000a
[b] Gorga et al, 2000

recommends that audiologists perform screening in this age range. Yin et al (2009) also found that TEOAE testing in preschools by school nurses was feasible. They reported a 5.5% refer rate; however, they did not report follow-up statistics on the children who referred or passed the screening. Finally, large-scale studies in school-age children have concluded that traditional behavioral screening is preferred over OAE screening (Krueger & Ferguson, 2002; Sabo, Winston, & Macias, 2000; Śliwa et al, 2011; Taylor & Brooks, 2000). In summary, OAEs have potential use as a screening tool for children, but further research is necessary to determine the accuracy of using OAEs to detect hearing loss in this population.

OAEs in the Diagnostic Test Battery

In the diagnostic test battery, TEOAEs and DPOAEs are used differently than for newborn hearing screening. For hearing screening, the goal is to identify the presence of hearing loss. In the diagnostic test battery, OAEs are used to provide ear-specific and frequency-specific information that can assist with site-of-lesion determination and also serve as a cross-check against other results of the test battery.

Once again, the question arises: "What are the best criteria to use as part of a diagnostic test battery for infants and children?" In starting to address this question, clinicians should consider applying more stringent criteria for test battery use than they employ in their newborn hearing screening programs. The prevalence of hearing loss is higher in the population of patients that come to an audiology clinic than in general populations of newborns or children. Infants and children are brought to the audiology clinic because there is a concern about their hearing, which is a risk indicator for hearing loss (JCIH, 2007). Second, when infants and children are being tested at an audiology clinic, the recording conditions are likely to be more optimal than they are in a screening setting. While there are no clear

OAE criteria to be used for infants and children in a diagnostic setting, there are studies that can guide us in choosing reasonable OAE criteria and lead us in developing our own norms. Numerous studies have been published about OAEs in ears with hearing loss, but only a few selected studies are presented in this chapter. These studies included ears with normal hearing and ears with hearing loss, as it is important to know the range for OAEs in ears with normal hearing as well as whether OAEs from ears with hearing loss fall within that "normal" range. Furthermore, these studies used measures obtainable from the equipment. Finally, the population under study included children.

The use of a template that included DPOAEs from ears with normal hearing and hearing loss, which could be used clinically, was pioneered by Gorga et al (1997). In the study, DPOAEs were measured in a total of 1267 ears from 806 participants ranging in age from 1.3 to 96.5 years. The f_2:f_1 ratio was 1.22, the level of f_2 was 55 dB SPL, and the f_1 level was 65 dB SPL. Rules based on ENR, minimum absolute DPOAE level, and test time were used in data collection (see Gorga et al, 1997, for details). Templates were constructed for both DPOAE level and ENR, with a replica of the template for DPOAE level presented in the left panel of **Fig. 13.3**.

The technique for making this type of template was adopted by Nicholson (2003) and Nicholson and Widen (2004) for TEAOEs measured with the ILO88 equipment in both FullScreen and QuickScreen modes (see Robinette & Glattke, 2007, for detailed information on these two types of stimulus/recording paradigms). The template for the FullScreen (middle panel) was based on OAEs measured from 240 ears of 135 participants aged 3.1 to 29.1 years. The template for the QuickScreen data was based on 84 ears of 49 participants aged 1.0 to 17.5 years. In both TEAOE templates, ENR in half-octave bands is plotted, rather than TEOAE level. For both of these templates, the stimulus was a click presented at 80±3 dB pSPL, and stimulus presentation and re-

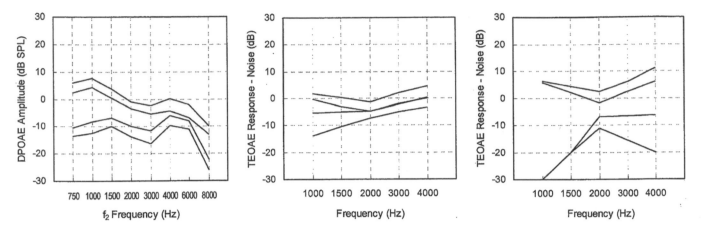

Fig. 13.3   Examples of clinical templates for DPOAEs (left panel), TEOAEs using the FullScreen option (middle panel), and TEOAEs using the QuickScreen option (right panel). Please see text for details. (From Nicholson, N., & Widen, J. E. (2007). Evoked otoacoustic emission in the evaluation of children. In M. Robinette & T. Glattke (Eds.), Clinical Applications of Otoacoustic Emissions (3rd ed.). New York, NY: Thieme, with permission.)

cording were done in the "nonlinear" mode. In addition, there had to be a minimum of 50 averages contributing to the final OAE.

On each of these templates, four solid lines on the graphs depict percentiles for populations of ears where normal hearing was defined as a behavioral threshold of ≤ 20 dB HL at the frequencies listed on the x-axis. The top solid line and the second solid line in each panel represent the 95th and 90th percentile (respectively) of DPOAE level (left panel) or TEAOE ENR (middle and right panels) from populations of ears with hearing loss. If you are testing a patient, and that patient's response is higher than the 95th percentile of OAE responses from ears with hearing loss, then there is reasonable confidence that the ear has normal hearing. The third and fourth solid lines from the top of the graph represent the 10th and 5th percentiles (respectively) of DPOAE levels (left panel) or TEOAE ENR (middle and right panels) from populations of ears with normal hearing. If you are testing a patient and that patient's response falls below the 5th percentile of responses from normally hearing ears, you can be reasonably confident that the ear has hearing loss. The most difficult interpretation of hearing status is if an individual's data fall between the second and third lines from the top. This area is below the 90th percentile of responses from ears with hearing loss and also higher than the 10th percentile of responses from ears with normal hearing. Said another way, the OAE response is within the overlapping range of response values from ears with hearing loss and those with normal hearing. In this case, you cannot be certain whether the ear has normal hearing or hearing loss, although there are examples of individual data with OAE responses in this range that have mild hearing loss (Gorga et al, 2005; Nicholson & Widen, 2007).

Although these templates are extremely useful for clinicians to determine whether an OAE is likely associated with normal hearing or with hearing loss, care must be taken to make sure the stimulus and recording parameters and patient population are similar to those used to construct the template. In addition, it is possible that equipment itself varies. There are currently no standards for acceptable equipment characteristics. Clinical equipment varies greatly in the frequency response of the probes, how the probes are calibrated, how responses are averaged, and how "noise" is defined. In addition, the ages and characteristics of the population on which the template was based must be similar to the patients in the clinician's practice. An example of how normative responses differ between two studies is shown in **Fig. 13.4**.

Fig. 13.4 illustrates cumulative distributions of DPOAE level for patients whose hearing thresholds were classified as normal based on behavioral (Gorga et al, 1997) or ABR (Prieve et al, 2008) threshold testing. The black lines depict data from Gorga et al (1997), in which the precursor of the Scout (Bio-Logic, Grenoble, France) was used to collect data from over 1200 ears in patients aged 1 to 96 years. The gray lines depict data collected using the Otodynamics equipment in 45 ears of infants aged 3 to 35 weeks [median = 10 weeks] from our clinic. The three line types represent data for three different f_2 frequencies. For every f_2 frequency, the DPOAE levels from the mixed population of children and adults are lower than those for the population composed only of infants. A horizontal line is drawn at the 10th percentile, demonstrating that it is quite different for the two populations. For example, at 2000 Hz, the 10th percentile from the study by Gorga et al (1997) is approximately –10 dB SPL, while that for the study

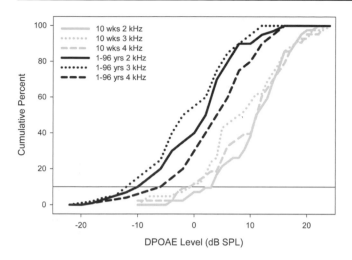

Fig. 13.4 Comparison of cumulative distributions of DPOAE levels from two studies. Data from Gorga et al (1997) are depicted by black lines, and those from Prieve, Calandruccio, Fitzgerald, Mazevski, & Georgantas (2008) in gray lines. See text for details.

by Prieve et al (2008) is ~ 4 dB SPL. Were an infant to be tested who had a DPOAE level of –8 dB SPL at 2000 Hz, that response would fall squarely within the region of "unknown" on the template shown in **Fig. 13.3**, but it actually falls below the 5th percentile of DPOAE levels from normally hearing ears if compared with infants the same age. The important point from this graph is that although the use of published templates is an excellent way to analyze individual clinical data, care must be taken to validate that the template is appropriate for your clinical population and equipment.

Pitfall

- When using normative data from other studies to guide your diagnostic decisions, make sure you know how your equipment, stimulus/recording parameters, and population ages compare.

A few final, important points are worth noting. The accuracy of identification of hearing loss is best from 2000 Hz to 4000 Hz, whether using TEOAEs (Hussain, Gorga, Neely, Keefe, & Peters, 1998; Prieve et al, 1993; Norton, Gorga, Widen, Folsom, et al, 2000; Nicholson, 2003) or DPOAEs (Gorga et al, 1997, 1999, 2000, 2005). At lower frequencies (750 Hz and 1000 Hz) as well as at higher frequencies (6000 Hz and 8000 Hz), identification of hearing loss is poorer. The identification of hearing loss at these frequencies can be improved by performing a multivariate statistical technique, such as logit or discriminant function

analyses. These techniques allow inclusion of OAE and noise levels for multiple frequencies to predict hearing loss at a single, chosen frequency (e.g., Dorn, Piskorski, Gorga, Neely, & Keefe, 1999; Hussain et al, 1998; Nicholson, 2003). Gorga et al (2005) provide "weights" and equations to calculate the logit function output for identification of hearing loss at a given frequency by DPOAEs. These weights and equations, calculated from a large clinical study (Gorga et al, 1997), were successfully applied to a smaller, clinical population using the Scout DPOAE system. Finally, it has also been shown that requiring DPOAEs or TEOAEs to meet criteria at more than one frequency (e.g., 4 out of 5 f_2 test frequencies) improves identification of hearing loss (Gorga et al, 1999, 2005).

Can the Middle Ear Affect OAEs?

Because the stimulus used to evoke OAEs must pass through the middle ear to get to the cochlea, and the OAE must travel back through the middle ear to be recorded in the ear canal, even minor pathologies can alter OAEs. Therefore, it is important to test middle ear function and/or determine the possibility of a conductive hearing loss if OAEs are absent in a diagnostic evaluation. TEOAE and DPOAE levels are reduced, but not usually to the point that they are absent, in infants and children having negative tympanometric peak pressure (measured from a tympanogram) ["Type C"] (Choi, Pafitis, Zalzal, Herer, & Patel, 1999; Hof, Anteunis, Chenault, & van Dijk, 2005; Hof, Dijk, Chenault, & Anteunism 2005; Lonsbury-Martin, Martin, McCoy, & Whitehead, 1994; Koike & Wetmore, 1999; Koivunen, Uhari, Laitakari, Alho, & Luotonen, 2000; Owens, McCoy, Lonsbury-Martin, & Martin, 1993; Prieve et al, 2008). The amount of OAE level reduction does not appear to be related to the severity of the negative pressure (Koike & Wetmore, 1999; Trine, Hirsch, & Margolis, 1993; Prieve et al, 2008). In a within-infant study, it was found that the mean TEOAE reduction was ~ 4 dB across frequency bands for mean changes in tympanometric peak pressure of –169 daPa (Prieve et al, 2008). While this was a significant change, it did not significantly change whether the infants passed a criterion of 6 dB ENR in all bands centered at 2000, 3000, and 4000 Hz. Small reductions in pass rate have been reported for children as well (Hof, Dijk et al, 2005; Koike & Wetmore, 1999). While reductions in OAE levels due to slight middle ear alteration are not a major problem for children undergoing a diagnostic test battery, middle ear status significantly affects the pass rates of newborn hearing screening programs (e.g., Chang, Vohr, Norton, & Lekas, 1993; Doyle et al, 2000; Keefe et al, 2003).

TEOAEs measured when tympanograms have no discernible peak pressure (flat, or "Type B") are dramatically reduced in amplitude and often are not measurable (Choi et al, 1999; Lonsbury-Martin et al,

1994; Koike & Wetmore, 1999; Koivunen et al, 2000; Owens et al, 1993). Some research advocates using absent OAEs as a tool to detect otitis media with effusion (e.g., Georgalas, Xenellis, Davilis, Tzangaroulakis, & Ferekidis, 2008). For children with otitis media, the two middle ear factors most highly associated with absent TEOAEs are viscosity (Amedee, 1995) and quantity of effusion (Koivunen et al, 2000). The clinician must realize that OAEs can still be present in infants and children with negative middle ear pressure and, sometimes, even in those with "flat" tympanograms. Negative tympanometric peak pressure on a tympanogram or a "flat" tympanogram should not preclude the audiologist from measuring OAEs as part of the test battery.

Another area for which OAEs can be helpful is monitoring for hearing loss due to ototoxicity. Hearing loss is a more prevalent side effect of cancer drug therapy in children than it is in adults (Li, Womer, & Silber, 2004). DPOAEs are used for ototoxicity monitoring because stimuli can be presented to 8000 Hz and above. Bhagat et al (2010) monitored 10 children undergoing carboplatin therapy for retinoblastoma. They found that, although mean changes in DPOAEs were not significant over 3–4 test sessions, children receiving higher doses of carboplatin had significant reductions of DPOAEs over several frequencies, which appears to be a common finding with adults (Reavis et al, 2011). Details about cochlear damage due to ototoxicity, as well as suggestions to include in an ototoxicity monitoring protocol, can be found in Prieve and Dreisbach (2011).

Pearl

- If the OAE measures do not meet criteria, and the tympanometric measures are abnormal, no decision can be made as to whether there is possible cochlear pathology.

How to Obtain Good Recordings

A proper probe fit is essential for good OAE recordings. A good probe fit keeps out unwanted room noise from the ear canal while maintaining the proper stimulus level and preventing reductions in measured OAE level. While measuring OAEs in a sound-treated booth is optimal, testing can easily be performed in a quiet room if the probe fit is good. The probe needs to be placed firmly into the ear, which can be done by grasping the back of the auricula while the probe is inserted. The probe assem-

bly can be clipped to the child's shoulder; however, it is often helpful to clip the assembly to the parent if the child is sitting on the parent's lap, or to the chair if the child is sitting quietly in the chair. Children can be coaxed to sit quietly by reading a book to the child with a low-level voice or having a video playing. Because identification of hearing loss is not as good below 1500 Hz and children are noisier than adults, recording time can be reduced by not testing low frequencies. The equipment should be calibrated according to the manufacturer's suggestions; many practitioners perform a test run in a standard cavity every day to ensure that there are no equipment artifacts that would affect OAE measurement. Finally, most equipment has a measure to determine the stability of the stimulus while the test is being conducted, which indicates if the probe is moving in the ear canal. A high stability measure (e.g., > 75%) as well as an acceptably low noise level, should be assessed to ensure that the OAE test was properly conducted. If the child is somewhat noisy, additional averaging may be needed to reduce the noise floor.

◆ Final Note

OAEs are excellent tools for use in identifying hearing loss in a screening situation and as site-of-lesion and cross-check measures in a diagnostic setting. Abnormal OAE measures, together with normal middle ear measures and hearing loss, lead us to suspect there is OHC loss. In this case, it is reasonable to suspect that the cochlear amplifier is compromised and hearing aids are an appropriate (re)habilitation strategy. Management is more difficult if the OAEs are robust but pure tone and speech audiometry indicate a hearing loss. These test outcomes, along with acoustic reflex and ABR test results, may be consistent with the diagnosis of ANSD. If the child has this diagnosis, the approach to (re)habilitation is not as clear and may include cochlear implants (e.g., Peterson et al, 2003).

Controversial Point

- Despite widespread clinical use for identification of hearing loss, researchers are investigating whether OAEs show change *before* behavioral thresholds change, especially with noise exposure and ototoxic drugs. This issue is not resolved for general and clinical populations.

Discussion Questions

1. What are the possible sources for changes in OAEs with development?

2. At what point in your diagnostic test battery should you measure OAEs? At the beginning? At the end? Before you measure tympanograms? Does it depend on the age of the child?

3. Speculate as to why OAEs are better at detecting mid- and high-frequency hearing loss than low-frequency hearing loss.

4. Patient scenario: You are performing a hearing screening for a child going through diagnostic testing for speech and language delay. You have measured minimal response levels in soundfield at 15 dB HL at 500, 1000, and 2000 Hz in a child aged 18 months. You also measure TEOAEs in both ears that have ENRs of 15 dB at bands centered at 2000 Hz, 3000 Hz, and 4000 Hz using the Otodynamics QuickScreen mode. Does this child have hearing sensitivity within normal limits? Do you need to perform more testing on this child?

◆ Acknowledgments

B.P. and L.L. were supported by a grant from the March of Dimes Birth Defects Foundation during the writing of this manuscript.

References

Amedee, R. G. (1995). The effects of chronic otitis media with effusion on the measurement of transiently evoked otoacoustic emissions. The Laryngoscope, 105(6), 589–595.

American Speech-Language-Hearing Association. (1997). Guidelines for audiologic screening. Rockville, MD: ASHA.

Beppu, R., Hattori, T., & Yanagita, N. (1997). Comparison of TEOAE with play audiometry for screening hearing problems in children. Auris, Nasus, Larynx, 24(4), 367–371.

Bhagat, S. P., Bass, J. K., White, S. T., Qaddoumi, I., Wilson, M. W., Wu, J., & Rodriguez-Galindo, C. (2010). Monitoring carboplatin ototoxicity with distortion-product otoacoustic emissions in children with retinoblastoma. International Journal of Pediatric Otorhinolaryngology, 74(10), 1156–1163.

Chang, K. W., Vohr, B. R., Norton, S. J., & Lekas, M. D. (1993). External and middle ear status related to evoked otoacoustic emission in neonates. Archives of Otolaryngology–Head & Neck Surgery, 119(3), 276–282.

Choi, S. S., Pafitis, I. A., Zalzal, G. H., Herer, G. R., & Patel, K. M. (1999). Clinical applications of transiently evoked otoacoustic emissions in the pediatric population. The Annals of Otology, Rhinology, and Laryngology, 108(2), 132–138.

Dhar, S. & Hall III, J. N. (2012). Otoacoustic emissions. Principles, procedures, and protocols. San Diego, CA: Plural Publishing.

Dorn, P. A., Piskorski, P., Gorga, M. P., Neely, S. T., & Keefe, D. H. (1999). Predicting audiometric status from distortion product otoacoustic emissions using multivariate analyses. Ear and Hearing, 20(2), 149–163.

Doyle, K. J., Rodgers, P., Fujikawa, S., & Newman, E. (2000). External and middle ear effects on infant hearing screening test results. Otolaryngology–Head and Neck Surgery, 122(4), 477–481.

Eiserman, W. D., Hartel, D. M., Shisler, L., Buhrmann, J., White, K. R., & Foust, T. (2008). Using otoacoustic emissions to screen for hearing loss in early childhood care settings. International Journal of Pediatric Otorhinolaryngology, 72(4), 475–482.

Georgalas, C., Xenellis, J., Davilis, D., Tzangaroulakis, A., & Ferekidis, E. (2008). Screening for hearing loss and middle-ear effusion in school-age children, using transient evoked otoacoustic emissions: a feasibility study. The Journal of Laryngology and Otology, 122(12), 1299–1304.

Gorga, M. P., Dierking, D. M., Johnson, T. A., Beauchaine, K. L., Garner, C. A., & Neely, S. T. (2005). A validation and potential clinical application of multivariate analyses of distortion-product otoacoustic emission data. Ear and Hearing, 26(6), 593–607.

Gorga, M. P., Neely, S. T., & Dorn, P. A. (1999). DPOAE test performance for a priori criteria and for multifrequency audiometric standards. Ear and Hearing, 20, 345–362.

Gorga, M. P., Neely, S. T., Ohlrich, B., Hoover, B., Redner, J., & Peters, J. (1997). From laboratory to clinic: a large scale study of distortion product otoacoustic emissions in ears with normal hearing and ears with hearing loss. Ear and Hearing, 18(6), 440–455.

Gorga, M. P., Norton, S. J., Sininger, Y. S., Cone-Wesson, B., Folsom, R. C., Vohr, B. R., et al. (2000). Identification of neonatal hearing impairment: distortion product otoacoustic emissions during the perinatal period. Ear and Hearing, 21(5), 400–424.

Hof, J. R., Anteunis, L. J. C., Chenault, M. N., & van Dijk, P. (2005). Otoacoustic emissions at compensated middle ear pressure in children. International Journal of Audiology, 44(6), 317–320.

Hof, J. R., Dijk, Pv., Chenault, M. N., & Anteunis, L. J. C. (2005). A two-step scenario for hearing assessment with otoacoustic emissions at compensated middle ear pressure (in children 1-7 years old). International Journal of Pediatric Otorhinolaryngology, 69(5), 649–655.

Hussain, D. M., Gorga, M. P., Neely, S. T., Keefe, D. H., & Peters, J. (1998). Transient evoked otoacoustic emissions in patients with normal hearing and in patients with hearing loss. Ear and Hearing, 19(6), 434–449.

Joint Committee on Infant Hearing. (1994). Position statement. American Speech-Language Hearing Association, 36, 38–41.

Joint Committee on Infant Hearing. (2007). Year 2007 position statement: Principles and guidelines for early hearing detection and intervention programs. Pediatrics, 120(4), 898–921.

Keefe, D. H., Gorga, M. P., Neely, S. T., Zhao, F., & Vohr, B. R. (2003). Ear-canal acoustic admittance and reflectance measurements in human neonates. II. Predictions of middle-ear dysfunction and sensorineural hearing loss. The Journal of the Acoustical Society of America, 113(1), 407–422.

Kemp, D. T. (1978). Stimulated acoustic emissions from within the human auditory system. The Journal of the Acoustical Society of America, 64(5), 1386–1391.

Koike, K. J., & Wetmore, S. J. (1999). Interactive effects of the middle ear pathology and the associated hearing loss on transient-evoked otoacoustic emission measures. Otolaryngology–Head and Neck Surgery, 121(3), 238–244.

Koivunen, P., Uhari, M., Laitakari, K., Alho, O. P., & Luotonen, J. (2000). Otoacoustic emissions and tympanometry in children with otitis media. Ear and Hearing, 21(3), 212–217.

Krueger, W. W., & Ferguson, L. (2002). A comparison of screening methods in school-aged children. Otolaryngology–Head and Neck Surgery, 127(6), 516–519.

Li, Y., Womer, R. B., & Silber, J. H. (2004). Predicting cisplatin ototoxicity in children: the influence of age and the cumulative dose. European Journal of Cancer, 40(16), 2445–2451.

Liberman, M. C., Gao, J., He, D. Z., Wu, X., Jia, S., & Zuo, J. (2002). Prestin is required for electromotility of the outer hair cell and for the cochlear amplifier. Nature, 419(6904), 300–304.

Liberman, M. C., Zuo, J., & Guinan, J. J., Jr. (2004). Otoacoustic emissions without somatic motility: can stereocilia mechanics drive the mammalian cochlea? The Journal of the Acoustical Society of America, 116(3), 1649–1655.

Lonsbury-Martin, B. L., Martin, G. K., McCoy, M. J., & Whitehead, M. L. (1994). Otoacoustic emissions testing in young children: middle-ear influences. The American Journal of Otology, 15, S13–S20.

Nicholson, N. (2003). Transient evoked otoacoustic emissions in relation to hearing loss: univariate and multivariate analyses. Dissertation Abstracts International, 64, 5432.

Nicholson, N., & Widen, J. E. (2004). Templates for diagnostic interpretation of TEOAEs. Poster presented at the 16th Annual American Academy of Audiology convention, Salt Lake, UT

Nicholson, N., & Widen, J. E. (2007). Evoked otoacoustic emissions in the evaluation of children. In M. Robinette & T. Glattke (Eds.), Otoacoustic emissions: clinical applications (3rd ed., pp. 365–399). New York, NY: Thieme.

Norton, S. J., Gorga, M. P., Widen, J. E., Vohr, B. R., Folsom, R. C., Sininger, Y. S., . . . Fletcher, K. A. (2000). Identification of neonatal hearing impairment: transient evoked otoacoustic emissions during the perinatal period. Ear and Hearing, 21(5), 425–442.

Norton, S. J., Gorga, M. P., Widen, J. E., Folsom, R. C., Sininger, Y., Cone-Wesson, B., . . . Fletcher, K. A. (2000). Identification of neonatal hearing impairment: evaluation of transient evoked otoacoustic emission, distortion product otoacoustic emission, and auditory brain stem response test performance. Ear and Hearing, 21(5), 508–528.

Owens, J. J., McCoy, M. J., Lonsbury-Martin, B. L., & Martin, G. K. (1993). Otoacoustic emissions in children with normal ears, middle ear dysfunction, and ventilating tubes. The American Journal of Otology, 14(1), 34–40.

Peterson, A., Shallop, J., Driscoll, C., Breneman, A., Babb, J., Stoeckel, R., & Fabry, L. (2003). Outcomes of cochlear implantation in children with auditory neuropathy. Journal of the American Academy of Audiology, 14(4), 188–201.

Prieve, B. A. (2007). Otoacoustic emissions in neonatal hearing screening. In M. Robinette & T. Glattke (Eds.), Otoacoustic emissions: clinical applications (3rd ed., pp. 343–364). New York, NY: Thieme.

Prieve, B. A., & Dreisbach, L. (2011). Otoacoustic emissions. In R. Seewald & A. M. Tharpe (Eds.), Comprehensive handbook of pediatric audiology (pp. 389–407). San Diego, CA: Plural.

Prieve, B. A., & Stevens, F. (2000). The New York State universal newborn hearing screening demonstration project: introduction and overview. Ear and Hearing, 21(2), 85–91.

Prieve, B. A., Calandruccio, L., Fitzgerald, T., Mazevski, A., & Georgantas, L. M. (2008). Changes in transient-evoked otoacoustic emission levels with negative tympanometric peak pressure in infants and toddlers. Ear and Hearing, 29(4), 533–542.

Prieve, B. A., Fitzgerald, T. S., & Schulte, L. E. (1997a). Basic characteristics of click-evoked otoacoustic emissions in infants and children. The Journal of the Acoustical Society of America, 102, 2860–2870.

Prieve, B. A., Fitzgerald, T. S., Schulte, L. E., & Kemp, D. T. (1997b). Basic characteristics of distortion product otoacoustic emissions in infants and children. The Journal of the Acoustical Society of America, 102, 2871–2879.

Prieve, B. A., Gorga, M. P., Schmidt, A. L., Neely, S., Peters, J., Schultes, L., & Jesteadt, W. (1993). Analysis of transient-evoked otoacoustic emissions in normal-hearing and hearing-impaired ears. The Journal of the Acoustical Society of America, 93(6), 3308–3319.

Prieve, B. A., Hancur-Bucci, C. A., & Preston, J. L. (2009). Changes in transient-evoked otoacoustic emissions in the first month of life. Ear and Hearing, 30(3), 330–339.

Reavis, K. M., McMillan, G., Austin, D., Gallun, F., Fausti, S. A., Gordon, J. S., . . . Konrad-Martin, D. (2011). Distortion-product otoacoustic emission test performance for ototoxicity monitoring. Ear and Hearing, 32(1), 61–74.

Ricci, A. (2003). Active hair bundle movements and the cochlear amplifier. Journal of the American Academy of Audiology, 14(6), 325–338.

Robinette, M., & Glattke, T. (2007). Otoacoustic emissions: clinical applications (3rd ed.). New York, NY: Thieme.

Sabo, M. P., Winston, R., & Macias, J. D. (2000). Comparison of pure tone and transient otoacoustic emissions screening in a grade school population. The American Journal of Otology, 21(1), 88–91.

Siegel, J. H., & Kim, D. O. (1982). Cochlear biomechanics: vulnerability to acoustic trauma and other alterations as seen in neural responses and ear-canal sound pressure. In D. Hamernik, D. Henderson, & R. Salvi (Eds.), New perspectives on noise-induced hearing loss (pp. 137–151). New York, NY: Raven.

Sininger, Y. S., Cone-Wesson, B., Folsom, R. C., Gorga, M. P., Vohr, B. R., Widen, J. E., . . . Norton, S. J. (2000). Identification of neonatal hearing impairment: auditory brain stem responses in the perinatal period. Ear and Hearing, 21(5), 383–399.

Śliwa, L., Hatzopoulos, S., Kochanek, K., Piłka, A., Senderski, A., & Skarżyński, P. H. (2011). A comparison of audiometric and objective methods in hearing screening of school children. A preliminary study. International Journal of Pediatric Otorhinolaryngology, 75(4), 483–488.

Smurzynski, J. (1994). Longitudinal measurements of distortion product and click-evoked otoacoustic emissions of preterm infants: preliminary results. Ear and Hearing, 15(3), 210–223.

Stover, L., Gorga, M. P., Neely, S. T., & Montoya, D. (1996). Toward optimizing the clinical utility of distortion product otoacoustic emission measurements. The Journal of the Acoustical Society of America, 100(2 Pt 1), 956–967.

Taylor, C. L., & Brooks, R. P. (2000). Screening for hearing loss and middle-ear disorders in children using TEOAEs. American Journal of Audiology, 9(1), 50–55.

Trine, M. B., Hirsch, J. E., & Margolis, R. H. (1993). The effect of middle ear pressure on transient evoked otoacoustic emissions. Ear and Hearing, 14(6), 401–407.

Vohr, B. R., Carty, L. M., Moore, P. E., & Letourneau, K. (1998). The Rhode Island Hearing Assessment Program: experience with statewide hearing screening (1993-1996). The Journal of Pediatrics, 133(3), 353–357.

Welch, D., Greville, K. A., Thorne, P. R., & Purdy, S. C. (1996). Influence of acquisition parameters on the measurement of click evoked otoacoustic emissions in neonates in a hospital environment. Audiology, 35(3), 143–157.

Wessex Universal Neonatal Hearing Screening Trial Group. (1998). Controlled trial of universal neonatal screening for early identification of permanent childhood hearing impairment. Lancet, 352(9145), 1957–1964.

Widen, J. E., Folsom, R. C., Cone-Wesson, B., Carty, L., Dunnell, J. J., Koebsell, K., . . . Norton, S. J. (2000). Identification of neonatal hearing impairment: hearing status at 8 to 12 months corrected age using a visual reinforcement audiometry protocol. Ear and Hearing, 21(5), 471–487.

Yin, L., Bottrell, C., Clarke, N., Shacks, J., & Poulsen, M. K. (2009). Otoacoustic emissions: a valid, efficient first-line hearing screen for preschool children. The Journal of School Health, 79(4), 147–152.

Chapter 14

The Role of the Audiology Assistant in Assessing Hearing in Children

Jane R. Madell

Key Points

- The audiology assistant is responsible for engaging the infant or child, keeping the child interested and attentive, and keeping family members at ease so they can cooperate with test protocols.

- In behavioral observation audiometry (BOA), the audiology assistant is responsible for monitoring the positioning of the child, observing responses and reporting observations to the audiologist, and monitoring the parent's or caregiver's behavior.

- In visual reinforcement audiometry (VRA), the audiology assistant's first responsibility is to assist in training the child to the task and then to keep the child focused at midline so that the child can make a conditioned head turn.

- With conditioned play audiometry (CPA), the audiology assistant teaches the child the listen-and-drop task and then assists the child in completing the test activities.

- An important responsibility for the audiology assistant is keeping the test room in order.

◆ The Audiology Assistant

An audiology assistant is a person who, after appropriate training and demonstration of competency, performs delegated duties and responsibilities that are directed and supervised by an audiologist. The role of the assistant is to support the audiologist by performing routine tasks and duties so that the audiologist is available for the more complex evaluative, diagnostic, management, and treatment services that require the education and training of a licensed audiologist (American Academy of Audiology [AAA], 2010). The AAA Guidelines require the audiology assistant to have a minimum of a high school diploma and competency-based training. The audiologist has the responsibility to provide training and to monitor performance of the audiology assistant.

The Audiology Assistant's Role in Testing Children

When evaluating infants and young children, testing is frequently more easily and accurately accomplished with two examiners. Both examiners may be audiologists, or one may be an audiologist and the other an audiology assistant or a parent. If there are two audiologists, they can alternate roles: one at the audiometer and one interacting with the child. If the second examiner is not an audiologist, alternating roles will not be possible.

Whether one or two audiologists are participating in testing, only one is in charge and "calling the shots." The "managing audiologist" (for want of a better term) will determine the test protocol, presentation mode, order of testing, and timing of presentations. The managing audiologist usually sits at the audiometer; sometimes, however, with a difficult-to-test child, the person working with the child may manage the session and give directions to the second audiologist, who is sitting at the audiometer and presenting test stimuli.

The purpose of this chapter is to describe the critical role of the audiology assistant during various pediatric tests. Please refer to Chapters 7 through 11 for detailed information about the specific behavioral assessments of infants and children.

◆ Working with Parents

The audiology assistant is responsible for engaging the infant or child, keeping him interested and attentive, and keeping family members at ease so that they can cooperate with test protocols. The audiology assistant needs first to be certain that family members understand exactly what is being tested, how testing is accomplished, and what their role will be. The child may be seated on a parent's lap or in an infant seat, a highchair, or a chair at a test table. The parent may be seated next to or slightly behind the child so as to be able to observe but not distract him. In other cases, especially if the child is uncomfortable with strangers, the parent may be the best person to play with him, with direction from the audiologist.

The first responsibility of the audiology assistant is to explain the test protocol to the family. The audiology assistant should describe what testing will consist of, what will be expected of the child, and what will be expected of the family. Family members need to understand they must appear interested, but must not respond to any test stimuli before the child responds, to be certain the responses obtained are measures of the child's hearing and not his ability to receive cues from the parents. It is frequently difficult for parents to sit still and not react when the child does not seem to be responding to the presentation of test stimuli. Parents may need to be instructed not to say "Did you hear that?," not to look expectantly when sounds are presented, not to look at the reinforcing toy during VRA, and not to suggest the child put the toy in the bucket when the parent hears the sound. When speech stimuli are used, the parents may need to be reminded that they must not repeat the tester's stimuli for the child (e.g., saying "baseball" if the tester said "baseball") when the child fails to respond. If the child is looking to the parent or audiology assistant for encouragement, it may be best to look away from the child. Look at the toy, the loudspeaker, or the floor so that the child understands he will not receive cues from adults in the room about when to respond.

Once family members understand that their distracting behaviors may make it difficult to obtain reliable results, they are usually willing to do whatever is needed to obtain an accurate test. The use of noise-canceling earphones may be effective in reducing extraneous behaviors from family members. Some parents, however, prefer to be able to hear the precise sounds the child can and cannot respond to; this is frequently very helpful when they receive counseling about test results.

◆ Behavioral Observation Audiometry

For BOA, both the managing audiologist and the audiology assistant need to have a good view of the infant so both can judge whether a response was made. If the infant is in an infant seat, either the audiology assistant or the parent may be holding the bottle, because, as detailed in Chapter 7, sucking is the primary reliably observed behavior. If the infant is being nursed

or is not comfortable in an infant seat, he will be in a parent's arms. If the parent is holding the infant or the bottle, the audiology assistant needs to be certain the parent is not changing the way she is holding the bottle or breast or moving it in or out of the infant's mouth when sound stimuli are presented.

The audiology assistant needs to be certain the infant is seated comfortably and not fidgeting. If may be helpful for the audiology assistant to hold and manipulate a bright toy or a light-emitting diode (LED) display in front of the infant to keep him focused straight ahead and to reduce fidgeting. If the audiology assistant is using a toy or light to distract the infant, the object should be placed so that the infant does not have to move his head up or down to see it.

When a sound is presented, both the audiology assistant and the managing audiologist need to judge the response. The audiology assistant needs to be careful about how to inform the managing audiologist about the observation. The testers need to work out a signal system such as a minor head nod indicating yes or no, or finger movement (one for yes, two for no). If the audiology assistant repeatedly says "No, I didn't see anything," such speech compromises the quiet test environment and is likely to be very disturbing to the family. Being right next to the baby, the audiology assistant will be able to make suggestions about when a rest or repositioning may be needed.

Pearl

- Before testing, audiologists should work out a way to communicate with each other without communicating to the family. A system to signal observation of responses or changes needed during testing might consist of head nods or finger taps.

◆ Visual Reinforcement Audiometry

In VRA, the audiology assistant's first responsibility is to help train the child to the task and then keep the child focused at midline so that the child can make a conditioned head turn. Positioning is especially important for young children and for children with neurological or developmental delays. The audiology assistant needs to be certain the child is comfortably seated, has sufficient neck support if needed, and is facing forward. If the child is turned toward one side and sound stimuli are being presented and reinforced from the other side, it may be difficult for the child to make a sufficient head turn to be counted as a response. Focusing the child at midline will be most easily accomplished if the audiology assistant is seated in front of the child but in a position that permits the managing audiologist to see the child as well. The distraction toys the audiology assistant selects should be easily manipulated, bright, and entertaining. As soon as the child starts to lose interest and look away, a new toy should be presented.

When training the child to the VRA task, the audiology assistant will keep the child's attention focused front. If the child does not turn and look on his own when the VRA toy is turned on, the audiology assistant will attract him to the reinforcing toy by waving at the toy or tapping the transparent box holding the toy to get the child's attention to the toy. Once the child is trained for the task, the audiology assistant is responsible for keeping him focused forward and away from the reinforcing toy. The child should be observing (not manipulating) the distracting toys, since physical play may be too engrossing, especially for young children and children with developmental issues. Older children may be able to play with some simple toys and still respond to sound. The audiology assistant needs to be alert and aware of how the child is responding and whether playing with a toy is interfering with attention. If it is, the tester will need to take the toys away from the child.

◆ Conditioned Play Audiometry

With CPA, the audiology assistant teaches the child the listen-and-drop task and assists him in completing the test activities. The audiology assistant must make a judgment about the child's motor skills so as to be able to select toys the child is capable of using, and must note when the child's interest is flagging and determine when a new toy is needed. For children who do not wish to cooperate, the audiology assistant will need to present a "firm but kind" attitude to increase cooperation. When the child is not cooperating, the audiology assistant will need to determine when it would be good to involve the parent in obtaining cooperation and when it is best to leave the parent out. As with VRA, the amount of interaction the tester and child will have will depend partly on the personality of the tester and partly on the child. However, because children who are able to engage in CPA are older, more interaction with the audiology assistant is to be expected.

◆ Speech Audiometry

The use of an audiology assistant can be critical for speech audiometry. If a closed-set task is being used, the audiology assistant will be responsible for turning pages and being certain the managing audiologist

knows how the child responded. If an open-set format is being used and the child is repeating the test stimulus, the audiology assistant may need to be the audiologist's "ears," especially if the child is responding in a very soft voice that is typical of many young children. The audiology assistant needs to find a way to let the audiologist know whether the child's response was correct and, if not, what the error was so that the audiologist can accurately score the response, especially when using phoneme scoring. It is important that the audiology assistant provide response accuracy information without making the child feel as if he is doing poorly at the task. The assistant can employ several strategies. The audiology assistant can simply repeat what the child says in a sufficiently loud voice for the audiologist to hear, or just repeat the error words. For example, if the stimulus item is "Say the word 'mouth'" and the child says "mouse," the audiology assistant can say "mouse" or "mouse, good job." The audiologist will know that an error was made and will be able to record what the error was, but the child will not feel he is failing at the task.

◆ Keeping Order in the Test Room

The test room does not have to be silent during testing, but it should be quiet. Conversations should be at a minimum. The amount of interaction between the tester and child will depend partly on the personality of the tester and partly on the child. For some children, smiling, clapping, and enthusiastic comments of "hurrah" will encourage longer attention to the VRA task. For other children, "cheerleading" will be intrusive and better results will be obtained if the audiology assistant is quieter or even silent. A silent audiology assistant is frequently valuable with a child with a pervasive developmental disorder (PDD) or other developmental disorders. The audiology assistant will need to observe the child and determine what behavior produces the best results.

An important responsibility for the audiology assistant is keeping the test room in order. When a child is brought into a test room, most of the toys should be out of sight. However, one or two toys could be visible to entice the child to enter the room and to sit in the test chair. Bringing a young child, especially a difficult-to-evaluate child, into a room that has toys all over the floor will make it difficult to seat the child and have him focus on the task. When toys are put away, they should be sorted appropriately. All parts of each toy should be placed in the correct box to facilitate moving quickly from one activity to the next. Using a peg board or a puzzle with a missing piece may result in annoyance or frustration for the child. Having toy cars mixed up with Lego pieces also can be problematic. Toy confusions often waste time while the child discusses what is missing and why things are in the wrong place. Some children need to examine each piece before using it to determine what it is and where it belongs. For some children, disorganization and missing pieces can interfere with testing.

◆ Conclusion

The audiology assistant is critical to obtaining accurate results in a timely manner. An enthusiastic, cheerful audiology assistant who enjoys children is likely to elicit good results.

When the audiology assistant and the managing audiologist disagree or are not communicating well, it is probably best if they take a moment to leave the test room and discuss how they want to proceed out of earshot of the family. It hardly encourages confidence if the testers cannot agree about what to do.

Pitfall

- Audiologists should not disagree in front of families. It can be distressing to the family and reduce trust about test results.

Communication between the audiologist and audiology assistant can be accomplished using a talk-back system with the audiometer in which the tester uses the audiometer microphone and the audiology assistant uses earphones. If the audiometer does not have a talk-back system, communication can be accomplished by using a frequency modulation (FM) system; the tester wears the microphone, and the audiology assistant wears the receiver. An experienced and professional team will make testing infants and children fun and enable results to be obtained efficiently and accurately.

Discussion Questions

1. What are some ways the audiologist and audiology assistant can communicate during testing?
2. What are the responsibilities of the audiology assistant during BOA, VRA, CPA, and speech audiometry?

Reference

American Academy of Audiology. (2010). Audiology assistant position statement. Retrieved from http://www.audiology.org/resources/documentlibrary/Documents/2010_AudiologyAssistant_Pos_Stat.PDF

Chapter 15

Auditory Evoked Response Testing in Infants and Children

Suzanne C. Purdy and Andrea Kelly

Key Points

- For auditory brainstem response (ABR) and auditory steady-state response (ASSR) testing, infants need to be well settled in a deep sleep for good-quality recordings.

- Electrode contacts need to be good (low and balanced impedances), and the environment should be free of electrical noise to obtain quality evoked response recordings.

- Frequency-specific testing is easy to do and is essential for fitting of hearing instruments for children whose hearing loss has been detected via universal newborn screening.

- Clinicians do not need to wait for confirmation of evoked response testing with behavioral data—hearing thresholds can be reliably estimated using evoked responses, although not for children with auditory neuropathy spectrum disorder.

- Bone conduction ABR should be performed when a hearing loss is identified using ABR or ASSR, to determine whether there is a conductive component to the hearing loss.

- Cortical evoked responses can be used for showing that amplified speech stimuli are audible for young infants who are not able to provide reliable behavioral responses to sound.

◆ What Are Auditory Evoked Responses and How Are They Recorded?

The auditory brainstem response (ABR) and the auditory steady-state response (ASSR) are the auditory evoked responses most commonly recorded in infants and children. Other less commonly recorded responses that also have clinical utility in pediatric audiology are the middle latency response (MLR), the electrocochleogram (ECoG), and the cortical auditory evoked potentials (CAEPs), also referred to as late latency response (LLR) or slow vertex response (SVR). These responses differ in terms of where they are generated in the auditory system and consequently occur at different times after presentation of an auditory stimulus. Optimal stimulus and recording parameters also differ. This chapter focuses on the evoked responses that are used most widely in pediatric audiology: the ABR and, to a lesser extent, ASSR. Clinical applications of CAEP, MLR, and ECoG are also discussed briefly.

All evoked responses represent summed auditory neural activity, usually recorded using sensors (electrodes) attached to the surface of the scalp. Each evoked response has a characteristic appearance and is usually described in terms of the timing (latency) and amplitude of particular peaks in the evoked response waveform. **Table 15.1** summarizes typical latencies and clinical applications of the evoked responses discussed here. **Fig. 15.1** shows a schematic diagram of an evoked response recording system. Typically, response averaging and stimulus generation occur within the same commercial system or computer. For some applications, however, such as cochlear implant (CI) recordings involving direct stimulation of electrodes, the stimuli are delivered via a separate system that has a "trigger" connected to the evoked response averaging computer (e.g., Runge-Samuelson, Drake, & Wackym, 2008).

With the exception of ASSR and screening (automated) ABR, most clinical evoked response recording systems enable clinicians to view a "time waveform" of the response (see example in **Fig. 15.2**). The time waveform is a plot of evoked response amplitude (voltage) as a function of time after stimulus presentation. **Fig. 15.2** shows a toneburst ABR recorded from a 4-month-old infant in response to a 4000 Hz toneburst. The infant has mild to severe hearing loss, thought to be caused by oxygen deprivation at birth.

Table 15.1 Characteristics of auditory evoked responses used clinically for testing children and clinical applications of these responses

Evoked response	Latency range	Clinical applications	Stimuli typically used
ABR	0–15 ms	Newborn hearing screening	Single-polarity clicks
		Diagnosis of ANSD	Single-polarity clicks
		Otoneurological investigation of retrocochlear pathology	Single-polarity clicks
		Objective estimation of pure tone hearing thresholds	Brief tonebursts
ASSR	0–15 ms	Objective estimation of pure tone hearing	Frequency and/or amplitude modulated continuous tones
ECoG	0–3 ms	Diagnosis of ANSD	Single-polarity clicks
		Objective estimation of pure tone hearing thresholds	Tonebursts
MLR	15–50 ms	Assessment of central auditory function	Clicks
CAEP	50–400 ms	Objective evaluation of hearing aids	Speech sounds
		Objective evaluation of hearing when ABR unreliable	Long duration tonebursts

Abbreviations: ABR, auditory brainstem response; ANSD, auditory neuropathy spectrum disorder; ASSR, auditory steady-state response; CAEP, cortical auditory evoked potentials; ECoG, electrocochleogram; MLR, middle latency response.

The time waveforms contain electrical noise plus the evoked response. The ABR peaks at 8 to 10 milliseconds, referred to as "wave V," can be seen at levels down to 90 dB, but wave V is not present at 80 dB normal hearing level (nHL). As the stimulus presentation level decreases, wave V amplitude decreases and latency increases slightly. This effect of stimulus level on response amplitude and latency is characteristic of all neural auditory evoked responses. At near-threshold levels, repeat recordings were obtained to verify the presence or absence of an evoked response and the two waveforms were overlaid.

Because auditory evoked responses, especially ABR, are very small compared with background electrical "noise," stimuli are presented multiple times and computer averaging is used to extract the response. The "noise" could be other brain or cardiac electrical activity generated by the child, or it could be electrical noise in the environment generated by equipment or the power supply to the room. In the ABR example in **Fig. 15.2**, the "baseline" recording at 80 dB nHL contains no repeatable ABR waveform but does contain electrical noise. It is important that clinicians recognize and minimize electrical noise in evoked response recordings to prevent interpretation errors, which can have serious consequences for children with hearing loss and their families. Competencies required for accurate evoked response audiometry have been described by the American Speech-Language-Hearing Association (ASHA) (2003).

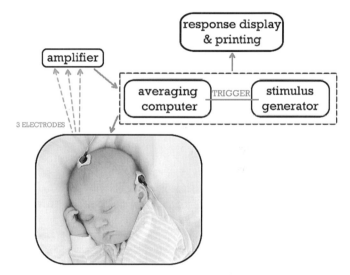

Fig. 15.1 Schematic diagram of evoked response recording equipment. Stimuli can be delivered to a range of transducers such as insert earphones, supraaural earphones, a bone conductor, or a loudspeaker. Three electrodes are required for a single-channel recording.

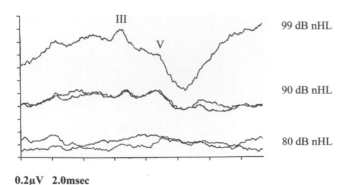

99 dB nHL

90 dB nHL

80 dB nHL

0.2µV 2.0msec

Fig. 15.2 Example of 4000 Hz toneburst ABR responses recorded to stimuli at decreasing presentation levels in a 4-month-old infant with severe high-frequency hearing loss. At stimulus levels of 90 and 80 dB normal hearing level (nHL), repeat recordings are overlaid.

◆ Auditory Brainstem Response

Neuromaturation and Response Generators

In older children and adults, the ABR to a high-level click stimulus consists of a series of positive and negative peaks occurring at 1.5 to 6 milliseconds (with each peak separated by ~ 1 millisecond), labeled as waves I, II, III, IV, V, and VI (Jewett & Williston, 1971). Waves IV and V are often merged and hence may appear as a "IV/V complex." Wave V is the most robust component in the waveform and may be the only identifiable peak, particularly at near-threshold levels. The right-hand panel in **Fig. 15.3** shows an adultlike ABR recorded to high-level click stimuli from a school-aged child.

Because of the complexity of ipsilateral and contralateral central auditory connections in the brainstem, a simple serial model of successive ABR peaks generated by successive brainstem nuclei is unlikely to be valid, but some knowledge of response generators is important, especially for children with neurological compromise that may affect interpretation of ABR results.

Pearl

- Current evidence indicates that ABR peaks represent summed activity of the auditory nerve and multiple fiber tracts and brainstem nuclei.

Waves I and II arise from the distal (i.e., close to the cochlea) and proximal (i.e., close to the brainstem) ends of the auditory nerve, and it is probable that wave III is largely from the cochlear nucleus, wave IV

is from the superior olivary complex, wave V is from the lateral lemniscus fiber tract, and the negativity following wave V (SN_{10}) is from the contralateral inferior colliculus (Moller, 2007).

Differences in the normal click ABR waveform of infants versus children are illustrated in **Fig. 15.3**, which shows the ABR evoked by 80 dB nHL clicks in a 3-month-old infant versus a 7-year-old child. The two overlaid waveforms show the stimulus artifact right at the beginning of the trace for both infant and child. For the infant, the cochlear microphonic (CM) is very evident before wave I. The CM waveform originates in the cochlea rather than in the nerve, as it inverts when the stimulus polarity reverses from rarefaction to condensation (Dallos, 1973). The neurogenic peaks (waves I to V) do not change greatly with stimulus polarity, making it possible to separate cochlear and neural components in the ABR waveform. The CM is present in infants with normal hearing (Starr et al, 2001) but is abnormally large and may be present in the absence of other ABR peaks in infants with auditory neuropathy spectrum disorder (ANSD) (Berlin et al, 1998). The ABR recording in **Fig. 15.3** may contain CM before wave I, but this is difficult to determine because the ABR was recorded with only one click polarity (rarefaction). Ipsilateral and contralateral recordings are shown, recorded with the noninverting (positive, "active") electrode on the vertex and the inverting (negative, reference) electrode on the same or opposite ear relative to the stimulus ear (ipsilateral versus contralateral). Later peaks are typically more robust than earlier peaks in contralateral recordings, as illustrated in **Fig. 15.3**, and show a clearer separation of waves IV and V than ipsilateral recordings do.

The maturation of the auditory system begins at the periphery, where it is relatively adultlike at birth. The cortical regions are not fully mature until late adolescence (Ponton, Don, Eggermont, Waring, & Masuda, 1996). During the first year of life, the ABR matures rapidly; morphology of the response and latencies reach adult values at around 24 months. In premature infants, the reliability of click-evoked ABR improves between 24 and 32 weeks gestational age; replicable waves I, III, and V are evident in the waveform at ~28 weeks gestational age (Eggermont & Salamy, 1988), hence automated ABR (AABR) will be unreliable in very young preterm infants, particularly for AABR screening systems with automatic waveform template-matching detection algorithms (van Straaten et al, 2003). Decreased latencies of waves III and V in the first 2 years of life are believed to be caused by decreased neural conduction time caused by completion of myelination in the proximal to distal direction in the central nervous system (Moore, Ponton, Eggermont, Wu, & Huang, 1996).

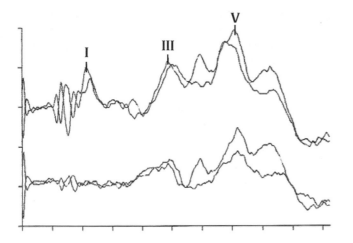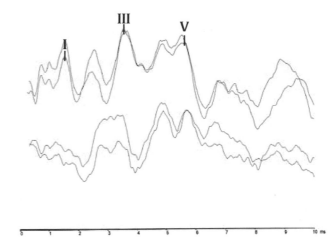

Fig. 15.3 Click-evoked (80 dB nHL, 17.1/s) ABR recordings for a 3-month-old infant (*left*) and a 7-year-old child (*right*), both of whom have normal hearing. For the infant, the overlaid waveforms are separate recordings for rarefaction and condensation clicks. For the child, the overlaid waveforms are repeat recordings for rarefaction clicks. In each case, two ABR channels were used to record both ipsilateral and contralateral waveforms. Ipsilateral recordings are shown above and contralateral recordings are shown below.

Pearl

- Because there are such pronounced changes in ABR latencies during the first 2 years, it is recommended that age-specific normative latency data be applied on a weekly basis during the preterm period, a biweekly basis during the 3-month period from term, and at monthly intervals thereafter until 18 to 24 months (Jacobson and Hall, 1994).

◆ Choice of Stimulus for ABR Recordings

For many years, clicks have been the favored stimulus for ABR recordings for neurological investigations of auditory pathways and estimating hearing sensitivity. A common misunderstanding has been that the click ABR reflects hearing only in the high frequencies because it is mainly generated by high-frequency cochlear regions in listeners with normal hearing (Coats & Martin, 1977; Hyde, 1985). Because of their rapid onset and short duration, clicks have a very broad frequency spectrum; hence, the click ABR can be generated from any cochlear region with good hearing sensitivity. Consequently, click ABR thresholds can indicate normal hearing or underestimate hearing thresholds when there is a significant hearing loss if the loss is restricted to part of the audiometric frequency range (Stapells & Oates, 1997; van der Drift, Brocaar, & van Zanten, 1987). Because there is well-established evidence for the limitations of click ABR for frequency-specific hearing threshold estima-

tion, protocols for diagnostic ABR testing of infants typically specify the use of frequency-specific stimuli (ASHA, 2004; Sininger, 2003; Stapells, 2002a).

Although toneburst ABR more accurately estimates pure tone thresholds than click ABR, click ABR continues to have an important role in screening and in the diagnosis of ANSD. Some authors suggest that clicks should still be used, alongside tonebursts, for ABR threshold assessment (Sauter, Douglas, & Speidel, 2012). If the child has a hearing loss, decisions about amplification and other treatments depend on information about hearing at specific audiometric frequencies. Hence it is recommended that frequency-specific stimuli be used for threshold estimation and that clicks be used only for screening and otoneurologic ABR. Janssen, Usher, & Stapells (2010) demonstrated that a considerable amount of clinically useful information can be obtained if this approach is adopted.

Clicks produce well-defined ABR waveforms because their rapid onset ensures optimal in-phase stimulation of high-frequency nerve fibers in the base of the cochlea (Kiang & Moxon, 1974). An alternative to the click stimulus, known as a "chirp," contains a wide range of frequencies, like the click, but the frequency content is swept from a low to a high frequency at a rate that simulates cochlear traveling wave speed, to achieve simultaneous activation across the cochlear partition and maximize evoked response amplitude (Bell, Allen, & Lutman, 2002; Wegner & Dau, 2002). Chirps evoke larger ABR amplitudes than clicks do (Kristensen & Elberling, 2012); hence, they are likely to be increasingly used for hearing screening and perhaps diagnostic purposes if efficient and reliable frequency-specific chirp protocols can be developed.

Choice of Stimulus Polarity

Table 15.2 summarizes recommended stimulus parameters for the two main applications of ABR recordings in children, namely, threshold estimation and otoneurologic investigations. More detailed information on specific toneburst ABR stimulus and recording parameters can be found in Stapells (2002b). The term *stimulus polarity* refers to the onset phase of the stimulus. For rarefaction onset polarity, there is an inward movement of the transducer diaphragm, negative onset pressure in the ear canal, and an initial upward movement of the basilar membrane (Brugge, Anderson, Hind, & Rose, 1969). Traditionally, clinicians have used rarefaction clicks, based on evidence for enhanced ABR amplitudes, including wave I and clearer wave IV and V separation. Alternating stimulus polarity is used for tonebursts to cancel stimulus artifact, because the relatively long duration of the stimuli means that the artifact may make it difficult to identify ABR peaks in the first part of the waveform (Foxe & Stapells, 1993). To screen for ANSD, separate rarefaction and condensation polarities should be used for otoneurologic click ABR recordings, to determine the presence of an abnormally large CM (Rance et al, 1999; Sininger, 2002). The phase of the CM will flip over with the change in stimulus polarity, but this does not occur for neurogenic peaks (waves I to V).

Toneburst ABR

Optimizing Test Efficiency

Most commonly, infants will be in a state of natural sleep for ABR testing (Janssen et al., 2010), although sometimes testing is done under general anesthesia (GA). The ABR is unaffected by sedation and can be recorded in comatose patients (Hall & Harris, 1994). Sedation or general anesthesia may be necessary to complete testing in a timely fashion in an infant with suspected hearing loss or if a child is difficult to test, despite the associated risks and the need for resuscitation equipment and appropriately qualified medi-cal staff. Chloral hydrate is widely used in clinics that perform ABRs under sedation; documented complications include vomiting, rash, hyperactivity, respiratory distress, and apnea (Avlonitou et al, 2011). Universal newborn hearing screening and early confirmation of hearing thresholds when infants are more likely to sleep naturally will reduce the need for GA and sedation; however, this will still be required for some children. ASHA has developed guidelines on the use of sedation for ABR testing (ASHA, 1992).

Regardless of whether the child is sleeping naturally or sedated, test efficiency is critical, and many authors have suggested a range of test protocols for ABR audiometry that maximize the information obtained per amount of time invested, since it may be necessary at any stage to abandon testing (Sutton & Lightfoot, 2013; Stapells, 2004). **Table 15.3** outlines some strategies for obtaining key information as quickly as possible so that, if the child wakes too soon, a decision can still be made about habilitation (hearing aids, cochlear implants, middle ear treatment, etc.).

The infant should be settled at the start of testing, ideally with insert earphones securely placed in each ear. It is best not to move the infant once testing begins, but it may be necessary to place a bone vibrator or reposition transducers. Advantages of insert earphones for pediatric ABR testing include reduced stimulus artifact caused by the greater distance between the transducer and the electrodes (assuming electrodes and transducers are carefully placed at a distance from each other), greater comfort, avoidance of ear canal collapse, and increased interaural attenuation. There is less need for contralateral masking, more reliable transducer placement, reduced interference from ambient noise if testing is not done in a sound booth, and improved infection control through use of disposable tips (Hall, 2007).

Special Consideration

- Supraaural earphones should be used only when inserts are not possible (e.g., ear canal atresia).

Table 15.2 Stimulus parameters commonly used for different ABR applications

Purpose of ABR testing	Stimulus type	Cycles	Rise, plateau, and fall times	Polarity	Durations for commonly used frequencies	Rate/s
Threshold estimation	Toneburst	5	2–1–2 cycles	Alternating	500 Hz = 10 milliseconds 1000 Hz = 5 milliseconds 2000 Hz = 2.5 milliseconds 4000 Hz = 1.25 milliseconds	39.1
Neurological investigation/ ANSD diagnosis	Click		Produced by delivering a "square" wave to transducer	Both rarefaction and condensation	100 µs	17.1

Table 15.3 Recommended diagnostic ABR protocol

Testing component	Minimum stimuli	Recommended additional stimuli	Recommendations for efficient ABR testing
AC toneburst stimuli	2000 Hz, 500 Hz	4000 Hz, 1000 Hz	• Test first at minimum (pass level), then increase level in 20–30 dB steps if no response • Once a response is obtained, establish threshold in 10 dB steps
BC toneburst stimuli	500 Hz, or at least one frequency where AC threshold is elevated	All frequencies where AC threshold is elevated	• If AC threshold is elevated, immediately check BC at that frequency before continuing with AC testing at other frequencies • As a minimum, BC at 500 Hz will facilitate interpretation of ABR results if there is a hearing loss, since most conductive hearing loss is low-frequency
High-level click	Rarefaction & condensation clicks, high stimulus intensity (always do this check for ANSD, even when AC toneburst ABR is present at minimal levels)		• If there are risk factors for ANSD, do high-level click ABR first; leave this check until the end if ANSD is not suspected • Note that the high-level click ABR may indicate ANSD even when toneburst ABR wave V responses are present, due to differences in neural synchrony underlying these responses

Note: Accurate threshold determination relies on bracketing of the threshold so that the minimum level at which the response is present can be determined, and ensuring wave V is replicable and larger than the residual noise in the waveform.

Examples of toneburst ABR recordings from an infant with normal hearing are shown in **Fig. 15.4**. Because the waveforms were very robust, it was possible to establish normal ABR thresholds at 500 and 2000 Hz very quickly in this infant. Repeat recordings are overlaid at the threshold levels. There is little noise in the recordings, and the waveforms are very robust, so a baseline recording was not performed. A baseline recording with an inaudible stimulus level (such as -20 dB nHL) is recommended if there is any doubt about response reproducibility or if it is difficult to determine threshold level.

Estimating Hearing Thresholds from Toneburst ABR

Toneburst ABR and pure tone thresholds show close agreement but are not exactly the same. This is not surprising given that the ABR is a "far-field" evoked potential, recorded on the surface of the scalp far away from the neural generators. Stapells and colleagues determined how many infants with normal hearing had toneburst ABR at near-threshold levels and found that, at 20 dB nHL or lower, 52% and 96% of infants had a toneburst ABR at 500 Hz and 2000 Hz, respectively (Stapells, Gravel, & Martin, 1995). Ninety-two percent of infants with normal hearing had a 500 Hz toneburst ABR at 30 dB nHL or lower. Thus, recommended pass levels for toneburst ABR are 30–40 dB and 20–30 dB nHL at 500 and 2000 Hz, respectively (ASHA, 2004).

Various authors have demonstrated excellent correlations between toneburst ABR and pure tone thresholds (Stapells et al, 1995; Stapells, Picton, Durieux-Smith, Edwards, & Moran, 1990). Toneburst ABR thresholds are generally within 5–10 dB of audiometric thresholds determined behaviorally (Hatton, Janssen, & Stapells, 2012). The relationship between ABR and pure tone thresholds is not exactly one to one, however, because there is closer agreement when hearing thresholds are more severe than for milder hearing loss (Stapells et al, 1995). The relationship between ABR and pure tone thresholds also varies across stimuli (Stapells, 2002b; Vander Werff, Prieve, & Georgantas, 2009). It is possible to have simple correction factors at each frequency when estimating the audiogram from the toneburst ABR (National Screening Unit [NSU], 2011). An alternative is to use a "lookup" table to estimate the audiogram, such as that shown in **Table 15.4** based on the regression equations reported by Stapells et al (1995).

Neurological Applications of ABR

The ABR is a sensitive indicator of brainstem status and has been used successfully to predict developmental outcomes in neonates who are at high risk for neurodevelopmental sequelae (Majnemer, Rosenblatt, & Riley, 1988). Abnormal findings associated with brainstem pathology or neuromaturational delay include absent or delayed waves, prolonged in-

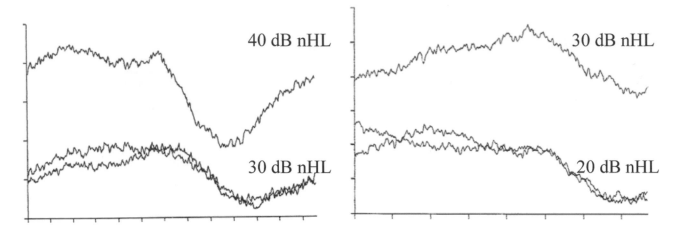

Fig. 15.4 Air conduction ABR recorded to 500 Hz (*left*) and 2000 Hz (*right*) tonebursts from a four-month-old infant with normal hearing. The time window differs between stimuli (25 milliseconds at 500 Hz versus 15 milliseconds at 2000 Hz). For tonebursts at 30 dB nHL, wave V occurs at ~ 12 milliseconds at 500 Hz and 9 milliseconds at 2000 Hz. This latency difference is expected based on cochlear travel times (Don, Eggermont, & Brackmann, 1979).

Table 15.4 Estimated pure tone thresholds (±10 dB) for three toneburst ABR frequencies

ABR threshold (dB nHL)	Estimated pure tone thresholds (dB HL)		
	500 Hz	2000 Hz	4000 Hz
30	23	29	31
35	27	34	36
40	32	38	40
45	36	43	45
50	40	47	49
55	45	52	54
60	49	56	58
65	53	61	63
70	58	66	67
75	62	70	72
80	66	75	76
85	71	79	81
90	75	84	85
95	79	88	90
100	84	93	94

Abbreviations: HL, hearing level; nHL, normal hearing level.
Source: Stapells et al (1995).

terwave intervals, and reduced wave V/I amplitude ratio (wave V small relative to wave I). Prolonged wave I–V intervals have been associated with brainstem pathology relating to perinatal asphyxia (Jiang & Tierney, 1996), prematurity and prenatal complications (Murray, 1988; Weber, 1982), and autism spectrum disorder (Wong & Wong, 1991). ABR may be useful for monitoring treatment or disease progression in children with medical conditions affecting the central auditory nervous system at the level of the brainstem (e.g., Spankovich & Lustig, 2007).

Using ABR to Diagnose ANSD

A subset of children with sensorineural hearing loss have ANSD, which is associated with unusual ABR findings. ANSD is characterized by abnormal hearing thresholds, absent (typically) acoustic reflexes, unexpectedly present otoacoustic emissions (OAEs), enlarged CM, and absent or abnormal ABR (Berlin, Hood, Morlet, Rose, & Brashears, 2003; Starr, Picton, Sininger, Hood, & Berlin, 1996). Speech recognition scores may be consistent with the audiogram or may be much poorer than the audiogram would predict (Rance et al, 1999). OAEs may or may not be present (Rance, Cone-Wesson, Wunderlich, & Dowell, 2002). The ABR findings are key to the diagnosis of ANSD. In children with ANSD, the ABR is absent or abnormal and contains evidence of cochlear activity (CM or abnormal positive potentials). **Fig. 15.5** shows an abnormal ABR recorded from the left ear of a 4-year-old with bilateral ANSD. This child developed encephalopathy and required resuscitation at age 4 and was subsequently referred to audiology because his

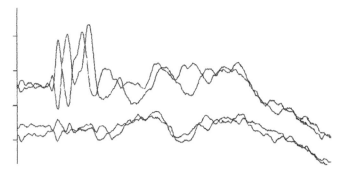

Fig. 15.5 Ipsilateral (*top*) and contralateral (*bottom*) ABR waveforms recorded in the left ear of a 4-year-old child with bilateral ANSD. Stimuli were 80 dB nHL clicks presented at 17.1/s to an insert earphone. Responses to rarefaction and condensation clicks are overlaid. There is a large CM at ~ 1–3 milliseconds in the early part of the ABR.

language had regressed. The ipsilateral ABR waveforms show a large CM and a late repeatable positive peak at ~8 milliseconds, which might be an abnormally delayed wave V.

Electrocochleography

Some clinics use ECoG as well as ABR for diagnosis of ANSD. Gibson and Sanli (2007) found that all 78 ears from 39 children with ANSD showed large CM and an abnormal positive potential (APP) when tested using ECoG with a round window recording electrode. ECoG is a technique used for "near-field" recording of cochlear and eighth-nerve potentials. This near-field technique enhances the amplitude of the cochlear potentials (CM and summating potential) and the whole nerve action potential (wave I of the ABR) because the recording electrodes are placed close to the generators of these responses. ECoG is performed either with a transtympanic electrode placed through the eardrum onto the promontory or in the round window niche or with an extratympanic electrode placed in the ear canal. ECoG recorded with tonal stimuli allows accurate estimation of pure tone thresholds (Fjermedal, Laukli, & Mair, 1988; Wong, Gibson, & Sanli, 1997). GA is required for transtympanic ECoG in children; hence, ABR is usually the preferred technique for diagnosis of ANSD and threshold estimation.

Bone Conduction ABR

When a hearing loss is detected using air conduction (AC) ABR, the next step is to determine whether there is a conductive component, as this may determine treatment. Tympanometry and acoustic reflexes are helpful but not entirely reliable. Reflexes will be ab-

sent when the hearing loss is more severe (Jerger, Harford, Clemis, & Alford, 1974). Tympanometry is not always reliable, especially in young infants, even when high-frequency probe tone tympanometry is used (Marchant et al, 1986). If tympanometry indicates the presence of middle ear disease, and ABR thresholds show a moderate or greater hearing loss, the size of the air-bone gap cannot be determined unless bone conduction (BC) ABR testing is performed.

Ears with conductive hearing loss show consistently delayed latencies across stimulus levels. However, this "typical" pattern may not occur when there is an unusually shaped hearing loss. For example, Gorga and colleagues reported a case of steep high-frequency sensorineural hearing loss that resulted in a latency-intensity function that looked like the classical pattern for conductive hearing loss (Gorga, Reiland, & Beauchaine, 1985). Current guidelines (ASHA, 2004) recommend BC-ABR testing to determine more reliably whether there is a conductive component.

Transducer placement and stimulus artifact cancellation are critical for successful BC-ABR recording (Foxe & Stapells, 1993). Another important consideration is the contribution of the opposite cochlea and whether masking is required. Stuart, Yang, and Botea (1990) and Yang, Rupert, and Moushegian (1987) investigated various bone vibrator placement options and determined that the best placement for BC-ABR is "supero-posterior," high on the mastoid, above and behind the auricula. This position optimizes ABR amplitude and minimizes stimulus artifact if the reference electrode is placed low on the mastoid. It is not possible to attach the bone vibrator comfortably using the usual headband; hence, various attachment options have been explored, including handheld placement or a Velcro/elastic headband. Handheld placement using a single finger in the center of the bone vibrator can provide the same signal quality as bone vibrator attachment with a conventional headband (Bachmann & Hall, 1998). Provided that sufficient care is taken to ensure consistent and appropriate placement, hand holding is an acceptable option for BC-ABR.

In young infants the bones of the skull are not fused, and there is greater interaural attenuation than in older children and adults (Yang et al, 1987). Thus, it is not always necessary to use masking, which can create masking dilemmas in children with bilateral atresia. The recommended approach when performing BC-ABR is to use two recording channels, with reference electrodes on the ipsilateral and contralateral ears. If, as is illustrated in **Fig. 15.6**, the response is larger and earlier in the ipsilateral recording channel, it must have been generated in the ipsilateral cochlea (Foxe & Stapells, 1993; Stapells & Ruben, 1989). **Fig. 15.6** shows an example of a BC-ABR recorded from a 3-month-old infant with unilat-

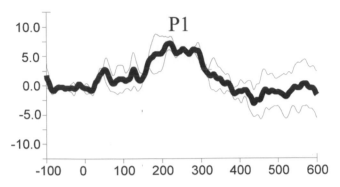

Fig. 15.8 CAEPs recorded to the speech sound /m/ in a 7-month-old infant with normal hearing. The stimulus (80 milliseconds duration, 1125 milliseconds interstimulus interval) was presented via a loudspeaker at 50 dB SPL to the infant who was listening binaurally seated on his mother's lap and distracted by toys during testing. In young infants, the CAEP waveform typically consists of a "P1" peak at ~ 200 milliseconds, with an amplitude of ~ 5–10 microvolts, as illustrated here.

researchers advocated the use of CAEPs to evaluate unaided versus aided hearing in children objectively (Gravel, Kurtzberg, Stapells, Vaughan, & Wallace, 1989; Rapin & Graziani, 1967). With the advent of universal newborn hearing screening, however, there is now much greater need for reliable, objective measures of hearing aid and cochlear implant success that can be used in infants. The ability to record aided CAEPs to a range of speech sounds is correlated with parental perceptions of aided hearing ability in infants with hearing loss (Golding et al, 2007). In children with hearing loss, CAEP presence reflects aided speech sound audibility (Chang, Dillon, Carter, van Dun, & Young, 2012).

Another potential application of CAEPs in children is in the area of ANSD. Children with ANSD who have poor speech perception outcomes have poor CAEPs for speech and tonal stimuli compared with those with relatively good speech perception (Rance et al, 2002). Sharma and coworkers found that CAEP P1 latencies in children with ANSD also correlate with parental ratings of auditory abilities in children with ANSD (Sharma, Cardon, Henion, & Roland, 2011). The relationship between CAEPs recorded early in infancy and later speech perception outcomes in children with ANSD is not yet known, however.

◆ Transducers and Stimulus Calibration

Insert earphones offer many advantages over supraaural earphones for evoked potential testing in children. Comfort and reliable placement are key

considerations when testing sleeping infants for prolonged periods. Output impedance values for evoked potential systems can be higher (e.g., 300 ohms) than values for pure tone audiometric equipment, so it is important to check that transducers are appropriately selected and calibrated. Insert earphones used repeatedly with sleeping infants in awkward positions may be dropped more often than those used to test awake adults, and frequent listening checks and regular calibration are important. The B-71 bone vibrator (Radioear Corp, New Eagle, PA) is most commonly used, complies with audiometric standards, and has a range of impedance options to suit different evoked potential systems. For soundfield delivery of stimuli (for example, for CAEP testing of aided hearing in infants), most clinical systems will require an external amplifier and loudspeaker. If that equipment is not purchased with the ABR system, care needs to be taken to ensure that impedances are matched, there is no distortion of the signal, and output levels are linear across a range of sound pressure levels.

Sound levels for evoked potential stimuli are specified in dB HL for longer-duration stimuli, such as those used for ASSR and CAEP testing. For these stimuli, the usual audiometric standards are relevant, although they do not specify reference levels for short speech sounds such as those used for aided CAEP testing in infants. For brief stimuli, such as clicks and tonebursts, stimulus levels are specified in dB nHL; this refers to the level of the stimulus relative to the normative threshold for otologically normal young adults. Calibration methods for clicks and tonebursts are described in the international standard IEC 60645–3 (*Audiometers–Part 3: Auditory test signals of short duration for audiometric and neuro-otological purposes*). This standard describes dB nHL levels and peak to peak equivalent sound pressure levels (dB ppeSPL) measurement techniques, but it does not specify reference threshold levels.

Several publications contain reference values for toneburst ABR (Sharma, Purdy, & Bonnici, 2003; Stapells, 2002b, 2004). Reference threshold levels (0 dB nHL) for clicks and tonebursts vary with stimulus frequency and repetition rate but are typically 20 to 35 dB ppeSPL for air conduction stimuli. Helpful guidelines for ABR stimulus calibration, including reference levels for clicks, tonebursts, and chirps, have been published by the United Kingdom's National Health Service Newborn Hearing Screening Program (NHSP) (2012). An international standard specifies reference levels for ABR stimuli (ISO 389–6:2007, *Acoustics–Reference zero for the calibration of audiometric equipment–Part 6: Reference hearing threshold levels for test signals of short duration*).

Pearls

Tips and Tricks for Successful Evoked Potential Recordings in Children

- Add waveforms to improve waveform quality. One or more repeat runs should be done at the level believed to be the ABR threshold to check for reliability of the response. Adding the two waveforms will normally improve the signal-to-noise ratio by enhancing wave V and reducing background noise, improving accuracy of peak identification.

- Use disposable electrodes or keep reusable electrodes in very good condition. The use of disposable electrodes ensures a consistent high-quality electrode surface. Occasionally, electrodes may need to be secured to the head with tape, particularly if the infant is hot and sweating. If reusable electrodes are used, it is possible to wear off the plating and expose the base metal, which will increase noise levels in evoked potential recordings. The same issues arise if reusable electrodes are tarnished or dirty.

- Braid electrode cables. The electrode cables act as an antenna and can pick up electromagnetic artifact that will degrade the quality of the evoked potential waveforms. Braiding the cables together will reduce the amount of electromagnetic artifact pickup. The most common source of this electromagnetic artifact is the transducer (bone vibrator, insert earphone, supraaural earphone), so cables should be placed as far as possible from the transducer. Potential sources of electrical artifact in the test environment should be kept away from the electrode cables (this includes mobile phones and other personal electronic devices).

- Place electrodes low on the mastoid so that the bone vibrator can fit if needed. In adults, the back of the earlobe and the mastoid are used interchangeably for ABR electrode placement. The mastoid is an easier location for electrode attachment in small infants, but it is also the place where the bone vibrator will be attached if BC-ABR is required. The negative electrode (also referred to as the noninverting or reference electrode) should be placed low on the mastoid so that, if BC-ABR is needed, the electrode is as far as possible from the electrode to minimize the chance of picking up electromagnetic artifact from the bone vibrator.

- Use a vertex electrode. ABR amplitudes are enhanced by having the positive electrode (also referred to as the noninverting or active electrode) on the vertex rather than the forehead (Beattie, Beguwala, Mills, & Boyd, 1986; Stuart et al, 1996). The vertex site is generally behind the fontanelle on most infants, so the fontanelle does not pose any problems for electrode attachment. Use of an abrasive paste such as NuPrep (Weaver and Company, Aurora, CO) on a cotton swab should ensure that skin impedances are sufficiently low (ideally lower than 5000 ohms; impedances are typically 2000 ohms or less with good-quality electrodes and good application technique). If an infant has thick hair, additional conductive paste may be needed to hold the electrode against the scalp and secure the electrode with tape.

- Use four electrodes routinely. Four electrodes should be attached routinely (positive on the vertex; negative electrodes on the two mastoids; common/ground on the forehead). If air conduction ABR testing indicates hearing loss and BC-ABR is required, it will then be easy to perform a two-channel (ipsilateral and contralateral) BC-ABR recording. Wave V amplitude and latency differences between channels, with ipsilateral earlier and larger than contralateral, provide confirmation that the BC-ABR is not a cross-heard response from the opposite cochlea (which would signal the need for masking).

- Use masking when testing at high stimulus levels for air conduction ABR. At high stimulus levels the recorded ABR may be a cross-heard response from the opposite cochlea (Hall, 2007). Interaural attenuation values for insert earphones are 55 dB or better (Etymotic Research, 2007). A delayed waveform recorded at high levels may be difficult to interpret, and a hearing loss asymmetry may not be evident if the clinician tested the poorer ear first, by chance, and then the infant woke up. To avoid this problem, contralateral broadband (white noise) masking should *always* be used when testing at stimulus levels of 70 dB nHL and higher.

- Use an external amplifier to get stimuli louder for more severe hearing losses. Commercial evoked potential systems typically have maximum stimulus levels for air conduction testing of 80 to 100 dB nHL, depending on the stimulus type and toneburst frequency and transducer type. Louder levels are needed for more accurate threshold estimation in children with severe or profound hearing loss. Toneburst levels up to ~110 dB nHL can be readily achieved without distortion if an additional external amplifier is used. If an external amplifier is used, care should be taken to ensure stimulus and masking levels are appropriately calibrated.

Jerger, J., Harford, E., Clemis, J., & Alford, B. (1974). The acoustic reflex in eighth nerve disorders. Archives of Otolaryngology, 99(6), 409–413.

Jewett, D. L., & Williston, J. S. (1971). Auditory-evoked far fields averaged from the scalp of humans. Brain, 94(4), 681–696.

Jiang, Z. D., & Tierney, T. S. (1996). Binaural interaction in human neonatal auditory brainstem. Pediatric Research, 39(4 Pt 1), 708–714.

John, M. S., Brown, D. K., Muir, P. J., & Picton, T. W. (2004). Recording auditory steady-state responses in young infants. Ear and Hearing, 25(6), 539–553.

Johnson, T. A., & Brown, C. J. (2005). Threshold prediction using the auditory steady-state response and the tone burst auditory brain stem response: a within-subject comparison. Ear and Hearing, 26(6), 559–576.

Kiang, N. Y., & Moxon, E. C. (1974). Tails of tuning curves of auditory-nerve fibers. The Journal of the Acoustical Society of America, 55(3), 620–630.

Kraus, N., & McGee, T. (1993). Clinical implications of primary and nonprimary pathway contributions to the middle latency response generating system. Ear and Hearing, 14(1), 36–48.

Kristensen, S. G. B., & Elberling, C. (2012). Auditory brainstem responses to level-specific chirps in normal-hearing adults. Journal of the American Academy of Audiology, 23(9), 712–721.

Kurtzberg, D., Hilpert, P. L., Kreuzer, J. A., & Vaughan, H. G., Jr. (1984). Differential maturation of cortical auditory evoked potentials to speech sounds in normal fullterm and very low-birthweight infants. Developmental Medicine and Child Neurology, 26(4), 466–475.

Lins, O. G., Picton, T. W., Boucher, B. L., Durieux-Smith, A., Champagne, S. C., Moran, L. M., . . . Savio, G. (1996). Frequency-specific audiometry using steady-state responses. Ear and Hearing, 17(2), 81–96.

Luts, H., & Wouters, J. (2004). Hearing assessment by recording multiple auditory steady-state responses: the influence of test duration. International Journal of Audiology, 43(8), 471–478.

Majnemer, A., Rosenblatt, B., & Riley, P. (1988). Prognostic significance of the auditory brainstem evoked response in high-risk neonates. Developmental Medicine and Child Neurology, 30(1), 43–52.

Marchant, C. D., McMillan, P. M., Shurin, P. A., Johnson, C. E., Turczyk, V. A., Feinstein, J. C., & Panek, D. M. (1986). Objective diagnosis of otitis media in early infancy by tympanometry and ipsilateral acoustic reflex thresholds. The Journal of Pediatrics, 109(4), 590–595.

Moller, A. R. (2007). Neural generators for auditory brainstem evoked potentials. In R. F. Burkard, M. Don, & J. J. Eggermont (Eds.), Auditory evoked potentials: basic principles and clinical application (1st ed.). Baltimore, MD: Lippincott Williams & Wilkins.

Moore, J. K., Ponton, C. W., Eggermont, J. J., Wu, B. J., & Huang, J. Q. (1996). Perinatal maturation of the auditory brain stem response: changes in path length and conduction velocity. Ear and Hearing, 17(5), 411–418.

Murray, A. D. (1988). Newborn auditory brainstem evoked responses (ABRs): prenatal and contemporary correlates. Child Development, 59(3), 571–588.

National Health Service Newborn Hearing Screening Program. (2012). NHSP recommended stimulus reference levels for ABR systems. Retrieved from http://hearing.screening.nhs.uk/audiologypublic

National Screening Unit. (2011). National Screening Unit Universal Newborn Hearing Screening And Early Intervention Programme (UNHSEIP) national policy and quality standards Appendix F: diagnostic and amplification protocols. Retrieved from http://www.nsu.govt.nz/files/F_word_2011.pdf

Picton, T. W., John, M. S., Dimitrijevic, A., & Purcell, D. (2003). Human auditory steady-state responses. International Journal of Audiology, 42(4), 177–219.

Ponton, C. W., Don, M., Eggermont, J. J., Waring, M. D., & Masuda, A. (1996). Maturation of human cortical auditory function: differences between normal-hearing children and children with cochlear implants. Ear and Hearing, 17(5), 430–437.

Purdy, S. C., Katsch, R., Dillon, H., Storey, L., Sharma, M., & Agung, K. (2005). Aided cortical auditory evoked potentials for hearing instrument evaluation in infants. Paper presented at A Sound Foundation through Early Amplification, Basel, Switzerland.

Purdy, S. C., Kelly, A. S., & Davies, M. G. (2002). Auditory brainstem response, middle latency response, and late cortical evoked potentials in children with learning disabilities. Journal of the American Academy of Audiology, 13(7), 367–382.

Purdy, S. C., Sharma, M., Munro, K. J., & Morgan, C. L. A. (2012). Stimulus level effects on speech-evoked obligatory cortical auditory evoked potentials in infants with normal hearing. Clinical Neurophysiology, 124(3), 474–480.

Rance, G., Beer, D. E., Cone-Wesson, B., Shepherd, R. K., Dowell, R. C., King, A. M., . . . Clark, G. M. (1999). Clinical findings for a group of infants and young children with auditory neuropathy. Ear and Hearing, 20(3), 238–252.

Rance, G., Cone-Wesson, B., Wunderlich, J., & Dowell, R. (2002). Speech perception and cortical event related potentials in children with auditory neuropathy. Ear and Hearing, 23(3), 239–253.

Rance, G., Tomlin, D., & Rickards, F. W. (2006). Comparison of auditory steady-state responses and tone-burst auditory brainstem responses in normal babies. Ear and Hearing, 27(6), 751–762.

Rapin, I., & Graziani, L. J. (1967). Auditory-evoked responses in normal, brain-damaged, and deaf infants. Neurology, 17(9), 881–894.

Runge-Samuelson, C. L., Drake, S., & Wackym, P. A. (2008). Quantitative analysis of electrically evoked auditory brainstem responses in implanted children with auditory neuropathy/dyssynchrony. Otology & Neurotology, 29(2), 174–178.

Sauter, B. T., Douglas, L. B., & Speidel, P. D. (2012). ABR and ASSR: challenges and solutions. Hearing Review, 19, 20–25.

Schochat, E., & Musiek, F. E. (2006). Maturation of outcomes of behavioral and electrophysiologic tests of central auditory function. Journal of Communication Disorders, 39(1), 78–92.

Sharma, A., & Dorman, M. F. (2006). Central auditory development in children with cochlear implants: clinical implications. Advances in Oto-Rhino-Laryngology, 64, 66–88.

Sharma, A., Cardon, G., Henion, K., & Roland, P. (2011). Cortical maturation and behavioral outcomes in children with auditory neuropathy spectrum disorder. International Journal of Audiology, 50(2), 98–106.

Sharma, M., Purdy, S. C., & Bonnici, L. (2003). Behavioural and electroacoustic calibration of air-conducted click and toneburst auditory brainstem response stimuli. Australian and New Zealand Journal of Audiology, 25, 54–60.

Sininger, Y. S. (2002). Identification of auditory neuropathy in infants and children. Seminars in Hearing, 23, 193–200.

Sininger, Y. S. (2003). Audiologic assessment in infants. Current Opinion in Otolaryngology & Head & Neck Surgery, 11(5), 378–382.

Small, S. A., & Stapells, D. R. (2006). Multiple auditory steady-state response thresholds to bone-conduction stimuli in young infants with normal hearing. Ear and Hearing, 27(3), 219–228.

Small, S. A., Hatton, J. L., & Stapells, D. R. (2007). Effects of bone oscillator coupling method, placement location, and occlusion on bone-conduction auditory steady-state responses in infants. Ear and Hearing, 28(1), 83–98.

Spankovich, C., & Lustig, L. R. (2007). Restoration of brain stem auditory-evoked potential in maple syrup urine disease. Otology & Neurotology, 28(4), 566–569.

Stapells, D. R. (2002a). The tone-evoked ABR: why it's the measure of choice for young infants. Hearing Journal, 55, 14–18.

Stapells, D. R. (2002b). Threshold estimation by the tone-evoked auditory brainstem response: a literature meta-analysis. Journal of Speech-Language Pathology and Audiology, 24, 74–83.

Stapells, D. R. (2004). Recommended recording parameters and stimulus parameters for clinical tone-evoked ABR in infants. Retrieved from http://www.courses.audiospeech .ubc.ca/haplab/TONE-ABR_PARAMETERS.html

Stapells, D. R., & Oates, P. (1997). Estimation of the pure-tone audiogram by the auditory brainstem response: a review. Audiology & Neuro-Otology, 2(5), 257–280.

Stapells, D. R., & Ruben, R. J. (1989). Auditory brain stem responses to bone-conducted tones in infants. The Annals of Otology, Rhinology, and Laryngology, 98(12 Pt 1), 941–949.

Stapells, D. R., Gravel, J. S., & Martin, B. A. (1995). Thresholds for auditory brain stem responses to tones in notched noise from infants and young children with normal hearing or sensorineural hearing loss. Ear and Hearing, 16(4), 361–371.

Stapells, D. R., Herdman, A., Small, S. A., Dimitrijevic, A., & Hatton, J. (2005). Current status of the auditory steady-state responses for estimating an infant's audiogram. In R. C. Seewald & J. M. Bamford (Eds.), A sound foundation through early amplification (pp. 43–59). Basel, Switzerland: Phonak.

Stapells, D. R., Picton, T. W., Durieux-Smith, A., Edwards, C. G., & Moran, L. M. (1990). Thresholds for short-latency auditory-evoked potentials to tones in notched noise in normal-hearing and hearing-impaired subjects. Audiology, 29(5), 262–274.

Starr, A., Picton, T. W., Sininger, Y., Hood, L. J., & Berlin, C. I. (1996). Auditory neuropathy. Brain, 119(Pt 3), 741–753.

Starr, A., Sininger, Y., Nguyen, T., Michalewski, H. J., Oba, S., & Abdala, C. (2001). Cochlear receptor (microphonic and summating potentials, otoacoustic emissions) and auditory pathway (auditory brain stem potentials) activity in auditory neuropathy. Ear and Hearing, 22(2), 91–99.

Stuart, A., Yang, E. Y., & Botea, M. (1996). Neonatal auditory brainstem responses recorded from four electrode montages. Journal of Communication Disorders, 29(2), 125–139.

Stuart, A., Yang, E. Y., & Stenstrom, R. (1990, Oct). Effect of temporal area bone vibrator placement on auditory brain stem response in newborn infants. Ear and Hearing, 11(5), 363–369.

Sutton, G., Lightfoot, G., Stevens, J., Booth, R., Brennan, S., Feirn, R., & Meredith, R. (2013). Guidance for auditory brainstem response in babies. NHSP Clinical Group. Retrieved from http://hearing.screening.nhs.uk/getdata.php?id=19345

Tucker, D. A., & Ruth, R. A. (1996). Effects of age, signal level, and signal rate on the auditory middle latency response. Journal of the American Academy of Audiology, 7(2), 83–91.

van der Drift, J. F., Brocaar, M. P., & van Zanten, G. A. (1987). The relation between the pure-tone audiogram and the click auditory brainstem response threshold in cochlear hearing loss. Audiology, 26(1), 1–10.

van Straaten, H. L. M., Hille, E. T. M., Kok, J. H., & Verkerk, P. H.; Dutch NICU Neonatal Hearing Screening Working Group. (2003). Implementation of a nation-wide automated auditory brainstem response hearing screening programme in neonatal intensive care units. Acta Paediatrica (Oslo, Norway), 92(3), 332–338.

Vander Werff, K. R., Prieve, B. A., & Georgantas, L. M. (2009). Infant air and bone conduction tone burst auditory brain stem responses for classification of hearing loss and the relationship to behavioral thresholds. Ear and Hearing, 30(3), 350–368.

Weber, B. A. (1982). Comparison of auditory brain stem response latency norms for premature infants. Ear and Hearing, 3(5), 257–262.

Wegner, O., & Dau, T. (2002). Frequency specificity of chirp-evoked auditory brainstem responses. The Journal of the Acoustical Society of America, 111(3), 1318–1329.

Wong, S. H., Gibson, W. P., & Sanli, H. (1997). Use of transtympanic round window electrocochleography for threshold estimations in children. The American Journal of Otology, 18(5), 632–636.

Wong, V., & Wong, S. N. (1991). Brainstem auditory evoked potential study in children with autistic disorder. Journal of Autism and Developmental Disorders, 21(3), 329–340.

Yang, E. Y., Rupert, A. L., & Moushegian, G. (1987). A developmental study of bone conduction auditory brain stem response in infants. Ear and Hearing, 8(4), 244–251.

Although there is no generally accepted comprehensive definition of auditory processing disorders, the challenges of the past have led the profession to current definitions that address, at least in part, these criticisms. ASHA (2005a) defines auditory processing as "the perceptual processing of auditory information in the CNS and the neurobiologic activity that underlies that processing and gives rise to electrophysiologic auditory potentials." Similarly, APD was defined in the recommendations of the Bruton conference as "a deficit in the processing of information in the auditory modality" (Jerger & Musiek, 2000). A critical issue that is not raised in either of these definitions but must be stated implicitly is that APD reflects deficits "in the formation and processing of audible signals not attributed to impaired hearing sensitivity or intellectual impairment," thus not resulting from peripheral hearing loss or cognitive disorders (DeConde-Johnson & Seaton, 2011). A simple yet functional description of an auditory processing disorder is a breakdown in auditory abilities resulting in diminished learning, or comprehension, or both, of auditory information through hearing, even though peripheral hearing sensitivity is normal. For the purposes of this description, normal hearing should be considered as detection thresholds of 15 dB hearing level (HL) or better by conventional audiometry for both ears, which has historically been referred to as the "low fence" for hearing in children. Despite controversies that persist in the area of auditory processing, years of evidence establish APD as a "true" clinical disorder (AAA, 2010).

Auditory processes may be described as the auditory system mechanisms responsible for the following behaviors: sound localization and lateralization, auditory discrimination, temporal aspects of audition, auditory performance decrements when competing acoustic information is present, and auditory performance decrements when the auditory signal is degraded (ASHA, 1996). According to the ASHA statement, deficits in one or more of these areas would constitute an APD. Auditory processing difficulties may be present for speech and nonspeech stimuli (Rosen, 2005). These types of deficits result in the auditory system being less flexible than required for effective listening in the wide variety of environments faced by most children each day. This is particularly true in the classroom environment, in which unfamiliar linguistic information is being introduced in an often less than optimal acoustic environment. This taxes an auditory system that cannot effectively rise to the challenge.

A strict definition of APD also has clinical relevance. In some ways, APD is a "field of dreams" for families looking for answers, when applied in its broadest definition. Parents or educators who are shopping for explanations for academic underachievement may cling to APD as a holy grail, since they may find this to be a more palatable diagnosis than other possible options, such as cognitive impairment or autism spectrum disorder (ASD). The ready availability of information and misinformation regarding auditory processing on the Internet also fuels referrals for testing. The audiologist is encouraged to base decision-making about auditory processing assessment on a strict definition of APD to minimize inappropriate referrals and to use time and resources most effectively.

In addition, APD is considered to be a low-incidence disorder, as a relatively small number of children are thought to have this type of exclusive condition. Chermak and Musiek (2007) estimate that as many as 2–5% of school-aged children who are identified as having a learning disorder have APD. However, there is limited epidemiological information about APD, mainly because there is no general agreement on diagnostic markers, a situation that is exacerbated by the potential overlap between the behavioral characteristics of APD and other types of neurobiologic disorders (Hind, 2006). As generally accepted definitions emerge and test batteries evolve, more accurate data about the prevalence of APD will become available.

Pitfall

- A complication in defining APD is that instead of a homogeneous disorder, the population of children with APDs is heterogeneous.

Since the disorder represents individual differences in the brain, APD is idiosyncratic because individual, subtle organizational abnormalities may have diverse presentations; therefore, APD can be as idiosyncratic as the individuals who experience it (Phillips, 2002). For most cases of APD in children, the actual etiology is unknown, but the disorder is attributed to poor underlying neurophysiologic representation of the auditory signal, a critical role of the central auditory nervous system (CANS) (Phillips, 1995). In some cases, the underlying etiology can be identified and may result from a head injury or neurologic disease. Delays in auditory development, related to factors such as chronic otitis media, may also be considered; however, some of the research in this area is contradictory, and the causal relationship may not always be clear (Hall, Grose, & Pillsbury, 1995). It is important to recognize that the processing of auditory information within the CANS is complex and involves both serial and parallel processing within the CANS as well as processing that is shared among other brain structures and systems, including those that govern language processing, attention, and executive control (AAA, 2010). These interactions underline the fact that the brain is not compartmentalized and that CANS dysfunction or pathology does not respect functional boundaries of the brain (Phillips, 2002). In addition, some of the criticisms of auditory processing theories of the past should not be surprising, based on the fact that the auditory system does not exist or function in isolation, but rather as part of complex interactions among other brain functions and structures. That being said, it is not surprising that behavioral manifestations and levels of impairment in children with auditory processing disorders are diverse and heterogeneous (AAA, 2010).

As noted previously, auditory processing may be considered on the continuum of hearing loss, and many of the behaviors noted in children with auditory processing disorders are similar to those in children with peripheral hearing loss, such as difficulty listening in the presence of background noise. A question that frequently arises is how to assess "auditory processing" skills in children with peripheral hearing loss. As established in this chapter, a generally accepted definition of auditory processing disorder addresses deficits in auditory behavior in the presence of normal peripheral hearing acuity. By definition, children with peripheral hearing losses would be expected to have difficulty with the processing of auditory information based on the nature of hearing loss alone. As established by Erber (1977), there is a hierarchy of auditory skills predicated on detection, or audibility, of sound. If audibility is compromised, as is the case with peripheral hearing loss, the child would experience difficulty with higher-level tasks, such as discrimination, identification, and comprehension. When asked about the idea of auditory processing deficits in a child with a peripheral hearing loss, the audiologist should explore the motivation for the question. Issues that should be assessed in this case include monitoring of peripheral hearing status, performance of speech-in-noise assessment, obtaining real ear measures to address audibility, and functional listening evaluation.

Assessment of an auditory processing disorder in a child with hearing loss is controversial and must be approached cautiously. The potential negative impact of peripheral hearing loss on the evaluation of auditory processing skills has been well established (Neijenhuis, Tschur, & Snik, 2004). The auditory processing skills of children with significant degrees of hearing loss cannot be accurately assessed; however, those with less significant degrees of hearing loss and good word recognition skills may potentially be assessed with tests that are less affected by cochlear hearing loss, such as the dichotic digits test (AAA, 2010). However, many of the tests with normative data that could be included in a behavioral test battery, such as the *SCAN-3: Tests for Auditory Processing Disorders,* provide specific cautions and caveats regarding using these tests on children with peripheral hearing loss. The relationship between periph-

eral hearing loss and auditory processing is complex; however, this relationship has been recognized as having a role in the definition of secondary APD. In this case, APD may occur as the result of a peripheral hearing loss, including transient hearing loss that has resolved, such as in the case of chronic otitis media (BAA, 2011). Based on the current state of the science, assessment of APDs in children is best reserved for children in whom normal peripheral hearing acuity has been established. However, a comprehensive assessment of listening skills in children with hearing loss should be performed, as outlined in Chapters 28 and 31 of this book.

◆ Assessment of Auditory Processing Skills in Children

The challenge in assessing APDs is to develop a comprehensive test battery that provides adequate information to describe the functional parameters of the child's skills across a variety of auditory behaviors, provides a differential diagnosis, and guides appropriate treatment and management. Historically, interest in assessing auditory processing skills arose from observations of adults who presented with complaints of difficulties listening in less than optimal environments, despite having normal peripheral hearing acuity. Sensitized speech tests, which reduced the external redundancy of the speech signal by distorting it (such as by filtering the stimuli) and reducing the intelligibility of the speech, were used to challenge the auditory system as part of a site-of-lesion assessment in adults with pathologies of the CANS (Bocca, Calearo, & Cassinari, 1954). Several tests, using various methods of distorting the signal and challenging the auditory system, were developed during this period, including the Staggered Spondaic Word test (Katz, 1962) and dichotic consonant-vowels (CVs) (Berlin, Lowe-Bell, Cullen, & Thompson, 1973), which are still used today. These tests are sensitive to detecting retrocochlear and central pathologies in adults.

Some children with normal peripheral hearing acuity were observed to present difficulties similar to those demonstrated by adults with known CANS lesions. This interest coincided with the introduction of the term *learning disabilities* into the realm of public education during the 1970s, along with the subsequent explosion in programs targeted at remediating learning disabilities, with a particular focus on processing and perceptual training (Hallahan & Mercer, 2002). Whether and where APD fits into the learning disability continuum is a discussion that continues today, as the impact of APD on children in the classroom environment continues to be of interest. The first tests designed specifically to assess APD the student in a classroom environment. If failure of communication occurs on the part of the listener, the speaker (or in this case, the teacher) should also be provided with strategies that can improve the child's comprehension. An example of such an intervention program targeted at the speaker is the concept of clear speech, a set of intervention techniques designed to address parameters of the speech signal that can enhance speech intelligibility for the listener (Krause & Braida, 2002; Tye-Murray & Schum, 1994).

The child may benefit from developing additional metacognitive abilities that empower him to implement small but significant accommodations in the classroom, which gives him control over his own listening and learning environment. Several techniques and skills, including use of a pocket calendar/organizer and guided notes provided by the teacher, provide accommodation under the metacognitive approach. A psychologist or speech-language pathologist in working with a child often addresses the development of these metacognitive skills.

Treatment by Direct Therapeutic Approaches

Historically, speech-language pathologists in the school setting have implemented auditory training programs for children with APD. Often these programs were implemented as part of a language therapy program and target a top-down approach to listening. Some of these programs also focused on addressing auditory aspects to build reading and literacy skills, such as the Orton-Gillingham or the Lindamood Phonemic Synthesis (LiPS) programs. These programs may include a multisensory approach to enhance auditory skills and often target global listening skills rather than addressing specific types of auditory processing skills that may be taught. In some cases, programming has been implemented from preprinted worksheets or handbooks that address listening skills. Although some of these programs may have efficacy, it has been difficult to measure changes in the auditory system following implementation of these programs or to accept that the focus of the program is anything beyond the development of compensatory skills.

Recent advances in auditory neuroscience have ignited renewed interest in the treatment of APDs. Phillips (2002) pointed out that changes in the auditory cortex, representing the neural plasticity of the system, are seen as a result of behavioral training, first noted in animal models and now seen in human auditory system development. Thompson (2000) described "representational plasticity" of the central auditory nervous system, engaging new growth in neural networks posttreatment. Although these theories have been in place for more than a decade, recent advances in clinical application of treatment programs have demonstrated advances in actual treatment of APD.

Although auditory training programs have historically been applied to intervention for children with APD, current programs attempt to capitalize on intensive adaptive training methods. Some have used specific types of stimuli presented in an adaptive manner and incorporated into a computer game format. One of the earliest such programs was Fast-ForWord, an auditory training program designed to address temporal processing (Tallal, Merzenich, Miller, & Jenkins, 1998). Although the efficacy of using FastForWord as a treatment program for children with APD was debated, the options for computer-assisted auditory training have grown because of an improved understanding of the principles that improve the efficacy and effectiveness with these types of programs and the ability to measure this efficacy.

Several treatment programs have incorporated the principles described above to address specific auditory processing deficits identified in the auditory processing assessment. One example is the dichotic interaural intensity difference (DIID) training for binaural integration deficits (Musiek, 2004). This training technique presents a stimulus to the dominant ear at a less intense level than a stimulus presented to the poorer ear. Improvement in left ear deficits has been reported (Musiek, 2004). Temporal processing deficits have been addressed using training on temporal ordering tasks, using the game SIMON (Hasbro, Pawtucket, RI) as the vehicle for auditory training (Musiek, 2005). Another example of a deficit-specific program is Auditory Rehabilitation for Interaural Asymmetry (ARIA), a program to strengthen the listening skills of the weaker ear in dichotic listening skills (Moncrieff & Wertz, 2008). Initial results for both programs were promising related to the ability to change the auditory system with treatment, based on behavioral changes observed in skills following treatment.

A new generation of treatment programs has emerged for APD, based on several trends, including linking assessment results to a treatment program and being able to document actual changes in the auditory system. One example of this is the LiSN and Learn auditory training program, developed by Cameron and Dillon at the National Acoustics Laboratories (2012). The software is targeted to remediate spatial processing disorders (SPD) as identified by the results of the LISN-S test, discussed earlier in this chapter. The program uses a game-based format with adaptive stimuli and is administered over a period of ~ 10 weeks, with the child "playing" two games a day, 5 days a week. Cameron and Dillon (2011) reported that children who participated in this program demonstrated a 10 dB post-treatment improvement at the conclusion of the 10-week treatment program with the LiSN and Learn program. These results demonstrated gains that resulted in typical listening skills at the end of treatment. The LiSN and Learn program is available through the National Acoustics Laboratories.

Speech-in-noise deficits, often considered the hallmark of auditory processing disorders, have been the recent focus of auditory training paradigms. As part of this process, the desire has been to improve the child's skills and to understand the underlying biological mechanisms mediating the improvements (Song, Skoe, Banai, & Kraus, 2012). This is another paradigm related to treating deficits identified in the evaluation process, in this case as identified by the cABR protocol discussed earlier in this chapter. The current research incorporates the use of the Listening and Communication Enhancement (LACE) auditory training program, which has a speech-in-noise training component (Sweetow & Henderson-Sabes, 2004). Early results suggest that the child's behavioral speech-in-noise skills improve with training, and changes in the cABR response correspond to the behavioral changes, supporting plastic changes in the auditory system as a result of treatment.

The role of musical training in the development of auditory processing skills has also received significant interest. The ability to focus on a particular sound of interest in a stream of "noise" has been described as a type of auditory attention and has been found to be strengthened in musicians (Kraus & Chandrasekaran, 2010). It has been hypothesized that these types of strengths will carry over to speech-in-noise perception and to the enhancement of auditory working memory (Kraus, 2011). Although it is too early to fully comprehend the implications of this research, it is clear that musical training appears to have positive and unique impacts on improving auditory processing skills, suggesting that musical training may be a recommendation for treating or preventing auditory processing deficits (Kraus, 2012).

Computerized auditory training programs will continue to grow as additional data are obtained about these programs and the ability to develop deficit-specific programs evolves. In addition, these computer programs are likely to have significant impact on developing auditory training as a means to build auditory processing skills in all younger children. However, the ability to generalize skills from auditory training programs to more global skills, such as reading or spoken language, has not been established. McArthur (2009) reviewed six studies in which children with APDs participated in auditory training programs that included nonspeech stimuli or simple speech sounds. The results indicated that both nonspeech training and simple speech sound training were effective in treating APDs in children; however, the training had little or no impact on reading, academic, and language skills. As computer training expands, it may be determined that this type of generalization is not possible or not necessary to make a difference in abilities. In addition, it is possible that auditory training programs will be better tailored to target both audi-

tory processing deficits and the ability to generalize to other communication and learning skills. It has been reported that transfer of training in treatment is optimized when some stimulus dimensions (e.g., speech, modulated noise, tonal frequency) in the treatment program are shared between the tasks and outcomes; outcome-specific materials for auditory training are recommended (Millward, Hall, Ferguson, & Moore, 2011).

◆ Summary

Assessment, treatment, and management of auditory processing skills in children are time- and labor-intensive, but a worthwhile investment on the part of the audiologist. Jerger (1998) states that "the reality of APD can no longer be doubted. It is a distinct entity across the entire age range." This chapter focuses on the pediatric patient; however, assessment and management of APD across the lifespan are certainly within the scope of practice of audiology, which recognizes the role of the brain in hearing and listening and acknowledges that hearing and listening do not stop at the level of the inner ear. The auditory system's ability to learn and change supports why audiologists enter the profession—the abilities to effectively identify an underlying disorder and to intervene to improve the quality of the person's life and communication are germane to the area of APDs.

Discussion Questions

1. How does the audiologist develop an interdisciplinary team to assess auditory processing skills in children?

2. What issues might an audiologist consider in developing an APD test battery? What specific test materials might be included in the test battery, based on the issues and the audiologist's philosophical approach?

3. What is the role of the audiologist in the management and treatment of APDs?

4. What impact is an APD likely to have on a child in the classroom and why? What types of interventions can address these types of deficits in the classroom environment?

5. What does the current model of auditory development and knowledge of neural plasticity suggest about the efficacy of treatments related to APDs?

6. What options for acoustic modifications are available in the classroom for the child with APD? Describe how each would be implemented and how the effectiveness of each would be determined.

◆ Appendix

Distributors for Auditory Processing Assessment Materials

Auditec of St. Louis
2515 South Big Bend Blvd
St. Louis, MO 63143
800-669-9065
auditecinfo@auditec.com (e-mail)
www.auditec.com (Website)

APD test materials include:
- Auditory Fusion Test—Revised
- Competing Sentences
- Dichotic Digits
- Dichotic Sentence Identification (DSI) Test
- Masking Level Difference
- Multiple Auditory Processing Assessment (MAPA)
- Pitch Pattern Sequence (PPS) Test
- Random Gap Detection Test (RGDT)
- Time Compressed Sentences Test (TCST)
- Time Compressed Sentences Test—Spanish version
- Selective Auditory Attention Test (SAAT)
- Staggered Spondaic Word Test—Spanish version

Educational Audiology Association
11166 Huron Street, Suite 27
Denver, CO 80234
800-460-7322
EAA@imigroup.org (e-mail)
www.edaud.org (Website)

APD materials include:
- Children's Auditory Performance Scale (CHAPs)
- Fisher's Auditory Checklist
- Listening Inventories for Education (LIFE)
- Screening Identification for Targeting Educational Risk Listening Inventories for Education (SIFTER)

National Acoustic Laboratories (NAL)
126 Greville Street
Chastwood, NSW 2067
Australia
+614–94126872
http://shop.nal.gov.au/store/lisn-learn.html

APD test materials include:
- LiSN and Learn auditory training program

Pearson
Attn: Inbound Sales & Customer Support
P.O. Box 599700
San Antonio, TX 78259
800-627-7271
http://www.pearsonassessments.com

APD test materials include:
- SCAN–3:A Tests for Auditory Processing Disorders in Adolescents and Adults (SCAN-3:A)
- SCAN–3:C Tests for Auditory Processing Disorders in Children (SCAN-3:C)
- Auditory skills assessment (ASA)

Precision Acoustics
505 NE 87th Ave., Ste 150
Vancouver, WA
360-892-9367

APD test materials include:
- Staggered Spondaic Word Test
- Phonemic Synthesis Test
- Competing Environmental Sounds (CES) Test

Phonak LLC
4520 Weaver Parkway
Warrenville, IL 60555–3927
800-777-7333
https://www.phonakpro.com/com/b2b/en/professional_tools/diagnostic/lisn-s/lisn-s_in_detail.html

APD test materials include:
- Listening in Spatialized Noise—Sentences (LISN–S)

References

American Academy of Audiology. (2010). Clinical practice guidelines. Diagnosis, treatment, and management of children and adults with central auditory processing disorder. Retrieved from http://www.audiology.org/resources/documentlibrary/Pages/CentralAuditoryProcessingDisorder.aspx

American National Standards Institute. (2002). ANSI S12.60–2002 American National Standard acoustical performance criteria, design requirements, and guidelines for schools. Melville, NY: ANSI.

American Speech-Language-Hearing Association. (1996). Central auditory processing: current status of research and implications for clinical practice. American Journal of Audiology, 5, 41–54.

American Speech-Language-Hearing Association. (1999). Guidelines for fitting and monitoring FM systems. ASHA desk reference. Rockville, MD: ASHA.

American Speech-Language-Hearing Association. (2004). Scope of practice in audiology [Scope of Practice]. Retrieved from http://www.asha.org/policy

American Speech-Language-Hearing Association. (2005a). (Central) auditory processing disorders. Retrieved from http://www.asha.org/members/deskref-journals/deskref/default

American Speech-Language-Hearing Association. (2005b). (Central) auditory processing disorders—the role of the audiologist [position statement]. Retrieved from http://www.asha.org/members/deskref-journals/deskref/default

Anderson, K. (1995). Screening Instrument for Targeting Educational Risk (SIFTER). Tampa, FL: Educational Audiology Association.

Anderson, K., Smaldino, J. J., & Spangler, C. (2011). The listening inventory for education—revised (LIFE-R). Tampa, FL: Educational Audiology Association.

Bamiou, D. E., Musiek, F. E., & Luxon, L. M. (2001). Aetiology and clinical presentations of auditory processing disorders—a review. Archives of Disease in Childhood, 85(5), 361–365.

Banai, K., & Kraus, N. (2008). The dynamic brainstem: implications for APD. In D. McFarland, & A. Cacace (Eds.), Current controversies in central auditory processing disorder (pp. 269–289). San Diego, CA: Plural.

Bellis, T. J., & Ferre, J. M. (1999). Multidimensional approach to the differential diagnosis of central auditory processing disorders in children. Journal of the American Academy of Audiology, 10(6), 319–328.

Berlin, C. I., Lowe-Bell, S. S., Cullen, J. K., Jr, & Thompson, C. L. (1973). Dichotic speech perception: an interpretation of right-ear advantage and temporal offset effects. The Journal of the Acoustical Society of America, 53(3), 699–709.

Besing, J. M., & Koehnke, J. (1995). A test of virtual auditory localization. Ear and Hearing, 16(2), 220–229.

Bocca, E., Calearo, C., & Cassinari, V. (1954). A new method for testing hearing in temporal lobe tumor. Acta Oto-Laryngologica, 44(3), 219–221.

Boothroyd, A. (2004). Room acoustics and speech perception. Seminars in Hearing, 25, 155–166.

British Academy of Audiology. (2011). Position statement. Auditory processing disorder (APD). Retrieved from http://www.thebsa.org.uk/images/stories/docs/BSA_APD_PositionPaper_31March11_FINAL.pdf

Cacace, A. T., & McFarland, D. J. (2005). The importance of modality specificity in diagnosing central auditory processing disorder. American Journal of Audiology, 14(2), 112–123.

Cameron, S., & Dillon, H. (2008). The Listening in Spatialized Noise-Sentences Test (LISN-S): comparison to the prototype LISN and results from children with either a suspected (central) auditory processing disorder or a confirmed language disorder. Journal of the American Academy of Audiology, 19(5), 377–391.

Cameron, S., & Dillon, H. (2011). Development and evaluation of the LiSN & Learn auditory training software for deficit-specific remediation of binaural processing deficits in children: preliminary findings. Journal of the American Academy of Audiology, 22(10), 678–696.

Chermak, G. D., & Musiek, F. E. (2007). Handbook of (central) auditory processing disorder: auditory neuroscience and diagnosis. San Diego, CA: Plural.

Clarke, E. M., Ahmmed, A., Parker, D., & Adams, C. (2006). Contralateral suppression of otoacoustic emissions in children with specific language impairment. Ear and Hearing, 27(2), 153–160.

Crandell, C. C., & Smaldino, J. J. (2000). Classroom acoustics for children with normal hearing and with hearing impairment. language, speech, and hearing services in schools. Language, Speech, and Hearing Services in Schools, 31, 362–370.

DeConde-Johnson, C., & Seaton, J. B. (2011). Educational audiology handbook (2nd ed.). Clifton Park, NY: Delmar Cengage Learning.

Downs, D., Schmidt, B., & Stephens, T. J. (2005). Auditory behaviors of children and adolescents with pervasive developmental disorders. Seminars in Hearing, 26, 226–240.

Egelhoff, K., Whitelaw, G., & Rabidoux, P. (2005). What audiologists need to know about autism spectrum disorders. Seminars in Hearing, 26, 202–209.

Emanuel, D. C., Ficca, K. N., & Korczak, P. (2011). Survey of the diagnosis and management of auditory processing disorder. American Journal of Audiology, 20(1), 48–60.

Erber, N. (1977). Evaluation speech perception ability in hearing impaired children. In F.H. Bess (Ed.), Childhood deafness: causation, assessment, and management (pp. 173–182). New York, NY: Grune & Stratton.

Fisher, L. I. (1978). Fisher's Auditory Checklist. Tampa, FL: Educational Audiology Association.

Geffner, D., & Goldman, R. (2010). Auditory skills assessment. San Antonio, TX: Pearson Education.

Gravel, J. W., Dunn, M., Lei, W. W., Ellis, M. A., & Hood, L. (2001). Indices of basic auditory processes in children with autism. Proceedings of the American Auditory Society Meeting.

Hall, J. W. & Grose, J. H. (1990). The masking level difference in children. Journal of the American Academy of Audiology, 1(2), 81–88.

Hall, J. W., III, Grose, J. H., & Pillsbury, H. C. (1995). Long-term effects of chronic otitis media on binaural hearing in children. Archives of Otolaryngology–Head & Neck Surgery, 121, 81–88.

Hall, J. W., III, Grose, J. H., Buss, E., & Dev, M. B. (2002). Spondee recognition in a two-talker masker and a speech-shaped noise masker in adults and children. Ear and Hearing, 23(2), 159–165.

Hallahan, D. P., & Mercer, C. D. (2002). Learning disabilities: historical perspective. Learning Disabilities Summit: Building a Foundation for the Future. Nashville, TN: National Research Center on Learning Disabilities. Retrieved from http://www.nrcld.org/resources/ldsummit/hallahan.pdf

Hind, S. (2006). Survey of care pathway of auditory processing disorder. Audiological Medicine, 4, 12–24. DOI:10.1080/16513860500534543

Hnath-Chisolm, T. E., Laipply, E., & Boothroyd, A. (1998). Age-related changes on a children's test of sensory-level speech perception capacity. Journal of Speech, Language, and Hearing Research: JSLHR, 41(1), 94–106.

Hornickel, J., Zecker, S. G., Bradlow, A. R., & Kraus, N. (2012). Assistive listening devices drive neuroplasticity in children with dyslexia. Proc. Natl. Acad. Sci. USA, 109(41), 16731–16736.

Intelligent Hearing Systems. (2012). SmartEP. Retrieved from http://www.ihsys.com/site/SmartEP.asp

Jerger, J. (1998). Controversial issues in central auditory processing disorders. Seminars in Hearing, 19(2), 393–398.

Jerger, J., & Musiek, F. E. (2000). Report of consensus conference on the diagnosis of auditory processing disorders in school-aged children. Journal of the American Academy of Audiology, 11(9), 467–474.

Jerger, J., & Musiek, F. E. (2002). On the diagnosis of auditory processing disorder: a reply to Clinical and research concerns regarding the 2000 APD consensus report and recommendations. Audiology Today, 14, 19–21.

Jirsa, R. E. (2002). Clinical efficacy of electrophysiologic measures in APD management programs. Seminars in Hearing, 23, 349–355.

Jirsa, R. E., & Clontz, K. B. (1990). Long latency auditory event-related potentials from children with auditory processing disorders. Ear and Hearing, 11(3), 222–232.

Johnson, C. E. (2000). Children's phoneme identification in reverberation and noise. Journal of Speech, Language, and Hearing Research: JSLHR, 43(1), 144–157.

Johnson, K. L., Nicol, T., & Kraus, N. (2005). The brainstem response to speech: a biological marker. Ear and Hearing, 26, 424–443.

Katz, J. (1962). The use of staggered spondaic words for assessing the integrity of the central auditory nervous system. The Journal of Auditory Research, 2, 327–337.

Katz, J., & Smith, P. S. (1991). The Staggered Spondaic Word Test. A ten-minute look at the central nervous system through the ears. Annals of the New York Academy of Sciences, 620(1), 233–251.

Katz, J., Stecker, N. A., & Henderson, D. (1992). Central auditory processing: a transdisciplinary view. St. Louis, MO: Mosby Year Book.

Keith, R. W. (2009). SCAN-3:C Tests for Auditory Processing Disorders for Children (SCAN-3:C). San Antonio, TX: Pearson.

Keith, R. W. (2000). Random gap detection test. St. Louis, MO: Auditec.

Knecht, H. A., Nelson, P. B., Whitelaw, G. M., & Feth, L. L. (2002). Background noise levels and reverberation times in unoccupied classrooms: predictions and measurements. American Journal of Audiology, 11(2), 65–71.

Kraus, N. (2011). Musical training gives edge in auditory processing. The Hearing Journal, 64(2), 10–16.

Kraus, N. (2012). Biological impact of music and software-based auditory training. Journal of Communication Disorders, 45(6), 403–410.

Kraus, N., & Chandrasekaran, B. (2010). Music training for the development of auditory skills. Nature Reviews. Neuroscience, 11(8), 599–605.

Krause, J. C., & Braida, L. D. (2002). Investigating alternative forms of clear speech: the effects of speaking rate and speaking mode on intelligibility. The Journal of the Acoustical Society of America, 112(5 Pt 1), 2165–2172.

Kuk, F., Jackson, A., Keenan, D., & Lau, C. C. (2008). Personal amplification for school-age children with auditory processing disorders. Journal of the American Academy of Audiology, 19(6), 465–480.

Lauter, J. L. (2004). New approaches to understanding the human brain: three theoretical models and a test battery. Seminars in Hearing, 25, 269–280.

Leavitt, R., & Flexer, C. A. (1991). Speech degradation as measured by the Rapid Speech Transmission Index (RASTI). Ear and Hearing, 12(2), 115–118.

Martin, N., & Brownell, R. (2010). Test of auditory processing skills-3. Novato, CA: Academy Therapy Publications.

McArthur, G. M. (2009). Auditory processing disorders: can they be treated? Current Opinion in Neurology, 22(2), 137–143.

Millward, K. E., Hall, R. L., Ferguson, M. A., & Moore, D. R. (2011). Training speech-in-noise perception in mainstream school children. International Journal of Pediatric Otolaryngology. 75(11), 1408–1417.

Moncrieff, D. W., & Wertz, D. (2008). Auditory rehabilitation for interaural asymmetry: preliminary evidence of improved dichotic listening performance following intensive training. International Journal of Audiology, 47(2), 84–97.

Muchnik, C., Ari-Even Roth, D., Othman-Jebara, R., Putter-Katz, H., Shabtai, E. L., & Hildesheimer, M. (2004). Reduced medial olivocochlear bundle system function in children with auditory processing disorders. Audiology & Neuro-Otology, 9(2), 107–114.

Musiek, F. E. (2004). The DIID: A new treatment for APD. Hearing Journal, 57, 50.

Musiek, F. E. (2005). Temporal (auditory) training for CAPD. Hearing Journal, 58, 46.

Musiek, F. E., Geurkink, N. A., & Kietel, S. A. (1982). Test battery assessment of auditory perceptual dysfunction in children. The Laryngoscope, 92(3), 251–257.

Musiek, F. E., Shinn, J. B., Jirsa, R., Bamiou, D. E., Baran, J. A., & Zaida, E. (2005). GIN (Gaps-In-Noise) test performance in subjects with confirmed central auditory nervous system involvement. Ear and Hearing, 26(6), 608–618.

Myklebust, H. R. (1954) Auditory disorders in children: a manual for differential diagnosis. New York, NY: Grune and Stratton.

National Acoustics Laboratories. (2012). NAL CAPD website. Retrieved from http://capd.nal.gov.au/

National Institutes of Health. (2001). Auditory processing disorder in children: what does it mean? NIH Publication No. 01–4949. Retrieved from http://www.nidcd.nih.gov/staticresources/health/healthyhearing/tools/pdf/audiprocdis.pdf

Neijenhuis, K., Tschur, H., & Snik, A. (2004). The effect of mild hearing impairment on auditory processing tests. Journal of the American Academy of Audiology, 15(1), 6–16.

Olsho, L. W., Koch, E. G., Carter, E. A., Halpin, C. F., & Spetner, N. B. (1988). Pure-tone sensitivity of human infants. The Journal of the Acoustical Society of America, 84(4), 1316–1324.

Phillips, D. P. (2002). Central auditory system and central auditory processing disorders: some conceptual issues. Seminars in Hearing, 23, 251–262.

Phillips, D. P. (1995). Central auditory processing: a view from auditory neuroscience. The American Journal of Otology, 16(3), 338–352.

Pinheiro, M. L., & Ptacek, P. H. (1971). Reversals in the perception of noise and tone patterns. The Journal of the Acoustical Society of America, 49(6), 1778–1783.

Prelock, P. A. (1993). Managing the language and learning needs of the communication-impaired preschool child. A proactive approach. Clinics in Communication Disorders, 3(1), 1–14.

Ptacek, P. H., & Pinheiro, M. L. (1971). Pattern reversal in auditory perception. The Journal of the Acoustical Society of America, 49(2), 2, 493–498.

Rosen, S. (2005). "A riddle wrapped in a mystery inside an enigma": defining central auditory processing disorder. American Journal of Audiology, 14(2), 139–142, discussion 143–150.

Schow, R. L., Seikel, A., Brockett, J. E., & Whitaker, M. M. (2007). Multiple auditory processing assessment. St. Louis, MO: Auditec.

Skoe, E., & Kraus, N. (2010). Auditory brain stem response to complex sounds: a tutorial. Ear and Hearing, 31(3), 302–324.

Smoski, W., Brunt, M., & Tannahill, J. (1998). Children's Auditory Performance Scale (CHAPS). Tampa, FL: Educational Audiology Association.

Song, J. H., Skoe, E., Banai, K., & Kraus, N. (2012). Training to improve hearing speech in noise: biological mechanisms. Cerebral Cortex, 22(5), 1180–1190.

Stein, R. (1998). Application of FM technology to the management of central auditory processing disorders. In M. Masters, N. Stecker, & J. Katz (Eds.), Central auditory processing disorders: mostly management (pp. 89–102). Needham Heights, MA: Allyn and Bacon.

Sweetow, R. W., & Henderson-Sabes, J. (2004). The case for LACE: listening and auditory communication enhancement training. The Hearing Journal, 57(3), 32–35, 38, 40.

Taber, M. V., Foulkes, E., & Whitelaw, G. M. (1999). Classroom Language and Auditory Strategies for Success. [Unpublished program.] Columbus: Ohio State University.

Tallal, P., Merzenich, M. M., Miller, S., & Jenkins, W. (1998). Language learning impairments: integrating basic science, technology, and remediation. Experimental Brain Research, 123(1–2), 210–219.

Tallal, P., Miller, S., and Fitch, R. (1993). Neurobiological basis of speech: a case for the preeminence of temporal processing. Annals of the New York Academy of Sciences, 682, 27–47.

Thompson, C. K. (2000). The neurobiology of language recovery in aphasia. Brain and Language, 71(1), 245–248.

Tremblay, K., Kraus, N., McGee, T. J., Ponton, C. W., & Otis, B. (2001). Central auditory plasticity: changes in the N1-P2 complex after speech-sound training. Ear and Hearing, 22(2), 79–90.

Tye-Murray, N., & Schum, L. (1994). Conversation training for frequent communication partners. Journal of the Academy of Rehabilitative Audiology, 27(Supplement), 209–222.

Willeford, J. A. (1977). Assessing central auditory behavior in children: a test battery approach. In R. Keith (Ed), Central auditory dysfunction (pp. 43–72). New York, NY: Grune and Stratton.

Chapter 17

Evaluation and Management of Vestibular Function in Infants and Children with Hearing Loss

Richard Gans

Key Points

- While we could survive without vision or hearing, as some species do, it would be impossible to survive without the ability to resist the pull of gravity or safely navigate within our environment.

- Recent investigators have reported as high as 90% abnormal vestibular evoked myogenic potentials (VEMP) responses in children with congenital sensorineural hearing loss.

- The majority of equilibrium problems that occur in infants and children manifest as delayed gross motor and balance problems, not as vertigo or dizziness.

- Muscle tone is another important aspect of an infant/child vestibular evaluation because it is closely associated with the integrity of the vestibular system.

Vestibular dysfunction, although not highly prevalent, does occur in children (O'Reilly et al, 2010). Numerous investigators have reported a higher incidence of vestibular problems in children with congenital and/or acquired sensorineural hearing loss than in the general pediatric population (Rine, O'Hare, Rice, Robinson, & Vergara, 1997; Kaga, 1999). Based on the well-known comorbidities of sensorineural hearing loss and vestibular deficits, it is equally as important to provide early identification and intervention for children with balance issues as it is for hearing loss. The global acceptance and success of early neonatal hearing testing has improved our ability to identify those infants who are also at risk for vestibular dysfunction.

Pearl

- All newborns and infants with identified congenital or acquired sensorineural hearing loss should be considered at risk for comorbidity of vestibular dysfunction.

In the literature, pediatric vestibular testing and normative data have focused primarily on school-age children, with modification of adult protocols utilizing videonystagmography (VNG), rotary chair, and computerized dynamic posturography (Cyr, 1980, 1983; O'Reilly et al, 2011; Valente, 2007; Weiss & Phillips, 2006). Given that these technologies are not available in most facilities, and even where they are, testing may not be obtained until the child is 3 years old or older, the focus of this chapter will be to provide the reader with an overview of vestibular function, common disorders, and evaluation methods for infants ranging from 3 months to 3 years of age. The good news is that, with a proper case history, interview of the parents, and understanding of the vestibular system's multiple reflex systems and their role in maturational motor milestones, most infants and young children can be identified as being at risk by most practitioners prior to comprehensive electrophysiologic examination.

Pearl

- Remember, the primary function of the inner ear is balance.

The Mechanisms of Equilibrium

The inner ear's contribution to equilibrium is significant. In fact, its primary function is equilibrium, not hearing. The vestibular labyrinth portion of the inner ear is the first sensory system to develop embryologically; it actually precedes cochlear development (the phylogenic development of the cochlea follows that of the saccule). As a species, we have developed an embryological hierarchy based on importance to survival. We could survive without vision or hearing, as some species do, but it would be impossible to survive without the ability to resist the pull of gravity or safely navigate within our environment. The labyrinth is fully developed anatomically in utero by 49 days' gestation. Its neural connections with the central pathways continue to develop through the eighth month of gestation (Wiener-Vacher, 2008). The system will continue to mature, myelinate, and evolve through childhood up to about 6 years of age.

Equilibrium requires more than just the vestibular labyrinth. It is a complex integration of the vestibular system, vision, the somatosensory system, proprioception, and the central nervous system. The vestibular system is the primary sensory modality, contributing approximately two-thirds of the critical data about where we are in space, including our sense of motion, speed, and direction. It is an internal reference, whereas vision and the somatosensory system are external reference systems, telling the brain about the status of the outside world. All sensory modalities must work together within several complex reflex arcs for accurate perception and response to the dynamic world. The four otoliths and six semicircular canals are the end organ receptors of the vestibular system. To begin to develop an understanding of methods available to evaluate the vestibular function of infants, a discussion of the underlying physiology and reflexes is presented.

Physiology of Equilibrium: Vestibular Reflexes

The vestibular system is a critical sensory component within multiple complex reflex arcs. As there are actually no direct tests of vestibular function, all established and commonly used vestibular function tests evaluate and record only the motor (output) portion of one or more of three vestibular reflex arcs. The test interpretation is an extrapolation of the influence of the inner ear on the results as to whether we have intact or dysfunctional vestibular participation. Ideally, for infants, just as with adults, we prefer to evaluate all three reflex arcs to obtain the best comprehensive picture of equilibrium function. The three distinct vestibular reflexes are the vestibuloocular (VOR), vestibulospinal (VSR), and vestibulocollic (VCR). Ideally, one or more, or preferably all three, may be evaluated even with behavioral techniques. The best test of the VCR is arguably the vestibular evoked myogenic potential (VEMP), which is an electrophysiological assessment tool.

The vestibuloocular reflex (VOR) allows stabilized vision with head movement. Without this function, the world would appear to jiggle or bounce each time the head was moved. This blurred vision or drop in visual acuity does occur with individuals who have a defect in the VOR and is termed oscillopsia. The VOR is an ascending pathway through the upper brainstem and contributes to the production of an accurate compensatory eye movement. For each and every head movement there must be equal and opposite eye movements. Adult VOR testing typically includes VNG, rotary chair, and dynamic visual acuity tests. Naturally, with infants these evaluation protocols will not be appropriate. The VOR receives some additional help to stabilize vision at lower movement frequencies provided by the optokinetic reflex. While the vestibular end organs are providing the brain with information about gravity and velocity, the optokinetic system produces eye movement based on motion of the external world. The eyes will follow in the direction of the movement and then quickly return to the center. This produces an involuntary eye movement, termed nystagmus, with a slow and fast phase. It is this integration that allows the individual to correctly perceive and respond to whether it is the individual or the world that is moving. It can be elicited at birth and is adultlike in its operation by about 6 months of age.

The vestibulospinal reflex (VSR) provides the antigravity muscles and musculoskeletal system with information through the lower brainstem and a descending motor tract to the extremities to correctly maintain our postural stability under both static and dynamic conditions. Vestibular signals interact in a complex manner with other systems to produce several postural reflexes. The cerebellum appears to play a key role in these interactions, which can involve limb and neck proprioception, touch, vision, and descending cortical influences relayed to the vestibular complex primarily via the reticular formation. Various sensory modalities interact to provide information to the postural control system from three frames of reference. These are (1) proprioception, the sense of position and movement of one part of the body relative to another, via muscle, joint, tactile, and visual receptors; (2) exteroception, the relationship of objects in the environment to each other, via primarily visual and tactile inputs; and (3) exproprioception, or information about the body parts relative to the external environment, from all types of sensory receptors. Because the vestibular system provides a purely exproprioceptive sense that reports velocity and acceleration of the head relative to gravity and inertia, it is especially helpful in correcting erroneous information from the other sensory inputs. Descending pathways responsible for postural reflexes include the vestibulospinal and reticulospinal tracts. Both receive signals from the vestibular end organ and both are strongly influenced by cerebellar efferents. Descending motor control of the neck musculature is more closely linked to the vestibular end organ and to the semicircular canals. Limb muscle reflexes are more closely linked to input from several sensory systems.

The vestibulocollic reflex (VCR) is considered to be a righting reflex. In essence, it is the gravity sensor within the inner ear communicating with the neck musculature keeping the head steady in response to body tilt. Originating within the saccule portion of the otolith mechanism, the reflex then courses through the lower brainstem in a descending pathway with its motor portion in cranial nerve XI, the accessory nerve innervating the sternocleidomastoid neck muscle. This reflex has gained much attention over the past decade; its measurement is the cervical VEMP (cVEMP).

Causes of Vestibular Dysfunction

Common causes of vestibular dysfunction in the pediatric population, both congenital and acquired, are outlined in **Fig. 17.1**. It is important to remember that the majority of causes result in overall equilibrium dysfunction secondary to bilateral loss or dysfunction rather than to acquired unilateral dysfunction resulting in vertigo or dizziness, as is the case with adult-onset vestibular disorders. This is likely why dizziness and vertigo have a low prevalence in the general pediatric population (Jahn, Langhagen, Schroeder, & Heinen, 2011; O'Reilly et al, 2011). With the exception of benign paroxysmal vertigo (BPV) of childhood, the infant or young child is not in apparent distress.

Pitfall

- Do not assume that children with "one good ear" are immune to bilateral vestibular labyrinthine dysfunction.

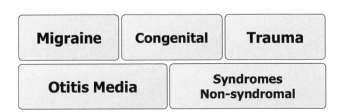

Fig. 17.1 Common causes of pediatric vestibular dysfunction.

Congenital disorders by far are the leading cause of pediatric vestibular dysfunction (Pikus, 2002). It is estimated that over 500 syndromes and nonsyndromes are known to have an audiovestibular expressivity (Pikus, 2002). Recent investigators have reported as high as 90% abnormal VEMP responses in children with congenital sensorineural hearing loss (SNHL). The emerging use of neonate and infant VEMP data suggests a much higher incidence of vestibular dysfunction than the 30–50% previously estimated (Kelsch, Schaefer, & Esquivel, 2006; Picciotti et al, 2007; Sheykholeslami, Megerian, Arnold, & Kaga, 2005; Zhou, Kenna, Stevens, & Licameli, 2009). Recent pediatric VEMP studies and their respective age ranges are presented in **Table 17.1**.

Syndromes with known and unspecified expressivity can be found in **Fig. 17.2**. A brief description of each syndrome is presented in **Table 17.2** to familiarize the reader with common expressivities associated with the conditions. It has been well established that audiovestibular anomalies are the most frequently found defect across all known mitochondrial diseases. In addition, there are nearly 70 identified different nonsyndromic loci for hereditary audiovestibular impairment. Of these, at least 30 are dominantly inherited, which means hearing loss may not be consistently seen. So, if there were no failure of a high-risk hearing screening at birth, but only the vestibular symptoms occurred, the vestibular loss would probably be missed. Autosomal recessive disorders in the nonsyndromic category account for over two dozen loci.

Table 17.1 Review of pediatric VEMP studies

Investigators	Study
Zhou et al, 2009	21/23 (91%) SNHL had abnormal amplitudes
Picciotti et al, 2007	Ages 3–15
Kelsch et al, 2006	Ages 3–11
Sheykholeslami et al, 2005	Neonates

known	unspecified
• Usher • Branchio-oto-renal/CHARGE • Pendred • Neurofibromatosis NF2 • CHARGE • Marshall • Spinocerebellar ataxias	• Waardenburg • Von Hippel-Lindau

Fig. 17.2 Syndromes with vestibular expressivity.

Table 17.2 Description of syndromes affecting the audiovestibular system

Usher syndrome	Type I: congential bilateral profound SNHL, retinitis pigmentosa
	Type II: mild–severe progressive high-frequency SNHL
Branchio-oto-renal (BOR) syndrome	Preauricular pits or tags, branchial cysts, hearing loss, and/or abnormal development of the kidneys
Pendred syndrome	Congenital, severe–profound SNHL, abnormality of bony labyrinth; abnormal thyroid development with goiter in early puberty or adulthood
Neurofibromatosis type 2 (NF2)	Bilateral vestibular schwannomas, tinnitus, hearing loss, and balance dysfunction; schwannomas of other peripheral nerves, meningiomas, and juvenile cataract
Waardenburg syndrome	Congenital SNHL, pigmentary disturbances of iris, hair, skin; vestibular disturbances without hearing loss
Von Hippel–Lindau syndrome	Hemangioblastomas of brain, spinal cord, and retina; renal cysts and renal cell carcinoma (40%); dizziness/imbalance and hearing loss may be initial symptoms, may mimic Meniere disease
CHARGE syndrome	Coloboma, heart anomaly, choanal atresia, retardation, genital and ear abnormalities; vestibular symptoms prevalent
Marshall syndrome	Saddle nose, myopia, early-onset cataracts, and short stature; vestibular symptoms prevalent
Spinocerebellar ataxia	Complex and progressive; 23 distinct genetic disorders; may also include hearing loss

Acquired conditions may include BPV of childhood, which generally is considered the leading cause of pediatric dizziness. BPV of childhood, a classification of migraine (Chang & Young, 2007), is the condition most likely to produce symptoms of vertigo in children (Gans, 2002). It could be argued that since this is a migraine variant, BPV of childhood is genetic. It is classified as one of the six subtypes of migraine by the International Headache Society (IHS) (2004). Basser coined the name in 1964 to describe brief bouts of vertigo, nausea, vomiting, and change in pallor (Basser, 1964). Onset usually occurs between ages 1 and 4, and it will virtually disappear in children by age 5 or 6. There are no lingering effects between episodes, and all radiographic and electroencephalographic (EEG) tests are unremarkable. So BPV of childhood is a diagnosis of exclusion, but because of its genetics and tone, more of the biological parents are likely to suffer from migraines. It is estimated that ~ 50% of these children will suffer migraines by puberty. BPV of childhood is defined as recurrent with at least five occurrences, which resolve spontaneously or within hours.

Head trauma may cause a form of positional vertigo, benign paroxysmal positional vertigo (BPPV), as seen in adults. BPPV is usually seen in older children and adolescents who are involved in soccer or other contact sports or activities where they are susceptible to even minor head bumps. Infants and children at any age, however, may experience BPPV with head trauma. These children can be quickly identified with appropriate modified Hallpike protocols and successfully treated with canalith repositioning maneuvers (CRM) and resume their normal activities without any restrictions, so long as there are no issues of concussion secondary to a head trauma to complicate their recovery.

Of great concern, particularly in emerging economies, is the overdosing with aminoglycosides for treatment of bacterial infections in infants and young children (Koyuncu et al, 1999). This has become a growing problem and is presently being addressed by a joint effort between the World Health Organization (WHO) and the American Academy of Otolaryngology–Head and Neck Surgery (AAO-HNS) Foundation. Educating attending physicians and healthcare providers in rural or remote regions has become a primary goal of these organizations.

Evaluation Techniques

Just as normal hearing is essential for acquisition of speech and language, intact vestibular function is critical to the infant's physical and motor development. The majority of equilibrium problems that occur in infants and children manifest as delayed gross motor and balance problems, not as vertigo or dizziness.

Pearl

- An infant's balance function may be evaluated as early as 3 months of age.

Delayed maturational motor milestones may be the earliest signs of a vestibular dysfunction. When interviewing parents of an infant with an identified hearing loss it is important to ask about the child's motor development timeline. Indicators of peripheral-central vestibular dysfunction may include the infant's inability to hold the head upright, and delayed crawling, standing, and walking.

Just as with auditory testing, there is an array of clinical-behavioral tests available. These are age specific with normative data in the form of maturational motor milestones, as shown in **Table 17.3** (Viholanen, Ahonen, Cantell, Tolvanen, & Lyytinen, 2006).

Pitfall

• Waiting until the child with hearing loss is 1 year old or more to see whether she starts to walk on time is too late to begin considering vestibular dysfunction.

One of the most commonly used developmental scales, the Denver Developmental Screening Test (Frankenburg & Dodds, 1967; Glascoe et al, 1992), is used by pediatricians and other health and social service providers to look at developmental problems in preschool children in the areas of social contact, fine motor skills, language, and gross motor skills. Gross motor skills involve the ability to use large muscles for movements like lifting the head, crawling, or walking. These skills begin to develop in infancy and early childhood.

Although delay in maturational milestones may indicate problems within the vestibular spinal reflex, infant's gross motor skills depend on both muscle tone and strength. Low muscle tone, or hypotonia, is a characteristic of several disabling conditions, such as Down syndrome, genetic or muscle disorders, or central nervous system disorders. These conditions may, of course, exist in conjunction with vestibular dysfunction secondary to congenital trauma or syndromes.

A good case history is essential in speaking with the parents and asking about when milestones were achieved. Likewise, spending time observing the infant playing, rolling, and interacting with a parent will provide a great deal of valuable information. Just as with hearing testing, much of the evaluation is child-directed. Vestibular evaluations can be accurately conducted as early as 3 months of age with neonates who are suspected of congenital hearing loss. Waiting until 3 months of age is preferable because time is needed for the neck musculature to mature enough for the child to begin to hold her own head upright. The neck muscles become stronger during these first few months of life. At first, newborns can hold their heads up only for a couple of seconds while on their stomachs. The muscles are strengthened each time the head is held up. By 3 months of age, infants lying on their stomachs can support their heads and chests up to their forearms.

Pitfall

• Concerns based solely on observations related to episodes of dizziness or vertigo will not identify vestibular problems in children.

Once infants can lift up their heads, they will push up using their arms and arch their back to lift up the chest. These movements help strengthen the upper body and are in preparation for sitting up. Infants may also rock while on their stomachs, kick their legs, and swim with their arms. These movements are necessary for rolling over and crawling. By the end of this period, infants should be able to roll over from stomach to back and back to stomach and probably are able to sit without any support.

By 8 months of age, most infants can sit up without support. They also figure out how to roll down to their stomachs and return to a sitting position again. Some infants are in constant motion; they arch their

Table 17.3 Summary of maturational motor milestones

3 months	7 months	9 months	12 months	24 months
• Raises head and chest when lying on stomach • Starts to use eyes and hands in coordination • Begins to support head • Pushes down with legs when feet placed on floor • Moves eyes in all directions	• Sits with and then without support of hands • Supports weight on legs • Ability to track moving objects improves • Rolls over • Supports head when sitting	• Crawling on hands and knees • Walking with assistance • Upper body-turns from sitting to crawling position	• Sits without assistance • Crawls forward on belly by pulling with arms and pushing with legs • Creeps on hands and knees and supports trunk • Pulls self up to standing position • Walks holding on to furniture • Stands momentarily without support	• Walks alone by 18 months • Begins to run • Can push a wheeled toy

necks and look around while on their stomachs and grab at their feet or objects while on their backs. All this activity is preparing them for crawling, which is usually mastered between 7 and 10 months of age. Crawling is important for the development of integrated communication between the two sides of the brain. Some infants never crawl but rather scoot on their bottoms or move on their stomachs.

After crawling is mastered, infants will begin to pull themselves up to a standing position. They then begin to take some steps while holding on to something for support. This will change into cruising around the furniture. As their balance improves, infants may gradually take a few steps without holding on. Many infants' first steps are taken around 12 months, but earlier or later than this is completely normal.

Lifting the child in space or changing the child's position while on a variety of movable surfaces can test righting reflexes and equilibrium responses. An example of this can be seen in **Fig. 17.3**. The 4-month-old male is placed on an exercise ball, which is a dynamic surface. The infant's head and torso remain stable and centered even when he is perturbed in any direction. Lateral tilt, for example, activates utricular receptors, which in turn excite vestibulospinal neurons and influence the activity of limb muscles. Age guidelines for head righting, equilibrium responses, and other postural reactions that are dependent, at least in part, on vestibular processing have been documented by many developmental researchers and are well known to therapists who work in pediatrics.

Pearl

- Evaluation protocols may include motor milestones and optokinetic reflexes when advanced testing such as VEMP is not available.

Another clinical observation relates to the presence of tonic neck postures. Problems in integration of tonic neck reflexes may implicate related vestibular dysfunction because labyrinthine receptors indicate body position only in conjunction with neck receptors. **Figs. 17.4** and **17.5** show a righting response. The 4-month-old boy is comfortably and safely placed on his mother's lap. The infant is then gently pointed downward. As can be seen in the second photo, there is a clear upturn of the head away from the floor.

Muscle tone is another important aspect of the evaluation, as it is closely associated with the integrity of the vestibular system. Loss of vestibular input may result in prolonged muscular debility that may even extend to the visceral muscles.

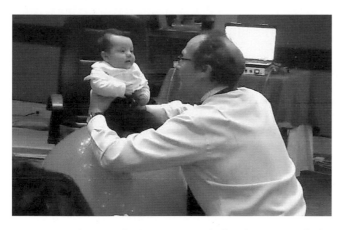

Fig. 17.3 Placing infant on exercise ball creates a vestibular reponse.

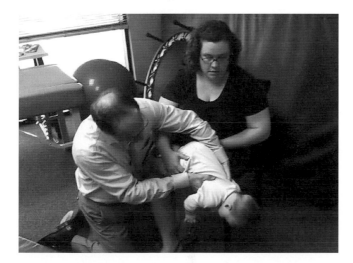

Fig. 17.4 Righting response places the infant toward the ground.

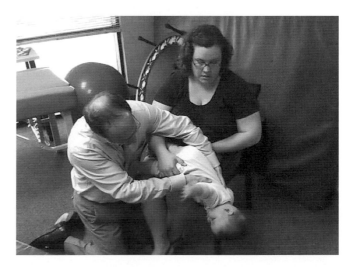

Fig. 17.5 Infant produces an upward head turn as part of the intact vestibular righting reflex.

The visual observation of optokinetic nystagmus (OKN) utilizing a rotating drum, which fills the infant's visual field (at least 80%) is also an excellent method of assessing the VOR. It has been demonstrated that its appearance is as early as 1 month and it is nicely developed at 3 months of age. Conditions where there is a bilateral vestibular dysfunction (BVD) will not produce a binocular bidirectional response. In those cases where there may be a noncompensated unilateral vestibular dysfunction (UVD), it will be asymmetrical, with no or reduced response with the moving stimuli in the direction of the involved labyrinth. It is this author's experience that it is rare to see infants or young children with noncompensated UVD secondary to an acquired otologic lesion.

◆ Summary

Infants with vestibular, equilibrium, and delayed maturational motor control disorders can now be identified at an earlier age, thanks to the success of

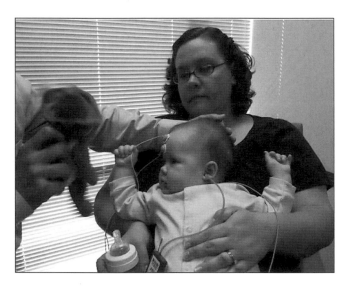

Fig. 17.6   VEMP testing may be reliably obtained at 3 months of age.

newborn hearing screening. Unlike older children or adults with acquired UVDs, infants with BVD will not benefit from traditional vestibular rehabilitation strategies. They will benefit, however, from ongoing sensory integration, substitution, and conditioning therapy with trained pediatric physical and occupational therapists. The knowledge of the status of vestibular modality will provide the therapists with valuable information about therapy protocols and ultimately the child's prognosis over time. Although it does require at least two intact sensory modalities to produce normal equilibrium function, an early vestibular therapy jump-start will be critical in providing infants and children with a more normal and active lifestyle during their formative years.

It is well documented that the audiovestibular system in infants is just as susceptible to vestibular deficits as it is to hearing deficits. Audiologists can play an important role in the early identification of infants, especially those with hearing loss, who may be at risk for balance problems as well. Young infants as early as 3 months of age can undergo VEMP testing, as shown in **Fig. 17.6**, but they are not candidates for VNG, posturography, or rotary chair examinations, even if the technologies are available. Therefore, an understanding of the vestibular system's role in postural and motor coordination performance can serve as an invaluable aid for early identification and intervention of vestibular problems.

Discussion Questions

1. Embryologically, in what timeframe does the vestibular labyrinth develop?
2. What is the relationship between congenital sensorineural hearing loss and vestibular dysfunction?
3. Is it possible for children to have BPPV? If so, how should they be treated?
4. What is the relationship between migraine and BPV of childhood?
5. What is the best intervention strategy for children identified with balance dysfunction?

References

Basser, L. S. (1964). Benign paroxysmal vertigo of childhood: A variety of vestibular neuritis. Brain, 87, 141–152.

Chang, C. H., & Young, Y. H. (2007). Caloric and vestibular evoked myogenic potential tests in evaluating children with benign paroxysmal vertigo. International Journal of Pediatric Otolaryngology. 71(3), 495–499.

Cyr, D. G. (1980). Vestibular testing in children. The Annals of Otology, Rhinology, and Laryngology, 89(5 Pt 2), 63–69.

Cyr, D. G. (1983). The vestibular system: pediatric considerations. Seminars in Hearing, 4(1), 33–45.

Frankenburg, W. K., & Dodds, J. B. (1967). The Denver Developmental Screening Test. The Journal of Pediatrics, 71(2), 181–191.

Gans, R. E. (2002). Classification of audiovestibular symptoms related to migraine, part 3: benign paroxysmal vertigo of childhood (BPVC). The Hearing Review, 36, 38.

Glascoe, F. P., Byrne, K. E., Ashford, L. G., Johnson, K. L., Chang, B., & Strickland, B. (1992). Accuracy of the Denver-II in developmental screening. Pediatrics, 89(6 Pt 2), 1221–1225.

International Headache Society. (2004). The international classification of headache disorders. Cephalalgia, 24 Supplement 1, 9–160.

Jahn, K., Langhagen, T., Schroeder, A. S., & Heinen, F. (2011). Vertigo and dizziness in childhood—update on diagnosis and treatment. Neuropediatrics, 42(4), 129–134.

Kaga, K. (1999). Vestibular compensation in infants and children with congenital and acquired vestibular loss in both ears. Int J Pediatr Otolaryngology, 49(3), 215–224.

Kelsch, T. A., Schaefer, L. A., & Esquivel, C. R. (2006). Vestibular evoked myogenic potentials in young children: test parameters and normative data. The Laryngoscope, 116(6), 895–900.

Koyuncu, M., Saka, M. M., Tanyeri, Y., Seşen, T., Ünal, R., Tekat, A., & Yilmaz, F. (1999). Effects of otitis media with effusion on the vestibular system in children. Otolaryngology—Head and Neck Surgery, 120(1), 117–121.

O'Reilly, R. C., Greywoode, J., Morlet, T., Miller, F., Henley, J., Church, C., . . . Falcheck, S. (2011). Comprehensive vestibular and balance testing in the dizzy pediatric population. Otolaryngology—Head and Neck Surgery, 144(2), 142–148.

O'Reilly, R. C., Morlet, T., Nicholas, B. D., Josephson, G., Horlbeck, D., Lundy, L., & Mercado, A. (2010). Prevalence of vestibular and balance disorders in children. Otology & Neurotology, 31(9), 1441–1444.

Picciotti, P. M., Fiorita, A., Di Nardo, W., Calò, L., Scarano, E., & Paludetti, G. (2007). Vestibular evoked myogenic potentials in children. International Journal of Pediatric Otorhinolaryngology, 71(1), 29–33.

Pikus, A. (2002). Heritable vestibular disorders. Seminars in Hearing, 23(2), 129–142.

Rine, R. M., O'Hare, T., Rice, M., Robinson, E., & Vergara, K. (1997). Relationship of vestibular function, motor and postural control ability in children with hearing impairment—a preliminary study. Pediatric Physical Therapy, 9, 194.

Sheykholeslami, K., Megerian, C. A., Arnold, J. E., & Kaga, K. (2005). Vestibular-evoked myogenic potentials in infancy and early childhood. The Laryngoscope, 115(8), 1440–1444.

Valente, M. (2007). Maturational effects of the vestibular system: a study of rotary chair, computerized dynamic posturography, and vestibular evoked myogenic potentials with children. Journal of the American Academy of Audiology, 18(6), 461–481.

Viholanen, H., Ahonen, T., Cantell, M., Tolvanen, A., & Lyytinen, H. (2006). The early motor milestones in infancy and later motor skills in toddlers: a structural equation model of motor development. Physical & Occupational Therapy in Pediatrics, 26(1-2), 91–113.

Weiss, A. H., & Phillips, J. O. (2006). Congenital and compensated vestibular dysfunction in childhood: an overlooked entity. Journal of Child Neurology, 21(7), 572–579.

Wiener-Vacher, S. R. (2008). Vestibular disorders in children. International Journal of Audiology, 47(9), 578–583.

Zhou, G., Kenna, M. A., Stevens, K., & Licameli, G. (2009). Assessment of saccular function in children with sensorineural hearing loss. Archives of Otolaryngology–Head & Neck Surgery, 135(1), 40–44.

Chapter 18

Interpreting Audiologic Test Results and Using the Test Information to Plan Management

Jane R. Madell and Carol Flexer

Key Points

- We establish degree of hearing loss not for its own sake, but to assist in selecting technology.

- Whenever a test is used as part of diagnostic protocol, the validity and reliability measures of the test are important because we are relying on the results of tests to determine technological and therapeutic management.

- All behavioral and electrophysiological audiologic tests are valid only if we are using correct test protocols on the appropriate populations.

- Validation of the hearing aid fitting is critical if we want to know what a child is actually hearing.

- Children speak what and how they hear.

- Interpreting audiologic test results includes estimating the child's performance outside of the test situation and making appropriate recommendations.

The only reason to perform audiologic diagnostic assessment is to determine recommendations and management protocols. The audiologist should constantly be considering management while testing is in progress. It is best if the audiologist who is making recommendations is the audiologist who conducted the assessments. Observing a child during testing provides much more information than simply obtaining test results. Observing a child's latency of response, response posture, and auditory attention provides information about how comfortable the child is when attending to auditory stimuli. For example, two children with hearing loss may have similar thresholds, but the first child is having a very difficult time attending and responding during the test situation while the second child is very auditorally attentive and responds quickly and with assurance. Their different response behaviors show the children are taking in auditory information in very different ways. So the audiologist's recommendations likely would be an expression of concern for the first child's auditory difficulties. That is, the audiologist might question how well the child can attend in the classroom. If the child is using technology, the audiologist may question how often the child wears the technology and how intensive the auditory therapy and parent practice are, and offer recommendations accordingly.

We establish degree of hearing loss not for its own sake, but to assist in selecting technology. We know that if a child has a mild hearing loss, appropriately set hearing aids will provide auditory brain access to soft speech throughout the frequency range. We also know that a child with a profound hearing loss cannot receive sufficient auditory brain access from hearing aids but could receive access to the entire speech spectrum through cochlear implants (Leigh, Dettman, Dowell, & Sarant, 2011). There are nuances involved in the selection and interpretation of appropriate pediatric tests that lead to the determination of management strategies.

The purpose of this chapter is to discuss issues in the interpretation of audiologic test results as the foundation of management strategies for children with all degrees of hearing loss. Accordingly, this chapter will provide an overview of validity and reliability issues and discuss how these issues affect test selection and interpretation. Case studies will be utilized to exemplify interpretation of assessment data.

◆ Validity and Reliability

Whenever a test is used as part of diagnostic protocol, the validity and reliability measures of the test are important because we are relying on the results of tests to determine technological and therapeutic management.

Validity

Validity is the degree to which a test measures what it purports to measure (Dillon, 2012). For a test to be accurately applied and interpreted, the test must be valid. Validity is determined by a body of research demonstrating the relationship between the test and the behavior it is intended to measure. For example, one would not want to use a math test to determine linguistic competency. Audiologists would not use a broadband noise stimulus to obtain frequency-specific information.

Reliability

Reliability is the consistency of a measure (Demorest & Walden, 1984). Tests are considered reliable if we obtain the same results repeatedly. In particular, test–retest reliability is the consistency of the results among different administrations of a test. Reliability assumes that there will be no change in the quality or construct being measured. For example, if we cannot obtain repeatable pure tone thresholds during one test session, we question the reliability of the test results.

Application of Reliability and Validity to Pediatric Testing

We need to ask ourselves the following questions: Are we measuring what we think we are measuring? Are we using the appropriate test for the child who is in front of us? Are we performing the test accurately? Are we interpreting test results correctly?

All behavioral audiologic tests are valid only if we use correct test protocols on the appropriate populations. To the extent that the appropriate procedures are not followed, or the test is performed on populations other than those for whom it was intended, the results cannot be accurately interpreted. (See Chapters 7, 8, 9, and 11 in this text for a discussion of pediatric behavioral test protocols.)

When performing pure tone assessments, there are pediatric procedures that are specific to certain developmental age levels. For example, visual reinforcement audiometry (VRA) is an appropriate test for a child who is cognitively between 6 and 36 months of

age, and conditioned play audiometry (CPA) is typically the appropriate test for children beginning at ~ 30–36 months of age. If VRA is used to test a child who is cognitively 64 months of age, the child will likely become bored with the test and stop responding. Would it then be correct to conclude that this child has a hearing loss? Obviously not. On the other hand, if we are evaluating a child who is cognitively 18 months of age but chronologically 64 months of age, would it be appropriate for us to evaluate that child based on his chronological age? Again, obviously not. While both VRA and CPA are valid test protocols to obtain pure tone thresholds when administered correctly, the results in the cases just described would not be valid. Some toddlers younger than 30 months are capable of reliably performing the CPA task, but results can be considered accurate only if they are repeatable. Results obtained only once cannot be considered reliable.

> **Pearl**
>
> - For test results to be interpreted accurately and appropriately, the correct test must be selected, and it must be administered according to the protocol that was used to validate the test.

For more information about hearing test protocols for children, see Chapter 6.

◆ Interpreting Test Results

Case 1: Speech Perception Interpretation Issues

Mark is 12 years old and in sixth grade in a mainstream educational setting. He has a severe to profound sensorineural hearing loss and has had bilateral implants since age 2 years. He recently had an audiological evaluation at his implant center. Threshold testing with the implants revealed excellent benefit, with implant thresholds between 15–20 dB hearing level (HL) throughout the frequency range. Speech perception testing was performed using the Phonetically Balanced Kindergarten (PBK) word lists in a monitored live-voice (MLV) format at 50 dB HL. Mark had excellent speech perception test results with scores of 96% bilaterally, in two separate test sessions.

Are these test results valid and reliable? This is an example of both a reliability and validity problem. We might assume that these results are reliable because they were obtained on two different occasions. However, repeated testing with a different examiner, or on a different day when the first examiner has a cold, might very well yield significantly different test results. The use of the PBK test is clearly not a valid protocol for this child. Every child needs to be tested with an age- and linguistically appropriate test. The PBK test is designed for and standardized on children 5–7 years of age (Haskins, 1949) and, therefore, would be too easy for a 12-year-old, so results would overestimate his speech perception skills. A child who is 12 years old and enrolled in a mainstream educational setting needs to be assessed using a test that is designed for a 12-year-old, so that the audiologist can make a judgment about how this child is likely to perform in a classroom setting. In fact, when Mark was retested using recorded consonant–nucleus–consonant (CNC) words presented at 50 dB HL, test results indicated scores of 66%, demonstrating that Mark is missing a great deal of speech information, thus justifying the need for accommodations in the classroom.

Case 2: Making Recommendations Based on Insufficient Information

Joan is 3 years old. Her parents bring her in for evaluation because her preschool teacher is reporting concern about Joan's ability to hear in the classroom and her poor speech. Joan is frightened and won't permit the use of either insert earphones or supraaural earphones. After attempting to coax her, the audiologist decides to begin with soundfield testing and obtains thresholds indicating a moderate hearing loss. Joan returned for follow-up testing but still refused to put anything in her ears, whether insert earphones, a tympanometric probe, or an otoacoustic emissions (OAE) probe. Otologic evaluation by the ear, nose, and throat (ENT) physician finds no medical concerns, and he clears her for hearing aids. Because the audiologist cannot obtain earphone testing, she proceeds to fit hearing aids based on soundfield data, recognizing that the results can apply only to the best-hearing ear. Real-ear testing was performed and verified that targets were met based on soundfield thresholds that were entered for each ear. Binaural aided soundfield testing performed at subsequent visits validated that Joan is able to detect the entire speech spectrum at soft conversational levels when wearing both hearing aids.

At a later date, when Joan is finally tested with insert earphones, results reveal that she has a moderate hearing loss in her right ear and a profound hearing loss in her left ear. Soundfield testing with hearing aids separately indicated that she is not receiving sufficient benefit in her left ear, which has the profound hearing loss. Joan has spent considerable time without appropriate auditory access. The real-ear data could not be accurate for the left ear because targets were based on data that were not valid. Management has not been adequate because the left ear has not received auditory access; technology needs to be changed for that ear (i.e., a more powerful hearing aid or a cochlear implant). In addition, auditory therapy needs to add a focus on improving listening skills for the left ear alone once appropriate technology is obtained.

Both the audiologist and the auditory therapist share the responsibility for not identifying the sensitivity discrepancy between the right and left ears early on. Even if the audiologist was unable to put earphones on Joan, she should have tested each hearing aid separately in the sound room by obtaining aided thresholds or speech perception information, which would have identified the difference in auditory access between the ears. The auditory therapist should have done some auditory work with each ear separately, which would also have identified that there was a problem. The child has lost significant time in auditory brain development. It is essential that everyone now working with the child move quickly to try to improve auditory access and build auditory/linguistic skills.

Case 3: Verification and Validation of Hearing Aid Fitting

José is a 7-year-old child with a bilateral moderate to severe sensorineural hearing loss. He comes into the clinic for his annual audiological evaluation. When updating the case history, the audiologist learns that José is in second grade and earning average grades. His auditory therapist and speech-language pathologist report that José is having difficulty both hearing and producing high-frequency consonants ([s], [f], and [q]) and word endings. Unaided testing confirms that his hearing loss continues to be stable. Middle ear evaluation indicates no middle ear disease. Acoustic reflexes are absent, consistent with his degree of hearing loss. After completing unaided testing, the audiologist decides to verify the hearing aid fitting. She performs real-ear measures and determines that the hearing aids are meeting target gain. However, even though high-frequency targets appear to be achieved as determined by real-ear protocols, the audiologist observes that the reports of the auditory therapist and speech-language pathologist are correct; José is not producing high-frequency consonants and is missing many word endings.

Should the audiologist assume the hearing aid settings are correct and remediation will need to be escalated by the auditory therapist and the speech-language pathologist, or is there additional testing the audiologist should perform? Real-ear measures are a verification technique confirming the hearing aids are acoustically working, but without validation it is not possible to know what the child is actually hearing (Humes, 2012). To validate the auditory performance of the hearing aids, the audiologist takes José back into the test booth to assess his aided performance. She obtains aided noise band thresholds and speech perception measures for normal and soft conversational speech in quiet and with competing noise. Speech perception testing was difficult to accomplish because José's speech production was poor. It was not always possible to determine whether José misheard a word or could not produce the word. The most desirable test would be an open-set recorded test, but José's speech production would make such a test invalid. The purpose of speech perception testing is to evaluate the child's ability to perceive speech sound distinctions accurately, not to assess his speech production. We should never assume that the error is a production error. A child's speech production errors may actually be auditory perception errors. There is no way we can know what the child is hearing unless the child can accurately repeat the word or write or spell the answer.

Table 18.1 reports the narrowband noise thresholds obtained for José and indicates that with hearing aids, José is not hearing high-frequency sounds at sufficiently soft levels.

Since speech perception testing could not be accomplished with the PBK recorded test because of José's speech production errors, a picture-pointing task was considered. The NU-CHIPS task, while easy for José to accomplish, is not an appropriate test because it has a vocabulary level of 3–5 years, which would be far too easy and could overestimate José's speech perception

capabilities. The decision was made to test him with the Western Ontario Plurals Test using a recorded picture-pointing format (Glista & Scollie, 2012) (**Table 18.2**). The test assesses the ability of the child to identify the presence of high-frequency stimuli (e.g., *shoe* versus *shoes*).

Testing confirmed that José is having difficulty hearing high frequencies even though real-ear measures indicated that José's hearing aid settings were meeting targets. It is important to remember that real-ear is an estimate and may not be accurate for an individual child. Validation of the hearing aid fitting is critical if we want to know what a child is actually hearing.

The audiologist adjusted the hearing aid settings to provide more high-frequency gain (above recommended target). José was retested, and results indicated both improved thresholds and speech perception scores. The audiologist obtained uncomfortable loudness thresholds (UCLs) and José demonstrated no UCLs at softer-than-expected levels.

Children speak what and how they hear. In José's case, his therapists had been working on the high-frequency sounds while sitting very close to his ear, so he was familiar with high-frequency consonants even though he did not hear them consistently. Improvement in José's auditory brain access resulted in immediate improvement in speech perception capabilities since he was already familiar with the sounds. If he had not been familiar with the consonants, even though aided thresholds would have improved immediately, speech perception improvement would have required additional auditory therapy.

Table 18.1 José's aided narrowband noise thresholds

	250 Hz	500 Hz	1000 Hz	2000 Hz	3000 Hz	4000 Hz	6000 Hz
Right HA (original settings)	20 dB	15 dB	20 dB	25 dB	35 dB	45 dB	50 dB
Left HA (original settings)	20 dB	10 dB	15 dB	25 dB	35 dB	45 dB	50 dB
Right HA (adjusted settings)	20 dB	15 dB	20 dB	20 dB	20 dB	25 dB	25 dB
Left HA (adjusted settings)	20 dB	10 dB	15 dB	20 dB	20 dB	20 dB	25 dB

Table 18.2 José's speech perception test results

	Right Aid	Left Aid	Binaural
50 dB HL (original settings)	56%	60%	60%
35 dB HL (original settings)			32%
50 dB HL + 5 SNR (original settings)			44%
50 dB HL (adjusted settings)	84%	76%	88%
35 dB HL (adjusted settings)			72%
50 dB HL + 5 SNR (adjusted settings)			76%

◆ Recommendations

Audiologic management is complex and involves more than reporting test results. Audiologists are not technicians; we have more responsibility than simply administering the tests. We do need to determine the validity and reliability of the procedures, but that is not enough. Interpreting test results includes estimating the child's performance outside of the test situation and making appropriate recommendations. That is, what are the implications of the child's sound room results on his real-world speech-language, academic, literacy, and social-emotional performance? For example, if a child's speech perception is poor at a typical conversational level (50 dB HL), he will not be able to understand people standing within 6 feet of him in a quiet setting. If speech perception is poor at 35 dB HL, he will not understand people more than 3 feet away and will have difficulty hearing in most classroom situations. While he might hear what the teacher speaks into the frequency modulation (FM) microphone, he will not hear the comments of his classmates, and missing them will significantly reduce his ability to participate in classroom discussions and to learn from others.

Types of Recommendations

Diagnostic Recommendations

If testing indicates conductive hearing loss, we know we need to refer for medical evaluation. If observations of the child suggest developmental concerns, referrals need to be made to appropriate practitioners (e.g., pediatrician, developmental pediatrician, pediatric neurologist, speech-language pathologist, and physical or occupational therapist).

Technology Recommendations

Technology evaluation should ensure that the child is hearing soft speech throughout the frequency range in each ear. If not, technology must be adjusted. Such adjustments might include changing the settings of the current hearing aids in each ear, changing to more powerful hearing aids, or considering cochlear implantation. Almost every child will benefit from FM use outside of the classroom for after-school activities, travel in the car, and dinnertime conversations. Therefore, a recommendation for home use of FM should be considered.

Speech/Language/Literacy Recommendations

If speech perception testing indicates anything less than excellent speech perception with technology that is providing optimal auditory access, the child needs to be referred to the appropriate practitioner for auditory/linguistic skill development. If the child is already in a therapy program, the practitioner should be alerted to any speech perception problems observed and documented by the audiologist.

Because a child's academic and social success depends on literacy skills, and literacy skills are based on auditory brain development, audiologists should always include literacy recommendations in the report (Cole & Flexer, 2011). Examples of literacy recommendations include:

- For an infant, read aloud 10–20 books per day.
- For older children, continue to read aloud to them at least 30 minutes per day. Once children begin reading themselves, we should select books to read aloud that are above their own reading level to expand word and conceptual knowledge, auditory attention, and auditory memory and to teach children to love literature.
- Sing to and with the child every day. (Adult-directed singing is an important aspect of auditory brain development and the paralinguistic aspects of language development.)

Educational Recommendations

See the Appendix for an extensive list of possible recommendations that include the topics of FM use, classroom noise accommodations, strategic seating, teaching accommodations, test accommodations, and other services.

Special Considerations

- Recommendations should not be made based on degree of hearing loss; they should be made based on formal and informal assessments.

Profound Hearing Loss

A child with a profound hearing loss who receives an implant at 9 months of age is in a completely different situation than a child with a profound hearing loss who receives an implant at age 4 or 5 years (Boons et al, 2012). Although both children should have good auditory brain access through the technology, the child who was implanted later will have had a longer period of auditory deprivation. As a result, it will take him much longer to obtain the necessary auditory exposure and practice for auditory/linguistic development. A child with a profound hearing loss who is not implanted until age 10 or 12 years and who did not have access to auditory information prior to receiving an implant is dealing with an extremely difficult situation because of cross-modal reorganization of the auditory cortex, a process that will make auditory skill development very difficult.

Mild and Unilateral Hearing Loss

A mild hearing loss in a child does not pose a simple, "mild" problem. A mild hearing loss can have substantial social, emotional, developmental, and academic implications. Most studies suggest that children with a mild hearing loss are more likely to have to repeat a grade then their typically hearing peers and to have academic and/or cognitive deficits. They score more poorly on standardized tests, including tests of reading vocabulary, language mechanics, phonological short-term memory and discrimination, and word analysis. Teachers have observed higher levels of dysfunction in classroom settings for children with mild hearing loss compared with their typically hearing peers. Bess, Dodd-Murphy, and Parker (1998) and Tharpe (2006) reported that younger children with mild hearing loss rated themselves as having less energy than their typically hearing peers, which may be the result of increased listening effort. Because of difficulty listening in anything other than an ideal acoustic environment, children with a mild hearing loss may not hear or may mishear their peers in a social situation, resulting in inappropriate behaviors.

Noise presents a significant problem for any child with a hearing loss, even a mild hearing loss. The effect of hearing loss in a classroom may result in problems with word recognition and spelling, distinguishing morphological markers, and hearing indicators of plurality, possession, and tense (Anderson & Arnoldi, 2011).

Evaluation should include assessment of speech perception in sound field at normal and soft conversational levels in quiet, and in competing noise to accurately assess a child's ability to hear in daily living situations and to make appropriate management recommendations.

◆ Summary

The audiologist has a responsibility to evaluate fully all aspects of a child's performance before finalizing audiologic recommendations. That is, the audiologist should be studying the whole child: the child's language, educational performance, and social-emotional functioning. By considering all aspects of a child's performance, the audiologist has a key role in ensuring the child's developmental progress.

◆ Appendix

The following was adapted from Madell, J. R. (2012). Acoustic accessibility: the role of the clinical audiologist. In J. J. Smaldino and C. Flexer (Eds.), *Handbook of acoustic accessibility: best practices for listening, learning, and literacy in the classroom* (Chapter 9). New York, NY: Thieme Medical Publishers. Used with permission.

Educational Recommendations

Personal FM Systems

1. FM for use during all academic subjects
2. Teacher training in appropriate use of the FM system
3. Troubleshooting information for FM system
4. Develop a system for the teacher to verify that the FM is working daily
5. Assign responsibility for charging the system daily
6. Loaner FM available should the child's system break
7. Assign responsibility for having FM system returned to the factory for servicing over the summer

Classroom Noise Accommodations

1. No open classrooms
2. Select a classroom away from lunchroom, toilets, and playground to reduce noise
3. Carpeting in noisy places like the block corner
4. Acoustic tiles on walls and ceilings as possible
5. Tennis balls or hush-ups on chair and table legs to reduce noise
6. Monitor noise from heating and ventilation system and repair as needed

Strategic Seating

1. Seating in the front third of the classroom near the side to allow the student to see the teacher and also other students
2. Permission to move around the room as needed to hear and see

Teaching Accommodations

These accommodations can make a significant difference in a child's success.

1. Work to keep the classroom quiet to facilitate listening and learning for all children.
2. Teacher's rate, pitch, articulation make speech easy to understand.
3. Teacher faces student when speaking to facilitate receiving information.
4. The classroom should encourage verbal communication, with the opportunity for children to speak with each other.
5. Repeat comments of other students into the FM microphone to be sure the student with hearing loss hears them.
   a. Use pass mic for FM to allow each student in the classroom to speak for herself.
6. Call the student by name to be sure she knows you are talking to her.
7. Confirm that the child with hearing loss hears and understands by asking questions (not "Did you hear that?" or "Do you understand?").
8. Reword, rather than repeat, if the message is not understood.
9. Encourage the student to ask for clarification when information is not clear.
10. Write assignments on the board or in a handout to be certain that the child receives the assignment accurately.
11. Consider assigning a buddy who can help the student with hearing loss get assignments, know what page to turn to, and so forth.
12. Observe what the student does and does not hear and report this information to the audiologist, Teacher of Deaf (TOD), and speech-language pathologist to modify treatment.
13. Activities requiring critical listening should be interspersed with activities that do not require listening.
14. Provide listening breaks during the day to reduce the stress of listening.

Test Accommodations

1. Testing should take place in a quiet room away from noise and interference.
2. Directions should be provided clearly and the tester should verify that the student understands.
3. Spelling tests should include a sentence so words that sound similar will not be confused.

Other Services to Be Considered

1. Regular audiological evaluations to monitor unaided and aided hearing
2. Auditory-based speech-language therapy with a therapist experienced in working with children with hearing loss
3. Teacher of Deaf or Hard of Hearing students to assess academic skills and preview and review academic material
4. Other tutoring as needed
5. Resource room as needed
6. Therapy or tutoring services conducted in a quiet place to facilitate learning
7. System for connecting to computers or other media in "smart classrooms"
8. Team meetings for all staff working with the child with hearing loss to discuss concerns and plan remediation

Discussion Questions

1. What is validity as applied to audiologic tests?
2. What is reliability as applied to audiologic tests?
3. What is the distinction between verification and validation of hearing aid fittings?
4. How are speech perception data used in making educational recommendations for a child with hearing loss?

References

Anderson, K., & Arnoldi, K. A. (2011). Building skills for success in the fast-paced classroom. Hillsboro, OR: Butte.

Bess, F. H., Dodd-Murphy, J., & Parker, R. A. (1998). Children with minimal sensorineural hearing loss: prevalence, educational performance, and functional status. Ear and Hearing, 19(5), 339–354.

Boons, T., Brokx, J. P., Dhooge, I., Frijns, J. H., Peeraer, L., Vermeulen, A., . . . van Wieringen, A. (2012). Predictors of spoken language development following pediatric cochlear implantation. Ear and Hearing, 33(5), 617–639.

Cole, E., & Flexer, C. (2011). Children with hearing loss: developing listening and talking, birth to six (2nd ed.). San Diego: Plural.

Demorest, M. E., & Walden, B. E. (1984). Psychometric principles in the selection, interpretation, and evaluation of communication self-assessment inventories. The Journal of Speech and Hearing Disorders, 49(3), 226–240.

Dillon, H. (2012). Hearing aids (2nd ed.). New York, NY: Thieme.

Glista, D., & Scollie, S. (2012). Development and evaluation of an English language measure of detection of word-final plurality markers: the University of Western Ontario Plurals Test. American Journal of Audiology, 21(1), 76–81.

Haskins, H. (1949). A phonetically balanced test of speech discrimination for children. Master's thesis, Northwestern University, Evanston, IL.

Humes, L. E. (2012). Verification and validation: The chasm between protocol and practice. The Hearing Journal, 65(3), 8–12. Retrieved from http://audiology.com/Cover_story__Verification_and_Validation__The.1.pdf

Leigh, J., Dettman, S., Dowell, R., & Sarant, J. (2011). Evidence-based approach for making cochlear implant recommendations for infants with residual hearing. Ear and Hearing, 32(3), 313–322.

Tharpe, A. M. (2006). The impact of minimal and mild hearing loss on children. Paper presented at the 4th Widex Congress of Paediatric Audiology, Ottawa, Canada, May 19–21, 2006.

Part III

**Hearing Access Technologies
for Infants and Children**

Chapter 19

The Acoustic Speech Signal

Arthur Boothroyd

Key Points

- An essential first step in auditory-oral intervention is the provision and adjustment of hearing aids or cochlear implants to give audibility of the sound patterns of speech.

- Conversational speech, when it reaches the listener's ear, has an overall level around 60 dB sound pressure level (SPL).

- The speech signal covers a range from around 100 Hz to higher than 8000 Hz; most of the energy is in the frequencies below 1000 Hz.

- Within each one-third-octave band, amplitude fluctuates from moment to moment over a range from around 15 dB above the average to 15 dB below it.

- This 30 dB range is responsible for the configuration of the normal performance versus intensity function, which rises from 0 to 100% over a range of 30 dB as the speech signal emerges from below threshold.

- Transferring the amplitude and frequency distribution of speech to the audiogram form produces the well-known speech banana.

- The utility of the speech banana is enhanced by an indication of the distribution of speech information within it—quantitatively, phonetically, and phonemically.

- The greatest concentration of useful information is found between 1000 and 3000 Hz. This is the region of the second vocal tract formant, which conveys information about place of articulation.

- Comparing the speech banana with a child's audiogram gives an impression of the audibility of speech and the potential benefits of hearing aids or cochlear implants.

- Difficulties of discrimination and noise susceptibility may remain even after the sound patterns of speech have been made audible.

◆ The Acoustic Speech Signal

Hearing and Spoken Language

Among the many requirements for acquisition of a first language, three are basic:

- Interaction with fluent users of that language
- Full sensory access to the symbols of that language
- Feedback to the child, via the same sense, of his own efforts to reproduce those symbols

For the hearing child of hearing parents, these three needs are met in relation to spoken language. For the deaf child of signing deaf parents, they are met in relation to signed language. For the deaf child of hearing parents, however, the second and third needs are not met. Without professional intervention, the developmental consequences of the resulting language deficits can be serious and far-reaching. However, these consequences begin with a simple fact: the child cannot hear (or cannot hear well) the sound patterns of speech, either her own or others'. It follows that, once spoken language has been adopted as a goal of intervention, a first step is to give the child sensory access to the sounds of speech—in other words, to optimize hearing. At the time of this writing, the principal tools are hearing aids and cochlear implants. Their effective use, however, requires an awareness of the possibilities and limitations of the child's assisted hearing. Part of that understanding calls for some knowledge of the acoustic properties and informational content of the speech signal. In short, if our goal is for the child to develop spoken language, it behooves us to understand something about the acoustic speech signal.

Overall Amplitude and the Effect of Distance

Overall amplitude, measured in decibels, is one of the basic properties of the speech signal. A typical talker, speaking with conversational effort, at a distance of around 4 feet, generates speech with an overall level of around 60 dB SPL (roughly 50 dB above the normal threshold of hearing). This level, however, falls by 6 dB for every doubling of distance (and increases by 6 dB for every halving of distance)[1] as shown in **Fig. 19.1**.

The Long-Term-Average Spectrum of Speech

The overall level of speech represents a summing of energy across frequency. If we examine the average level within narrow frequency bands, each one-third of an octave wide,[2] we find that:

- Most of the energy is contained in the lower frequencies, below ~ 1000 Hz.
- The level falls at the rate of ~ 5 or 6 dB per octave for frequencies above 500 Hz.

A plot of speech level as a function of frequency is known as the long-term-average spectrum of speech (LTASS) and is used as a basis for the prescriptive fitting of hearing aids.[3]

Fig. 19.2 shows an example of a LTASS derived from a 20-second sample of speech from a woman talker. Also shown, for reference, is the normal soundfield

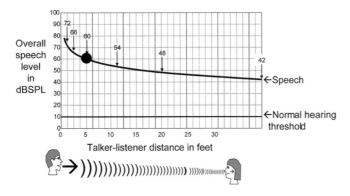

Fig. 19.1   Effect of distance on the overall level of the acoustic speech signal (disregarding the effects of room acoustics). The black circle continues in **Fig. 19.2**.

hearing threshold (Robinson & Dadson, 1956; Sivian & White, 1933).

Variation of Amplitude with Time

The LTASS in **Fig. 19.2** is averaged over time and does not, therefore, reflect the short-term variations of speech amplitude. **Fig. 19.3** shows both the long-term average level and the maximum level as functions of frequency. The maximum levels are measured over short periods lasting around 0.5 second. Also shown are the minimum levels below which there is unlikely to be any useful information. These levels are placed 30 dB below the maximum levels.[4] The result is an area on the amplitude-versus-frequency graph representing the boundaries of the distribution of useful information in the acoustic speech signal. This area is shown in **Fig. 19.3** along with the normal threshold of hearing.

The Performance versus Intensity Function

The 30 dB intensity range of speech is responsible for the 30 dB range of the normal performance versus intensity (P/I) function. This function records the percentage of speech units recognized as the average speech level rises from below threshold. The speech units can be phonemes (vowels and consonants), monosyllables in isolation, spondees in isolation, words in sentences, or other chosen units. **Fig. 19.4** shows the P/I function for phonemes in consonant–vowel–consonant (CVC) words. Phoneme recognition begins to rise above zero as the speech area first peeps above threshold and approaches 100% when the whole area is above threshold. Note that the speech area has been restricted to the region between 300 and 6000 Hz in **Fig. 19.4**, this being the region that contains most of the acoustic cues responsible for phoneme recognition. Note, also, that when roughly 50% of the speech area is above threshold, phoneme recognition is already around 80%—reflecting the ability of normally hearing users of spoken language to take advantage of phonemic and lexical redundancy to compensate for an incomplete signal.[5]

---

[1] Indoors, the 6 dB rule only applies up to a certain distance. Beyond this distance, the useful energy reaching the listener is determined by reflections from the room's boundaries. Unfortunately, these useful early reflections are accompanied by later reflections, or reverberation, which can have a negative effect on perception of the received signal (Boothroyd, 2004). The effects of room acoustics on the effectiveness of hearing aids and cochlear implants is an important and complex topic and beyond the scope of the present chapter.

[2] An octave band is a range of frequencies in which the highest frequency is twice the lowest. In a one-third-octave band, the highest frequency is 1.26 times the lowest. The ear integrates energy over roughly one-third of an octave.

[3] This spectrum is different for men, women, and children; it varies with talker within each of these groups; it changes with vo-

cal effort; it changes with orientation of the talker with respect to the listener; and it changes somewhat with distance when close to the talker's mouth (Pittman, Stelmachowicz, Lewis, & Hoover, 2003).

[4] It is difficult to specify a meaningful minimum level because speech can contain breaks and pauses. It is generally accepted, however, that the useful information at any frequency is uniformly distributed over a range of around 30 dB. This assumption is incorporated into the computation of Speech Intelligibility Index (American National Standards Institute [ANSI], 1997).

[5] Young children with hearing loss cannot be assumed to have the skills or knowledge needed to compensate for an incomplete signal. They need full access if they are to acquire them.

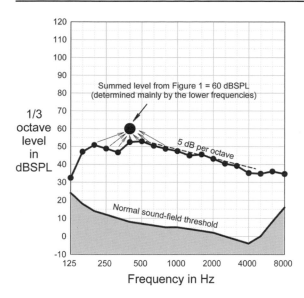

Fig. 19.2   Long-term average speech spectrum, in one-third-octave bands, derived from a 20-second sample of a woman's speech. Talker distance is assumed to be 4 feet (**Fig. 19.1**). The line continues in **Fig. 19.3**.

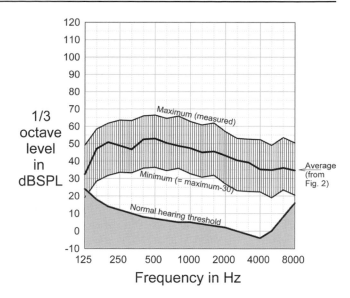

Fig. 19.3   The speech level in any frequency band varies over a range of around 30 dB, from 15 dB above the average to 15 dB below it. The resulting speech area is shown here with vertical shading, in relation to the threshold of normal hearing. The shaded area continues in **Fig. 19.4**.

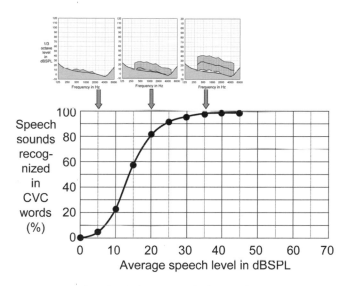

Fig. 19.4   The decibel range of the performance-versus-intensity function reflects the short-term amplitude range of the speech signal. CVC: consonant–vowel–consonant.

Representing Speech on the Audiogram Form

So far, all representations of amplitude have been in SPL, with sound level increasing as we move upward on the amplitude-versus-frequency graphs. This approach is widely used when dealing with hearing aid testing and fitting. In the intervention world, however, clinicians and educators are more familiar with the audiogram form. On this form, amplitude is measured in relation to the normal hearing threshold, and sound level increases as we move downward. The transformation is

illustrated in **Fig. 19.5**. In this context, the speech area is commonly referred to as the speech banana. In the current example, the banana looks a little crumpled. These data, however, were derived from a 20-second sample of the speech of a specific talker. The more familiar representation shows the average of many talkers and is somewhat smoother, as shown in subsequent figures.

Information and Frequency

The information in speech is distributed unevenly across frequencies.

Pearl
• The highest concentration of information is found between ~ 1000 and 3000 Hz, with progressively less at higher and lower frequencies.

This point is illustrated by the concentration of dots in **Fig. 19.6**. There are 100 dots, so a little counting serves to identify the percentage of useful information in different frequency regions.[6] Also shown in **Fig. 19.6** are the frequency ranges of certain acoustic and phonetic features, discussed subsequently.

---

[6] This way of representing the relative importance of different frequencies is based on the "count the dots" approach of Mueller and Killion (1990).

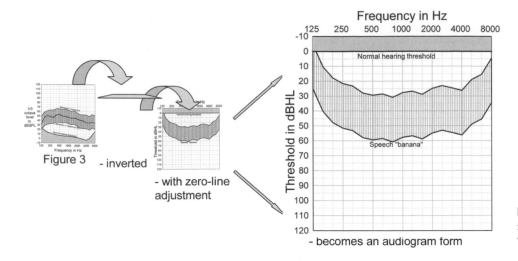

Figure 3   - inverted

- with zero-line adjustment

- becomes an audiogram form

Fig. 19.5 Conversion from a sound pressure level representation to a hearing level representation.

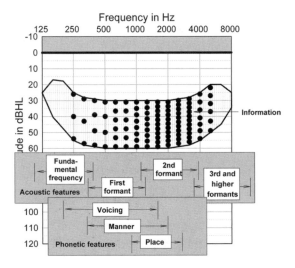

Fig. 19.6 The relative importance of different parts of the speech banana is shown here by the distribution of dots. Also shown are the frequency ranges covered by some acoustic and phonetic features of the speech signal.

Acoustic Properties and Frequency

The concentration of information in the 1000 to 3000 Hz region is by no means coincidental. This is the region covered by the second vocal tract formant. A formant is a peak in the short-term spectrum of speech caused by resonance in the oral cavities (Pickett, 1999). There are many formants, and they are numbered in order of increasing frequency. The second formant is produced by resonance of the cavity at the front of the mouth—from tongue to lips. For an adult male talker, its frequency varies over a 3:1 range from around 900 to 2700 Hz. (In women and children the values are somewhat higher.) The

frequency at any moment is determined by a combination of the size of the lip opening and the location of the narrowest portion of the oral cavity, which depends mainly on the position and shape of the tongue. The frequency of the second formant (and the way it changes over time) provides the listener with information about the positions, shapes, and movements of tongue and lips. These articulators are responsible for many of the distinctions among the sound patterns of spoken language—hence the major importance of the frequency region covered by the second formant.

Of somewhat less importance, but also useful, is the first formant. This is produced by resonance of the whole oral cavity—from larynx to lips. For an adult male talker, its frequency varies over a 3:1 range from around 300 to 900 Hz. (Once again, in women and children the values are somewhat higher.) The frequency at any moment is determined by the vertical size of the oral cavity. The frequency of the first formant and the way it changes over time provide the listener with information about the raising and lowering of the jaw and tongue as well as the opening and closing of the lips.

The higher formants carry information about fricative sounds such as [ʃ] ("sh") and [s] ("s"), as well as bursts, such as [tʃ] ("ch") and [t] ("t"). They also help the listener identify the talker.

The melodic pattern of speech is determined by voice fundamental frequency. This is the frequency at which the vocal folds vibrate. It covers a range of ~ 3:1, with an average around 100 Hz for men, 200 Hz for women, and higher for children. The value of fundamental frequency and its variation over time provide the listener with information not just about talker age and sex, but also about such things as syllable and word stress, phrase and sentence boundaries, and the talker's emotional state.

- Interestingly, the listener does not need to hear the fundamental frequency but can acquire information about it from higher frequencies, especially from the region of the first formant.

Information about the frequency ranges covered by these acoustic cues is included in **Fig. 19.6**.

◆ Phonetic Features and Frequency

The acoustic properties mentioned above carry information about articulatory features that are responsible for defining the sound system of the language. Three features of consonant articulation are of special interest to clinicians and educators. These are voicing, manner of articulation, and place of articulation. Miller and Nicely (1955) published the results of a series of experiments on the effects of filtering on consonant confusions. From their data, Boothroyd (1978) determined, for each consonant feature, the frequency ranges containing the bulk of the useful information. This information is included in **Fig. 19.6**. The most striking feature of these data are that the range for identification of place of consonant articulation is very close to the range containing the highest concentration of information. This is not a coincidence. Consonants contribute considerably to intelligibility, and place of articulation carries more information about

consonant identity than does either of the other two features. Moreover, the second vocal tract formant is the primary cue for place of articulation.

Phonemes, Amplitude, and Frequency

Spoken vowels and consonants are identified by acoustic patterns. These patterns involve components that cover a wide range of frequencies, they change over time, and they are influenced by the sounds that precede and follow them. It is, therefore, difficult to allocate specific phonemes to specific locations within the speech banana. There are a few sounds, however, whose key acoustic cues are restricted to a relatively small frequency region, and we can be reasonably certain that they will not be recognized if those regions are inaudible. A sample of such sounds is shown in **Fig. 19.7**, which is based on experimental data (Boothroyd, Erickson, & Medwetsky, 1994).[7] Some of these sounds are used in the Ling 5- or 6-sound test to confirm that a child can hear and identify speech patterns over an appropriate range of frequencies (Ling, 1989).

The Audiogram and the Speech Banana

When pure tone thresholds are recorded on an audiogram form, the result is an audiogram. The line joining the Os or Xs divides the form into two regions. Above the line are inaudible sounds—the lost hearing. Below the line are audible sounds—the remaining or residual hearing. By examining the audiogram in relation to the speech banana, we can obtain a sense of the acoustic cues, the percent information, the consonant features, and even the types of speech sound that are available to the child through the sense of hearing. Consider, for example, the audiogram represented in **Fig. 19.8**. If we assume that this is the child's better ear, we can see that she should be able to recognize those sounds whose identity depends on low-frequency patterns, but she will be unable even to hear high-frequency sounds, such as [ʃ] and [s] (also [tʃ] and [t]), let alone recognize them. And

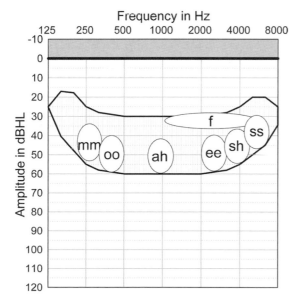

Fig. 19.7 The locations of the key acoustic cues needed for recognition of selected speech sounds.

---

[7] Illustrations like this must be interpreted with caution. For example, the frequency range of the key resonance in the sound [s] tends to be much higher for women than for men; it varies within each gender group; and it is highly dependent on the preceding or following vowels (Boothroyd & Medwetsky, 1992). Recognition of the sound [iː] ("ee") depends on audibility of the second formant (around 2500 Hz), but detection depends mainly on the first formant, which is almost identical to that of the sound [uː] ("oo"). If the second formant of [iː] is inaudible, [iː] and [uː] tend to be confused. More importantly, simple audibility of a given speech sound is no guarantee that it will be recognized or distinguished from similar sounds.

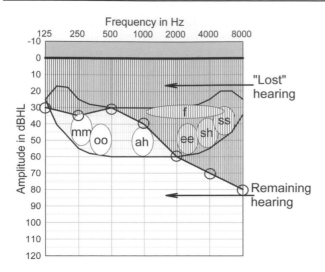

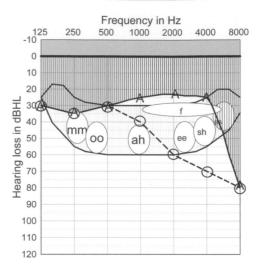

Fig. 19.8 Examining a child's audiogram in relation to the speech banana provides insights into the child's access to acoustic speech information.

Fig. 19.9 The effect of amplification on audibility of the speech signal is illustrated by showing the speech banana in relation to the aided soundfield threshold.

even though she will hear the [i:] ("ee") sound, it will be indistinguishable from an [u:] ("oo"). If we were also to overlay this audiogram on **Fig. 19.6**, we would see that only ~ 30% of the useful acoustic information in the acoustic speech is available to this child—basically, that contained in the first formant and the variations of amplitude and fundamental frequency over time. We would also conclude that she will have great difficulty identifying (and, therefore, reproducing) place of consonant articulation.

The Aided Audiogram and the Speech Banana

Now contrast **Fig. 19.8** with **Fig. 19.9**, in which we compare the speech banana with the aided audiogram.[8] Most of the phonemes shown here have been rendered audible. There is, however, a restriction on the audibility of the highest frequencies, particularly of the sound [s]. This restriction occurs because current hearing aids are incapable of providing substantial gain at the higher frequencies (Stelmachowicz. Pittman, Hoover, & Lewis, 2001, 2002). One must also be very cautious when interpreting an illustration like this one. The damage to the hearing mecha-

nism that produces the threshold shift also causes a loss of spectral and temporal resolution. As a result, the child may still have difficulty identifying and differentiating sounds, even when they have been made audible. In addition, reduced spectral and temporal resolution renders the listener highly susceptible to the interfering effects of background noise—a complaint of all hearing aid users. To emphasize these limitations, the higher-frequency sounds in **Fig. 19.9** are shown with reduced font size.

The Speech Banana and Cochlear Implants

---

[8] The difference between the aided and unaided thresholds reflects the gain of the hearing aid, at least for very low inputs. With the introduction of wide-dynamic-range-compression hearing aids, the aided audiogram has become inappropriate as a way of estimating effective hearing aid gain. Because gain falls with increasing input, illustrations like **Fig. 19.9** tend to overestimate gain for realistic speech inputs. Nevertheless, this remains a valid technique for deciding whether a given sound is audible via aided hearing—providing one keeps a clear distinction between audibility and recognition.

Instead of the upper frequency limit imposed by the physical construction of a hearing aid, the spectral resolution available with a cochlear implant depends on such things as the number of electrodes and their location in relation to independently stimulable auditory nerve cells. With modern implants, there is every reason to expect that temporal resolution will be preserved. The small number of independent channels of stimulation, however, are unable to provide normal spectral resolution. Appropriate mapping can usually provide audibility over a wide frequency range, including the high frequencies typically unavailable to the hearing aid user, as shown in **Fig. 19.10**. Because of reduced spectral resolution, however, the resulting hearing will exhibit problems of discrimination and noise susceptibility similar to those experienced by children with moderately severe hearing loss who use hearing aids. Again, this effect is emphasized in **Fig. 19.10** by a reduction of font size.

◆ Summary

A first step in auditory-oral intervention is to optimize hearing so that the child has access to as much of the information as possible in the acoustic speech signal. This signal, which has an overall level of around 60 dB SPL when measured at a conversational distance, contains components that are distributed across a wide frequency range, from around 100 Hz to higher than 8000 Hz. Most of the energy is in frequency regions below 1000 Hz but the maximum concentration of useful information is between around 1000 and 3000 Hz. This is the range covered by the second vocal-tract formant, which conveys considerable information about place of articulation. At any frequency, the short-term amplitude varies between 15 dB above and below the average. The resulting range of 30 dB is reflected in the normal performace versus intensity (P/I) function, in which recognition of speech elements rises from 0 to 100% over a range of ~ 30 dB as speech emerges from inaudibility to full audibility. Expressing levels in relation to normal hearing threshold, and transferring them to an audiogram form, results in the speech banana. Examination of this area in relation to a child's audiogram can provide insights into the acoustic cues, phonetic cues, and phonemes that are likely to be accessible to the child through the unaided sense of hearing. The same technique can be used to show the potential benefits of assistance with hearing aids or cochlear implants, providing one recognizes that the resulting hearing is not perfect and that difficulties of discrimination and noise susceptibility are likely to remain. Providing access to the information contained in the acoustic patterns of speech is an essential first step in auditory-oral intervention, but it is only the first step.

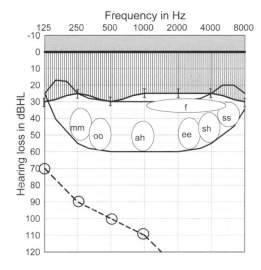

Fig. 19.10 Modern multichannel cochlear implants can provide profoundly and totally deaf children with audibility of the speech spectrum over a wide range of frequencies. Unlike hearing aids, the implant is not constrained in terms of an upper frequency limit and it is not susceptible to acoustic feedback. The limited number of independent channels of stimulation, however, still leads to reduced spectral resolution when compared with normal hearing.

◆ Acknowledgments

Preparation of this chapter was supported, in part, by NIH grant no. DC006238 to the House Ear Institute.

Discussion Questions

1. Discuss the configuration of the normal P/I function.
2. Describe the utility of the speech banana.
3. Detail the difficulties that a child with a mild hearing loss will have discriminating speech in the presence of noise.
4. Why is a cochlear implant not an amplifier?

lished, the use of coupler gain measures to verify that REAG targets are matched in hearing aids, and the use of parental observations and electrophysiologic measures in evaluating the effectiveness of hearing aids. Third, children rely on amplification to develop speech and language and to acquire knowledge of the world around them. They need better signal-to-noise ratios (SNRs) than adults do for perceiving speech, and they need access to sounds in their environment for incidental learning. Hearing aid technologies should be selected to meet the special needs of children.

◆ Selection of Hearing Aids: New Technologies

Wireless Compatibility

The passage of sound across a room inevitably degrades its quality. A hearing aid microphone detects the original sound, the reverberation of that sound around the room, noise from any other sources inside the room and possibly outside the room, and reverberation of the noise. Only the first of these signals helps the child understand speech; the rest degrade understanding. (As an exception, the very early echoes can also enhance intelligibility by increasing the level of speech, but most reverberant energy is detrimental to intelligibility.) By contrast, the wireless transmission of sound by using it to control electromagnetic energy (at radio frequencies or at infrared frequencies) can pass over huge distances with little or no degradation of sound quality. The most common transmission methods have previously involved frequency modulation (FM) of the electromagnetic waves, hence these systems are mostly referred to as FM systems. Increasingly, various digital modulation methods are being used, and a more general name for these systems is wireless remote-microphone hearing aids.

Consequently, children are likely to benefit from wireless transmission of speech whenever they have to listen to someone from a distance of, say, 1 m or farther. The greater the hearing loss and the greater the difficulty in understanding speech, the greater will be the benefit that wireless transmission offers. The primary limitation is achieving the cooperation of the person or persons talking. When there is just one talker, the situation is clear: the talker wears a transmitter, including a microphone mounted as close as possible to the mouth, and the child wears a receiver coupled to, or integral with, hearing aids. In many situations, however, there are several people to whom the child needs to listen, including himself or herself. The hearing aid must therefore appropriately combine the signal detected by the wireless receiver with the signal detected by the hearing aid microphone. Here the difficulties start, because mixing the

two signals can adversely affect the intelligibility of each, whereas a wireless signal can easily offer as much as a 20 dB improvement in SNR over acoustic reception. This will be substantially degraded (but still be beneficial) if the wireless and microphone paths are adjusted to have similar sensitivity.

The best mixing solution is when the receiver and hearing aid combination automatically gives high priority to the wireless signal whenever it recognizes voice activity in the wireless channel, and turns off the wireless channel when no voice activity is detected. Sadly, although such speech-operated switching systems have been available for at least 20 years, most wireless systems on the market do not have this feature. Consequently, the clinician must ensure that the hearing aid and receiver are adjusted to achieve the desired relativity between the wireless and hearing aid microphone signals. This is a difficult choice: too little and the advantage of the wireless system is largely lost; too great and the child will have inadequate audibility when someone other than the user of the transmitter is talking. Reflecting the difficulty of this choice, the ratio of wireless to microphone level at the output of the hearing aid has been recommended by different people (for a summary, see Dillon, 2012) to be from 5 to 15 dB.

Wireless transmission to hearing aids has been available for three decades. The major change in this technology is that the receivers available are now small enough to clip onto the hearing aid or be entirely contained within the hearing aid, rather than as large external devices.

Compression

There is no doubt that compression (nonlinear amplification) should be prescribed for children, and it is particularly beneficial for children too young to use a volume control. The major advantages of compression are that, relative to a linear amplifier with a fixed gain-frequency response, gain is increased for lower-level sounds (increasing intelligibility) and decreased for higher-level sounds (increasing comfort and acoustic safety). Although an adult or older child can achieve a similar result by using a volume control, an infant or younger child cannot. Fortunately, the gains prescribed by both major generic prescription rules—NAL-NL2 (National Acoustic Laboratories, Macquarie University, New South Wales, Australia) and DSLm[i/o] (National Centre for Audiology, University of Western Ontario, London, Ontario, Canada)—and by all proprietary prescription rules, inherently contain compression. Consequently, the clinician does not explicitly have to choose compression if hearing aids are adjusted to match these prescriptions.

Some clinicians have precociously chosen not to provide compression for people (of any age) with severe to profound hearing loss. This choice may be based on some early research indicating that compression was mostly detrimental for people with such losses (Boothroyd, Springer, Smith, & Schulman, 1988). More recent research, aimed at discovering the optimal degree of compression, indicates it is appropriate to provide compression for even these greater degrees of hearing loss (Keidser, Dillon, Dyrlund, Carter, & Hartley, 2007). In extensive listening trials in real-life conditions, a low compression ratio, particularly for the low frequencies, was preferred to either linear amplification or higher compression ratios. Compression in moderation for severe or profound loss therefore appears to be the key. It is not known whether children should be prescribed fast- or slow-acting compression. Gatehouse, Naylor, and Elberling (2006) have shown that for adults, the more alert the person and the more dynamic the listening environment, the greater the advantage of fast-acting compression over slow-acting, on average. The application of this to children remains unknown. The use of wide-dynamic-range compression for all children is no longer debated. There is, however, still some uncertainty over the maximum compression ratios that should be used and how fast the compression should be.

Adaptive Noise Reduction and Speech Enhancement

Adaptive noise reduction (also known as speech enhancement) systems in hearing aids work by reducing the gain in a frequency region where the SNR is poorer than in other frequency regions, or poorer than some preset criterion amount. Some hearing aids are designed to be sufficiently fast-acting that the gain changes in the gaps between the syllables of speech; others are designed to be sufficiently slow-acting that the gain fluctuates over periods of seconds or tens of seconds. In both cases, the result is that those frequency regions where noise dominates are deemphasized relative to other regions where speech is more dominant. Many studies over the decades (for a summary, see Dillon, 2012) have shown that adults prefer noise suppression on the grounds that listening comfort is greater, and that noise is less salient, even though noise reduction has little or no effect on intelligibility. Evaluations on children are consistent with this: noise reduction mostly has no effect on intelligibility but, in a few circumstances, can improve it (Marcoux, Yathiraj, Côté, & Logan, 2006; Pittman, 2011; Stelmachowicz et al, 2010). There does not seem to be any compelling reason why adaptive noise reduction should not be used for all children. Some have argued that the spectrum presented to children should not be altered while children are still learning to understand speech. However, the audible spectrum alters every time a different person talks, or the talker and listener move to a dif-

ferent room, or a different masking noise occurs. The spectral changes caused by noise suppression are relatively small compared with these and are always in the direction of making speech more salient. We therefore recommend that noise reduction systems in hearing aids be routinely enabled for children of all ages, just as they are for adults. Increasingly, manufacturers are linking control of the adaptive noise reduction to the hearing thresholds for which the hearing aid is programmed. With such systems, there seems almost no possibility that adaptive noise reduction systems could inadvertently reduce the audibility of speech signals.

A second form of noise suppression available in hearing aids is transient suppression. This processing strategy recognizes when the waveform is changing at a rate so high it cannot be the result of a speech signal, and it reduces the gain of the signal during this portion of rapid change. The result is that the loudness of impulsive sounds such as doors slamming or hammering is greatly reduced (Keidser, O'Brien, Latzel, & Convery, 2007). The processing has no adverse effect on speech and can be left permanently activated.

Directional Microphones

It is clear from physical principles that if a child is looking at a sound source, if the distance from the child to the source is not too much greater than the critical distance of the room, and if there is noise or reverberation in the environment, directional microphones will offer an improved SNR. Notwithstanding the ample evidence on the benefits of directional amplification for adults, this technology has been little used in the fitting of infants and young children. This has been the case because of clinicians' concerns that directional microphones will decrease SNR when the talker to whom the child is listening is to the side or rear of the child. In particular, clinicians may be concerned that fitting directional amplification will limit children's access to incidental learning that results from sounds arriving from nonfrontal directions.

In laboratory settings, the benefit of directional microphones for school-aged children has been demonstrated by presenting speech from 0° azimuth and noise from 180° azimuth (Gravel, Fausel, Liskow, & Chobot, 1999). The children tested, ranging in age from 4 to 11 years, obtained an improvement of 5 dB on average when they used directional microphones to listen to words and sentences presented in multitalker babble than when they used omnidirectional amplification. Consistent with findings in earlier studies, children younger than 7 years required better SNR than older children to achieve the same level of performance. Ching et al (2009) studied the real-life looking behavior of children aged 11 to 78 months. They found that the amount of time the children looked at, versus away from, the prier is to adjust a control until the sound is clearest. This is little different in complexity from performing a paired-comparison task either in the clinic or at home with a two-program hearing aid. Children (with hearing impairment but no other developmental delay) aged 8 years or older are able to do both of these tasks reliably. Children of this age are also able to take direct responsibility for selecting between wireless input and combined wireless/hearing aid input, another task of similar complexity. It therefore seems reasonable to use trainability for children aged 8 years or older. Although there is no reason to expect that children will train the hearing aid to produce output levels intense enough to damage their remaining hearing, it would be beneficial if manufacturers provided the ability to limit the degree to which the hearing-aid gain could be increased above the prescribed settings at each frequency, particularly for the gain applied to higher-level sounds.

Earmolds

Earmolds for older children are little or no different from those for adults, but earmolds for infants are small! The very small size has several implications. First, when an impression is taken, a very small cotton block is needed if a sufficient insertion depth is to be achieved. Best results can be achieved with blocks custom made (from cotton-wool and thread) to best suit each ear, rather than the often-too-large ready-made ones. Second, the small size usually makes it impossible to fit in a vent or acoustic horn. Infants whose hearing loss is detected at birth usually have a sufficiently large loss that vents are not needed. If one is required, an external vent can be created by grinding a slit down the outside of the earmold. Far more commonly, the clinician would like to be able to stop leakage around the mold (rather than create it with a vent). The third issue arising from small ear canal size is that small ear canals grow rapidly, causing the earmold to become loose and leak, in turn causing feedback oscillation or causing the earmold to fall out. Earmolds are likely to have to be made monthly up to 6 months of age, bimonthly up to 12 months, and three to four times per year up to the age of 3 years.

Earmolds for infants and younger children are usually made of soft materials, either because the softer materials are thought to have less leakage or because they are inherently safer if the child's activities are likely to result in an accidental blow to the ear. Unfortunately, soft materials degrade faster, but this is not such a problem when they have to be regularly replaced because of ear canal growth. For ears prone to discharge, hard materials, and a spare set of molds to enable cleaning and drying, are advantageous.

Retaining hearing aids in place on small ears can be a problem. Devices that assist with this problem include double-sided sticky tape, extra-small earhooks, extra-stiff (moisture resistant) tubing, and Huggies to hold the hearing aid to the auricula. Finally, hypoallergenic coatings are available, and brightly colored earmolds are extremely popular.

◆ Prescription of Hearing Aids

Once the diagnosis of hearing loss is confirmed, tympanometry, or high-frequency tympanometry, should be performed (Purdy & Williams, 2000; Feeney & Sanford, Chapter 12, this volume) to obtain information about middle ear function. In addition, acoustic reflex testing and otoacoustic emissions (OAE) testing should be used to determine if further review for auditory neuropathy or retrocochlear pathology (Purdy & Kelly, Chapter 15; Neault, Chapter 32 this volume) is necessary. To proceed with aiding, it is necessary to determine an audiogram, to adopt an approach that caters to the special needs of children, and to fit bilateral amplification according to a prescriptive procedure.

Audiogram

An optimal hearing aid fitting starts with an accurate audiogram. An important consideration in determining an audiogram for fitting is that the small ear canal sizes of infants and young children influence the validity of conventional audiometric measures. Because audiometers are conventionally calibrated such that an average adult has normal hearing thresholds of 0 dB hearing level (HL), constant across transducers, the same will not be true for children, whose ear canals are shorter and narrower than those of adults. If insert earphones are used in determining thresholds, the volume of the ear canal directly affects the sound pressure level generated at the eardrum. As a child grows, the canal volume increases and the sound pressure level (SPL) generated at the eardrum decreases. This in turn causes apparent hearing thresholds to "deteriorate" with increase in age. If soundfield assessment is used, the length of the ear canal determines its resonance properties, or REUG, and hence affects the threshold expressed as level in the undisturbed field. If headphones are used, both the volume and the length of the ear canal will affect thresholds. These effects render the audiometer dial readings inaccurate when measuring thresholds of anyone who does not have an average adult ear canal, which clearly includes infants and small children. A consequence is that hearing thresholds measured using different audiometric transducers (insert earphones, soundfield loudspeakers, supra-aural headphones) are not equivalent. To resolve this anomaly, there are two possible solutions. First, children's thresholds can be expressed in terms of dB SPL at the eardrum (Seewald & Scollie, 2003). This method involves measuring a child's real-ear-to-coupler difference (RECD) (i.e., the difference between the level of a signal in the ear canal and the level of the same signal in a coupler). The RECD can be used to convert hearing thresholds in dB HL to ear canal SPL. The equations used in the transformations are given in Bagatto et al (2005), and the calculation is done automatically in the DSL fitting software (Seewald et al, 1997; Scollie et al, 2005). This representation allows easy comparison of threshold levels with aided speech levels in the real ear. Second, an equally effective solution is to express thresholds in terms of adult equivalent hearing level. This is the threshold level that an average adult would have if the adult had the same threshold in dB SPL at the eardrum as the child (Dillon, 2012). The same techniques (using RECD) are used to determine the threshold SPL in the ear canal, but these thresholds are then converted to average equivalent hearing level by subtracting the average adult RECD (Ching & Dillon, 2003). The calculation is done automatically in the NAL fitting software (Dillon, 1999). As hearing loss is represented in terms of the familiar dB HL, the magnitude of the hearing loss is more easily grasped.

A second consideration in determining an audiogram for fitting arises from the fact that behavioral thresholds are often not available for children diagnosed with hearing loss soon after birth. Instead, auditory evoked potentials, which provide frequency-specific information for each ear, are used to estimate hearing thresholds. (Chapter 7 describes a behavioral evaluation technique that can successfully be used with infants.) The available electrophysiologic measures include auditory brainstem responses (ABRs; Stapells, Gravel, & Martin, 1995), auditory steady-state responses (ASSRs; Rance et al, 2005), and electrocochleography (ECoG; Wong, Gibson, & Sanli, 1997). Threshold estimations obtained from auditory evoked potentials are referenced in dB normalized HL (dB nHL). This normative reference is defined differently across systems, but the calibration of systems invariably is based on obtaining behavioral thresholds from adults for the stimuli used in evoking auditory potentials (Stapells et al, 1995; see Bagatto et al, 2005, for a discussion). Correction figures for estimating behavioral thresholds in dB HL from ABR-derived thresholds in dB nHL have been derived by relating measured behavioral thresholds to ABR-derived thresholds of adults and older children with stimuli presented under headphones (Stapells 2000a, 2000b) or insert earphones (Sininger, Abdala, & Cone-Wesson, 1997). It is assumed that the normative reference defined by adults' hearing sensitivity would apply similarly to infants, were it possible to measure behavioral thresholds for establishing a normative reference for infants. However,

this is not likely to be a good assumption, because the adult and the infant ear canals differ in volume and length. The same stimulus level presented via a headphone will result in different sound pressure levels at the eardrum, of the order of 2 to 7 dB lower in the infant's than in the adult's ear for high frequencies (Voss & Herrmann, 2005). If insert earphones are used, the volume of the ear canal directly affects the sound pressure level generated at the eardrum. Higher sound pressure levels will be generated in the infant's than in the adult's ear for the same input level. The error implicit in assuming that the infant's behavioral threshold is 0 dB HL needs to be modified by incorporating the difference in RECDs between an adult and an infant in the correction figures.

Once estimates of behavioral thresholds for at least one low (e.g., 500 Hz) and one high (e.g., 2 kHz) frequency are available, amplification should be provided immediately to support early language development (see Thompson et al, 2001, for a review, and Stredler-Brown, Chapter 27 in this text). As thresholds at additional frequencies are obtained, the hearing aid can be adjusted if needed. The estimated thresholds should be confirmed by ear-specific audiometry to establish air conduction thresholds when reliable behavioral responses can be obtained. If a child has a chronic conductive hearing loss, bone conduction thresholds have equal priority with air conduction thresholds. The effectiveness of amplification for providing auditory information to the child should be evaluated and monitored over time.

RECD/REAG/CG Adjustment Method

To achieve a consistent SPL at the eardrum, prescriptive targets should be specified in terms of REAG. This is the increase in signal level when aided, relative to the level in the soundfield (Dillon, 2012, provides a detailed discussion). For a REAG prescription, the corresponding coupler gain (CG) targets are affected only by the difference between the coupler-measured gain and the real-ear gain, that is, the RECD. Therefore, an effective method to allow for differences in ear canal size is to measure the RECD (Moodie, Seewald, & Sinclair, 1994) before prescribing hearing aids and to use the RECDs to calculate the CGs that will result in the target REAG. As a child grows, changes in the ear canal acoustics result in decreases in RECD (Feigin, Kopun, Stelmachowicz, & Gorga, 1989), and higher coupler gains will be required to provide the same REAG targets. If measurement of individual RECD is not possible, age-appropriate values may be used (Feigin et al, 1989; Bagatto, Scollie, Seewald, Moodie, & Hoover, 2002; Bagatto et al, 2005; Dillon, 2012) to derive coupler gain targets. Hearing aids can be adjusted and verified in a 2 cc (2 cm³) coupler to match the prescribed viding more gain in hearing aids, but the increased audibility may result in more frequent saturation or in an increase in loudness without any increase in speech intelligibility. The contribution of audibility to speech intelligibility depends on the amount of speech information that can be extracted from an audible signal. This decreases as hearing loss increases (Ching, Dillon, & Byrne, 1998; Ching, Dillon et al, 2001; Hogan & Turner, 1998) and as the population of functioning inner hair cells in the cochlea diminishes (Moore, 2001). For this reason, audibility displays may be used to suggest the amount of audible information available to a child with mild or moderate hearing loss, but they should not be relied upon for estimating the information available to a child with more severe loss. The effectiveness of amplification in providing auditory information to a child has to be established by evaluating aided performance.

Aided Thresholds

The measurement of soundfield aided thresholds has traditionally been used to demonstrate a child's ability to detect the presence of sound in an audiometric test booth when the child is aided. However, aided thresholds do not provide information about a child's hearing ability at suprathreshold levels or about sensation levels of amplified speech. Nevertheless, aided thresholds are useful for establishing whether a child's unaided thresholds are vibrotactile when hearing loss is profound. In such cases, aided and unaided thresholds will be approximately the same. When aided thresholds are used to supplement the RECD/CG approach to verifying hearing aids, the thresholds obtained should be compared with those prescribed by the prescription procedure used. The NAL prescription for nonlinear hearing aids includes aided threshold targets that can be used for this purpose.

Speech Tests

A realistic method to demonstrate aided improvement of a child with hearing loss to the family is to establish the child's speech reception threshold (SRT) and to compare the child's performance in aided and unaided conditions. For older children, a range of speech tests are available for assessing performance (see Pediatric Working Group, 1996, for a review; see Dillon & Ching, 1995, and Madell, Chapter 11 in this book, for a discussion of selection and use of speech tests).

For assessing the binaural processing ability of children, the SRT for speech and noise presented from the same loudspeaker positioned at 0° azimuth can be compared with the SRT for speech presented at 0° azimuth and noise at ±90° azimuth (Ching, van Wanrooy et al, 2006; Ching, van Wanrooy, Dil-

lon, & Carter, 2011). Children with normal hearing will display a 3 dB advantage from spatial separation, whereas some children with congenital hearing loss will commonly display no advantage.

For evaluating alternative amplification schemes to see which one is most effective, speech testing is not the method of choice despite its face validity. Not only are speech tests very time-consuming to perform, they are also limited in sensitivity to differences in hearing aid characteristics (Studebaker, 1982). If speech tests are administered for evaluating the effectiveness of amplification, they should be supplemented by assessments of functional performance in everyday situations.

Paired-Comparison Testing

The paired-comparison technique allows several schemes to be compared in pairs so that a listener can select the most preferred scheme for amplifying speech. Previous research with adults has shown that this method is more sensitive than speech perception tests to differences in amplification characteristics (Studebaker, 1982; Byrne, 1986). It can be used with school-aged children to compare the relative intelligibility of speech amplified with alternative frequency responses (Eisenberg & Levitt, 1991; Ching, Hill, Birtles, & Beecham, 1999). More reliable judgments can be obtained with audiovisual than with auditory-alone presentation of speech stimuli (Ching et al, 1994). The optimal frequency response for speech intelligibility was found to be the same, irrespective of the mode of stimuli presentation. Paired-comparisons testing, like speech testing, can be used only with older children. For young children, the available options for evaluating the effectiveness of amplification include subjective reports and objective electrophysiologic assessments.

Pearl

- Effectiveness of amplification is best determined by evaluating aided performance using subjective reports and objective electrophysiologic measures.

Subjective Reports

Infants and young children are limited in their ability to provide verbal comment on the relative effectiveness of amplification for speech intelligibility and sound quality. Although self-reports are useful for adults and possibly some older children (see Stelmachowicz, 1999, for a review), they are not applicable to young children. A variety of subjective report tools that rely on the observations of parents and teachers have been developed to guide audiologic intervention for young children, but these are limited in the range of ages and degrees of hearing loss to which they can be applied (see Ching & Hill, 2007, for a review). To address the need to evaluate amplification for children of a wide range of age and hearing loss, the Parents' Evaluation of Aural/Oral Performance of Children (PEACH) has been developed (Ching & Hill, 2007). The PEACH questionnaire, which is shown in the Appendix and may be copied for use, consists of items that relate to usage of device, loudness comfort, functional performance in quiet and in noise, and alertness to environmental sounds. Parents are requested to observe and record their child's auditory and oral behaviors in everyday life situations in a diary, and the examples are solicited in a structured interview for scoring. PEACH can be used with children as young as 1 month through to school age, and for all degrees of hearing loss. Test-retest reliability is high, and critical difference values are published. There is evidence to indicate that PEACH scores are significantly correlated with language development of children at 3 years of age (Ching, Crowe et al, 2010). Details of administration, together with instructions, questionnaire forms, and score sheets, are available on the NAL website (http://www.nal.gov.au). Normally hearing children achieve near-perfect scores by ~ 3 years of age, but children with hearing loss exhibit deficits compared with their normal-hearing peers. By using the PEACH, the relative effectiveness of amplification for a child can be quantified in terms of deviations of his score from the normative mean. In addition, the scale also provides a "quiet" and a "noise" subscale score based on groups of items. In clinical applications, the "noise" subscale score is particularly useful in indicating the need for fitting FMs to individual children.

The Meaningful Auditory Integration Scale (MAIS; Robbins, Renshaw, & Berry, 1991) and its version for infants and toddlers (IT-MAIS; Zimmerman-Phillips, Osberger, & Robbins, 1997) are other commonly used methods for collecting parent reports about functioning in everyday life. They are particularly suited for children with severe and profound hearing loss.

Obligatory Cortical Auditory Evoked Potential

With the rise of early identification of hearing loss programs, the need to evaluate hearing aid fittings in very young infants has gained increasing importance. In infants or older children with significant developmental delay, estimates of behavioral thresholds that are based on electrophysiologic thresholds are often used to derive target gain, but the need to evaluate the appropriateness of the fit remains. The recording of cortical auditory evoked potentials (CAEPs) to

speech stimuli has the potential to provide such verification in these cases.

Various objective methods for evaluating the appropriateness of the hearing aid fit have been proposed over the years (for discussions on the application of ABRs, see Beauchaine, Gorga, Reiland, & Larson, 1986; Hecox, 1983; Kiessling, 1982; and for discussions on the application of ASSRs in the evaluation of hearing aid fittings, see Dimitrijevic, John, & Picton, 2004; Picton et al, 1998; Picton, Dimitrijevic, & John, 2002). CAEP testing, however, offers a rather unusual opportunity to present speech stimuli and record an electrophysiologic response from the cortical region. The advantages of CAEP testing for hearing aid evaluation include the following:

- In contrast to ABR, the test stimuli can have the same length as occurs for phonemes in natural speech, enabling hearing aids to respond to the sounds in a more realistic manner.
- In contrast to ASSR, the response is not dependent on a particular amplitude modulation of the stimulus, which is advantageous because room acoustics will always decrease amplitude modulation before it reaches the listener.
- In contrast to ABR and probably ASSR, signals have to pass through the entire auditory system before a response is generated, rather than just reach the brainstem.

A difference that is sometimes an advantage and sometimes a disadvantage is that CAEP testing is best done while the client is awake.

Stimuli

Obligatory CAEPs (cortically generated responses to any audible stimulus of an appropriate length) can be reliably evoked by virtually any suprathreshold speech sound or tonal stimuli in infants and adults (Agung et al, 2006). For most clinical purposes, it seems reasonable to limit the choice of stimuli, bearing in mind the practicalities of keeping test time to a minimum. As an example, the spectra for the stimuli [m], [g], and [t] are shown in **Fig. 20.1**.

They have a spectral emphasis in the low-, mid-, and high-frequency regions, respectively, and therefore have the potential to give diagnostic information about the perception of speech sounds in different frequency regions.

Parameters for Recording CAEPs in Infants

Table 20.1 shows parameters suitable for eliciting CAEPs in infants. The free-field test environment should regularly be calibrated to ensure the test-speakers and room acoustics give a flat frequency response and hence do not distort the test signals, and

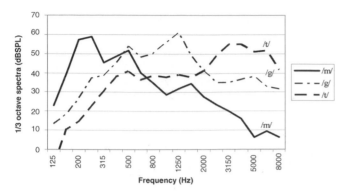

Fig. 20.1 The one-third-octave spectra for the three speech stimuli [m], [g], and [t] are shown. They were extracted from continuous discourse that was spoken by a female with an average Australian accent and which had been filtered to match the International Long-Term Average Speech Spectrum.

Table 20.1 Parameters suitable for recording cortical auditory evoked potentials in infants

Analysis time: 100 milliseconds (or longer) prestimulus and 600 milliseconds (or longer) poststimulus onset

Filters: 0.1 to 30 Hz

Interstimulus interval: 1125 milliseconds

Electrode sites: Vertex to mastoid

Artifact reject: ± 100 to 150 m V

Number of accepted epochs: 100–200

Stimuli: Speech segments presented in the free field at suprathreshold levels

Infant state: Awake but settled

that the intensity of the stimuli at the test position (a comfortable lounge chair for the parent, who then holds the infant, is ideal) is correct. The employment of a colleague as a distractor is highly desirable to ensure that the child is occupied but quiet enough for quality recording to occur.

Infant Responses and Maturation

CAEPs can be reliably recorded in infants and children in response to speech stimuli in aided and unaided conditions (Cone-Wesson & Wunderlich, 2003; Gravel, Kurtzberg, Stapells, Vaughan, & Wallace, 1989; Pang & Taylor, 2000), and a relationship between CAEPs and receptive language skills has been demonstrated by Kurtzberg (1989), who reported that infants with normal CAEPs (defined as age-appropriate morphology, latency, and amplitude) to suprathreshold stimuli were more likely to show normal receptive language function than those with abnormal responses at 1 year of age. There are, however, substantial differences between the average infant CAEP and adult CAEP waveforms. The newborn infant CAEP to speech stimuli is dominated by a prominent peak at 200 to 300 milliseconds when recorded at the midline (Kurtzberg, 1989; Sharma, Dorman, & Spahr, 2002; Stapells & Kurtzberg, 1991). Grand averaged CAEPs from 10 infants aged 3 to 7 months are shown in **Fig. 20.2**.

In **Fig. 20.2**, the addition of a precortical response is also evident in response to [t]. This is consistent with a brainstem-generated postauricular muscle response (PAMR), which is sensitive to abrupt-onset stimuli (Agung, Purdy, Patuzzi, O'Beirne, & Newall, 2005). As infants with normal hearing mature, cortical responses change significantly with respect to the shape and latency of the major components over the first 14 to 16 years of life (Hyde, 1997; Pasman, Rotteveel, Maassen, & Visco, 1999; Rotteveel et al, 1986). These morphological changes with age likely reflect underlying developmental changes in the response generators, such as improved synaptic efficiency arising from increased axon myelination and maturation of intra- and interhemispheric connections throughout the cortex (Cunningham, Nicol, Zecker, & Kraus, 2000; Eggermont & Ponton, 2003).

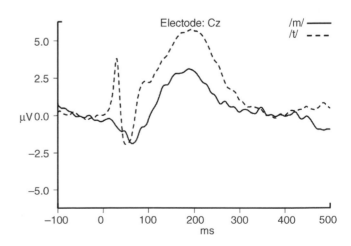

Fig. 20.2 Grand averaged CAEP responses from 10 normal hearing infants are shown. The stimuli were [t] and [m] (durations of 31 milliseconds and 32 milliseconds, respectively) presented at 65 dB SPL in the soundfield.

Pearl

- Obligatory CAEPs can be reliably recorded in young infants at suprathreshold levels, but inter-subject variability of the response shape is high.

Response Detection

In common with most auditory evoked potentials, two or more averaged CAEP responses are often overlaid and inspected for repeatability before the examiner will conclude that a response has been detected. In addition, the latency of key response components may also be reviewed and compared with age-appropriate normative data before the response is considered to be normal. Age-appropriate normative data can, however, be misleading. First, substantial intersubject differences in wave morphology are not uncommon in CAEPs from infants with normal-hearing CAEPs, even when tested in an ideal state (Wunderlich & Cone-Wesson, 2006). Second, latencies that are greater than normal occur in children who have had inadequate auditory stimulation for the early years of their lives (Bauer, Sharma, Martin, & Dorman, 2006; Sharma et al, 2002; Sharma et al, 2005). The rigid application of waveform templates to the individual CAEP response is therefore less reliable in defining abnormal and normal CAEP outcomes than is experienced in ABR testing. Given this intersubject variability, the clinical expertise required to identify a CAEP response in infants can be daunting, so the addition of a statistical test to aid in detection is highly desirable. The application of statistical measures in evoked potential detection is not new (for an excellent review of automated and machine scoring methods, see Hall,1992), but techniques that assume a certain waveshape are not likely to be successful in detecting CAEPs from infants or young children, particularly those who have previously been deprived of auditory stimulation. An objective technique involving the application of the Hotelling's T2 statistic (Flury & Riedwyl, 1988) has been shown to be at least as accurate as expert observers (Golding, Dillon, Seymour, Purdy, & Katsch, 2007; Carter, Golding, Dillon, & Seymour, 2010). The technique requires minimal assumptions about the waveshape. The result of this analysis is the probability that the observed average waveform arises just from random sources unrelated to the timing of the stimulus. The clinician can use this statistical outcome in combination with the displayed averaged response waveform to decide whether a response to auditory stimulation has been detected.

The Relationship between Cortical Auditory Evoked Potential Detection and Behavioral Measures

In cooperative older children and adults, the CAEP threshold to tonal stimulation closely approximates the pure tone audiometric threshold. The difference between the two is, on average, 0 to 10 dB (Davis, 1965; Rickards, DeVidi, & McMahon, 1996). In infants, the difference may be similar if they can be kept quiet and unwanted physiologic noise can be kept to a minimum during recording (Cone-Wesson & Wunderlich, 2003), but few data support this hypothesis. For speech stimuli presented at conversational level, aiding a child can often lead to a CAEP response where none existed when the child was unaided (Gravel et al, 1989).

> **Pearl**
>
> - Researchers reported in the 1960s that CAEPs generated from a hearing-impaired infant were better defined when hearing aids were fitted (Rapin & Graziani, 1967).

Golding, Pearce, et al (2007) studied 28 aided infants and children age 6 weeks to 3 years 5 months (mean age 8 months, standard deviation 8.6) to compare the presence or absence of CAEPs for three speech stimuli to observed auditory behaviors that were recorded using the PEACH questionnaire (Ching & Hill, 2007). A positive correlation between the number of detected CAEPs to these speech stimuli (i.e., none to a maximum of three) and the age-corrected PEACH score was found. These results were significant using human expert and statistical detection methods. Gardner-Berry, Ching, Purdy, and Dillon (in preparation) found that infants with auditory neuropathy who had cortical responses when aided had higher PEACH scores than those for whom no cortical responses were recorded. Rance, Cone-Wesson, Wunderlich, and Dowell (2002) found that older children with auditory neuropathy who had cortical responses had better understanding of speech than those for whom no cortical response is observable.

> **Pearl**
>
> - Although the correlation between CAEP and questionnaire outcomes was not perfect, the results do suggest that detection of CAEPs to speech stimuli is a valid measure of aided functional performance in infants and young children.

Cortical Auditory Evoked Potential Detection and Aided Performance

Research to date suggests that the recording of CAEPs may assist in verifying hearing aid fitting in infants. Once the aid has been prescribed using electrophysiologic estimates of threshold to determine gain across the frequency range, it seems appropriate to confirm that selected speech stimuli are detected, with hearing aids fitted, at the cortical level. If detection cannot be shown, one of several strategies may be required.

- As with any electrophysiologic measure, the quality of testing should be reviewed. Apart from system checks (e.g., electrode integrity, stimulus intensity accuracy, functional performance of the hearing aids), the child may have been particularly restless during the assessment, leading to high response rejection rates that will undoubtedly obscure weak cortical responses, and a retest may be warranted.
- The original threshold estimates that were used in the prescription of the hearing aid should be checked in case the hearing aids were prescribed to have insufficient gain (Korczak, Kurtzberg, & Stapells, 2005).
- The CAEP test outcomes should be reviewed in the light of all other available information about the child, both behavioral and electrophysiologic, before deciding on a course of action. The clinician may decide to adjust the hearing aid gain-frequency response, even if this means departing from the hearing aid prescription, or may choose to use the CAEP test outcomes to guide a behavioral test session if the child is nearing this stage of development. If the CAEPs were present to some but not all stimuli, for example, it may be appropriate to focus behavioral testing on stimulus presentations within frequency regions that did not elicit a CAEP response. An absence of CAEP responses, even when aided, is a particularly important piece of information when implantation is being considered, especially given the importance of implantation occurring within the first year of life (Ching et al, 2006c).
- In some cases of auditory neuropathy spectrum disorders (ANSD), CAEP responses may be detected when ABRs are absent (Hood, 1999; Rance et al, 2002). Pearce, Golding, and Dillon (2007) reported the case study of two infants who had been diagnosed with ANSD. Both had otoacoustic emissions but lacked ABR responses to tonal stimuli at the time of diagnosis. One of the infants had repeatable CAEPs to speech stimuli presented at conversation levels. In this case, the severity of loss suggested by the ABR outcomes was inaccurate and could have led to overprescription of hearing aid gain. For children like this, a more conservative approach to the prescription of hearing aid gain that still enables detection of speech sounds, as evidenced by the CAEP responses, is appropriate. This will minimize the risk that the outer hair cells are damaged by amplified sound (Hood, 1998; Stredler-Brown, 2002). The child's progress should be monitored regularly.

Pearl

- Recording CAEPs to speech stimuli in the aided infant provides evidence that the stimuli are detected at the cortex and therefore strongly suggests that the stimuli are audible to the infant.

Obligatory Cortical Auditory Evoked Potential and the Discrimination of Speech Stimuli

The presence of CAEPs to speech stimuli provides physiologic evidence that these stimuli have arrived at the cortex and are potentially audible to the infant with hearing aids fitted (Korczak et al, 2005). Detection is, however, the first step in the cognitive processes associated with discrimination of speech. Various studies have shown that the latency and amplitude of CAEP components may differ with changes in a feature of the stimulus (Hyde, 1997), such as voice onset time (Tremblay, Billings, Friesen, & Souza, 2006; Tremblay, Friesen, Martin, & Wright, 2003). Similarly, a cortical response to the change in spectrum during the transition from a fricative to a vowel in a consonant–vowel (CV) syllable (Ostroff, Martin, & Boothroyd, 1998) provides evidence that information sufficient to differentiate the two phonemes has made it to the auditory cortex. This suggests that examination of the latency and amplitude of the CAEP components and the detection of response differences by a statistical test may provide some evidence that differing perceptual processes are occurring for different speech sounds, and such differences may augur well for the development of speech discrimination ability. Much more work is needed in this area to understand fully how CAEPs might reflect these perceptual processes, particularly when the speech stimuli used to generate the responses are delivered through hearing aids with various signal processing characteristics (Tremblay et al, 2006). The latency of the positive peak has been shown to be a strong indicator of functional hearing ability in young children with ANSD (Sharma, Cardon, Henion, & Roland, 2011).

Special Consideration

- To ensure that an infant or young child is quiet but alert during testing, a variety of noiseless toys should be on hand. DVDs (without sound) can also be very useful forms of occupation.

Appendix Parents' evaluation of aural/oral performance of children

Child's Name:					D.O.B.:		Sex:	
Respondent:					Interviewer:		Date:	

Frequency of reported behavior:

Preinterview questions:			Never 0%	Seldom 25%	Sometimes 50%	Often 75%	Always >75%
Child's use of hearing aids/cochlear implants			0	1	2	3	4
Is your child upset by loud sounds?			4	3	2	1	0

PEACH items:

No	Scale	Item	Never 0%	Seldom 25%	Sometimes 50%	Often 75%	Always >75%
1	Q	Respond to name in quiet	0	1	2	3	4
2	Q	Follow verbal instructions in quiet	0	1	2	3	4
3	N	Respond to name in noise	0	1	2	3	4
4	N	Follow verbal instructions in noise	0	1	2	3	4
5	Q	Follow story read aloud	0	1	2	3	4
6	Q	Participate in conversation in quiet	0	1	2	3	4
7	N	Participate in conversation in noise	0	1	2	3	4
8	N	Participate in conversation in transport	0	1	2	3	4
9	Q	Recognize voice of familiar persons	0	1	2	3	4
10	Q	Converse on the phone	0	1	2	3	4
11	N	Recognize sounds in the environment	0	1	2	3	4

Discussion Questions

1. Which features in hearing aids intended for adults should be disabled when fitted to children younger than 3 years?

2. What effects do small ear canals have on measured hearing thresholds?

3. What effects do small ear canals have on the REAG provided to infants?

4. How is the RECD measurement applied in pediatric audiology?

5. What are the options for, and advantages of, different methods of evaluating the aided performance of children for (1) children younger than 12 months, (2) children age 4 to 5 years, (3) children age 6 years or older?

6. Should the recording of CAEPs be performed routinely in the assessment of all infants referred for hearing testing?

7. How might the detection of CAEPs form part of a routine evaluation of hearing aid fitting in infants?

8. If an infant is found to have CAEPs to speech stimuli but his ABRs to tonal stimuli are absent, what procedures should be followed?

References

Agung, K., Purdy, S. C., McMahon, C. M., & Newall, P. (2006, Sep). The use of cortical auditory evoked potentials to evaluate neural encoding of speech sounds in adults. Journal of the American Academy of Audiology, 17(8), 559–572.

Agung, K., Purdy, S. C., Patuzzi, R. B., O'Beirne, G. A., & Newall, P. (2005). Rising-frequency chirps and earphones with an extended high-frequency response enhance the post-auricular muscle response. International Journal of Audiology, 44(11), 631–636.

Bagatto, M., Moodie, S., Scollie, S., Seewald, R., Moodie, S., Pumford, J., & Liu, K. P. (2005). Clinical protocols for hearing instrument fitting in the Desired Sensation Level method. Trends in Amplification, 9(4), 199–226.

Bagatto, M. P., Scollie, S. D., Seewald, R. C., Moodie, K. S., & Hoover, B. M. (2002). Real-ear-to-coupler difference predictions as a function of age for two coupling procedures. Journal of the American Academy of Audiology, 13(8), 407–415.

Bauer, P. W., Sharma, A., Martin, K., & Dorman, M. (2006). Central auditory development in children with bilateral cochlear implants. Archives of Otolaryngology–Head & Neck Surgery, 132(10), 1133–1136.

Beauchaine, K. A., Gorga, M. P., Reiland, J. K., & Larson, L. L. (1986). Application of ABRs to the hearing-aid selection process: preliminary data. Journal of Speech and Hearing Research, 29(1), 120–128.

Blamey, P. J., Sarant, J. Z., Paatsch, L. E., Barry, J. G., Bow, C. P., Wales, R. J., . . . Tooher, R. (2001). Relationships among speech perception, production, language, hearing loss, and age in children with impaired hearing. Journal of Speech, Language, and Hearing Research: JSLHR, 44(2), 264–285.

Boothroyd, A., & Eran, O. (1994). Auditory speech perception capacity of child implant users expressed as equivalent hearing loss. The Volta Review, 96, 151–168.

Boothroyd, A., Springer, N., Smith, L., & Schulman, J. (1988). Amplitude compression and profound hearing loss. Journal of Speech, Language, and Hearing Research: JSLHR, 31(3), 362–376.

Byrne, D. (1986). Effects of frequency response characteristics on speech discrimination and perceived intelligibility and pleasantness of speech for hearing-impaired listeners. The Journal of the Acoustical Society of America, 80(2), 494–504.

Byrne, D., & Ching, T. Y. C. (1997). Optimising amplification for hearing impaired children, I: Issues and procedures. Australian Journal of Education of the Deaf, 3, 21–28.

Byrne, D., & Dillon, H. (1986). The National Acoustic Laboratories' (NAL) new procedure for selecting the gain and frequency response of a hearing aid. Ear and Hearing, 7(4), 257–265.

Byrne, D., Newall, P., & Parkinson, A. (1991). Modified hearing aid selection procedures for severe/profound hearing losses. In G. Studebaker, F. Bess, & L. Beck (Eds.), The Vanderbilt Hearing Aid Report II. Parkton, MD: York.

Carter, L., Golding, M., Dillon, H., & Seymour, J. (2010). The detection of infant cortical auditory evoked potentials (CAEPs) using statistical and visual detection techniques. Journal of the American Academy of Audiology, 21(5), 347–356.

Ching, T. Y. C., & Dillon, H. (2003). Prescribing amplification for children: adult-equivalent hearing loss, real-ear aided gain, and NAL-NL1. Trends in Amplification, 7(1), 1–9.

Ching, T. Y. C., & Hill, M. (2007). The Parents' Evaluation of Aural/Oral Performance of Children (PEACH) scale: normative data. Journal of the American Academy of Audiology, 18(3), 220–235.

Ching, T. Y. C., & Incerti, P. (2012). Bimodal fitting or bilateral cochlear implantation? In L. Wong & L. Hickson (Eds.), Evidence based practice in audiologic intervention (Chapter 9). San Diego, CA: Plural.

Ching, T.Y.C., Britton, L., Dillon, H., & Agung, K. (2002). RECD, REAG, NAL-NL1: accurate and practical methods for fitting non-linear hearing aids to infants and children. Hearing Review, 9, 12–20, 52.

Ching, T. Y. C., Crowe, K., Martin, V., Day, J., Mahler, N., Youn, S., . . . Orsini, J. (2010). Language development and everyday functioning of children with hearing loss assessed at 3 years of age. International Journal of Speech-Language Pathology, 12(2), 124–131.

Ching, T. Y. C., Dillon, H., & Byrne, D. (1998). Speech recognition of hearing-impaired listeners: predictions from audibility and the limited role of high-frequency amplification. The Journal of the Acoustical Society of America, 103(2), 1128–1140.

Ching, T. Y. C., Dillon, H., Day, J., van Wanrooy, E., Massie, R., Van Boynder, P., . . . Leigh G. (2006). Outcomes of children with hearing impairment: early vs later-identified. Paper presented at the British Academy of Audiology Conference, Telford UK, November 22–24, 2006.

Ching, T.Y.C., Dillon, H., Hou, S., Zhang, V., Day, J., Crowe, K., . . . Thomson, J. (2012). A randomized controlled comparison of NAL and DSL prescriptions for young children: Hearing-aid characteristics and performance outcomes at 3 years of age. International Journal of Audiology. [Electronic publication ahead of print].

Ching, T. Y. C., Dillon, H., Katsch, R., & Byrne, D. (2001). Maximizing effective audibility in hearing aid fitting. Ear and Hearing, 22(3), 212–224.

Ching, T. Y. C., Hill, M., Birtles, G., & Beecham, L. (1999). Clinical use of paired comparisons to evaluate hearing aid fitting of severely/profoundly hearing impaired children. Australian and New Zealand Journal of Audiology, 21, 51–63.

Ching, T.Y.C., Hill, M., Dillon, H., & van Wanrooy, E. (2004). Fitting and evaluating a hearing aid for recipients of unilateral cochlear implants: the NAL approach. Part 1. Hearing Review, 11, 14–22, 58.

Ching, T. Y. C., Newall, P., & Wigney, D. (1994). Audio-visual and auditory paired comparison judgments by severely and profoundly hearing impaired children: reliability and frequency response preferences. Australian Journal of Audiology, 16, 99–106.

Ching, T. Y. C., O'Brien, A., Dillon, H., Chalupper, J., Hartley, L., Hartley, D., . . . Hain, J. (2009). Directional effects on infants and young children in real life: implications for amplification. Journal of Speech, Language, and Hearing Research: JSLHR, 52(5), 1241–1254.

Ching, T. Y. C., Psarros, C., Hill, M., Dillon, H., & Incerti, P. (2001). Should children who use cochlear implants wear hearing aids in the opposite ear? Ear and Hearing, 22(5), 365–380.

Ching, T. Y. C., Scollie, S. D., Dillon, H., & Seewald, R. (2010a, Jan). A cross-over, double-blind comparison of the NAL-NL1 and the DSL v4.1 prescriptions for children with mild to moderately severe hearing loss. International Journal of Audiology, 49(Suppl 1), S4–S15.

Ching, T. Y. C., van Wanrooy, E., & Dillon, H. (2007). Binaural-bimodal fitting or bilateral implantation for managing severe to profound deafness: a review. Trends in Amplification, 11(3), 161–192.

Ching, T. Y. C., van Wanrooy, E., Dillon, H., & Carter, L. (2011). Spatial release from masking in normal-hearing children and children who use hearing aids. The Journal of the Acoustical Society of America, 129(1), 368–375.

Ching, T. Y. C., van Wanrooy, E., Hill, M., & Incerti, P. (2006). Performance in children with hearing aids or cochlear implants: bilateral stimulation and binaural hearing. International Journal of Audiology, 45(Suppl 1), S108–S112.

Cone-Wesson, B., & Wunderlich, J. (2003). Auditory evoked potentials from the cortex: audiology applications. Current Opinion in Otolaryngology & Head & Neck Surgery, 11(5), 372–377.

Cunningham, J., Nicol, T., Zecker, S., & Kraus, N. (2000). Speech-evoked neurophysiologic responses in children with learning problems: development and behavioral correlates of perception. Ear and Hearing, 21(6), 554–568.

Davis, H. (1965). Slow cortical responses evoked by acoustic stimuli. Acta Oto-Laryngologica, 59, 179–185.

Dillon, H. (1999). NAL-NL1: a new prescriptive fitting procedure for non-linear hearing aids. Hearing Journal, 52, 10–16.

Dillon, H. (2012). Hearing aids (2nd ed.). Sydney, Australia: Boomerang.

Dillon, H., & Ching, T. (1995). What makes a good speech test? In G. Plant & K.-E. Spens (Eds), Profound deafness and speech communication (pp. 305–344). London, UK: Whurr.

Dillon, H., Zakis, J., McDermott, H., Keidser, G., Dreschler, W., & Convery, E. (2006). The trainable hearing aid: what will it do for clients and clinicians? Hearing Journal, 59, 30–36.

Dimitrijevic, A., John, M. S., & Picton, T. W. (2004). Auditory steady-state responses and word recognition scores in normal-hearing and hearing-impaired adults. Ear and Hearing, 25(1), 68–84.

Eggermont, J. J., & Ponton, C. W. (2003). Auditory-evoked potential studies of cortical maturation in normal hearing and implanted children: correlations with changes in structure and speech perception. Acta Oto-Laryngologica, 123(2), 249–252.

Eisenberg, L. S., & Levitt, H. (1991). Paired comparison judgments for hearing aid selection in children. Ear and Hearing, 12(6), 417–430.

Feigin, J. A., Kopun, J. G., Stelmachowicz, P. G., & Gorga, M. P. (1989). Probe-tube microphone measures of ear-canal sound pressure levels in infants and children. Ear and Hearing, 10(4), 254–258.

Flury, B., & Riedwyl, H. (1988). Multivariate statistics: a practical approach. London, UK: Chapman and Hall.

Gardner-Berry, K., Ching, T. Y. C., Purdy, S. C., & Dillon, H. In preparation. The audiological journey and early outcomes of infants with auditory neuropathy spectrum disorder from birth to 3 years of age. International Journal of Pediatric Otorhinolaryngology.

Gatehouse, S., Naylor, G., & Elberling, C. (2006). Linear and nonlinear hearing aid fittings—2. Patterns of candidature. International Journal of Audiology, 45(3), 153–171.

Glista, D., Scollie, S., Bagatto, M., Seewald, R., Parsa, V., & Johnson, A. (2009). Evaluation of nonlinear frequency compression: clinical outcomes. International Journal of Audiology, 48(9), 632–644.

Golding, M., Dillon, H., Seymour, J., Purdy, S., & Katsch, R. (2007). Obligatory CAEP testing in infants: a five year review. Annual Report of the National Acoustic Laboratories, 2005–2006, 14–17. Retrieved from http://www.NAL.gov.au

Golding, M., Pearce, W., Seymour, J., Cooper, A., Ching, T. Y. C., & Dillon, H. (2007). The relationship between obligatory cortical auditory evoked potentials (CAEPs) and functional measures in young infants. Journal of the American Academy of Audiology, 18(2), 117–125.

Gravel, J. S., Fausel, N., Liskow, C., & Chobot, J. (1999). Children's speech recognition in noise using omni-directional and dual-microphone hearing aid technology. Ear and Hearing, 20(1), 1–11.

Gravel, J. S., Kurtzberg, D., Stapells, D. R., Vaughan, H. G., & Wallace, I. F. (1989). Case studies. Seminars in Hearing, 10, 272–287.

Hall, J. W. (1992). Handbook of auditory evoked responses. Needham Heights, MA: Allyn and Bacon.

Hecox, K. E. (1983). Role of auditory brain stem response in the selection of hearing aids. Ear and Hearing, 4(1), 51–55.

Hogan, C. A., & Turner, C. W. (1998). High-frequency audibility: benefits for hearing-impaired listeners. The Journal of the Acoustical Society of America, 104(1), 432–441.

Hood, L. J. (1998). Auditory neuropathy: What is it and what can we do about it? Hearing Journal, 51, 10–18.

Hood, L. J. (1999). A review of objective methods of evaluating auditory neural pathways. The Laryngoscope, 109(11), 1745–1748.

Hyde, M. (1997). The N1 response and its applications. Audiology & Neuro-Otology, 2(5), 281–307.

Keidser, G., Dillon, H., Dyrlund, O., Carter, L., & Hartley, D. (2007). Preferred low- and high-frequency compression ratios among hearing aid users with moderately severe to profound hearing loss. Journal of the American Academy of Audiology, 18(1), 17–33.

Keidser, G., O'Brien, A., Latzel, M., and Convery, E. (2007b). Evaluation of a transient noise reduction algorithm. Hearing Journal, 60, 29, 32, 34, 38–39.

Kiessling, J. (1982). Hearing aid selection by brainstem audiometry. Scandinavian Audiology, 11(4), 269–275.

Korczak, P. A., Kurtzberg, D., & Stapells, D. R. (2005). Effects of sensorineural hearing loss and personal hearing AIDS on cortical event-related potential and behavioral measures of speech-sound processing. Ear and Hearing, 26(2), 165–185.

Kuk, F., Keenan, D., Peeters, H., Lau, C., & Crose, B. (2007). Critical factors in ensuring efficacy of frequency transposition. Part 1. Individualizing the start frequency. Hearing Review, 14, 60–67.

Kurtzberg, D. (1989). Cortical event-related potential assessment of auditory system function. Seminars in Hearing, 10, 252–261.

Leijon, A., Lindkvist, A., Ringdahl, A., & Israelsson, B. (1990). Preferred hearing aid gain in everyday use after prescriptive fitting. Ear and Hearing, 11(4), 299–305.

Litovsky, R. Y. (2005). Speech intelligibility and spatial release from masking in young children. The Journal of the Acoustical Society of America, 117(5), 3091–3099.

Litovsky, R. Y., Johnstone, P. M., & Godar, S. P. (2006). Benefits of bilateral cochlear implants and/or hearing aids in children. International Journal of Audiology, 45(Suppl 1), S78–S91.

Marcoux, A. M., Yathiraj, A., Côté, I., & Logan, J. (2006). The effect of a hearing aid noise reduction algorithm on the acquisition of novel speech contrasts. International Journal of Audiology, 45(12), 707–714.

Moodie, K. S., Seewald, R. C., & Sinclair, S. T. (1994). Procedure for predicting real-ear hearing aid performance in young children. American Journal of Audiology, 8, 23–31.

Moore, B. C. J. (2001). Dead regions in the cochlea: diagnosis, perceptual consequences, and implications for the fitting of hearing aids. Trends in Amplification, 3, 1–34.

Nittrouer, S., & Chapman, C. (2009). The effects of bilateral electric and bimodal electric–acoustic stimulation on language development. Trends in Amplification, 13(3), 190–205.

Offeciers, E., Morera, C., Müller, J., Huarte, A., Shallop, J., & Cavallé, L. (2005). International consensus on bilateral cochlear implants and bimodal stimulation. Acta Oto-Laryngologica, 125(9), 918–919.

Ostroff, J. M., Martin, B. A., & Boothroyd, A. (1998). Cortical evoked response to acoustic change within a syllable. Ear and Hearing, 19(4), 290–297.

Pang, E. W., & Taylor, M. J. (2000). Tracking the development of the N1 from age 3 to adulthood: an examination of speech and non-speech stimuli. Clinical Neurophysiology, 111(3), 388–397.

Pasman, J. W., Rotteveel, J. J., Maassen, B., & Visco, Y. M. (1999). The maturation of auditory cortical evoked responses between (preterm) birth and 14 years of age. European Journal of Paediatric Neurology, 3(2), 79–82.

Pearce, W., Golding, M., & Dillon, H. (2007). Cortical auditory evoked potentials in the assessment of auditory neuropathy: two case studies. Journal of the American Academy of Audiology, 18(5), 380–390.

Pediatric Working Group. (1996). Amplification for infants and children with hearing loss. American Journal of Audiology, 5, 53–68.

Picton, T. W., Dimitrijevic, A., & John, M. S. (2002). Multiple auditory steady-state responses. The Annals of Otology, Rhinology, and Laryngology, 189, 16–21.

Picton, T. W., Durieux-Smith, A., Champagne, S. C., Whittingham, J., Moran, L. M., Giguère, C., & Beauregard, Y. (1998). Objective evaluation of aided thresholds using auditory steady-state responses. Journal of the American Academy of Audiology, 9(5), 315–331.

Pittman, A. (2011). Age-related benefits of digital noise reduction for short-term word learning in children with hearing loss. Journal of Speech, Language, and Hearing Research: JSLHR, 54(5), 1448–1463.

Purdy, S. C., & Williams, M. (2000). High frequency tympanometry: a valid and reliable immittance test protocol for young infants. New Zealand Audiological Society Bulletin, 10, 9–24.

Rance, G., Cone-Wesson, B., Wunderlich, J., & Dowell, R. (2002). Speech perception and cortical event related potentials in children with auditory neuropathy. Ear and Hearing, 23(3), 239–253.

Rance, G., Roper, R., Symons, L., Moody, L. J., Poulis, C., Dourlay, M., & Kelly, T. (2005). Hearing threshold estimation in infants using auditory steady-state responses. Journal of the American Academy of Audiology, 16(5), 291–300.

Rapin, I., & Graziani, L. J. (1967). Auditory-evoked responses in normal, brain-damaged, and deaf infants. Neurology, 17(9), 881–894.

Rickards, F. W., DeVidi, S., & McMahon, D. S. (1996). Cortical evoked response audiometry in noise induced hearing loss claims. Australian Journal Otolaryngology, 2, 237–241.

Robbins, A. M., Renshaw, J. J., & Berry, S. W. (1991). Evaluating meaningful auditory integration in profoundly hearing-impaired children. The American Journal of Otology, 12(Suppl), 144–150.

Rotteveel, J. J., Colon, E. J., Notermans, S. L., Stoelinga, G. B. A., de Graaf, R., & Visco, Y. M. (1986). The central auditory conduction at term date and three months after birth. IV. Auditory cortical responses. Scandinavian Audiology, 15(2), 85–95.

Scollie, S. D., Ching, T. Y. C., Seewald, R. C., Dillon, H., Britton, L., Steinberg, J., & King, K. (2010). Children's speech perception and loudness ratings when fitted with hearing aids using the DSL v.4.1 and the NAL-NL1 prescriptions. International Journal of Audiology, 49(Suppl 1), S26–S34.

Scollie, S., Seewald, R., Cornelisse, L., Moodie, S., Bagatto, M., Laurnagaray, D., . . . Pumford, J. (2005). The Desired Sensation Level multistage input/output algorithm. Trends in Amplification, 9(4), 159–197.

Seewald, R. C., & Scollie, S. D. (2003). An approach for ensuring accuracy in pediatric hearing instrument fitting. Trends in Amplification, 7(1), 29–40.

Seewald, R., Ching, T., Dillon, H., Joyce, J., Britton, L., & Scollie, S. (2002). Hearing aid selection procedures for children: Report of a collaborative study. Paper presented at the International Hearing Aid Research Conference, Aug 21–25, Lake Tahoe, NV.

Seewald, R. C., Cornelisse, L. E., Ramji, K. V., Sinclair, S. T., Moodie, K. S., & Jamieson, D. G. (1997). DSL v4.1 for Windows: a software implementation of the desired sensation level (DSL[i/o]) method for fitting linear gain and wide-dynamic-range compression hearing instruments. Users' manual. London, ON: Hearing Health Care Research Unit.

Sharma, A., Cardon, G., Henion, K., & Roland, P. (2011). Cortical maturation and behavioral outcomes in children with auditory neuropathy spectrum disorder. International Journal of Audiology, 50(2), 98–106.

Sharma, A., Dorman, M. F., & Spahr, A. J. (2002). A sensitive period for the development of the central auditory system in children with cochlear implants: implications for age of implantation. Ear and Hearing, 23(6), 532–539.

Sharma, A., Martin, K., Roland, P., Bauer, P., Sweeney, M. H., Gilley, P., & Dorman, M. (2005). P1 latency as a biomarker for central auditory development in children with hearing impairment. Journal of the American Academy of Audiology, 16(8), 564–573.

Simpson, A., Hersbach, A. A., & McDermott, H. J. (2005). Improvements in speech perception with an experimental nonlinear frequency compression hearing device. International Journal of Audiology, 44(5), 281–292.

Sininger, Y. S., Abdala, C., & Cone-Wesson, B. (1997). Auditory threshold sensitivity of the human neonate as measured by the auditory brainstem response. Hearing Research, 104(1–2), 27–38.

Stacey, P. C., Fortnum, H. M., Barton, G. R., & Summerfield, A. Q. (2006, Apr). Hearing-impaired children in the United Kingdom, I: Auditory performance, communication skills, educational achievements, quality of life, and cochlear implantation. Ear and Hearing, 27(2), 161–186.

Stapells, D. R. (2000a). Frequency-specific evoked potential audiometry in infants. In R. C. Seewald (Ed.), A sound foundation through early amplification: proceedings of an international conference (pp. 13–32). Stäfa, Switzerland: Phonak AG.

Stapells, D. R., & Kurtzberg, D. (1991). Evoked potential assessment of auditory system integrity in infants. Clinics in Perinatology, 18(3), 497–518.

Stapells, D. R. (2000b). Threshold estimation by the tone-evoked auditory brainstem response: a literature meta-analysis. Journal of Speech-Language Pathology and Audiology, 24, 74–83.

Stapells, D. R., Gravel, J. S., & Martin, B. A. (1995). Thresholds for auditory brain stem responses to tones in notched noise from infants and young children with normal hearing or sensorineural hearing loss. Ear and Hearing, 16(4), 361–371.

Stelmachowicz, P. G. (1999). Hearing aid outcome measures for children. Journal of the American Academy of Audiology, 10(1), 14–25, quiz 66.

Stelmachowicz, P., Lewis, D., Hoover, B., Nishi, K., McCreery, R., & Woods, W. (2010). Effects of digital noise reduction on speech perception for children with hearing loss. Ear and Hearing, 31(3), 345–355.

Stredler-Brown, A. (2002). Developing a treatment program for auditory neuropathy. Seminars in Hearing, 23, 239–249.

Studebaker, G. A. (1982). Hearing aid selection: an overview. In G. A. Studebaker & F. H. Bess (Eds.), The Vanderbilt Hearing Aid Report: State of the art—research needs. Upper Darby, PA: Instrumentation Associates.

Thompson, D. C., McPhillips, H., Davis, R. L., Lieu, T. L., Homer, C. J., & Helfand, M. (2001). Universal newborn hearing screening: summary of evidence. Journal of the American Medical Association, 286(16), 2000–2010.

Tremblay, K. L., Billings, C. J., Friesen, L. M., & Souza, P. E. (2006). Neural representation of amplified speech sounds. Ear and Hearing, 27(2), 93–103.

Tremblay, K. L., Friesen, L., Martin, B. A., & Wright, R. (2003). Test-retest reliability of cortical evoked potentials using naturally produced speech sounds. Ear and Hearing, 24(3), 225–232.

Voss, S. E., & Herrmann, B. S. (2005). How does the sound pressure generated by circumaural, supra-aural, and insert earphones differ for adult and infant ears? Ear and Hearing, 26(6), 636–650.

Wong, S. H., Gibson, W. P. R., & Sanli, H. (1997). Use of transtympanic round window electrocochleography for threshold estimations in children. American Journal of Otolaryngology, 18(5), 632–636.

Wunderlich, J. L., & Cone-Wesson, B. K. (2006). Maturation of CAEP in infants and children: a review. Hearing Research, 212(1–2), 212–223.

Zakis, J. A., Dillon, H., & McDermott, H. J. (2007). The design and evaluation of a hearing aid with trainable amplification parameters. Ear and Hearing, 28(6), 812–830.

Zimmerman-Phillips, S., Osberger, M. J., & Robbins, A. M. (1997). Infant Toddler: Meaningful Auditory Integration Scale (IT-MAIS). Sylmar, CA: Advanced Bionics.

Chapter 21

Bone-Anchored Implants for Children

Lisa Vaughn Christensen

Key Points

- Bone-anchored implants are a viable option for children with bilateral conductive or mixed hearing losses.

- Bone-anchored implants are FDA-approved for implantation in children 5 years of age and older.

- While bone-anchored implants have primarily been used for the treatment of atresia, there are many other special populations that might benefit from this particular implant.

- The use of a softband can be achieved as soon as hearing loss is confirmed, even in young infants.

- Implantation must be carefully discussed with families preoperatively; as with any surgical procedure, there are special considerations and potential complications that should be detailed.

- Many children with profound unilateral hearing losses have educational delays, and the use of a bone-anchored implant can help with their understanding of speech in background noise.

◆ History

Bone-anchored hearing aid implants were first introduced as a viable surgical option for bilateral conductive or mixed hearing loss in 1977 (Tjellström & Håkansson, 1995) and were commercially available in 1987 (Abramson et al, 1989). The first commercially developed systems were developed in Gothenburg, Sweden, and the first patients were implanted in Nijmegen, The Netherlands, in June 1988. However, it was 1996 before the Food and Drug Administration (FDA) approved the device for use in the United States (FDA, 1995). In the United States, the device was initially approved by the FDA for bilateral conductive or mixed hearing losses. Other approvals from the FDA soon followed; pediatric approval for implantation in children 5 years of age or older in 1999 (FDA, 1999), bilateral implantation in 2001 (FDA, 2001), and implantation for unilateral or single-sided deafness in 2002 (FDA, 2002).

When these devices were first introduced, they were referred to as bone-anchored hearing aids, with the acronym BAHA. Shortly after purchasing the rights to the system from Entific Medical Systems in 2005, however, Cochlear Limited (Sydney, Australia) made "Baha" into a registered trademark. Now, with the appearance of additional bone-anchored devices, such as the Ponto (Oticon Medical, Askim, Sweden), cleared by the FDA in 2008, terminology has changed once again. Terms like "osseointegrated implants" and "bone conduction hearing devices" have emerged to describe this type of implantable device. In this chapter, they are referred to as bone-anchored implants (BAIs).

◆ Overview

The BAI is a semi-implantable percutaneous bone conduction hearing device that is secured to the skull by an osseointegrated titanium fixture. A BAI system consists of three main components: sound processor, abutment, and implant (**Fig. 21.1**).

The detachable sound processor and abutment are the external components, and the implant is the internal component. The external component connects percutaneously to the internal component when implanted in the skull bone behind the ear. Both the abutment and the implant are made of titanium and are compatible with magnetic resonance imaging (MRI) and computed tomography (CT). The BAI provides an alternative pathway for sound to reach the brain through bone conduction instead of air conduction, utilizing the process of osseointegration (**Fig. 21.2**).

Osseointegration was first introduced for the concept of direct bone conduction with hearing aids by Tjellström and coworkers in 1980. The titanium oxide

228

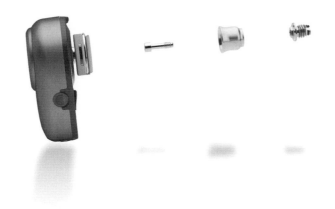

Fig. 21.1 Parts of a BAI. Used with permission from Oticon Medical.

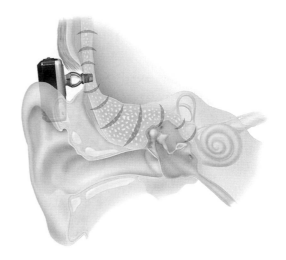

Fig. 21.2 Anatomical view: implant with abutment and processor. Used with permission from Cochlear Americas.

surface on the implant is highly compatible with osteocytes, which integrate with the surface of the titanium to form a stable connection. This connection in turn forms a long-term stability and an ability to withstand load and stress from various directions (Brånemark et al, 1983; Tjellström & Håkansson, 1995).

◆ Candidacy

Beginning in 1996, the FDA outlined BAI as a device to be used by patients who have a conductive hearing loss (CHL) or mixed hearing loss (MHL) and can still benefit from sound amplification (**Table 21.1**).

Table 21.1 BAI candidacy criteria

	Criteria
Softband	• Bilateral conductive hearing loss • Bilateral mixed hearing loss (bone conduction PTA of 45 dB or less or equal to 60% speech discrimination scores) • SSD or unilateral CHL recommended only after 1 year of age when proper verification and placement can be achieved
Bilateral implants	• Symmetric bone conduction thresholds less than 10 dB difference on average (0.5, 1, 2, and 3 kHz) or less than 15 dB at individual frequencies 5 years of age or older.
SSD implants	• Profound unilateral hearing loss • MHL or CHL with a PTA greater than 50 dB • Better-hearing ear must be normal (15 dB or less in children) • 5 years of age or older

For MHL, the pure tone average (PTA) for bone conduction thresholds should be less than or equal to 45 dB hearing level (HL). In 1999, the FDA cleared usage of the BAI system in children 5 years of age and older. The better the bone conduction thresholds, the closer to the normal range the aided thresholds will be, increasing the ability to give the proper amount of amplification, which is critical when working with children in the process of acquiring speech and language skills. Both manufacturers of BAI, Cochlear and Oticon, now offer "power" devices, enabling patients with greater degrees of bone conduction loss (up to 45 dB HL) to be fitted properly.

While the most common use of BAI in children has been for treatment of atresia, especially in children with Treacher-Collins syndrome, many other cases of CHL and MHL in children can be treated with a BAI. Children with Down syndrome are another special population who have documented benefit with BAI. Specifically, McDermott, Williams, Kuo, Reid, and Proops (2008) found BAI to be successfully and consistently used with 15 children with Down syndrome who had shown inconsistent use of traditional hearing aids and who had received repeated insertions of ventilation tubes. Other common indications for BAI include, but are not limited to, chronic otitis media that is unable to be medically resolved, hearing loss following cholesteatoma removal, chronic middle ear dysfunction, and middle ear disease.

Any child with a CHL or MHL that is inoperable may be a potential BAI candidate. A critical factor to consider when determining candidacy for a BAI is family choice. Even if the hearing loss is operable, after receiving complete medical information, a family may decide a BAI is the best option. To explain, surgical intervention to cosmetically repair the auricula and restore hearing has been shown to have mixed outcomes. Problems may include the need for multiple surgeries, the high cost of ongoing surgeries, surgical difficulty, poor audiological outcomes, and surgical complications (de Alarcon & Choo, 2007; Patel & Shelton, 2007; Evans & Kazahaya, 2007; De la Cruz & Teufert, 2003; Digoy & Cueva, 2007). Poor surgical outcomes are especially likely in patients who experience syndromes in which the middle ear is grossly malformed. A BAI may involve less surgical intervention and result in better hearing. Therefore the audiologist and surgeon should present all potential treatments for conductive and mixed hearing loss to the family so that children and their families know the risks and potential number of surgical interventions involved with each procedure.

Preoperative Testing

Perhaps the most unique part of a BAI system is the ability to conduct preoperative testing that can closely predict postoperative results. There are three ways to conduct testing preoperatively. The first is by using a small plastic coupler called the test rod. The sound processor can be connected to the rod and then held tightly to the mastoid; through bone conduction, the patient will be able to hear via the sound processor. When working with children, the test rod is best used as a listening check tool for audiologists, teachers, parents, or other professionals who may need to conduct a daily listening check for the child. To use the test rod as a listening check device, simply plug both ears and put the test rod with the processor in place either on the mastoid or on the jaw/tragus area. This placement will allow listening through the BAI to occur and determination of sound quality, similar to performing listening checks on traditional amplification.

The other preoperative testing apparatus is the testband, a metal headband that has the coupling to allow a sound processor to be snapped into the headband. The testband allows the patient to try the sound processor in different listening environments. Because the testband is made of metal, long periods of wear time may provide some discomfort. For longer periods of wear time, especially during extended trial periods, the use of a softband is often recommended (**Fig. 21.3**). The softband is an adjustable band containing a snap coupler that enables the sound processor to be snapped in place for preoperative testing, trial periods, and for young children to wear prior to being old enough for surgery.

Preoperative testing protocols differ with the age of the patient and the indications for the BAI. For children with bilateral, conductive, or mixed hearing losses, behavioral testing can be completed in sound-field using age-appropriate audiometry, with and without a softband (or testband). The sound quality

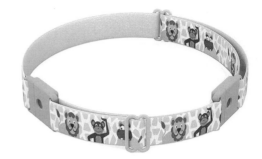

Fig. 21.3 Softband. Used with permission from Oticon Medical.

of the testband or softband is slightly reduced compared with the osseointegrated implant, especially in higher frequencies, where attenuation through skin is greatest (Christensen, Smith-Olinde, Kimberlain, Richter, & Dornhoffer, 2010; van der Pouw, Snik, & Cremers, 1999; Browning & Gatehouse, 1994; Håkansson, Carlsson, Tjellström, & Lidén, 1994).

◆ Counseling

Preoperative Expectations

As with any implantable device or even traditional amplification, it is important to give the family and child a realistic expectation of the BAI. The child and family should be well informed and have the proper expectations prior to implantation. The poorer the bone conduction thresholds, the greater chance there will be for less than desirable aided thresholds. Poorer aided thresholds, therefore, signal the absolute necessity of performing preoperative behavioral testing utilizing the testband or softband. This preoperative behavioral testing allows aided thresholds to be obtained that can predict acoustic access to speech and language following BAI surgery.

Because of the percutaneous nature of a BAI, it is important that a family member, guardian, or the child be able to care for the abutment and the skin around the abutment. This health care should be discussed at length with the family prior to implantation. Otherwise complications can result, such as infection, skin overgrowth, or extrusion of the abutment or implant. Also of importance when implanting children with congenital malformations is sufficient bone volume and bone quality—a necessary condition for successful implantation and proper osseointegration. Extreme sensory issues and developmental delays that would affect the child's ability to keep the site properly cleaned and maintained daily should also be considered. In addition, developmental delays that prevent efficient head control or balance/stability for walking and potential falls should also be considered prior to implantation. These conditions can pose potential problems for implant extrusion or the ability to keep the sound processor snapped on the abutment consistently.

◆ Surgical Procedures

BAIs can be surgically implanted utilizing either a one-stage surgery or a two-stage surgery. Exact procedures will vary from surgeon to surgeon. When using a one-stage surgery, the placement of the implant and typically premounted abutment are completed in one surgical procedure. During the same surgery, soft tissue and hair follicles may be removed around the abutment. This is typically done as an outpatient day surgery.

During a two-stage surgical procedure, the implant is placed and a cover screw is put over the implant. The implant is left to osseointegrate with the bone before the abutment is attached. The time for osseointegration varies but is typically 3 to 6 months. After osseointegration has occurred, the second-stage surgery is conducted in which the abutment is placed. Tissue and hair follicle reduction may be done in either surgery stage but is most commonly completed during the first stage of the surgery; therefore, only a skin biopsy punch is needed to expose the implant instead of another full surgical incision.

One-stage surgeries are typically reserved for adults with good bone quality as assessed by the surgeon. Two-stage surgeries are typically considered for children, individuals with poor bone quality, or irradiated patients. Often during pediatric surgeries, a "sleeper" or "rescue" implant is used. The sleeper implant is simply an additional implant placed in the bone that does not receive the second-stage surgery in which the abutment is attached. It is simply there as a "rescue" implant should the initial implant become harmed in any way, allowing a second abutment to be placed on the sleeper implant as soon as possible without waiting for an additional osseointegration period if the first implant fails or is damaged.

Postoperative Appointments

Sound processor fitting dates are determined by the surgeon and are typically based on single- or two-stage surgery, osseointegration, and the healing processes of the patient. Typically, one-stage surgeries have sound processor fittings between 3 and 6 months after the surgery. Two-stage surgeries are typically fitted with the sound processor between 2 and 6 weeks after the second surgery.

During the sound processor fittings, the following topics should be discussed and demonstrated for the child and family: daily cleaning of the abutment us-

ing the soft brush provided by the manufacturer plus a mild soap and water; proper removal and replacement of the sound processor; battery information; and operation of the sound processor. Also, at this time the audiologist should perform aided behavioral testing (**Table 21.2**).

There are a variety of pediatric-friendly options for programming and arranging the sound processors, such as lockable battery doors, lockable volume controls, the ability to add frequency modulation (FM) systems (**Fig. 21.4**), and retention clips that help prevent the sound processors from being lost or dropped and damaged. Also available are direct audio input cords that can be used for MP3 players or computers.

Subsequent appointments should include audiological testing for changes in hearing (especially bone conduction thresholds), aided behavioral testing to ensure the BAI is functioning properly, and abutment checks for cleanliness and stability. Examination of the condition of the child's skin around the abutment should be conducted by the surgeon or audiologist every 3 months for the first year. Subsequent appointments after the first year can generally be reduced to 6 month intervals for the following year and, eventually, to yearly appointments with the audiologist and surgeon.

◆ Softband

When children are born with a conductive or mixed hearing loss, they may be candidates for a BAI; however, current FDA regulations restrict implantation of the device before 5 years of age (FDA, 2001). For

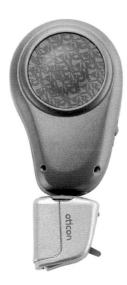

Fig. 21.4 FM Receiver: Oticon Medical Ponto with Amigo receiver. Used with permission from Oticon Medical.

Table 21.2 Suggested testing protocol for BAI

Appointment	Tasks

Preoperative	• Full audiological evaluation to determine candidacy for BAI
	• Trial in-office with processor on testband or softband (device may be sent home for extended trial if deemed necessary by the audiologist)
	• Evaluation with BAI
	  – For bilateral CHL or MHL, complete functional gain testing with processor on softband or testband
	  – For unilateral CHL or MHL, complete functional gain testing with processor on softband or testband and masking in the better-hearing ear
	  – For SSD, obtain speech-in-noise testing in soundfield and age-appropriate outcome measure to assess daily listening skills
	• ENT visit to assess skull thickness (usually by CT scan) and other surgical considerations deemed necessary by the surgeon

Postoperative/fitting	• Counseling with patient and family on use of BAI to include, but not limited to, the following:
	  – How and when to clean the abutment
	  – Battery size, life, and safety
	  – Removing and replacing processor
	  – Functions of processor
	  – Child-friendly accessories
	  – Full-time wearing of the processor
	  – Determine need for speech/language therapy or educational audiological needs
	  – Speech-in-noise testing with processor in place

3 months postoperative	• Check abutment for tightness, skin irregularities, or swelling; if any noted, contact surgeon • Make any necessary programming adjustments • Speech-in-noise testing • Repeat the outcome measures given preoperatively
6 months postoperative	• Abutment check: can be completed by audiologist, surgeon, or nurse
9 months postoperative	• Check abutment for tightness, skin irregularities, or swelling; if any noted, contact surgeon • Make any necessary programming adjustments • Speech-in-noise testing • Repeat the outcome measures given preoperatively
Maintenance appointments (frequency of these appointments should be determined by the audiologist based on the length of time since implant and age of the child)	• Full audiological evaluation • Check abutment for tightness, skin irregularities, or swelling; if any noted, contact surgeon • Make any necessary programming adjustments • Speech-in-noise testing • Repeat the outcome measures given preoperatively • ENT appointment

children under the age of 5, the use of a softband has been demonstrated to deliver results similar to the implantation of the BAI. The softband can be fitted, in the same manner as traditional amplification, as soon as the hearing loss is confirmed. The softband is a transcutaneous (across the skin) application of the BAI, consisting of an adjustable band and a snap coupler that connects the sound processor to the band, holding the device to the skin. Previous softbands were comprised of an elastic band with a Velcro fastener, however, now both BAI manufactures have changed to a latex-free and Velcro-free softband to prevent the allergic reactions and skin irritations that were sometimes seen with the previous version of the softband (**Fig. 21.3**). The new version of softbands also includes a safety release feature that is designed to release if the softband is ever caught or snagged so that the child is not in danger of being harmed. Also available is an option that enables the wearing of two sound processors on one softband for a bilateral fit. Both manufacturers offer a variety of color options to appeal to children and their families.

Softband Efficacy

Hol, Cremers, Coppens-Schellekens, and Snik (2005) studied two children with bilateral congenital aural atresia fitted with the Baha softband. The results of their study demonstrated that Baha use with a softband was at least comparable with, if not slightly more favorable than, conventional bone conduction hearing aids for the two children studied. More recently, Nicholson, Christensen, Dornhoffer, Martin, and Smith-Olinde (2011) found similar results when studying 25 children aged 6 months of age to 18 years of age. In this study, the use of the Baha softband coupled to the Baha Compact provided a viable treatment for children with congenital conductive hearing loss, resulting in an average of 40 dB of functional gain across the speech spectrum.

Softband Fitting and Verification

Bone conduction devices at the present time are unable to be verified electroacoustically in a clinical setting. Children born with atresia and microtia are unable to wear air conduction hearing aids, which are typically verified clinically using electroacoustical measures. The Pediatric Amplification Protocol, published by the American Academy of Audiology (AAA) (2003), stated that aided soundfield thresholds may be useful in verification of audibility of the speech spectrum for bone conduction devices. Therefore, to verify that proper auditory access is achieved using softbands, behavioral testing must be completed in a soundbooth while the child is wearing the properly functioning processor and softband (functional gain testing). Testing is performed, like any other behavioral testing on children, using developmentally appropriate audiological protocols. Even for infants and toddlers, soundfield verification must be completed when fitting a softband using behavioral observation audiometry (BOA) or visual reinforcement audiometry (VRA) as appropriate. See Chapters 7 and 8, respectively, for more information on testing children using BOA and VRA.

To ensure proper fitting of the softband, families must be counseled on appropriate fitting strategies. The softband should fit tightly enough to make good contact with the skin/skull but not so tight that it causes discomfort for the child. When fitting infants, it is important to remember and note head control, because head movement is limited and the majority of an infant's day is spent lying on a portion of her head. For infants, it is recommended that the processor on the softband be put more on the temporal or forehead region to ensure that the microphone is not covered, to allow more comfort for the infant, and to keep the processor attached to the softband. The retention clip can be used with the softband, clipped to the softband or to the child's shirt to ensure that the processor is not lost. When the infant begins to sit up well and has better head control, the softband should be moved to the mastoid area. Changing sides of the processor, if using a single-processor softband,

or repositioning slightly, if using a bilateral softband, a couple of times a day can help keep discomfort or irritation to a minimum for these young children.

Because each individual head is different in respect to size and shape, it is important that behavioral testing be conducted to make sure all speech sounds are completely audible for the child. It is important for aided thresholds to be as near as possible to the normal range of hearing for children (15 dB HL), to ensure that the child has access to the entire speech spectrum. Other means of verification should include speech-language assessments and outcome measures for the family to monitor overall progress.

◆ Implantation

Prior to the development of BAI, children and adults with conductive and mixed hearing losses wore traditional bone conduction hearing aids if surgical intervention did not yield favorable results. The traditional bone conduction hearing aids were worn throughout the entire lifespan. Now, because of the good results provided by softbands, some surgeons, many audiologists, and most insurance providers ask whether implant surgery should be considered. Do the risk and potential benefit warrant the monetary difference between a softband and implantation?

When looking at aided thresholds of traditional bone conduction hearing aids compared with aided thresholds of the softband, a statistically significant improvement with softband aided thresholds has been noted (Christensen, Smith-Olinde et al, 2010). The Baha coupled to the abutment has also been found to be superior to preoperative testbands (Verstraeten, Zarowski, Somers, Riff, & Offeciers, 2009). Also previously noted was that an implanted Baha had statistically as much gain as a bone conduction transducer at 500, 1000, 2000, and 4000 Hz (Christensen, Richter, & Dornhoffer, 2010). These data demonstrate the benefit of BAI either on a softband or implanted. Based on these positive results, a BAI system should be strongly considered for intervention, rather than seen as the last option for children with conductive or mixed hearing losses.

Prior to the FDA ruling on bilateral implantation in 2001, selection of the side of implant was very important. Now most BAI candidates with symmetrical bilateral conductive or mixed losses can be implanted bilaterally, and many of these cases are completed with a simultaneous implantation. Symmetrical bone conduction thresholds are defined by the FDA as less than 10 dB difference on average at 500, 1000, 2000, and 3000 Hz or less than 15 dB at individual frequencies (**Table 21.1**). Some contraindications to bilateral implantation are poor bone density on one side and asymmetrical hearing. Bilateral BAI in children was first studied by Priwin, Jönsson, Hult-crantz, and Granström (2007). Twenty-two children and adolescents with either unilateral or bilateral CHL were studied on their abilities to localize and understand speech in noise. When the children with bilateral conductive losses were given an additional BAI, there was improved localization and improved speech recognition in noise.

◆ Unilateral Hearing Loss/ Single-Sided Deafness

The incidence of profound unilateral sensorineural hearing loss (USNHL), otherwise known as single-sided deafness (SSD), in children ranges from 0.1 to 3% (Prieve, 2000; Bess, Dodd-Murphy, & Parker, 1998). Evidence suggests that children with profound USNHL tend to perform poorly in school, display learning difficulties, and have behavioral problems relative to their normal-hearing peers (Bess & Tharpe, 1986; English & Church, 1999; McKay, Gravel, & Tharpe, 2008). These problems can be attributed to the inability of individuals with SSD to perform well in noise, and they may require some school support; see Chapters 29 and 31 in this text (Welsh, Welsh, Rosen, & Dragonette, 2004; Sargent, Herrmann, Hollenbeak, & Bankaitis, 2001; Ruscetta, Arjmand, & Pratt, 2005).

Despite evidence that children with unilateral hearing loss benefit from FM systems and hearing aids, there remains limited compliance in using these devices (Davis, Reeve, & Bamford, 2001; Updike, 1994). Soundfield FM/infrared systems, especially, do not work outside the classroom, and personal FM systems are not ideal for daily activity with multiple speakers. The use of contralateral routing of signals (CROS) amplification for unilateral hearing loss in children is not recommended (AAA, 2003; American Academy of Pediatrics, Joint Committee on Infant Hearing (JCIH), 2007). Thus, treatment options for profound unilateral hearing loss in children are limited, thereby creating a source of frustration and a need for alternative treatments.

Results for 23 children with profound sensorineural hearing loss in one ear and normal hearing in the other (i.e., SSD) with an average age of 12.6 years demonstrated significant improvements on the Hearing in Noise Test (HINT) (Nilsson, Soli, & Sullivan, 1994) and Children's Home Inventory of Listening Difficulties (CHILD) (Anderson & Smaldino, 2000; Christensen, Richter et al, 2010) when wearing a BAI. All children showed significant improvements in HINT scores and CHILD scores. Preimplant mean scores for the CHILD were 4.49 for the children and 4.60 for the parents. Postimplant mean scores were 6.90 for the children

and 7.10 for the parents. These improvements in understanding speech in background noise with the HINT and daily listening abilities make the BAI a viable treatment for children with SSD.

Unilateral Losses/SSD and Softbands

Young children with SSD or unilateral conductive or mixed hearing losses due to atresia or microtia can also be candidates for BAI utilizing a softband. It is important to be able to verify the benefit for these children. Although infants with bilateral hearing loss can be tested for functional gain in soundfield, when a child has a unilateral hearing loss (SSD or atresia) the better-hearing ear will always respond. In cases with unilateral hearing loss due to atresia or other issue that causes a conductive or mixed hearing loss, the better ear can be masked and aided thresholds can be obtained in soundfield utilizing the BAI through either a softband or a testband. For older children, speech-in-noise testing is recommended to demonstrate even more benefit of binaural hearing.

When there is SSD in a young child, simply masking the better-hearing ear will not demonstrate good aided benefit. If only one cochlea is properly functioning, the use of masking and functional gain to test the child is not appropriate. In these cases, outcome measures and speech-in-noise testing (see Chapter 11 for information about speech testing) must be used. Outcome measures (typically paper-and-pencil forms) should be ones that evaluate the child's listening abilities. For infants and toddlers, these functional tools should be handed to parents, guardians, or other caregivers to fill out. A detailed list of functional assessments can be found in Chapter 22.

In addition, if an infant or toddler with a unilateral hearing loss or SSD does not have enough head control to keep a processor on a softband near or on the mastoid, the fitting of the softband should wait until that head control can be achieved. Placing the processor on a softband on the forehead for SSD or unilateral conductive/mixed loss will not yield a binaural effect as well as when the processor is properly placed on the mastoid process. Recommended fitting time for unilateral hearing losses utilizing softbands is typically at least 1 year of age.

SSD Preimplant Counseling

When working with children with SSD and their families, it is important to remember the following preimplant counseling topics. First, a BAI is not a cure for SSD; it will not make hearing normal or even near normal in the implanted ear. It is important to explain how bone conduction works and how the BAI transfers the sound from the SSD ear quickly through bone conduction to the better ear, thus imitating binaural hearing.

It is beneficial to have demonstration devices for these children and families to utilize during preimplantation counseling. This is an excellent opportunity to show the child and her family exactly what the device looks like and how it works. The child can wear a testband or a softband with the sound processor attached for a few minutes in the clinic, while walking around the clinic, or during an extended trial period set by the audiologist, allowing the child to listen to an approximation of the implanted device.

During this preimplant counseling appointment, it is important to document what difficulties the child is having due to the hearing loss. This process not only gives the audiologist documentation on difficulties to consider in counseling the family or the child's school, but also gives some tangible information to document for insurance providers regarding reimbursement. Speech-in-noise testing in soundfield and functional outcome measures that specifically look at daily listening situations should be completed at this time. By utilizing speech-in-noise testing and outcome measures in the preimplant condition, the level of auditory difficulty experienced by the child can be demonstrated and BAI can be recommended if appropriate.

SSD Postimplantation

When the processor is fitted, it is important to discuss care and maintenance of the processor, similarly to a hearing aid fitting, but the audiologist must also include BAI specifics, such as care and cleaning of the abutment, proper placement and removal of the processor, specific processor features, and any accessories needed. The timeframe for fitting in SSD is identical to the timeframe for basic BAI implantation. At the processor fitting, speech-in-noise testing can be completed. However, postfitting functional outcome measures should not be completed until the child has had an adequate amount of time to experience listening with the BAI on a consistent basis. As with any typical BAI implantation, the goal is to see the child often during the first year, because that is when most complications occur to the skin around the abutment (**Table 21.2**).

◆ Complications

When using a percutaneous implant, complications can occur. There are two main categories of postoperative complications: adverse skin reactions and osseointegration failures (OIF), which cause the implant to extrude (McDermott, Williams, Kuo, Reid, & Proops, 2009; Lloyd, Almeyda, Sirimanna, Albert, & Bailey, 2007). Lee, Christensen, Richter, and Dornhoffer (2011) found complications to be more likely in children. Fifty-seven devices were implanted in 42 children, and 20 were implanted in 18 adults. All implants were completed by a single surgeon using the same technique and yet yielded vastly different rates of implant extrusions. The adult extrusion rate was 0%, but the pediatric implants had an extrusion rate of 21%. Five of the 12 implant failures involved two patients; both were identified as having specific syndromes and one had known vestibular issues. Of the 12 OIFs in the children, four experienced trauma to the abutment, three had skin infections around the abutment prior to the extrusion, and the remaining four had no known cause for the extrusion.

In previous studies, pediatric osseointegration failure rates ranged from 5 to 29%. (Jacobsson, Albrektsson, & Tjellström, 1992; Stevenson et al, 1993; Papsin, Sirimanna, Albert, & Bailey, 1997; Béjar-Solar, Rosete, de Jesus Madrazo, & Baltierra, 2000; Tietze & Papsin, 2001; Zeitoun, De, Thompson, & Proops, 2002; Lloyd et al, 2007; McDermott et al, 2009). Lee et al (2011) recorded higher OIFs in children with syndromes and noted that activity and play levels of most children place the BAI at risk of forceful extrusion, if it is not anchored firmly. They concluded that there is a need for routinely implanting a sleeper fixture for pediatric patients in the event of OIF. Often the sleeper implant can be uncovered in the clinic under local anesthesia without the additional operating room visit that may require the use of a general anesthetic.

◆ Conclusion

The effectiveness of BAI usage in children has been demonstrated. Special considerations for working with children, as with any other amplification device, need to be designed, and audiologists need to follow protocols, FDA regulations, national pediatric guidelines, and state licensure laws. When these guidelines are followed, BAI use for children shows great promise for improvements in auditory access and listening skills. More research is needed to offer additional evidence to assist in future reimbursement for softbands, bilateral implants, and unilateral hearing losses that do not occur only with craniofacial anomalies. For now, audiologists must be clear in their recommendations and provide documentation and research evidence to support the use of BAI.

Discussion Questions

1. When considering a BAI, what is the role of the (1) pediatric audiologist? (2) surgeon? (3) family?

2. When fitting softbands on infants and young children, what are some of the verification measures that can be used for these populations?

3. What are some ways to determine potential benefit of BAIs when working with unilateral hearing losses?

4. What are some possible advantages to using bilateral softbands?

5. What are the main components of the BAI system, and which of these components are MRI compatible?

6. How does the BAI differ from: (1) traditional bone conduction hearing aids? (2) traditional hearing aids? (3) cochlear implants?

References

Abramson, M., Fay, T. H., Kelly, J. P., Wazen, J. J., Liden, G., & Tjellstrom, A. (1989). Clinical results with a percutaneous bone-anchored hearing aid. The Laryngoscope, 99(7 Pt 1), 707–710.

American Academy of Audiology. (2003). Pediatric amplification protocol. Reston, VA: AAA. Retrieved from www.audiology.org/NR/rdonlyres/53D26792-E321-41AF-850F-CC253310F9DB/0/pedamp.pdf

American Academy of Pediatrics, Joint Committee on Infant Hearing. (2007). Year 2007 position statement: Principles and guidelines for early hearing detection and intervention programs. Pediatrics, 120(4), 898–921.

Anderson, K. L., & Smaldino, J. J. (2000). Children's home inventory of listening difficulties (CHILD). Tampa, FL: Educational Audiology Association. Retrieved from http://successforkidswithhearingloss.com/

Béjar-Solar, I., Rosete, M., de Jesus Madrazo, M., & Baltierra, C. (2000). Percutaneous bone-anchored hearing aids at a pediatric institution. Otolaryngology–Head and Neck Surgery, 122(6), 887–891.

Bess, F. H., Dodd-Murphy, J., & Parker, R. A. (1998). Children with minimal sensorineural hearing loss: prevalence, educational performance, and functional status. Ear and Hearing, 19(5), 339–354.

Bess, F. H., & Tharpe, A. M. (1986). Case history data on unilaterally hearing-impaired children. Ear and Hearing, 7(1), 14–19.

Branemark, P. I., Adell, R., Albrektsson, T., Lekholm, U., Lundkvist, S., & Rockler, B. (1983). Osseointegrated titanium fixtures in the treatment of edentulousness. Biomaterials, 4, 25–28.

Browning, G. G., & Gatehouse, S. (1994). Estimation of the benefit of bone-anchored hearing aids. The Annals of Otology, Rhinology, and Laryngology, 103(11), 872–878.

Christensen, L., Richter, G. T., & Dornhoffer, J. L. (2010). Update on bone-anchored hearing aids in pediatric patients with profound unilateral sensorineural hearing loss. Archives of Otolaryngology–Head & Neck Surgery, 136(2), 175–177.

Christensen, L., Smith-Olinde, L., Kimberlain, J., Richter, G. T., & Dornhoffer, J. L. (2010). Comparison of traditional bone-conduction hearing aids with the Baha system. Journal of the American Academy of Audiology, 21(4), 267–273.

Davis, A., Reeve, S.H, Bamford, J. (2001). Children with mild and unilateral hearing impairment. In R. Seewald & J. Gravel (Eds.), A sound foundation through early amplification, Proceedings of the Second International Conference (pp. 179–186). Warrenville, IL: Phonak.

de Alarcon, A., & Choo, D. I. (2007). Controversies in aural atresia repair. Current Opinion in Otolaryngology & Head & Neck Surgery, 15(5), 310–314.

De la Cruz, A., & Teufert, K. B. (2003). Congenital aural atresia surgery: long-term results. Otolaryngology–Head and Neck Surgery, 129(1), 121–127.

Digoy, G. P., & Cueva, R. A. (2007). Congenital aural atresia: review of short- and long-term surgical results. Otology & Neurotology, 28(1), 54–60.

English, K., & Church, G. (1999). Unilateral hearing loss in children: an update for the 1990s. Language, Speech, and Hearing Services in Schools, 30, 26–31.

Evans, A. K., & Kazahaya, K. (2007). Canal atresia: "surgery or implantable hearing devices? The expert's question is revisited." International Journal of Pediatric Otorhinolaryngology, 71(3), 367–374.

Food and Drug Administration. (1995). Summary of Safety and Effectiveness [Initial FDA Approval] K955713. Retrieved from http://www.accessdata.fda.gov/cdrh_docs/pdf/K955713.pdf

Food and Drug Administration. (1999). Summary of Safety and Effectiveness [Pediatric Use] K984162. Retrieved from http://www.accessdata.fda.gov/cdrh_docs/pdf/k984162.pdf

Food and Drug Administration. (2001). Summary of Safety and Effectiveness [Bilateral Fitting] K011438. Retrieved from http://www.accessdata.fda.gov/cdrh_docs/pdf/k011438.pdf

Food and Drug Administration. (2002). Summary of Safety and Effectiveness [Single Sided Deafness] K021837. Retrieved from http://www.accessdata.fda.gov/cdrh_docs/pdf2/k021837.pdf

Håkansson, B. E., Carlsson, P. U., Tjellström, A., & Lidén, G. (1994). The bone-anchored hearing aid: principal design and audiometric results. Ear, Nose, and Throat Journal, 73(9), 670–675.

Hol, M. K., Cremers, C. W., Coppens-Schellekens, W., & Snik, A. F. (2005). The BAHA Softband. A new treatment for young children with bilateral congenital aural atresia. International Journal of Pediatric Otorhinolaryngology, 69(7), 973–980.

Jacobsson, M., Albrektsson, T., & Tjellström, A. (1992). Tissue-integrated implants in children. International Journal of Pediatric Otorhinolaryngology, 24(3), 235–243.

Lee, C. E., Christensen, L., Richter, G. T., & Dornhoffer, J. L. (2011). Arkansas BAHA experience: transcalvarial fixture placement using osseointegration surgical hardware. Otology & Neurotology, 32(3), 444–447.

Lloyd, S., Almeyda, J., Sirimanna, K. S., Albert, D. M., & Bailey, C. M. (2007). Updated surgical experience with bone-anchored hearing aids in children. The Journal of Laryngology and Otology, 121(9), 826–831.

McDermott, A. L., Williams, J., Kuo, M., Reid, A., & Proops, D. (2009). The Birmingham pediatric bone-anchored hearing aid program: a 15-year experience. Otology & Neurotology, 30(2), 178–183.

McDermott, A. L., Williams, J., Kuo, M. J., Reid, A. P., & Proops, D. W. (2008). The role of bone anchored hearing aids in children with Down syndrome. International Journal of Pediatric Otorhinolaryngology, 72(6), 751–757.

McKay, S., Gravel, J. S., & Tharpe, A. M. (2008). Amplification considerations for children with minimal or mild bilateral hearing loss and unilateral hearing loss. Trends in Amplification, 12(1), 43–54.

Nicholson, N., Christensen, L., Dornhoffer, J., Martin, P., & Smith-Olinde, L. (2011). Verification of speech spectrum audibility for pediatric BAHA softband users with craniofacial anomalies. The Cleft Palate-Craniofacial Journal, 48(1), 56–65.

Nilsson, M., Soli, S. D., & Sullivan, J. A. (1994). Development of the Hearing in Noise Test for the measurement of speech reception thresholds in quiet and in noise. The Journal of the Acoustical Society of America, 95(2), 1085–1099.

Papsin, B. C., Sirimanna, T. K. S., Albert, D. M., & Bailey, C. M. (1997). Surgical experience with bone-anchored hearing aids in children. The Laryngoscope, 107(6), 801–806.

Patel, N., & Shelton, C. (2007). The surgical learning curve in aural atresia surgery. The Laryngoscope, 117(1), 67–73.

Prieve, B. A. (2000). Identification of neonatal hearing impairment: a cornerstone for newborn hearing screening. Ear and Hearing, 21(5), 345.

Priwin, C., Jönsson, R., Hultcrantz, M., & Granström, G. (2007). BAHA in children and adolescents with unilateral or bilateral conductive hearing loss: a study of outcome. International Journal of Pediatric Otorhinolaryngology, 71(1), 135–145.

Ruscetta, M. N., Arjmand, E. M., & Pratt, S. R. (2005). Speech recognition abilities in noise for children with severe-to-profound unilateral hearing impairment. International Journal of Pediatric Otorhinolaryngology, 69(6), 771–779.

Sargent, E. W., Herrmann, B., Hollenbeak, C. S., & Bankaitis, A. E. (2001). The minimum speech test battery in profound unilateral hearing loss. Otology & Neurotology, 22(4), 480–486.

Stevenson, D. S., Proops, D. W., Wake, M. J., Deadman, M. J., Worrollo, S. J., & Hobson, J. A. (1993). Osseointegrated implants in the management of childhood ear abnormalities: the initial Birmingham experience. The Journal of Laryngology and Otology, 107(6), 502–509.

Tietze, L., & Papsin, B. (2001). Utilization of bone-anchored hearing aids in children. International Journal of Pediatric Otorhinolaryngology, 58(1), 75–80.

Tjellström, A., & Håkansson, B. (1995). The bone-anchored hearing aid. Design principles, indications, and long-term clinical results. Otolaryngologic Clinics of North America, 28(1), 53–72.

Updike, C. D. (1994). Comparison of FM auditory trainers, CROS aids, and personal amplification in unilaterally hearing impaired children. Journal of the American Academy of Audiolology. 5(3), 204–209.

van der Pouw, C. T., Snik, A. F., & Cremers, C. W. (1999). The BAHA HC200/300 in comparison with conventional bone conduction hearing aids. Clinical Otolaryngology and Allied Sciences, 24(3), 171–176.

Verstraeten, N., Zarowski, A. J., Somers, T., Riff, D., & Offeciers, E. F. (2009). Comparison of the audiologic results obtained with the bone-anchored hearing aid attached to the headband, the testband, and to the "snap" abutment. Otology & Neurotology, 30(1), 70–75.

Welsh, L. W., Welsh, J. J., Rosen, L. F., & Dragonette, J. E. (2004). Functional impairments due to unilateral deafness. The Annals of Otology, Rhinology, and Laryngology, 113(12), 987–993.

Zeitoun, H., De, R., Thompson, S. D., & Proops, D. W. (2002). Osseointegrated implants in the management of childhood ear abnormalities: with particular emphasis on complications. The Journal of Laryngology and Otology, 116(2), 87–91.

Chapter 22

Cochlear Implants for Infants and Children

René H. Gifford

Key Points

- Behavioral assessment of hearing should be completed prior to determining cochlear implant candidacy.

- Cochlear implant candidacy is based on audiometric thresholds as well as lack of progress on auditory skills development and language.

- Age at implantation significantly affects postoperative outcomes.

- If a child is not making at least month-for-month auditory and speech-language developmental progress with appropriately fitted hearing aids and intervention, cochlear implantation should be considered.

- The most influential factors affecting postoperative outcomes are (1) full-time use of the cochlear implant(s), (2) early and consistent intervention focusing on listening and spoken language, and (3) time spent talking to the child in the home.

Cochlear implant criteria have expanded over time since the Food and Drug Administration (FDA) first approved multichannel cochlear implants for children in June 1990. Candidacy criteria, also referred to as labeled indications, vary with age and etiology as well as across the different manufacturers. In addition, there are several auditory-related milestones that, when not met, may suggest implant candidacy regardless of whether the child meets the typical candidate profile.

There are several elements of the candidate selection process as well as postoperative management that require careful consideration and coordination between members of the interdisciplinary cochlear implant team. Some elements fall within the domain of the audiologist and are related to the audiologic evaluation, including behavioral assessment of hear-

ing and auditory capabilities. Other elements are within the domain of the speech-language pathologist (SLP) and are related to speech and language development. There are also medical, radiologic, and psychological elements requiring consideration both pre- and postoperatively. This chapter will discuss pediatric cochlear implantation, including aspects to be considered from the perspective of the audiologist, SLP, deaf educator, social worker, and psychologist as well as the medical/surgical team. This chapter will further describe the elements of cochlear implant candidate selection for children with hearing loss as it stands today, as well as discuss those elements that, as a field, we may want to consider in the expansion of criteria for future evaluation processes.

◆ Audiologic Evaluation

Assessment of Hearing Status

Pediatric cochlear implant evaluations generally begin in the audiology clinic. The cochlear implant evaluation is ordinarily preceded by numerous appointments in the diagnostic audiology clinic for objective assessment of auditory function, including otoacoustic emissions (OAE) and auditory brainstem response (ABR) as well as behavioral hearing assessment. It is generally the case that the cochlear implant evaluation does not involve the initial diagnosis of a severe to profound hearing loss, as children and their families will present to the evaluation with a confirmed diagnosis and hearing aid experience. For those audiologists engaging in all aspects of pediatric audiologic care, a patient and family will likely be followed from initial diagnosis to hearing aid fitting, follow-up, and assessment of auditory progress through determination of candidacy as well as postoperatively.

Even if a family presents to the implant evaluation with prior audiograms and objective estimates of auditory function, it is still recommended that comprehensive audiometric testing be completed. This affords an opportunity to gain additional ear-specific pure tone and speech awareness information—particularly for those frequencies that prior audiograms may have been missing—and permits the cochlear implant team to get to know the child better and to be able to determine how best to obtain the child's cooperation. The audiologic evaluation also gives the child the opportunity to get to know members of the implant team so that the child's first experience with the team is not conducive to distress. It is also recommended that tympanograms and, at a minimum, ipsilateral acoustic reflex testing be attempted (see Chapter 12 for further information regarding guidelines for middle ear measurements in infants and children). Multiple assessments of behavioral hearing status are recommended prior to *finalizing* candidate selection. This is possible as newborns identified with hearing loss are generally not seen by the cochlear implant team for comprehensive behavioral evaluation/assessment until 6 months age—the age at which behavioral assessment of hearing using visual reinforcement audiometry (VRA) can be completed. Thus the earliest implant evaluation/workup appointments will involve VRA, behavioral observation audiometry (BOA), or both. Behavioral audiometry becomes more complicated when assessing infants and children with additional diagnoses that may delay sitting up, independent head and neck control, and more global developmental and/or cognitive abilities.

OAEs can provide valuable information for the cochlear implant evaluation (see Chapter 13). Although most newborn hearing screening programs in well-baby nurseries utilize OAEs as a first-pass tool for screening (e.g., National Institutes of Health [NIH], 1993; White, Behrens, & Strickland, 1995; Gravel et al, 2005; American Academy of Pediatrics, Joint Committee on Infant Hearing [JCIH], 2007), not all chil-

dren will have been screened prior to discharge, and not all babies are born in medical facilities. Further, many experienced pediatric audiologists working with implants have at least one story about a patient presenting for an evaluation who is diagnosed with auditory neuropathy spectrum disorder (ANSD; see Chapter 32) during the course of the implant evaluation appointment. Although it is true that ANSD does not preclude a patient from cochlear implantation (e.g., Shallop, Peterson, Facer, Fabry, & Driscoll, 2001; Peterson et al, 2003; Rance & Barker, 2008; Teagle et al, 2010; Breneman, Gifford, & Dejong, 2012), it is still important to have an accurate diagnosis in place as well as to explore all possible habilitative options prior to recommending surgical intervention.

Audiometric Criteria for Implantation

Children < 24 Months

> **Pearl**
>
> - Critical language learning occurs during the first year of life. Infants with severe to profound hearing loss—even if fitted with hearing aids—will miss many of these opportunities. Thus, it is reasonable to expect that future pediatric implant indications will expand to include infants under 12 months of age.

Audiometric criteria for pediatric cochlear implantation differ across implant manufacturers. For pediatric candidacy, there is an additional element of age-specific criteria with respect to severity of hearing loss. **Table 22.1** lists the audiometric criteria for pediatric implantation for all three implant manufacturers

Table 22.1 Current indications for pediatric cochlear implantation

	Audiometric criteria		Speech recognition criteria	
Advanced Bionics	Profound SNHL, ≥ 90 dB HL		< 4 years old < 20% open-set words (e.g., MLNT) via MLV at 70 dB SPL	4+ years old < 12% for difficult, recorded open-set words (e.g., PBK) or < 30% open-set sentences (e.g., HINT-C) at 70 dB SPL
Cochlear	< 24 months Profound SNHL	24+ months Severe-to-profound SNHL	≤ 30% on open-set words MLNT or LNT	
MED-EL	Profound SNHL, 90+ dB HL at 1 kHz		< 20% for MLNT or LNT words	

Abbreviations: HINT-C, Hearing-in-Noise Test for Children; LNT, Lexical Neighborhood Test; MLNT, Multisyllabic Lexical Neighborhood Test; MLV, monitored live-voice; PBK, Phonetically Balanced Kindergarten; SNHL, sensorineural hearing loss; SPL, sound pressure level.

who have FDA approval in the United States: Cochlear (Sydney, Australia), Advanced Bionics (Sylmar, CA), and MED-EL (Innsbruck, Austria). The current labeled criteria specify bilateral *profound* sensorineural hearing loss (SNHL) for children aged 12 to 24 months (Cochlear America package insert; Advanced Bionics package insert; MED-EL package insert). This is not to imply that children with less severe hearing losses would not benefit from cochlear implantation; rather, the historical concern has been that obtaining reliable behavioral thresholds for the youngest children was more difficult than for older children, and thus the criteria were set to be most stringent for the youngest candidates. Such concern may not be as pertinent in our current environment, given the audiologic checks and balances that are at our disposal for both behavioral assessment of hearing and physiologic estimation of auditory function. In fact, this is also an argument for lowering the FDA-approved age for cochlear implantation from 12 months to slightly younger—perhaps in the 6- to 9-month range (e.g., Cosetti & Roland, 2010; Kim, Jeong, Lee, & Kim, 2010). Research suggests that children implanted earlier exhibit higher levels of word and language acquisition (Bergeson, Houston, & Miyamoto, 2010; Houston & Miyamoto, 2010; Houston, Stewart, Moberly, Hollich, & Miyamoto, 2012; Niparko et al, 2010; Moog & Geers, 2010), speech perception (Tajudeen, Waltzman, Jethanamest, & Svirsky, 2010), speech production intelligibility (Habib, Waltzman, Tajudeen, & Svirsky, 2010), and vocabulary development (Hayes, Geers, Treiman, & Moog, 2009; Houston & Miyamoto, 2010; Houston et al, 2012; Tomblin, Barker, Spencer, Zhang, & Gantz, 2005)—even when considering those children implanted under 12 months as compared with children implanted in the second year of life.

Pearl

- Regular administration of validated auditory questionnaires will provide us with information about auditory skills development and point out red flags that audiologists may miss during the limited audiology appointments and standard parental interview.

For the infant with severe-to-profound hearing loss receiving little to no benefit from full-time use of amplification, there are several developmental changes and language learning opportunities occurring within the first year of life that will be missed without cochlear implants. This is true even for infants with appropriately fitted hearing aids, given that audibility may not be sufficient to en-

able consistent auditory access to spoken language at various levels. Some of these developmental changes occurring during the first year of life are word segmentation abilities, auditory memory, and phonological/lexical/semantic representation. Word segmentation—the process of dividing connected discourse into meaningful units, such as individual words—has been to shown to develop rapidly between 7.5 and 10.5 months (e.g., Jusczyk, 2002). Further, infants have demonstrated the capacity for auditory memory and long-term storage of new words—an important prerequisite for auditory-based language learning—by 8 months of age (Jusczyk & Hohne, 1997; Houston & Jusczyk, 2003). Development of phonological, lexical, and semantic representations is also known to influence word-learning abilities (e.g., Gupta & MacWhinney, 1997; Hollich, Jusczyk, & Luce, 2002; Soja, Carey, & Spelke, 1991) and is emerging within the first year of life as a child acquires new words both expressively and receptively (e.g., Storkel, 2009). Thus the infant with severe to profound SNHL and limited aided audibility is missing out on the development of critical auditory-based language learning opportunities.

Pearl

- Recent research has shown that children implanted under 12 months of age demonstrate greater word-learning abilities and audiovisual integration than children implanted between 12 and 24 months of age.

Children Aged 2 Years and Older

For children over 2 years of age, audiometric criteria for implantation with a Nucleus implant are slightly more lenient, including bilateral severe to profound SNHL—allowing slightly more residual acoustic hearing for candidacy qualification (Cochlear America package insert). Both Advanced Bionics and MED-EL, however, continue to specify bilateral profound SNHL in the labeled indications even for children over 2 years of age. Audiometric criteria for FDA labeled indications are listed in **Table 22.1** for all three manufacturers.

Cochlear Implant Criteria: The Role of the FDA

Cochlear implant labeled indications (i.e., candidacy criteria) can be found in the physician's package insert that is included in the packaging for each internal device. The FDA is not responsible for designating the criteria or indications for cochlear implantation. Rather, the manufacturer submits an application for FDA approval, outlining the proposed criteria for their device. Thus, it is the role of the FDA to either approve or reject the submitted application for approval and the *manufacturer-defined indications* typically following an approved clinical trial. If ultimately approved, the manufacturer-defined indications/criteria for implantation are then listed as the FDA labeled indications for use of that device.

What is important for the clinician to recognize in this process is that *the FDA governs industry, not the individual clinician or implant center*. Industry is strictly prohibited from promoting off-label usage of a device. What this means is that, despite considerable evidence in support of expanded cochlear implant candidacy criteria, the manufacturers are absolutely not allowed to recommend implantation for individuals not meeting labeled indications. Clinicians, on the other hand, are afforded the professional judgment to make appropriate clinical recommendations for their patients about the suitability of cochlear implant candidacy. For this reason, the FDA has published *Off-Label and Investigational Use of Marketed Drugs, Biologics, and Medical Devices* (Food and Drug Administration [FDA], 2011), which details the conditional approval of off-label usage of medical devices, drugs, and biologics as recommended by professional, licensed clinicians. This document explicitly endorses the off-label usage of a marketed biomedical device when the intent is for clinical practice (i.e., excluding research applications). The FDA states that, should clinicians recommend off-label usage of a device, they have the responsibility to ensure the following:

- They are well informed about the product.
- They base its use on firm scientific rationale and on sound medical evidence.
- They maintain records of the product's use and effects.

Thus, it is within the domain of the clinicians on the cochlear implant team to provide professional, clinical determinations regarding candidacy. If an infant is not making auditory progress with full-time use of appropriately fitted hearing aids and compliance with the recommended intervention and therapy schedule, that child meets cochlear implant candidacy—based upon the professional clinical judgment of the cochlear implant team. In the same vein, if a child has moderate sloping to profound SNHL and is not making auditory progress with appropriately fitted hearing aids and intervention, the cochlear implant team should still consider recommending implantation.

◆ Speech Recognition Testing

The Importance of Using Recorded Materials

A vital component of pediatric cochlear implant evaluations for the older child involves the behavioral assessment of auditory-based speech understanding. Many children with hearing loss rely heavily on visual cues, such as lip reading and global nonverbal communication. Thus, to gain an understanding of an individual's auditory-based abilities, speech stimuli are presented without visual cues.

Given the variability in performance associated with monitored live voice (MLV) presentation of speech stimuli (Roeser & Clark, 2008), the presentation of recorded stimuli is needed for assessment of pediatric cochlear implant candidacy in a standardized manner. Of interest is that, at the time of this chapter's preparation, Advanced Bionics' package insert specifies administration of the Multisyllabic Lexical Neighborhood Test (Kirk, Pisoni, & Osberger, 1995) using MLV. Given that the MLNT and its monosyllabic analog, the Lexical Neighborhood Test (Kirk et al, 1995), are available in recorded format, MLV presentation would be contraindicated by best practices for pediatric audiology (see Chapters 6 and 11).

Despite the variability in performance for speech recognition stimuli administered via MLV, depending on the child's age and developmental status, MLV may be required to elicit reliable responses. Live voice from a familiar, trusted clinician certainly represents a simpler speech recognition task than using a recorded stimulus. The recorded voice is unfamiliar and often lacks the affect that is found in the speaking style of an individual who works with children. Should a child respond only to MLV stimulus presentation and continue to exhibit poor recognition, it is reasonable to determine implant candidacy, as speech recognition with standardized, recorded stimuli will be either equivalent or poorer (Roeser & Clark, 2008).

Presentation Levels

An important consideration for speech recognition testing in the determination of cochlear implant candidacy involves the presentation level of the speech stimuli. For many years, audiologists used 70 dB sound pressure level (SPL); however, 70 dB SPL is no longer considered an acceptable presentation level, as it does not represent average conversational level speech (Pearsons, Bennett, & Fidell, 1977; Olsen, 1998). Though there is not currently a best practices recommendation for pediatric implant assessment, the existing adult recommendations—as found in the adult minimum speech test battery (MSTB)—include the use of recorded speech materials presented at 60 dBA[1] for assessment of speech recognition performance in both pre- and postimplant testing. Thus, it would also follow that 60 dBA should be the *highest* presentation level used for pediatric candidacy assessment. Data exist in support of even lower presentation levels for both adults and children, given that average, casual speech levels for children and women range from 50 to 56 dBA (Pearsons et al, 1977; Olsen, 1998). Thus, to gauge a child's understanding of both women and other children, lower presentation levels should also be considered for speech recognition testing, such as 50 dBA.

Pitfall

- Assessing speech recognition abilities with high stimulus levels (> 60 dB SPL) and live voice stimuli has the potential to inflate a child's performance. This is particularly important when determining cochlear implant candidacy for the older child, who is able to complete speech recognition testing.

◆ Speech Recognition Test Materials and Cochlear Implant Candidacy

Children ≤ 3 Years

Auditory skills development and speech understanding for younger children in this age range will most generally be gauged via auditory questionnaire data, parental report, and speech/language assessment. This is particularly true for the youngest children with severe to profound SNHL, for whom we anticipate poor progress on auditory skills and auditory-oral language development. The obvious exception to this rule is younger children with acquired hearing loss or progressive hearing loss. The FDA labeled criteria for children in this age range with respect to "speech understanding" are rather vague; however, all manufacturers make reference to limited benefit from appropriately fitted hearing aids and habilitation as evidenced by lack of progress in the development of simple auditory skills.

Current labeled indications for pediatric cochlear implantation do not make reference to the use of closed-set metrics of speech perception for determining implant candidacy for the toddler age group, though this does not mean that closed-set metrics are not valuable instruments for assessing speech recognition performance and progress prior to determining implant candidacy. These metrics should be used to assess speech recognition for our youngest patients, if for no other reason than to provide a baseline measurement against which preoperative progress with hearing aids or postoperative progress with cochlear implants can be gauged. For more detailed information regarding closed-set tests of speech recognition that are available for use in this population, see Chapter 11.

Children Aged 3 Years and Up

Current implant candidacy criteria for older children are based on either mono- or multisyllabic word recognition, depending on which is developmentally appropriate for the child being evaluated. The tests listed by the cochlear implant manufacturers in the FDA labeled indications are as follows (presented in order of developmentally appropriate progression): Early Speech Perception (ESP) test (Moog and Geers, 1990), MLNT (Kirk et al, 1995), LNT (Kirk et al, 1995), Phonetically Balanced Kindergarten (PBK) word recognition test (Haskins, 1949), and Hearing-in-Noise Test for Children (HINT-C) (Gelnett, Sumida, Nilsson, & Soli, 1995).

Older children for whom these metrics are considered developmentally appropriate are required to exhibit considerably lower performance than even that listed for adult implant criteria (**Table 22.1**). Word recognition candidacy criteria for older children range from 12 to 30% correct in the best-aided condition across all three manufacturers. Advanced Bionics further lists performance up to 30% correct for HINT-C sentences when developmentally appropriate for children over 4 years. This same manufacturer has set its HINT sentence recognition criteria for adult candidacy at 50% correct. Of interest is that pediatric implant criteria—with respect to speech recognition—are disproportionally restrictive even though children are in the process of acquiring auditory language. Thus, the need for the expansion of labeled pediatric cochlear implant criteria has been and continues to be a hot topic. This is another area in which children may be implanted using "off label" criteria. Indeed, there have been several reports of highly successful outcomes for nontraditional pediatric implant recipients who were either under 12 months of age or exhibited less severe hearing losses, asymmetric hearing loss, or higher-than-criterion-level performance on measures of speech recognition (Dettman et al, 2004; Dowell, Hollow, & Winton, 2004; Leigh, Dettman, Dowell, & Sarant, 2011; Sunderhaus, Hedley-Williams, & Gifford, 2012). There

---

[1] The use of A weighting for sound level meter measurements is recommended because linear weighting—which is implied in an SPL reference unless otherwise specified—provides noisier recordings due to flat frequency response through the lower frequency region. In contrast, the A-weighted frequency response rolls off for lower frequencies having reached 20 dB of attenuation (relative to the passband) at 100 Hz.

are increasing data emerging that suggest a relatively narrow critical period for cochlear implantation for the development of listening and spoken language (Hayes et al, 2009; Moog & Geers, 2010; Bergeson et al, 2010; Niparko et al, 2010; Habib et al, 2010; Houston & Miyamoto, 2010) as well as auditory pathway maturation (Ponton et al, 2000; Sharma, Dorman, & Spahr, 2002; Eggermont & Ponton, 2003; Gordon, Tanaka, & Papsin, 2005; Kral, Tillein, Heid, Klinke, & Hartmann, 2006; Sharma & Dorman, 2006; Gilley, Sharma, & Dorman, 2008; Sharma, Nash, & Dorman, 2009). It seems reasonable that the combined fields of otology, audiology, and speech-language pathology are questioning the reasoning behind labeling the most stringent candidacy criteria for the youngest auditory language learners and that criterion-level performance should more closely approximate what is outlined for adult implant candidate selection.

Another consideration in pediatric implant selection is the assessment of speech recognition in noise. Assessing speech recognition in noise is a reasonable consideration given that children are rarely in quiet listening environments.[2] Educational acoustic research has reported occupied classroom noise ranging from 48 dBA to 69 dBB, with mean levels approximating 65 dBA for an early elementary classroom (e.g., Sanders, 1965; Nober & Nober, 1975; Bess, Sinclair, & Riggs, 1984; Finitzo-Hieber, 1988). Considering that a child's typical listening day takes place both inside and outside the classroom, equivalent continuous noise level (LEq) 24-hour levels of a child's environment reveal that average levels range from 87.3 dBA for all students to as high as 95.5 dBA for fifth-graders (Clark & Govett, 1995). Given that a child's everyday listening environment is *much noisier* than even that encountered by the typical adult, it follows in the process of determining implant candidacy that speech recognition in noise should be standard practice. It is likely that a pediatric minimum speech test battery will soon emerge, providing pediatric implant audiologists with best practice recommendations for the minimum testing to be conducted at both pre- and postimplant intervals.

◆ Evaluation of Auditory Skills and Progress in Infants and Younger Children

Birth to 3 Years

Determining a child's auditory skills and progress with amplification prior to determining implant candidacy goes well beyond the audiogram. It is common clinical knowledge that similar audiograms do not necessarily yield similar levels of benefit from amplification across a range of hearing losses and configurations. Given that speech recognition performance cannot be completed for infants or even for some toddlers, it is vital that the candidacy evaluation include assessment of auditory skills, development, and progress with hearing aids. Working within the domain of the audiologist, these skills will most likely be assessed via parental history and administration of validated questionnaires that are designed to gauge a child's auditory-based responsiveness to sounds in the environment.

Perhaps the most frequently used questionnaires for children from birth to 3 years is the IT-MAIS, the Infant-Toddler version of the Meaningful Auditory Integration Scale (MAIS) (Zimmerman-Phillips, Robbins, & Osberger, 2000). All cochlear implant manufacturers reference the MAIS (Robbins, Renshaw, & Berry, 1991) and/or IT-MAIS for the assessment of auditory progress with amplification. For children up to 3 years, the 10-item IT-MAIS is commonly used, given its widespread familiarity as well as its ease and the short time required for administration. The IT-MAIS was developed to be administered via structured parental interview and thus requires that the clinician interpret open-ended responses and assign numerical scores ranging from 0 (never) to 4 (always).

There are other parental questionnaires designed for use with infants and toddlers that are becoming increasingly popular in the busy cochlear implant clinic. The LittlEARS from MED-EL (Weichbold, Tsiakpini, Coninx, & D'Haese, 2005; Coninx et al, 2009) includes 35 yes/no questions that assess auditory-based responsiveness to different sounds and environments. The questionnaire was organized in a hierarchical fashion with a progression of difficulty so that after six consecutive 'no' answers, no further answers are required. The LittlEARS was designed for normal-hearing children up to 24 months or for administration 24 months following implant activation—though a typically developing child implanted early who is making full-time use of the implant processors will often reach ceiling levels prior to that test point. Completion of the LittlEARS takes 5 to 7 minutes, and because it was not designed for parental interview, its administration does not need to take up valuable appointment time.

The Auditory Skills Checklist (ASC) (Meinzen-Derr, Wiley, Creighton, & Choo, 2007) is a 35-item questionnaire that gauges detection, discrimination, identification, and comprehension. Similar to the IT-MAIS, the ASC was developed for parental interview and/or clinician observation, for which the parent/administrator assigns a score from 0 to 2 as follows: 0, child does not have the skill; 1, child has emerging skill development; 2, child consistently demonstrates the skill. The ASC can be given along with the

---

[2] Current FDA indications for cochlear implantation do not suggest the use of speech-in-noise testing for determining either adult or pediatric implant candidacy.

IT-MAIS and/or LittlEARS, as the ASC may be reused over a longer period of time (for children implanted up to 3 years of age) and will provide a multidimensional assessment revealing smaller increments in auditory skills development.

Another relatively new questionnaire is the Functioning After Pediatric Cochlear Implantation (FAPCI) questionnaire (Lin et al, 2007). Though the FAPCI was designed primarily for use following implantation, it can offer valued information when administered during the candidacy process, thereby serving as a baseline measurement. The 23-item FAPCI was designed for children aged 2 to 5 years and does not require parental interview. The FAPCI assesses a child's behaviors as related to auditory-based responsiveness and expressive verbal communication and takes 5 to 10 minutes for completion.

The Functional Auditory Performance Indicators (FAPI) (Stredler-Brown & DeConde Johnson, 2003) was designed to gauge sound awareness, meaningful sounds, auditory feedback, sound localization, discrimination, short-term auditory memory, and linguistic auditory processing. The clinician will assign a score for each of the seven categories of auditory development as emerging (0–35%), in process (36–79%), or acquired (80–100%). The FAPI can be administered to families with children as young as a few months of age and can continue to be administered until "acquired" scores are obtained for all categories.

The Early Language Milestone (ELM) scale (Coplan, 1987) contains 43 items that assess language development in children from birth to 3 years. The ELM has three sections that focus on expressive, receptive, and visual language. This instrument is generally administered via parental interview. There are sections, however, for which clinician observation may also be used for scoring purposes. ELM administration takes 3 to 10 minutes depending upon the age of the child, level of development, and scoring method (i.e., pass/fail or point scoring).

Individual implant programs can determine which questionnaires best meet the needs of their patient population and their families. More important than the chosen questionnaire(s) is that the clinicians within a given program be consistent across all patients, thus adhering to the clinic protocol. Protocol adherence allows each implant program to generate its own normative data for patient outcomes, which significantly aids family counseling. This also provides clinics with the data needed to compare their outcomes to average patient performance in the literature. Further, since most implant programs have multiple clinicians, adherence to protocol allows clinician substitution without sacrificing assessment accuracy.

Pitfall

- Some clinicians are reluctant to recommend cochlear implantation for a child not making expected progress with hearing aids despite full-time use and adherence to the recommended schedule of intervention, if the child does not meet the "typical" audiologic profile. The audiogram provides only one piece of information and does not reflect a child's functional auditory performance.

Preschool and School-Age Children

As mentioned for infants and toddlers, auditory skills and development for older children may also not be well predicted by the audiogram. Although behavioral assessment of a child's auditory skills should always be attempted for preschool and school-age children, due to several factors, behavioral assessment may not be possible or only very limited information may be obtained at any given appointment. For this reason, there are several auditory questionnaires designed for supplementary use with preschool and school-age children.

The MAIS (Robbins et al, 1991) is a 10-item parental interview–style questionnaire aimed at the assessment of auditory skills, including spontaneous responses to sounds, for children aged 3 to 5 years. All implant manufacturers make reference to this questionnaire for determining auditory progress—or lack thereof—with appropriately fitted hearing aids.

The Parents' Evaluation of Aural/oral performance of CHildren (PEACH) is a 13-item questionnaire that was designed for parents' estimation of their child's functional aural and oral abilities in everyday life (Ching & Hill, 2007). The PEACH is considered appropriate for children aged 3 to 7 years. The PEACH requires parents to reflect on their child's listening behavior over the previous week and assigns a numerical value to parental answers ranging from 0 (Never or 0%) to 4 (Always or 75 to 100%). The PEACH includes questions that gauge listening behaviors in both quiet and noisy surroundings.

The 23-item FAPCI questionnaire (Lin et al, 2007) can be administered to parents of children aged 2 to 5 years. As stated previously, although the FAPCI was originally intended to track postoperative progress, administration during the candidacy evaluation can provide clinicians and families with a baseline against which future growth in auditory skills can be gauged.

There are other more general parent-based questionnaires available for use with children who have severe-to-profound sensorineural hear-

Table 22.2 Parental questionnaires gauging auditory skills prior to and following pediatric cochlear implantation

Measure name	Length; est. time to complete	Domains assessed	Age range	Administration
LittlEARS	35 yes/no items; 5–7 minutes	Age appropriateness of auditory behaviors (e.g., responsiveness to acoustic rituals, looking for sound sources)	0–24 months	Independent parental completion; parent report
Auditory Skills Checklist	35 items; < 10 minutes	Detection, discrimination, identification and comprehension	0–36 months	Parental interview; clinician observation
Early Language Milestones (ELM)	43 items; < 10 minutes	Auditory-based language behaviors: expressive, receptive, and visual	0–36 months	Parental report; direct observation
Infant-Toddler Meaningful Auditory Integration Scale (IT-MAIS)	10 items; 5–10 minutes	Device bonding, alerting to sound, vocalization, deriving meaning from sound	0–36 months	Parental interview
Functioning After Pediatric Cochlear Implantation (FAPCI)	23 items; 5–10 minutes	Speech intelligibility, auditory responsiveness, real-world verbal communication	2–5 years	Independent parental completion; parent report
Functional Auditory Performance Indicators (FAPI)	33 items; 10–15 minutes	Auditory awareness, feedback and integration, discrimination, comprehension, memory and linguistic processing	3 months until "acquired" is obtained for all categories	Parental interview; parent report; direct observation
Meaningful Auditory Integration Scale (MAIS)	10 items; 5–10 minutes	Device bonding, alerting to sound, vocalization, deriving meaning from sound	3–5 years	Parental interview
Parents' Evaluation of Aural/Oral Performance of Children (PEACH)	13 items; 5–10 minutes	Aural/oral speech communicative behaviors in quiet and noisy situations	3–7 years	Independent parental completion; parent report

ing loss, including the Meaningful Use of Speech Sounds (MUSS) (Robbins et al, 1991); Children's Home Inventory for Listening Difficulties (CHILD) (Anderson & Smaldino, 1999); and Developmental Index of Audition and Listening (DIAL) (Palmer & Mormer, 1999). The questionnaires listed in **Table 22.2** are those most frequently used with children during both pre- and postimplantation assessment. As stated previously, more importantly than the chosen questionnaires, individual clinics will determine the appropriateness of the different instruments and appropriateness for their patient population and must strive to maintain consistency across clinicians and patients. This allows individual clinics to track the typical performance for children implanted at their center as well as transparency across clinicians for families' experience with audiologic management.

◆ Hearing Aid Trial and Verification as Related to the Development and Evaluation of Speech and Language

When beginning a hearing aid trial for infants and children who are thought to meet cochlear implant candidacy based on the severity of the hearing loss, it is critical to schedule a speech-language assessment as well to determine baseline language skills against which future development can be measured. The specific metrics used by the SLP will be dependent upon both the chronologic age as well as the "hearing" age of the child. During the trial period, it is expected that a child demonstrate *at least* month-for-month auditory progress as well as speech and language developmental progress with amplification. What that means is that, if a child has been using amplification for 3 months, the child should make *at least* 3 months of progress in auditory skills and speech-language development. If this is not the case for a child making full-time use of amplification and appropriate habilitation, cochlear implantation should be considered. All three manufacturers specify the need for a 3- to 6-month trial with amplification prior to determining implant candidacy. The length of the trial, however, may be compressed in cases of meningitis, for which concerns about cochlear ossification and electrode insertion are present.

Prior to the diagnostic speech-language evaluation, the child's hearing aid settings must first be verified. According to the Pediatric Amplification Protocol (AAA, 2003), best practices require that hearing aids be verified using either probe microphone measurements or test box verification with patient-specific real-ear to coupler difference (RECD) measurements. Given that nonlinear hearing aid circuitry is generally used to attain audibility at various input levels for both adult and pediatric hearing aid fittings, a prescriptive formula, such as DSL*m*[i/o] (Seewald, Ross, & Spiro, 1985; Cornelisse, Seewald, & Jamieson, 1995; Scollie et al, 2005), should be used to verify target audibility at speech input levels corresponding to soft, average, and loud, such as 50, 60, and 70 dB SPL. For further information regarding hearing aid verification, see Chapter 20. In addition, behavioral testing of performance with the hearing aids should be performed.

It is best that a child receive at least two diagnostic speech-language evaluations during the candidacy selection process when the child is participating in the hearing aid trial. Although it may not be possible to administer norm-referenced measures over such a short time period (see Chapter 28), there are available criterion-referenced measures that can provide vital clinical information about a child's progress with hearing aids. These measures may be more reflective of a child's abilities than data gleaned from parental questionnaires (e.g., Hedley-Williams, Bagatto, Boscini, & Gifford, 2012).

Early intervention (including home visits from a member of the early intervention team) and regular speech-language therapy, as well as active parental involvement supplementing therapy with accurate modeling of spoken language, are absolutely critical for a child's speech and language development. The cochlear implant team can gather considerable clinically relevant information from parental compliance not only with full-time use of hearing aids, but also with the recommended intervention schedule. Family adherence to the therapy schedule during the candidacy process establishes an important behavioral precedent for what is expected following cochlear implantation. All clinicians realize the intensive nature of postoperative intervention and therapy that is required in order for a child to take full advantage of the audibility provided by the implant; however,

most families report that, although they had been counseled, they had not realized the full extent of the commitment required to achieve the communication goals outlined for their child.

◆ Beyond the Audiologist and Speech-Language Pathologist: Other Critical Members of the Cochlear Implant Team

Social Workers and Psychologists

Social workers and psychologists play an essential role in the process of candidate selection. A psychological or developmental psychological evaluation may be recommended should concerns arise regarding the child's overall cognitive and global development. A psychologist and/or social worker can also provide families with assistance with the acceptance of the hearing loss and the implications of having a child who will be dependent upon technology for lifelong communication. Also within the scope of practice for the psychologist or social worker is the evaluation of family dynamics and level of family dedication to the recommended postoperative therapy schedule. This guidance may also be recommended following cochlear implantation, as needed.

Social workers are trained to provide counseling and support for families in terms of the financial requirements for their child's medical care. This service may be of particular importance for families of children who will be undergoing surgical implantation of auditory prostheses. Many families are unaware of the financial resources available for insurance coverage of the implant as well as for the required therapy and other assistive listening devices, such as amplified telephones and FM systems. Social workers not only provide financial counseling but can also assist with the required paperwork, helping families navigate through the application process. In some instances, social workers are able to assist families by coordinating medical and therapy appointments as well as by reviewing completed and future appointments to ensure that all medical specialties and evaluations have been either scheduled or completed.

Otologists and Neuro-otologists

The cochlear implant surgeon is most generally an otologist or neuro-otologist—an otolaryngologist who has completed a 2-year, postresidency fellowship in otology and skull-based surgery. The implant surgeon plays an obvious significant role in the candidate selection process, as she completes a thorough preimplant evaluation and is also responsible for the implant surgical procedure and postoperative otologic care. The implanting surgeon and her medical team are also responsible for ensuring that implant candidates are current regarding the recommended immunization schedule prior to surgery. This is especially critical given that children with cochlear implants and children with temporal bone anatomic anomalies are both at increased risk for contracting meningitis. The recommended immunizations and associated schedule for children undergoing cochlear implant surgery can be found on the Centers for Disease Control (CDC) Web site and includes—at a minimum—an age-specific pneumococcal vaccination (CDC, 2012).

Prior to surgery, the otologist orders a preanesthetic medical evaluation or preoperative evaluation to ensure that the child is medically able to undergo surgery and the associated anesthetic risk. Otologists will also typically refer children to ophthalmology as well as medical genetics given that ~ 40% of children with SNHL have other medical or developmental comorbidities, including cognitive, visual, motor, behavioral, and learning issues (Fortnum, Marshall, & Summerfield, 2002; Gallaudet Research Institute, 2008; Roberts & Hindley, 1999; Van Naarden, Decouflé, & Caldwell, 1999). Additional medical specialties, such as neurology, physical medicine and rehabilitation, and developmental pediatrics, are also consulted when determined necessary for an individual child.

Otologists routinely order imaging studies to determine cochlear patency as well as to rule out cochlear or other temporal bone abnormalities that could affect the surgical procedure. Cochlear and temporal bone abnormalities, however, do not necessarily mean cochlear implantation is contraindicated, though it is critical that the surgical team be aware of such issues. High-resolution computed tomography (CT) is generally ordered for all patients having met audiological criteria for cochlear implantation. Magnetic resonance imaging (MRI) is generally ordered for pediatric patients who either have exhibited no hearing via behavioral audiometry or may be suspect for cochlear nerve deficiency. Many cochlear implant programs obtain preoperative MRI for all pediatric patients prior to implantation. The reason is that since postoperative MRI above 0.3 tesla is contraindicated in the United States *without* magnet removal (see physician package inserts), many otologists consider preoperative MRI to be the last chance to obtain detailed imaging information regarding the cochleovestibular nerve.

Factors Affecting Postoperative Outcomes

Once cochlear implant candidacy has been determined, in-depth counseling and education are absolutely critical. Educating the family about the function of cochlear implants and what they can do is just as important as focusing on what implants *cannot* do. For example, clinicians should counsel families that cochlear implants cannot restore "normal" hearing and auditory function nor do they change the underlying diagnosis of sensorineural deafness.

Perhaps the number one question that families will ask regarding cochlear implantation for their child is how well he or she will be able to communicate via listening and spoken language. There are several factors that have the potential to have an impact on postoperative outcomes, including wear time, intervention, integrity of cochlear and neural structures, and etiology.

Age at Implantation

As mentioned earlier in this chapter, there are several studies documenting a relatively narrow critical period for cochlear implantation for the development of listening and spoken language (Hayes et al, 2009; Moog & Geers, 2010; Bergeson et al, 2010; Niparko et al, 2010; Habib et al, 2010; Houston & Miyamoto, 2010) as well as auditory pathway maturation (Ponton et al, 2000; Sharma et al, 2002; Eggermont & Ponton, 2003; Gordon et al, 2005; Kral et al, 2006; Sharma & Dorman, 2006; Gilley et al, 2008; Sharma et al, 2009). Houston and colleagues have shown significantly higher levels of word learning in children implanted under 13 months of age (Houston et al, 2012; Houston and Miyamoto, 2010) as compared with children implanted between 16 and 23 months of age. Other studies have shown that children implanted between 18 and 24 months of age demonstrate significantly greater language and vocabulary development—both expressive and receptive—than children implanted after 2 years of age (Hayes et al, 2009; Niparko et al, 2010; Markman et al, 2011; Boons et al, 2012).

Though it has been demonstrated that younger is better for a child's auditory-oral language outcomes, children implanted after 2 years of age still derive *significant benefit*. The issue is that family counseling and education regarding realistic expectations need to consider the age at activation as a critical variable. Further, clinicians will inform families that more aggressive intervention may be needed for the child implanted after 2 years of age for whom the family's goal remains listening and spoken language with high levels of speech intelligibility.

Implant Use During All Waking Hours

While cochlear implants provide access to sound, the processor(s) must be worn all waking hours to derive maximum benefit. The Alexander Graham Bell Association for the Deaf and Hard of Hearing provides specific examples emphasizing the need for consistent device wear time. They report that an infant with normal hearing listens for ~ 10 hours each day, totaling at least 3,650 hours of listening over the first year of life. On the other hand, for the infant with part-time use of hearing aids during the candidacy process—estimated at just 4 hours per day—it would take 6 years to provide as much listening experience as the baby with normal hearing or the baby wearing hearing aids or implant sound processors all waking hours (Stovall, 1982; Rossi, 2003). A toddler/preschooler with normal hearing is estimated to be listening ~ 12 hours per day. Over the course of one year, that totals to 4,380 hours of listening. If a toddler/preschooler wears the implant sound processors part time—such as 2.75 hours per day while at preschool—it would take 9 years to provide the listening experience gained over a single year for the child with normal hearing or for the child making full-time use of the sound processors (Rossi, 2003).

Age at implantation is just one critical variable regarding outcomes. Regardless of the age at implantation, if full-time use of the sound processor(s) is not enforced, *a child will not make progress*. The importance of wear time is a critical pre- and postimplant counseling point and one that bears repetition at multiple visits with the family and all caregivers.

Intervention

The best outcomes are not achieved simply with early implantation and wear time. The highest auditory-oral language outcomes are achieved in conjunction with early and consistent intervention (e.g., Hayes et al, 2009; Nicholas & Geers, 2007; Moeller, 2000; Moog & Geers, 2010). Early enrollment in comprehensive intervention programs, incorporating parental/family involvement and focusing on listening and spoken language, is associated with higher levels of receptive and expressive language for school-age children with cochlear implants (Moeller, 2000; Moog & Geers, 2010). The best outcomes will be achieved with regular and intensive habilitation, including regular speech-language therapy, continuation of infant and family services with home-based infant/family specialists, enrollment in parent-infant programs, and later involvement in a preschool program focusing on listening and spoken language. Cochlear implantation and activation represent the first steps in the hearing journey, with the majority of the "work" occurring thereafter.

An auditory-oral (listening and spoken language) approach to communication may not be the goal of every family, nor may it be a reasonable goal based on factors such as the age of identification, age at implantation, family dynamics, and/or other developmental delays associated with the underlying etiology or other diagnoses. There are modes of communication that incorporate signing, cued speech, augmentative communication, or any combination thereof that may ultimately serve as a better fit for a given child. Though the family's goal for communication and education should be paramount, considering child-specific expectations that may change over time allows for the highest level of family-centered counseling and service delivery.

Anatomy of Cochlear and Neural Structures

Anatomic anomalies involving the bony labyrinth, cochlear lumen, or internal auditory canal have the potential to affect postoperative outcomes. Up to 35% of children with SNHL also have cochleovestibular structural abnormalities (Papsin, 2005). Structural abnormalities that may be uncovered in the pediatric population include Mondini dysplasia, common cavity, enlarged vestibular aqueduct (EVA), and atretic or absent internal auditory canal. Structural abnormalities such as these would be observed via CT imaging and would thus be diagnosed prior to implantation, provided that temporal bone CT had been completed.

Cochlear nerve deficiency (CND) is another possible, though rare, neural structural abnormality that may be uncovered for a child with profound SNHL. CND is associated with an absent or hypoplastic auditory nerve. For children with CND and absent auditory nerve, cochlear implantation is contraindicated. The reason is that the primary auditory neurons (i.e., spiral ganglion cells located within the modiolus) are the neural targets for cochlear implant stimulation. Children with auditory nerve hypoplasticity tend to achieve poorer postoperative outcomes with cochlear implantation, yet implants can still offer significant communicative benefit (Breneman et al, 2012; Teagle et al, 2010; Buchman et al, 2011; Seymour et al, 2010). CND is diagnosed via MRI imaging and would be diagnosed prior to implantation.

Auditory neuropathy is yet another diagnosis that has the potential to impact outcomes. A diagnosis of auditory neuropathy can be associated with a true neuropathy of the auditory branch of cranial nerve VIII, which is typically associated with other peripheral neuropathies. Auditory neuropathy can also involve auditory neuropathy spectrum disorder (ANSD), which is typically associated with pediatric diagnoses (see Chapter 32). A diagnosis of ANSD includes variable levels of audiometric thresholds, poorer than expected speech recognition, generally absent acoustic reflexes, presence of OAEs that are incongruent with the audiogram, and presence of cochlear microphonic with either absent or abnormal auditory brainstem response (ABR) (e.g., Starr, Picton, Sininger, Hood, & Berlin, 1996; Berlin, Hood, Cecola, Jackson, & Szabo, 1993; Berlin et al, 2005, 2010.)

A true auditory nerve neuropathy is important to diagnose prior to considering cochlear implantation, as it can significantly affect outcomes. The term "neuropathy" implies neural damage or dysfunction. Cochlear implantation is generally contraindicated in cases of auditory neuropathy in which the integrity of the auditory nerve is significantly compromised. True auditory nerve neuropathy is rarely diagnosed in childhood and, when present, is most frequently a diagnosis secondary to a primary peripheral neuropathy, as in Charcot–Marie–Tooth disease.

Etiology

The underlying etiology of hearing loss for a large proportion of pediatric patients will be unknown. Approximately half of all congenital hearing losses have an underlying genetic component—though this estimate will likely increase as advances in human genomic research are realized (Rehm, 2005). For most pediatric patients, concerns about etiology will not affect counseling for postoperative outcomes—at least not at the time of implantation. There are, however, some etiologies associated with poorer postoperative outcomes for pediatric implant recipients. Some of the more common etiologies and associated concerns follow.

Meningitis

Bacterial meningitis accounts for ~ 6% of cases involving acquired SNHL in infancy and childhood (Smith, Bale, & White, 2005). Though the pneumococcal conjugate vaccine has significantly reduced the incidence of bacterial meningitis in children, ~ 5 to 10% of meningitic cases result in severe to profound SNHL (Baraff, Lee, & Schriger, 1993; Smith et al, 2005). The underlying cause of sensorineural hearing loss associated with bacterial meningitis is related to the development of labyrinthitis, loss of hair cells, spiral ganglion cell degeneration, and cochlear ossification (Lu & Schuknecht, 1994; Nadol & Hsu, 1991). More specifically, cochlear ossification and spiral ganglion degeneration can further result in bony obliteration of the cochlea, loss of auditory function, and poorer postoperative outcomes.

In cases of severe cochlear ossification, the surgeon may not be able to achieve a full insertion of the electrode array, resulting in a limited number of intracochlear electrodes that elicit auditory perception. In cases of shallow insertion depth or spiral ganglion cell degeneration, it is also possible that the implanted electrodes yield little to no auditory stimulation. Postoperative outcomes with meningitis and cochlear ossification are highly variable and therefore difficult to predict (Nichani et al, 2011). Not all cases of meningitis result in cochlear ossification, but for those children exhibiting evidence of preoperative ossification, counseling with respect to realistic expectations is vital.

Syndromic-Related Deafness

There are several syndromes for which various degrees of SNHL are expected. There are, however, many reports of successful cochlear implantation in children with syndromic hearing loss, including branchial-oto-renal (BOR) syndrome; coloboma, heart anomaly, choanal atresia, retardation, genital, and ear (CHARGE) syndrome; Pendred syndrome; Refsum disease; Usher syndrome; and Waardenburg syndrome (e.g., Loundon et al, 2003; Raine, Kurukulasuriya, Bajaj, & Strachan, 2008; Cullen et al, 2006; Vescan, Parnes, Cucci, Smith, & MacNeill, 2002; Arndt et al, 2010; Lina-Granade, Porot, Vesson, & Truy, 2010). Syndromes also known to be related to progressive loss of vision—such as Usher syndrome and Refsum disease—have considerable potential to affect outcomes, as speech-language therapy and everyday communication makes use of visual cues. Syndromes that may affect global development and cognition, such as CHARGE, may also affect outcomes and thus require extensive preimplant counseling regarding appropriate expectations and communication-related goals following implantation.

Chromosomal-Related Deafness

Trisomy 21, more commonly known as Down syndrome, is most commonly linked with SNHL. SNHL is observed in ~ 5 to 20% of cases, with severe to profound deafness present in 5% or fewer cases (Roizen, Wolters, Nicol, & Blondis, 1993; Hans, England, Prowse, Young, & Sheehan, 2010). Cochlear implantation is a viable treatment option for children with Down syndrome and significant SNHL (Hans et al, 2010; Cruz et al, 2012). Expectations for progress and communication following activation are heavily dependent upon the child's cognitive status as well as the increased risk for middle ear disease. Given that children with Down syndrome have a predisposition for recurrent middle ear disease, it is particularly important that appropriate vaccinations are up to date should a family pursue cochlear implantation.

Other Variables Affecting Postoperative Outcomes

Several multicenter longitudinal studies examining postoperative outcomes for pediatric implant recipients have demonstrated that the number of variables potentially affecting outcomes is large and includes age at implantation, type and frequency of early intervention, educational placement, and postoperative degree of audibility with implants, as well as several variables of familial and social relevance (e.g., Niparko et al, 2010; Barker et al, 2009; Geers,

Brenner, & Davidson, 2003; Szagun & Stumper, 2012). Family and social outcomes most likely to have an impact on postoperative outcomes for language development and speech recognition were family size, intelligence, socioeconomic status, maternal level of education, and the amount of time spent talking to the child at home. Obviously not all of these variables are appropriate to discuss during preoperative counseling, such as family size, maternal level of education, and socioeconomic status. One variable that needs considerable discussion during both the pre- and postactivation periods is the amount of time spent talking to the child at home. Such behaviors should commence well before the surgery date, as they foster a learned behavior/habit of incorporating language modeling and functional auditory-oral communication throughout the day for all family members living in the home.

◆ Outcomes

As discussed up to this point, postactivation outcomes for speech and language development and auditory-only speech understanding can be highly variable because of several hearing- and non-hearing-related issues. In the best cases, children with cochlear implants demonstrate a normal to near-normal trajectory of auditory-oral speech, language, and vocabulary growth (e.g., Niparko et al, 2010; Geers et al, 2003; Yoshinaga-Itano, Baca, & Sedey, 2010) and exhibit high levels of academic success within a mainstream educational placement. In cases where children are implanted at older ages, have additional diagnoses or comorbidities affecting cognition, behavior, or global development, or have incorporated manual communication, the rate of auditory-oral growth in speech, language, and vocabulary will expectedly be slower.

Communication goals are different for every family and should be set individually for every child based on ability, environment, and family goals for communication and quality of life. It is rare that a cochlear implant yields little to no discernible benefit for a child and his/her family. Nevertheless, there are children who ultimately become nonusers of their implants as a result of several factors that may include repeated device failure,[3] behavioral issues, old age at implantation, or changing family goals regarding mode of communica-

tion or educational placement (Raine, Summerfield, Strachan, Martin, & Totten, 2008).

◆ Conclusion

Cochlear implant candidate selection for the pediatric population is not necessarily a straightforward process. The determination of cochlear implant candidacy, implantation, activation, and postoperative management are truly a *process* that is accomplished via the collective teamwork of an interdisciplinary group of professionals. Many patients and their families are astonished at the intricacies involved in a cochlear implant evaluation and in the long-term management of the pediatric implant recipient. Given the expansion of cochlear implant criteria for children and increasing research in this area, the cochlear implant selection process and postoperative follow-up will undoubtedly continue to evolve and expand rapidly.

Cochlear implants have the potential to change the course of a child's life and, in the best cases, allow for normal development of audition, speech, and language. Even for children not able to achieve an auditory/oral (listening and spoken language) approach to speech and language, cochlear implants provide sound awareness, increasing safety and improving quality of life for the recipient (e.g., Loy, Warner-Czyz, Tong, Tobey, & Roland, 2010; Clark et al, 1987; Edwards, Hill, & Mahon, 2012). It is important to recognize that pediatric candidacy criteria have dramatically evolved over the past several decades and that cochlear implants are no longer only for children with bilateral profound deafness. The interdisciplinary cochlear implant team offers patients the highest level of care and information needed to progress from the candidacy selection process to a successful activation and postoperative development of auditory-based communication.

Discussion Questions

1. List the different disciplines that are typically part of a cochlear implant team.
2. Describe the candidacy evaluation process from the perspective of an audiologist.
3. How can you approach a child with moderate to severe sensory hearing loss who, despite making full-time use of amplification, is not making expected auditory and language development?
4. What variables affect outcomes? Over which variables do families have control?

---

[3] Cochlear implant device failure in pediatric populations has been estimated to range from 2.9% (Eskander et al, 2011) up to 10% over device analysis periods up to 18 years postimplant (Soli & Zheng, 2010).

References

American Academy of Audiology (AAA). (2003). Pediatric Amplification Protocol. www.audiology.org (accessed May 2, 2012).

American Academy of Pediatrics, Joint Committee on Infant Hearing. (2007). Year 2007 position statement: Principles and guidelines for early hearing detection and intervention programs. Pediatrics, 120(4), 898–921.

Anderson, K. L., & Smaldino, J. (1999). Listening inventories for education: A classroom measurement tool. The Hearing Journal, 52, 74–76.

Arndt, S., Laszig, R., Beck, R., Schild, C., Maier, W., Birkenhäger, R., . . . Aschendorff, A. (2010). Spectrum of hearing disorders and their management in children with CHARGE syndrome. Otology & Neurotology, 31(1), 67–73.

Baraff, L. J., Lee, S. I., & Schriger, D. L. (1993). Outcomes of bacterial meningitis in children: a meta-analysis. The Pediatric Infectious Disease Journal, 12(5), 389–394.

Barker, D. H., Quittner, A. L., Fink, N. E., Eisenberg, L. S., Tobey, E. A., Niparko, J. K.; CDaCI Investigative Team. (2009). Predicting behavior problems in deaf and hearing children: the influences of language, attention, and parent-child communication. Development and Psychopathology, 21(2), 373–392.

Bergeson, T. R., Houston, D. M., & Miyamoto, R. T. (2010). Effects of congenital hearing loss and cochlear implantation on audiovisual speech perception in infants and children. Restorative Neurology and Neuroscience, 28(2), 157–165.

Berlin, C. I., Hood, L. J., Cecola, R. P., Jackson, D. F., & Szabo, P. (1993). Does type I afferent neuron dysfunction reveal itself through lack of efferent suppression? Hearing Research, 65(1–2), 40–50.

Berlin, C. I., Hood, L. J., Morlet, T., Wilensky, D., St John, P., Montgomery, E., & Thibodaux, M. (2005). Absent or elevated middle ear muscle reflexes in the presence of normal otoacoustic emissions: a universal finding in 136 cases of auditory neuropathy/dys-synchrony. Journal of the American Academy of Audiology, 16(8), 546–553.

Berlin, C. I., Hood, L. J., Morlet, T., Wilensky, D., Li, L., Mattingly, K. R., . . . Frisch, S. A. (2010). Multi-site diagnosis and management of 260 patients with auditory neuropathy/dys-synchrony (auditory neuropathy spectrum disorder). International Journal of Audiology, 49(1), 30–43.

Bess, F. H., Sinclair, J. S., & Riggs, D. E. (1984). Group amplification in schools for the hearing impaired. Ear and Hearing, 5(3), 138–144.

Boons, T., Brokx, J. P., Dhooge, I., Frijns, J. H., Peeraer, L., Vermeulen, A., . . . van Wieringen, A. (2012). Predictors of spoken language development following pediatric cochlear implantation. Ear and Hearing, 33(5), 617–639.

Breneman, A. I., Gifford, R. H., & Dejong, M. D. (2012). Cochlear implantation in children with auditory neuropathy spectrum disorder: long-term outcomes. Journal of the American Academy of Audiology, 23(1), 5–17.

Buchman, C. A., Teagle, H. F., Roush, P. A., Park, L. R., Hatch, D., Woodard, J., . . . Adunka, O. F. (2011). Cochlear implantation in children with labyrinthine anomalies and cochlear nerve deficiency: implications for auditory brainstem implantation. The Laryngoscope, 121(9), 1979–1988.

Centers for Disease Control and Prevention. (2012). Use of vaccines to prevent meningitis in persons with cochlear implants. Retrieved from http://www.cdc.gov/vaccines/vpd-vac/mening/cochlear/dis-cochlear-gen.htm

Ching, T. Y., & Hill, M. (2007). The Parents' Evaluation of Aural/Oral Performance of Children (PEACH) scale: Normative data. Journal of the American Academy of Audiology, 18(3), 220–235.

Clark, W. W., & Govett, S. B. (1995). School-related noise exposure in children. Paper presented at the Association for Research in Otolaryngology Mid-Winter Meeting, St. Petersburg, FL.

Clark, G. M., Busby, P. A., Roberts, S. A., Dowell, R. C., Tong, Y. C., Blamey, P. J., Franz, B. K. (1987). Preliminary results for the Cochlear Corporation multielectrode intracochlear implant in six prelingually deaf patients. The American Journal of Otology, 8(3), 234–239.

Coninx, F., Weichbold, V., Tsiakpini, L., Autrique, E., Bescond, G., Tamas, L., . . . Brachmaier, J. (2009). Validation of the LittlEARS((R)) Auditory Questionnaire in children with normal hearing. International Journal of Pediatric Otorhinolaryngology, 73(12), 1761–1768.

Coplan, J. (1987). ELM Scale: The Early Language Milestone Scale (Revised). Austin, TX: Pro-Ed.

Cornelisse, L. E., Seewald, R. C., & Jamieson, D. G. (1995). The input/output formula: a theoretical approach to the fitting of personal amplification devices. The Journal of the Acoustical Society of America, 97(3), 1854–1864.

Cosetti, M., & Roland, J. T., Jr. (2010). Cochlear implantation in the very young child: issues unique to the under-1 population. Trends in Amplification, 14(1), 46–57.

Cruz, I., Vicaria, I., Wang, N. Y., Niparko, J., & Quittner, A. L.; CDaCI Investigative Team. (2012). Language and behavioral outcomes in children with developmental disabilities using cochlear implants. Otology & Neurotology, 33(5), 751–760.

Cullen, R. D., Zdanski, C., Roush, P., Brown, C., Teagle, H., Pillsbury, H. C., III, & Buchman, C. (2006). Cochlear implants in Waardenburg syndrome. The Laryngoscope, 116(7), 1273–1275.

Dettman, S. J., D'Costa, W. A., Dowell, R. C., Winton, E. J., Hill, K. L., & Williams, S. S. (2004). Cochlear implants for children with significant residual hearing. Archives of Otolaryngology–Head & Neck Surgery, 130(5), 612–618.

Dowell, R. C., Hollow, R., & Winton, E. (2004). Outcomes for cochlear implant users with significant residual hearing: implications for selection criteria in children. Archives of Otolaryngology–Head & Neck Surgery, 130(5), 575–581.

Edwards, L., Hill, T., & Mahon, M. (2012). Quality of life in children and adolescents with cochlear implants and additional needs. International Journal of Pediatric Otorhinolaryngology, 76(6), 851–857.

Eggermont, J. J., & Ponton, C. W. (2003). Auditory-evoked potential studies of cortical maturation in normal hearing and implanted children: correlations with changes in structure and speech perception. Acta Oto-Laryngologica, 123(2), 249–252.

Eskander, A., Gordon, K. A., Kadhim, L., Papaioannou, V., Cushing, S. L., James, A. L., Papsin, B. C. (2011). Low pediatric cochlear implant failure rate: contributing factors in large-volume practice. Archives of Otolaryngology–Head & Neck Surgery, 137(12), 1190–1196.

Finitzo-Hieber, T. (1988). Classroom acoustics. In R. Roeser (Ed.), Auditory disorders in school children (2nd ed., pp. 221–223). New York, NY: Thieme-Stratton.

Food and Drug Administration. (2011). "Off-Label" and investigational use of marketed drugs, biologics, and medical devices. Retrieved from http://www.fda.gov/RegulatoryInformation/Guidances/ucm126486.htm

Fortnum, H. M., Marshall, D. H., & Summerfield, A. Q. (2002). Epidemiology of the UK population of hearing-impaired children, including characteristics of those with and without cochlear implants–audiology, aetiology, comorbidity and affluence. International Journal of Audiology, 4, 170–179.

Gallaudet Research Institute. (2008). Regional and national summary report of data from the 2008 Annual Survey of Deaf and Hard of Hearing Children and Youth. Washington, DC: Gallaudet University.

Geers, A., Brenner, C., & Davidson, L. (2003). Factors associated with development of speech perception skills in children implanted by age five. Ear and Hearing, 24(1, Suppl), 24S–35S.

Gelnett, D., Sumida, A., Nilsson, M., & Soli, S. D. (1995). Development of the Hearing in Noise Test for Children (HINT-C). Annual Meeting of the American Academy of Audiology, Dallas.

Gilley, P. M., Sharma, A., & Dorman, M. F. (2008). Cortical reorganization in children with cochlear implants. Brain Research, 1239, 56–65.

Gordon, K. A., Tanaka, S., & Papsin, B. C. (2005). Atypical cortical responses underlie poor speech perception in children using cochlear implants. Neuroreport, 16(18), 2041–2045.

Gravel, J. S., White, K. R., Johnson, J. L., Widen, J. E., Vohr, B. R., James, M., ... & Meyer, S. (2005). A multisite study to examine the efficacy of the otoacoustic emission/automated auditory brainstem response newborn hearing screening protocol: recommendations for policy, practice, and research. American Journal of Audiology, 14(2), S217–S228.

Gupta, P., & MacWhinney, B. (1997). Vocabulary acquisition and verbal short-term memory: computational and neural bases. Brain and Language, 59(2), 267–333.

Habib, M. G., Waltzman, S. B., Tajudeen, B., & Svirsky, M. A. (2010). Speech production intelligibility of early implanted pediatric cochlear implant users. International Journal of Pediatric Otorhinolaryngology, 74(8), 855–859.

Hans, P. S., England, R., Prowse, S., Young, E., & Sheehan, P. Z. (2010). UK and Ireland experience of cochlear implants in children with Down syndrome. International Journal of Pediatric Otorhinolaryngology, 74(3), 260–264.

Haskins, H. L. (1949). A phonetically balanced test of speech discrimination for children. Master's thesis, Northwestern University, Evanston, IL.

Hayes, H., Geers, A. E., Treiman, R., & Moog, J. S. (2009). Receptive vocabulary development in deaf children with cochlear implants: achievement in an intensive auditory-oral educational setting. Ear and Hearing, 30(1), 128–135.

Hedley-Williams, A., Bagatto, M., Boscini, E., & Gifford, R. H. (2012). Outcome measures for pediatric cochlear implant recipients. Paper presented at the American Academy of Audiology, AudiologyNOW, March 26, 2012. Boston, MA.

Hollich, G., Jusczyk, P., & Luce, P. (2002). Lexical neighborhood effects in 17-month-old word learning. In Proceedings of the 26th Annual Boston University Conference on Language Development (pp. 314–323). Boston, MA: Cascadilla.

Houston, D. M., & Jusczyk, P. W. (2003). Infants' long-term memory for the sound patterns of words and voices. Journal of Experimental Psychology. Human Perception and Performance, 29(6), 1143–1154.

Houston, D. M., & Miyamoto, R. T. (2010). Effects of early auditory experience on word learning and speech perception in deaf children with cochlear implants: implications for sensitive periods of language development. Otology & neurotology: official publication of the American Otological Society, American Neurotology Society. European Academy of Otology and Neurotology, 31(8), 1248.

Houston, D. M., Stewart, J., Moberly, A., Hollich, G., & Miyamoto, R. T. (2012). Word learning in deaf children with cochlear implants: effects of early auditory experience. Developmental Science, 15(3), 448–461.

Jusczyk, P. W. (2002). Some critical developments in acquiring native language sound organization during the first year. The Annals of Otology, Rhinology & Laryngology. Supplement, 189, 11–15.

Jusczyk, P. W., & Hohne, E. A. (1997). Infants' memory for spoken words. Science, 277(5334), 1984–1986.

Kim, L. S., Jeong, S. W., Lee, Y. M., & Kim, J. S. (2010). Cochlear implantation in children. Auris, Nasus, Larynx, 37(1), 6–17.

Kirk, K. I., Pisoni, D. B., & Osberger, M. J. (1995). Lexical effects on spoken word recognition by pediatric cochlear implant users. Ear and Hearing, 16(5), 470–481.

Kral, A., Tillein, J., Heid, S., Klinke, R., & Hartmann, R. (2006). Cochlear implants: cortical plasticity in congenital deprivation. Progress in Brain Research, 157, 283–313.

Leigh, J., Dettman, S., Dowell, R., & Sarant, J. (2011). Evidence-based approach for making cochlear implant recommendations for infants with residual hearing. Ear and Hearing, 32(3), 313–322.

Lin, F. R., Ceh, K., Bervinchak, D., Riley, A., Miech, R., & Niparko, J. K. (2007). Development of a communicative performance scale for pediatric cochlear implantation. Ear and Hearing, 28(5), 703–712.

Lina-Granade, G., Porot, M., Vesson, J. F., & Truy, E. (2010). More about cochlear implantation in children with CHARGE association. Cochlear Implants International, 11(Suppl 1), 187–191.

Loundon, N., Marlin, S., Busquet, D., Denoyelle, F., Roger, G., Renaud, F., & Garabedian, E. N. (2003). Usher syndrome and cochlear implantation. Otology & Neurotology, 24(2), 216–221.

Loy, B., Warner-Czyz, A. D., Tong, L., Tobey, E. A., & Roland, P. S. (2010). The children speak: an examination of the quality of life of pediatric cochlear implant users. Otolaryngology–Head and Neck Surgery, 142(2), 247–253.

Lu, C. B., & Schuknecht, H. F. (1994). Pathology of prelingual profound deafness: magnitude of labyrinthitis fibro-ossificans. Otology & Neurotology, 15(1), 74–85.

Markman, T. M., Quittner, A. L., Eisenberg, L. S., Tobey, E. A., Thal, D., Niparko, J. K., Wang, N. Y.; CDaCI Investigative Team. (2011). Language development after cochlear implantation: an epigenetic model. Journal Neurodevelopmental Disorders, 3(4), 388–404.

Meinzen-Derr, J., Wiley, S., Creighton, J., & Choo, D. (2007). Auditory Skills Checklist: clinical tool for monitoring functional auditory skill development in young children with cochlear implants. The Annals of Otology, Rhinology, and Laryngology, 116(11), 812–818.

Moeller, M. P. (2000). Early intervention and language development in children who are deaf and hard of hearing. Pediatrics, 106(3), E43.

Moog, J. S., & Geers, A. E.(1990). Early speech perception test for profoundly hearing-impaired children. St. Louis, MO: Central Institute for the Deaf.

Moog, J. S., & Geers, A. E. (2010). Early educational placement and later language outcomes for children with cochlear implants. Otology & Neurotology, 31(8), 1315–1319.

Nadol, J. B., Jr, & Hsu, W. C. (1991). Histopathologic correlation of spiral ganglion cell count and new bone formation in the cochlea following meningogenic labyrinthitis and deafness. The Annals of Otology, Rhinology, and Laryngology, 100(9 Pt 1), 712–716.

National Institutes of Health. (1993). Early identification of hearing impairment in infants and young children. NIH Consensus Development Conference Statement. Retrieved from http://consensus.nih.gov/1993/1993HearingInfants Children092html.htm

Nichani, J., Green, K., Hans, P., Bruce, I., Henderson, L., & Ramsden, R. (2011). Cochlear implantation after bacterial meningitis in children: outcomes in ossified and nonossified cochleas. Otology & Neurotology, 32(5), 784–789.

Nicholas, J. G., & Geers, A. E. (2007). Will they catch up? The role of age at cochlear implantation in the spoken language development of children with severe to profound hearing loss. Journal of Speech, Language, and Hearing Research: JSLHR, 50(4), 1048–1062.

Niparko, J. K., Tobey, E. A., Thal, D. J., Eisenberg, L. S., Wang, N. Y., Quittner, A. L., Fink, N. E.; CDaCI Investigative Team. (2010). Spoken language development in children following cochlear implantation. Journal of the American Medical Association, 303(15), 1498–1506.

Nober, L., & Nober, E. (1975). Auditory discrimination of learning disabled children in quiet and classroom noise. Journal of Learning Disabilities, 8, 656–773.

Olsen, W. O. (1998). Average speech levels and spectra in various speaking/listening conditions: A summary of the Pearson, Bennett, & Fidell (1977) report. American Journal of Audiology, 7(2), 21.

Palmer, C. V., & Mormer, E. (1999). Goals and expectations of the hearing aid fitting. Trends in Amplification, 4, 61–71.

Papsin, B. C. (2005). Cochlear implantation in children with anomalous cochleovestibular anatomy. The Laryngoscope, 115(1 Pt 2, Suppl 106), 1–26.

Pearsons, K. S., Bennett, R. L., & Fidell, S. (1977). Speech levels in various noise environments. Washington, DC: Office of Health and Ecological Effects, Office of Research and Development, US EPA.

Peterson, A., Shallop, J., Driscoll, C., Breneman, A., Babb, J., Stoeckel, R., & Fabry, L. (2003). Outcomes of cochlear implantation in children with auditory neuropathy. Journal of the American Academy of Audiology, 14(4), 188–201.

Ponton, C. W., Eggermont, J. J., Don, M., Waring, M. D., Kwong, B., Cunningham, J., & Trautwein, P. (2000). Maturation of the mismatch negativity: effects of profound deafness and cochlear implant use. Audiology & Neuro-Otology, 5(3–4), 167–185.

Raine, C. H., Kurukulasuriya, M. F., Bajaj, Y., & Strachan, D. R. (2008). Cochlear implantation in Refsum's disease. Cochlear Implants International, 9(2), 97–102.

Raine, C. H., Summerfield, Q., Strachan, D. R., Martin, J. M., & Totten, C. (2008). The cost and analysis of nonuse of cochlear implants. Otology & Neurotology, 29(2), 221–224.

Rance, G., & Barker, E. J. (2008). Speech perception in children with auditory neuropathy/dyssynchrony managed with either hearing aids or cochlear implants. Otology & Neurotology, 29(2), 179–182.

Rehm, H. L. (2005). A genetic approach to the child with sensorineural hearing loss. Seminars in Perinatology, 29(3), 173–181.

Robbins, A. M., Renshaw, J. J., & Berry, S. W. (1991). Evaluating meaningful auditory integration in profoundly hearing-impaired children. Otology & Neurotology, 12(3, Suppl), 144–150.

Roberts, C., & Hindley, P. (1999). The assessment and treatment of deaf children with psychiatric disorders. Journal of Child Psychology and Psychiatry, and Allied Disciplines, 40(2), 151–167.

Roeser, R. J., & Clark, J. L. (2008). Live voice speech recognition audiometry—stop the madness! Audiology Today, 20(1), 32.

Roizen, N. J., Wolters, C., Nicol, T., & Blondis, T. A. (1993). Hearing loss in children with Down syndrome. The Journal of Pediatrics, 123(1), S9–S12.

Rossi, K. (2003). Learn to talk around the clock. Washington, DC: AG Bell.

Sanders, D. A. (1965). Noise conditions in normal school classrooms. Exceptional Children, 31, 344–353.

Scollie, S., Seewald, R., Cornelisse, L., Moodie, S., Bagatto, M., Laurnagaray, D., . . . Pumford, J. (2005). The Desired Sensation Level multistage input/output algorithm. Trends in Amplification, 9(4), 159–197.

Seewald, R. C., Ross, M., & Spiro, M. K. (1985). Selecting amplification characteristics for young hearing-impaired children. Ear and Hearing, 6(1), 48–53.

Seymour, F. K., Cruise, A., Lavy, J. A., Bradley, J., Beale, T., Graham, J. M., & Saeed, S. R. (2010). Congenital profound hearing loss: management of hypoplastic and aplastic vestibulocochlear nerves. Cochlear Implants International. 11(Suppl 1), 213–216.

Shallop, J. K., Peterson, A., Facer, G. W., Fabry, L. B., & Driscoll, C. L. (2001). Cochlear implants in five cases of auditory neuropathy: postoperative findings and progress. The Laryngoscope, 111(4 Pt 1), 555–562.

Sharma, A., & Dorman, M. F. (2006). Central auditory development in children with cochlear implants: clinical implications. Advances in Oto-Rhino-Laryngology, 64, 66–88.

Sharma, A., Nash, A. A., & Dorman, M. (2009). Cortical development, plasticity and re-organization in children with cochlear implants. Journal of Communication Disorders, 42(4), 272–279.

Sharma, A., Dorman, M. F., & Spahr, A. J. (2002). A sensitive period for the development of the central auditory system in children with cochlear implants: implications for age of implantation. Ear and Hearing, 23(6), 532–539.

Smith, R. J., Bale, J. F., Jr, & White, K. R. (2005). Sensorineural hearing loss in children. Lancet, 365(9462), 879–890.

Soja, N. N., Carey, S., & Spelke, E. S. (1991). Ontological categories guide young children's inductions of word meaning: object terms and substance terms. Cognition, 38(2), 179–211.

Soli, S. D., & Zheng, Y. (2010). Long-term reliability of pediatric cochlear implants. Otology & Neurotology, 31(6), 899–901.

Starr, A., Picton, T. W., Sininger, Y., Hood, L. J., & Berlin, C. I. (1996). Auditory neuropathy. Brain, 119(Pt 3), 741–753.

Storkel, H. L. (2009). Developmental differences in the effects of phonological, lexical and semantic variables on word learning by infants. Journal of Child Language, 36(2), 291–321.

Stovall, D. (1982). Teaching speech to hearing impaired infants and children. Springfield, IL: Charles C. Thomas.

Stredler-Brown, A., & DeConde Johnson, C. (2003). Functional auditory performance indicators: An integrated approach to auditory development. Colorado Department of Education, Special EducationServices Unit. Retrieved from http://www.cde.state.co.us/cdesped/SpecificDisability-Hearing.html

Sunderhaus, L., Hedley-Williams, A., & Gifford, R. H. (2012). Evidence for the expansion of pediatric cochlear implant criteria. Presented at the 12th International Conference on Cochlear Implants and Other Implantable Auditory Technologies, Baltimore, MD.

Szagun, G., & Stumper, B. (2012). Age or experience? The influence of age at implantation and social and linguistic environment on language development in children with cochlear implants. Journal of Speech, Language, and Hearing Research: JSLHR, 55(6), 1640–1654.

Tajudeen, B. A., Waltzman, S. B., Jethanamest, D., & Svirsky, M. A. (2010). Speech perception in congenitally deaf children receiving cochlear implants in the first year of life. Otology & Neurotology, 31(8), 1254–1260.

Teagle, H. F., Roush, P. A., Woodard, J. S., Hatch, D. R., Zdanski, C. J., Buss, E., . . . Wouters, J. (2010). Audiology & Neuro-Otology, 15(1), 7–17.

Tomblin, J. B., Barker, B. A., Spencer, L. J., Zhang, X., & Gantz, B. J. (2005, Aug). The effect of age at cochlear implant initial stimulation on expressive language growth in infants and toddlers. Journal of Speech, Language, and Hearing Research: JSLHR, 48(4), 853–867.

Van Naarden, K., Decouflé, P., & Caldwell, K. (1999, Mar). Prevalence and characteristics of children with serious hearing impairment in metropolitan Atlanta, 1991–1993. Pediatrics, 103(3), 570–575.

Vescan, A., Parnes, L. S., Cucci, R. A., Smith, R. J., & MacNeill, C. (2002). Cochlear implantation and Pendred's syndrome mutation in monozygotic twins with large vestibular aqueduct syndrome. The Journal of Otolaryngology, 31(1), 54–57.

Weichbold, V., Tsiakpini, L., Coninx, F., & D'Haese, P. (2005). Development of a parent questionnaire for assessment of auditory behaviour of infants up to two years of age [in German]. Laryngo- Rhino- Otologie, 84(5), 328–334.

White, K. R., Behrens, T. R., & Strickland, B. (1995). Practicality, validity, and cost-fficiency of universal newborn hearing screening using transient evoked otoacoustic emissions. Journal for Children with Communication Disorders, 17, 9–14.

Yoshinaga-Itano, C., Baca, R. L., & Sedey, A. L. (2010). Describing the trajectory of language development in the presence of severe-to-profound hearing loss: a closer look at children with cochlear implants versus hearing aids. Otology & Neurotology, 31(8), 1268–1274.

Zimmerman-Phillips, S., Robbins, A. M., & Osberger, M. J. (2000). Assessing cochlear implant benefit in very young children. The Annals of Otology, Rhinology & Laryngology. Supplement, 185, 42–43.

Chapter 23

Acoustic Accessibility: Room Acoustics and Remote Microphone Use in Home and School Environments

Joseph Smaldino and Carol Flexer

Key Points

- The classroom is an auditory verbal environment in which accurate transmission and reception of speech between the teacher and students, or between students and students, is critical for effective learning to occur.

- Speech intelligibility is based on the science of signal-to-noise ratio (SNR), the relationship of the desired signal to all background and competing noise; children need the desired signal to be 10 times, or 15 to 20 dB louder than, background noise to discriminate words clearly.

- Classroom Audio Distribution System (CADS) technology is an exciting educational tool that allows control of the acoustic environment in a classroom, thereby facilitating acoustic accessibility of teacher instruction for all children in the room.

- Efficacy of technology use may be measured through educational performance, behavioral speech perception analyses, direct measures of changes in brain development, or functional assessments.

- The purpose of all environmental and technological management strategies is to enhance the reception of clear and intact acoustic signals to access, develop, and organize the auditory centers of the brain. Accordingly, this chapter will discuss classroom acoustics and the frequency modulation (FM) and infrared (IR) technologies that are necessary to improve access to the learning environment for all children.

◆ Classroom Acoustics: An Overview

The classroom is an auditory verbal environment in which accurate transmission and reception of speech between the teacher and students and between students and students is critical for effective learning to occur. Since information is exchanged in a classroom, it can be modeled using an information theory approach. Modern information theory arose from Claude Shannon's 1948 paper, "A Mathematical Theory of Communication" (Shannon, 1948). By simplifying this theory, an understanding of the classroom acoustic environment and ways to maximize communication can occur. **Fig. 23.1** is an example of such an information transfer model.

In this model, the speaker and listener bring important variables to the communication process. The speaker must speak loudly enough for speech to be

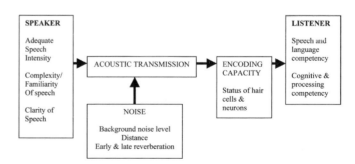

Fig. 23.1 A simplified version of Shannon's mathematical theory of communication.

audible. This audibility variable is influenced by the vocal effort of the speaker and the distance between the speaker and listener. The speaker must also present a clear, undistorted speech signal. Finally, the speaker can use speech that is either simple or complex, and the speech can be familiar or unfamiliar to the listener. The listener must have enough speech and language competency to use the efficiencies and redundancy resident in speech and language syntax, semantics, and phonology. In addition, the listener must have certain cognitive and processing competencies to retain and form auditory-linguistic linkages in the speech and language centers of the brain.

Separating the speaker and listener is the acoustic transmission path of the speech signal and encoding capacity of the listener. The transmission pathway can be quiet, or it can be noisy. If noisy, the noise can derive from loss of information caused by inaudibility, background noise that masks information, or reverberation that distorts and ultimately masks information. The encoding capacity of the listener is a measure of the intactness of the peripheral, brainstem, and central auditory mechanisms. Loss of hair cells or auditory neurons also can reduce the child's encoding capacity—the child's ability to perceive the message.

Any of these variables can influence the adequacy of the communication between speaker and listener and can occur in a multitude of combinations. The best-case scenario would be a speaker whose speech was audible and clear, using simple and familiar speech, standing close to a normal-hearing listener with fully developed and normal speech, language, and cognitive processes, in a room with little noise. The worst case would be a speaker whose speech is inaudible or distorted, using complex and unfamiliar speech, some distance from an individual who is severely hearing-impaired with incomplete speech, language, or cognitive processes, in a room with a lot of noise. Classroom communication environments are somewhere between these two extremes.

Although there has been much research on the effects of room acoustics on speech perception of individuals with hearing loss, **Fig. 23.1** shows that hearing impairment is one of several variables that can be managed to improve information transfer. The other variables can and should also be managed if inadequacy in a variable produces loss of information transfer. Management could include auditory processing therapy, speech therapy, cognitive therapy, hearing assistive devices, and management of the noise in the transmission path. Also, **Fig. 23.1** shows that breakdowns in information transfers are not solely dependent on hearing status. In other words, students with normal hearing but with weaknesses in any other of the highlighted variables will also have an information transfer problem. In addition, some of the variables, such as speech and language competency or cognitive competency, are developmental, so the younger the student, the more impact

these variables will have on information transfer, simply because they have not attained their final values. Each variable shown in **Fig. 23.1** is worthy of in-depth consideration, but this discussion will focus on the noise components.

> ### Pearl
>
> - The adequacy of the acoustic speech signal is an important variable in a classroom learning environment that can deleteriously affect accurate listening and successful learning.

The acoustic characteristics of the classroom mainly determine the adequacy of the speech signal received by the students. Of importance is the signal-to-noise ratio (SNR) of the teacher's speech received by the student and the reverberation time (RT) of the room. The SNR represents the relative intensity of the teacher's speech compared with the level of any background noise present in the classroom as measured at the location of the student. RT expresses the length of time a signal persists in a room after the original signal has ended. Sometimes this persistence of sound is referred to as sound reflection or echoes in the classroom. Research has demonstrated that inappropriate levels of classroom noise or reverberation can compromise not only speech perception but also reading scores, spelling ability, behavior, attention, and concentration in children with normal hearing and are even more deleterious to children with hearing loss or children who are at risk for listening and learning (see Crandell, Smaldino, & Flexer, 2005, and Smaldino & Flexer, 2012, for reviews of these studies).

Effects of SNR

Background noise in a room reduces speech recognition by covering up or masking important acoustic/linguistic cues in the message. This is especially true of the consonants, which carry most of the intelligibility of speech necessary for accurate perception. (See Chapter 19 for a discussion of speech acoustics.) Background noise in a room tends to mask the weaker consonant phonemes significantly more than it does the more intense vowel phonemes. The most important factor for accurate speech recognition, in this regard, is the ratio of the intensity of the desired signal to the intensity of the undesired signal or noise. This ratio is reported as the decibel difference between the two intensities. For example, if the speech was 15 dB louder than the background noise, the SNR would be +15 dB. Speech perception is generally better when speech is considerably louder than the noise and decreases as the SNR of the environment is reduced (Finitzo-Hieber & Tillman, 1978). Speech-recognition ability in adults with normal hearing is not significantly reduced until the SNR is below 0 dB (Bradley, 1986). Ample evidence indicates that children require a much better SNR than adults do (Boothroyd, 2004). The rationale for the better SNR is derived from the fact that children do not have fully developed auditory-linguistic and cognitive systems. Their immature systems limit the use of language redundancy and cognitive mechanisms, such as short-term memory, that can be used to overcome the masking effects on speech of too much background noise. To obtain speech recognition scores equal to those of normal hearers, listeners with sensorineural hearing loss (SNHL) require the SNR to be improved by 4 to 12 dB (Killion, 1997). An additional 3 to 6 dB are needed in rooms with moderate levels of reverberation (Hawkins & Yacullo, 1984). Based on these data, acoustic guidelines for populations who experience hearing loss suggest that SNRs should exceed +15 dB for accurate speech recognition.

Effects of RT

RT refers to the amount of time it takes for a steady-state sound to decrease 60 dB from its peak amplitude. In a reverberant room, speech is reflected from various hard room surfaces, so some of the speech elements are delayed in reaching the ear of the listener. The reflected speech overlaps with the direct speech signal (the signal not reflected before reaching the listener's ear) and covers up or masks certain acoustic speech components (Valente, Plevinsky, Franco, Heinrichs-Graham, & Lewis, 2012). Because vowels are more in-tense than consonants, a long RT tends to produce a prolongation of the spectral energy of vowels, which then covers up less intense consonant components. A reduction of consonant information can have a significant effect on speech recognition, as most acoustic information that is important for speech recognition is provided by consonants (French & Steinberg, 1947). Speech recognition, therefore, tends to decrease with increases in RT. Speech recognition in adults with normal hearing is not significantly degraded until the RT exceeds ~ 1 second. Listeners with SNHL, however, need considerably shorter RT (0.4 to 0.5 seconds) for optimal communication (Crandell et al, 2005). Because of this increased difficulty, acoustic guidelines for populations who experience hearing loss suggest that RT should not exceed 0.4 to 0.5 seconds in communication environments frequented by these individuals (American Speech-Language-Hearing Association [ASHA], 1995, 2005).

Effects of SNR and RT Together

The effects of RT and SNR interact. That is, when the factors are combined (which is the case in virtually all real-world listening environments), the combination affects speech recognition more than either of the factors alone does. Finitzo-Hieber and Tillman (1978) eloquently demonstrated this combination effect. A summary of their findings is shown in **Table 23.1**.

Table 23.1 shows the mean speech recognition scores of children with normal hearing and children with SNHL for monosyllabic words across various SNRs

Table 23.1 Mean speech recognition scores (% correct) by children with normal hearing and children with SNHL for monosyllabic words across various SNR and RT values

RT	SNR	Normal hearing	Hearing impaired
0.0 seconds	Quiet	94.5	83.0
	+12 dB	89.2	70.0
	+6 dB	79.7	59.5
	0 dB	60.2	39.0
0.4 seconds	Quiet	92.5	74.0
	+12 dB	82.8	60.2
	+6 dB	71.3	52.2
	0 dB	47.7	27.8
1.2 seconds	Quiet	76.5	45.0
	+12 dB	68.8	41.2
	+6 dB	54.2	27.0
	0 dB	29.7	11.2

Abbreviation: RT, reverberation time; SNR, signal-to-noise ratio.
Source: Table adapted from Finitzo-Hieber and Tillman (1978).

and RTs. At an SNR of +12 dB and RT of 0.4 seconds, children with normal hearing do not recognize speech perfectly (83%), and children with hearing impairment perform even more poorly (60%). As the SNR decreases or as the RT lengthens, speech recognition decreases to the worst case studied (SNR = 0 dB; RT = 1.2 seconds), where children with normal hearing achieve a 30% score and children with hearing loss recognize virtually none of the speech (11%). Both of these listening conditions have been reported in classroom environments. Imagine trying to succeed in school perceiving only 11% of what the teacher presents orally!

Another dramatic example of the interplay between classroom acoustics and speech was reported by Leavitt and Flexer (1991). Using the Rapid Speech Transmission Index (RASTI), they demonstrated that 83% of the speech energy, delivered in the front of a classroom, was available to a listener in the front row of a typical classroom-sized environment. However, in the back row of the same classroom, only ~ 50% of the speech energy was available. RASTI is a measure of speech energy as it traverses a room and is an index of the amount of energy available to be perceived when influenced by SNR and RT, not the amount actually perceived. Even less of the signal would be available if the listener has hearing loss or reduced auditory and language processing. These factors would hamper the student's actual perception of the available speech energy. That is, add the impact of the classroom acoustical environment to the distortion imposed by a damaged auditory or linguistic system, and it becomes apparent why simply using a hearing aid is not likely to result in satisfactory communication in the classroom (Wróblewski, Lewis, Valente, & Stelmachowicz, 2012).

◆ Classroom Acoustic Guidelines and Standards

The American National Standards Institute (ANSI) issued Standard S12.60 for classroom acoustics, including performance criteria, design requirements, and guidelines (ANSI, 2002, 2009, 2010). As most recently revised, this standard recommends background noise level of no more than 35 dB(A) (ANSI, 2009, 2010). The newer standard provides a phase-in of background noise level criteria for relocatable classrooms. Studies have reported that these acoustic criteria are infrequently achieved in the academic setting (Crandell & Smaldino, 1995; Knecht, Nelson, Whitelaw, & Feth, 2002; Nelson, Smaldino, Erler, & Garstecki, 2008).

Noise Effects on Student and Teacher Performance

In addition to affecting speech recognition directly, background noise can also compromise academic achievement, literacy, and attendant listening and learning behaviors in the classroom (Anderson, 2001). Rosenberg (2005) completed a comprehensive review of studies that have explored the effects of undesirable levels of background noise. What is striking from reading these studies is that, no matter what the variable under study, a better performance was obtained as the SNR improved in virtually every case.

The widespread nature of excessive noise in the classroom was underscored in a 1998 survey of school administrators. The General Accounting Office found that inappropriate classroom acoustics was the most commonly cited problem that affected the learning environment (Access Board, 1998). In addition, the negative effects of undesirable levels of background noise on teachers have been reported. Sapienza, Crandell, and Curtis (1999) showed that teachers exhibit a significantly higher incidence of vocal problems than the general population. It is reasonable to assume that these vocal difficulties are caused, at least in part, by teachers' having to increase vocal output to overcome the effects of classroom noise during the school day (Blair, 2006).

Effects of Reverberation

As previously discussed, speech recognition in adults with normal hearing is not significantly affected until the RT exceeds ~ 1.0 second. For listeners with SNHL, most investigators have recommended that RTs for listening environments should not exceed ~ 0.4 second (through the speech frequency range: 500, 1000, and 2000 Hz) to provide optimum communicative efficiency (Wróblewski et al, 2012). For permanent buildings, the current American national classroom acoustics standard (ANSI, 2010) recommends an RT of 0.6 seconds or less for average-sized classrooms and 0.4 seconds if the classroom contains children who are hearing-impaired. A review of the literature suggests that appropriate RTs for persons with hearing loss are rarely achieved (Crandell & Smaldino,1995; Knecht et al, 2002).

Status of the ANSI S12.6 Acoustic Standard

Compliance with the ANSI classroom performance criteria is, at this writing, completely voluntary. It is hoped that, in the future, adequate acoustics will be thought of as a necessary requirement in a learning environment, not a luxury. In the future, universal building codes might be modified to include good acoustics, making the classroom listening environment no less important than items already in the codes, such as adequate lighting and ventilation. Every effort should be made to meet the background noise and reverberation stipulations of the standard as a first step in improving listening and learning environments for all children. Because of expense, meeting the ANSI stipulations is often not possible by physical room modification alone.

Pearl

- Meeting the ANSI acoustic performance stipulations does not guarantee adequate classroom acoustic accessibility for children with special listening and learning needs. Other SNR-enhancing technologies must also be considered.

◆ Assistive Listening Devices: Hearing Loop, Personal FM, and Classroom Audio Distribution Systems

Even though hearing aids are the initial form of amplification for infants and children with hearing loss, they are not designed to deal with all listening needs (Dillon, 2012). Their biggest limitation is their inability to make the details of spoken communication available when there is competing noise, when the listener cannot be physically close to the speaker, or both. Because a clear and complete speech signal greatly facilitates the development of oral expressive language and reading skills, some means of improving the SNR must be provided in all of a child's learning domains (Anderson, 2004; Estabrooks, 2006; Ling, 2002; Smaldino & Flexer, 2012).

The term *Hearing Assistive Technology (HAT)* denotes a range of products designed to solve the problems of noise, distance from the speaker, and room reverberation or echo that cannot be solved with a hearing aid alone (Boothroyd, 2002; Dillon, 2012). HATs enhance the SNR to improve the intelligibility of speech, expand the baby's or child's distance hearing, and enable incidental learning.

There are many categories of HATs, ranging from listening devices (which will be discussed in this section) to telephone devices and alert/alarm devices. The types of HATs most relevant to children might

be referred to as SNR-enhancing devices, which include hearing loop systems, personal FM systems, and wide area classroom amplification systems. By enhancing the SNR, these devices can augment the audibility and intelligibility of the speaker's voice.

Special Consideration

- A pediatric or educational audiologist must be involved in the recommendation and fitting of all hearing aids and assistive listening devices.

Hearing Loop Systems

Also known as electromagnetic analog induction loop amplification systems, hearing loop systems are one of the oldest forms of room amplification. In a loop system, a microphone is connected (via hard wire or wirelessly) to an amplifier. The amplifier transmits the electrical signal from the microphone to a length of insulated copper wire encircling the room. The electrical current flowing through the wire creates an electromagnetic field that can be picked up by any device using a telecoil, a thin conductive wire wound around a ferrous metal core. When electricity passes through the wire, a magnetic field is created that can be picked up by the device containing the telecoil and converted into an acoustic signal.

Many hearing aids and cochlear implants include a telecoil option, and separate telecoil receivers can be worn by individuals who do not have hearing aids. Incremental improvements have been made in analog inductance systems, with the newer systems being less prone to interference and better able to maintain consistent signal strength. A major improvement in analog inductance systems has come from a standard that specifies proper installation and performance rather than an emerging technology. A new inductance loop standard, published by the International Electrotechnical Commission (IEC) (2006), specifies reference magnetic field strength levels and coverage as well as acceptable background SNR levels. Compliance with the standard should equalize the performance of analog inductance systems in terms of useful listening volume and frequency response of the system. Inductance systems installed without regard to the standard may provide unpredictable and possibly substandard performance.

The primary advantages of loops over other classroom options are lower purchase and maintenance costs. The primary limitations are that each student needs a functional telecoil to benefit from the system, that the functionality of the system can be variable and requires verification, that not all reception devices include the capability to allow the telecoil and internal device microphone to function simultaneously, and finally, that the loop system, if poorly designed and installed, can be subject to electromagnetic interference.

Personal FM Units

A personal FM unit is a wireless personal listening device that includes a remote wireless microphone placed near the desired sound source (usually the speaker's mouth, but it could also be a tape recorder or TV) and a receiver for the listener, who can be situated anywhere within ~ 50 feet of the talker. No wires are required to connect the talker and listener, because the unit is really a small FM radio that transmits and receives on a single frequency.

Because the talker wears the remote microphone within 6 inches of her mouth, the personal FM unit creates a listening situation that is comparable to a parent or teacher being within 6 inches of the child's ear at all times, thereby providing a positive and constant SNR (Sexton, 2003). The close proximity to the microphone also eliminates the effects of reverberation, because only direct (not reflected) sound reaches the microphone for transmission. Personal FM systems, therefore, offer a direct communication connection between the talker and listener in any communication situation (American Academy of Audiology [AAA], 2008; Anderson, Goldstein, Colodzin, & Inglehart, 2005; Launer, 2003). Personal FM units are essential for a child with any type and degree of hearing loss, from minimal to profound, who is in any classroom or group learning situation (Anderson & Arnoldi, 2011; Flynn, Flynn, & Gregory, 2005). Several models of personal FM equipment are available. In the most common styles, the FM receiver is built into the ear-level hearing aid case, or a small FM receiver boot is attached directly to the bottom of the ear-level hearing aid or to a cochlear implant speech processor.

Most recently, wearable personal FM systems, designed for children with normal hearing but who are challenged by poor SNRs (e.g., children with central auditory processing disorders [CAPD]) have become available. The iSense by Phonak (**Fig. 23.2**) was designed specifically for listeners with normal hearing sensitivity. The iSense is a miniaturized FM receiver that can be used with a variety of FM transmitters. The discreet, ear-level receiver is easily fitted by an audiologist. Its primary purpose is to improve listening and attention skills and perhaps the academic abilities of children with attention deficit/hyperactivity disorder (ADHD) and CAPD by improving the SNR

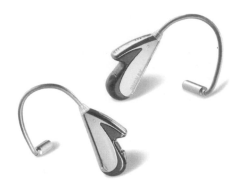

Fig. 23.2   The iSense, a miniaturized FM receiver, was designed for listeners with normal hearing sensitivity and can be used with a variety of FM transmitters. Photo courtesy of Phonak.

and enhancing signal saliency. Studies conducted to date support the effectiveness of these personal FM systems for children with CAPD in attaining short-term and long-term objectives. Short-term results include better auditory focus, increased attention span, longer time on task, and fewer disruptive behaviors (Hall, 2011; Johnston, John, Kreisman, Hall, & Crandell, 2009). Long-term results are based on learning and practicing new skills and strategies and may include measurable changes in auditory neurophysiology (Hornickel, Zecker, Bradlow, & Kraus, 2012).

A sampling of manufacturer Web sites is offered at the end of the chapter for product information about wireless personal FM systems and other classroom products. The AAA's clinical practice guidelines are discussed in the following section.

HAT Guidelines from the AAA

The AAA (2008) provides a rationale and comprehensive protocol for devices that use remote microphones, such as personal FMs and loop systems. These guidelines apply not only to children with all degrees of hearing loss but also to children with normal hearing who have special listening requirements, including children with CAPD.

The AAA protocol contains a core statement that addresses the complex process of HAT selection, fitting, and management, plus supplements that outline procedures for fitting and verification of ear-level FM (Supplement A) and classroom audio distribution systems (CADS) (Supplement B). A third supplement for personal neck loops is under development.

The guidelines discuss regulatory considerations and qualifications of personnel as well as candidacy, fitting, and verification protocols. Monitoring and managing equipment is discussed in detail, including procedures for checking systems to be sure they are working. Strategies for implementing guidelines in the schools are offered.

Use of a Personal FM at Home

Traditionally, personal FM systems coupled to hearing aids have been used for school-age children in the classroom setting, but growing evidence suggests that children of all ages can also benefit from personal FM systems used at home. Moeller, Donaghy, Beauchaine, Lewis, and Stelmachowicz (1996) compared two groups of children; one group was encouraged to use an FM system at home, and another group used hearing aids alone. The families who used the FM systems at home were provided with training about how to operate the units. Subjective reports from parents suggested that appropriate use of the FM at home facilitated effective communication in a variety of listening situations. Some parents of young children report that having the FM transmitter around their neck is a reminder to "talk, talk, talk" to their children, increasing the auditory input the child receives. Another reported advantage was that two of the children felt an increased sense of security when they could hear their parents from a distance.

In another study about home FM use, Gabbard (2003) reported preliminary information that was gathered from the Colorado Loaner FM Project. The project used the FM Listening Evaluation for Children as a way to gain an understanding of the use and benefit of hearing aids and FM systems with children. Parents were asked to complete the evaluation form at least 3 to 6 months following FM fitting and then again at quarterly intervals. Some of the parents' comments regarding perceived benefit of the FM included "being mobile while continuing to hear," "consistent sound whether noisy or not," "provides the best amplification to help auditory skills," and "keeps him focused on the speaker." Flynn et al (2005) agreed that FM use at home improved speech understanding as measured by functional auditory assessment tools.

Classroom Audio Distribution Systems

Soundfield technology, now referred to as Classroom Audio Distribution Systems (CADS), is an exciting educational tool that allows control of the acoustic environment in a classroom, thereby facilitating acoustic accessibility of teacher instruction for all children in the room (Crandell et al, 2005; Smaldino & Flexer, 2012). CADS look like a wireless public address (PA) system, but they are designed specifically to ensure that the entire speech signal, including the weak high-frequency consonants, reaches every child in the room (see **Fig. 23.3a,b**). In addition, other audio sources (e.g., computer, MP3 player, DVD player, or smart phone) can be channeled through CADS.

By using this technology, an entire classroom can be amplified through the use of one to four wall- or ceiling-mounted loudspeakers.

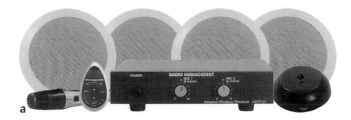

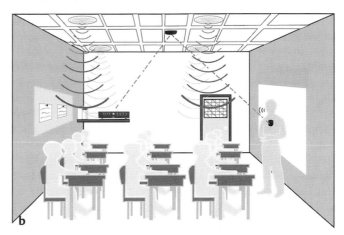

Fig. 23.3a–b   **(a)** A CAD system used in the classroom has a wireless microphone worn by the teacher, a pass-around microphone for students, an amplifier, and evenly dispersed ceiling-mounted loudspeakers. This IR-2007 Dual Channel Infrared Receiver System by Audio Enhancement has a student handheld pass-around microphone, an all-in-one teacher "pendant-style" microphone, four speakers, and ceiling-mounted dome sensor. Photo is provided courtesy of Audio Enhancement. **(b)** Infrared is a commonly used mode of transmission, where the infrared signal is sent *(emitted)* from the teacher microphone to the diode in the center of the ceiling, from there to the amplifier on the wall, and thence to the four loudspeakers in the ceiling. (Photo and schematic from Audio Enhancement; used with permission.)

The teacher wears a wireless microphone transmitter, and the voice is sent via radio waves (FM) or infrared light waves (IR) to an amplifier that is connected to the loudspeakers. There are no wires connecting the teacher with the equipment. The radio or optical link allows the teacher to move about freely, unrestricted by wires. The loudspeakers are designed and positioned to improve the SNR uniformly throughout the areas where instruction occurs in the room.

Who Might Benefit from CADS?

It could be argued that virtually all children benefit from CADS because the improved SNR creates a more favorable learning environment. Studies continue to show that CADS facilitate opportunities for improved academic performance (Crandell et al, 2005; Flexer & Long, 2003; Mendel, Roberts, & Walton, 2003; Smaldino & Flexer, 2012).

If children could hear better, more clearly, and more consistently, they would have an opportunity to learn more efficiently (Edwards & Feun, 2005; Rosenberg & Blake-Rahter, 1999). No one disputes the necessity of creating a favorable visual field in a classroom. A school building would never be constructed without lights in every classroom. Recognizing the positive impact of better SNR in classrooms, some school systems have as a goal the amplification of every classroom in their districts (Knittel, Myott, & McClain, 2002).

Pitfall

- Because "adequate acoustics" is an invisible and ambiguous concept, the necessity of creating a favorable acoustic environment may be questioned by school personnel.

The populations that seem to be especially in need of SNR-enhancing technology include children with fluctuating conductive hearing loss (ear infections), unilateral hearing loss, "minimal" permanent hearing loss, auditory processing problems, cochlear implants, cognitive disorders, learning disabilities, attention problems, articulation (speech) disorders, and behavior problems.

Teachers who use CADS report that they also benefit. Many state that they need to use less energy projecting their voices; they have less vocal abuse and are less tired by the end of the school day (Blair, 2006; Morrow & Connor, 2011). Teachers also report that the unit increases their efficiency as teachers, requiring fewer repetitions, thus allowing for more actual teaching time. With more and more school systems incorporating principles of inclusion, children who previously would have been educated in self-contained classrooms are in the mainstream classroom. CADS offer a way of enhancing the classroom learning environment for the benefit of all children, creating a win-win situation.

Pearl

- About 90% of today's population of children who are identified with hearing loss at birth likely will go directly into general education classrooms by 5 or 6 years of age. Those classrooms must be acoustically ready for them.

To summarize, CADS facilitate the reception of consistently more intact signals than those received in an unamplified classroom, but signals are less complete than those provided by using a personal FM unit (Anderson et al, 2005; Smaldino & Crandell, 2004; Smaldino & Flexer, 2012). The equipment, especially the loudspeakers, must be installed appropriately; teachers must be trained about the rationale for, and effective use of, the technology; and acoustics must be managed as much as possible prior to installation (Wilson, Marinac, Pitty, & Burrows, 2011).

Pearl

- A primary value of CADS is that the better SNR can focus the students and facilitate attention to relevant information. To that end, the clever use of the sound system's microphone can be a powerful teaching tool. Teachers need to be trained about how to use the microphones and their voices to create a listening attitude in the room; the purpose of the improved SNR is to quiet and focus the room, not to excite or distract the children.

Desktop or portable soundfield systems have been introduced to provide improved soundfield conditions for individual students. **Fig. 23.4** depicts a small loudspeaker placed on a student's desk. Usually, students with exceptional listening needs (e.g., students with cochlear implants or students with more severe central auditory processing problems) use this form of soundfield amplification (Anderson et al, 2005). Obviously, other students in the classroom do not benefit from this kind of system, because the sound improvements are localized to that student's immediate area, not broadcast uniformly throughout the classroom.

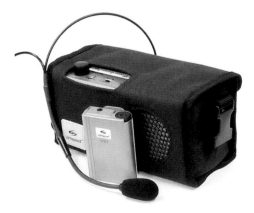

Fig. 23.4 A small loudspeaker (*desktop system*) placed on a student's desk can increase the loudness of the teacher's speech, thereby improving the SNR, for that particular student. (LES-391 desktop speaker, courtesy of LightSPEED Technologies.)

A Universal Design Rather Than a Treatment Perspective

Historically, amplification technologies such as hearing aids, personal FM systems, and now cochlear implants have been recommended as treatments for hearing loss. Because there certainly are populations for whom an enhanced SNR can mean the difference between passing and failing in school, CADS came to be recommended as a treatment for hearing problems. If viewed as a treatment, CADS are recommended for a particular child and managed through the special education system. When recommended for a specific child with hearing problems, CADS fit in the treatment category.

However, with the recognition that all children require an enhanced SNR comes the necessity of moving beyond thinking of CADS as a treatment. CADS need to be integrated into the general education arena. The concept of *universal design* can be useful in this regard.

The concept of universal design originated in the architectural domain with the common examples of curb cuts, ramps, and automatic doors. After years of use, it was found that the modifications that were originally believed to be relevant for only a few people turned out to be useful and beneficial for a large percentage of the population (Gargiulo & Metcalf, 2013).

In terms of learning, universal design means that the assistive technology is not specially designed for an individual student but rather for a wide range of students. Universally designed approaches are implemented by general education teachers rather than by special education teachers (Gargiulo & Metcalf, 2013). It is critical to note that implementation of CADS is shifting from the special education to the general education arena (Smaldino & Flexer, 2012).

◆ Practical Issues for Assistive Listening Device Selection

Many issues need to be evaluated when selecting CADS or when an audiologist recommends CADS rather than a personal FM system for a particular child, and few data are available to guide these decisions (Crandell et al, 2005; Flexer, 2004). Following is a list of questions that an audiologist should consider in making decisions about classroom amplification.

- What steps can be taken to improve the classroom's acoustics by reducing noise and reverberation?
- Have teachers been given thorough in-service training about the auditory basis of classroom instruction and subsequent rationale for the use of CADS?
- What type of microphone should be used: lapel microphone, boom (head worn) microphone, or collar microphone?
- Who will be the contact person in the district or building to troubleshoot and maintain equipment and manage spare parts?
- Is there administrative support for project coordination?
- How many loudspeakers should be installed in a given room?
- Where should the loudspeakers be installed?
- What is the best SNR made possible by the equipment?
- What is the carrier frequency for the radio signal of the unit and the potential for interference (from cellular phones, pagers, etc.)?

Should an Audiologist Recommend a Personal FM System, CADS, or Both for a Given Child?

Once it is determined that a child has a listening problem that interferes with acoustic accessibility, the first step is to try to modify the physical characteristics of the classroom to approximate the ANSI classroom acoustics standards. The next step involves recommending, fitting, and using some type of SNR-enhancing technology.

Pitfall

- "Preferential seating" may improve visual accessibility to speech in some situations but does not control the background noise and reverberation in the classroom, stabilize teacher and pupil position, or provide for an even and consistent SNR. Rather, think "strategic seating" for best acoustic access to the *entire* classroom.

In many instances, the best listening and learning environment can be created by using both a CADS FM or IR and a personal FM system at the same time. The CADS FM or IR unit, appropriately installed in a mainstreamed classroom, improves acoustic access for all students in the classroom. For children especially challenged by the effects of poor SNR and reverberation, such as hearing loss or auditory processing problems, a personal FM system might be more effective. The teacher need wear only a single transmitter if the child's personal FM transmitter is coupled to the audio-out port of the CADS, using an appropriate patch cord. The child with hearing loss (or who is otherwise listening-challenged) greatly benefits from having access to the two microphones of the CADS. He also benefits from having a quiet environment in the classroom and a specific auditory focus. Because of the added complexity of using two technologies, teachers do require training about both technologies, including how to troubleshoot and use them.

Whatever type of SNR-enhancing technology is selected, the following common-sense tips could facilitate use and function of the technology:

- *Try the equipment.* People must experience SNR-enhancing equipment for themselves; they cannot speculate about function.
- *Be mindful of appropriate microphone placement.* Microphone placement dramatically affects the output speech spectrum. Specifically, high frequencies are weaker in off-axis positions. A head-worn microphone provides the best, most complete, and most consistent signal. A collar microphone, worn around the teacher's neck, also allows some level of control of microphone distance. If a lapel microphone is worn, it should be placed midline on the chest ~ 6 inches from the mouth.
- *Check the batteries first if any malfunction occurs.* Weak battery charge can cause interference, static, and intermittent signals.
- *Audiologists should write clear recommendations.* For FM or IR equipment, specify the rationale, type of SNR-enhancing technology needed, equipment characteristics, coupling arrangement chosen, parent and teacher training, and follow-up visits.

Measuring Efficacy of Fitting and Use of Technology

Efficacy can be defined as the extrinsic and intrinsic value of a treatment (Crandell et al, 2005). The recent focus on evidence-based practice underscores the importance of demonstrating that interventions work. Even though the literature shows that the uses of FM and IR technologies clearly have value (Rosenberg, 2005; John & Kreisman, 2012), some efficacy measurements need to be made to show that the individual baby or child in question is obtaining benefit. Benefit can be measured through educational performance, behavioral speech perception tests, direct measures of changes in brain development, or through functional assessments (Tharpe, 2004).

Functional Assessments as a Measure of Efficacy of FM and IR Technology

Functional assessments as a measure of efficacy are typically conducted by having the teacher, student, or parent complete a questionnaire before and after use of the personal FM or CADS (Cole & Flexer, 2011). The following functional assessment tools are readily available and are widely used as efficacy measures for classroom interventions.

SIFTER (Screening Instrument for Targeting Educational Risk)

The SIFTER is a one-page form that is easily filled out by the teacher or teachers at multiple intervals during a school year (Anderson, 1989). The form allows the teacher to observe and rate the student's performance compared with typical students in the class according to the five content areas: academic, attention, communication, class participation, and school behavior. The total score in each area is recorded as pass, marginal, or fail. Even though the SIFTER was originally developed to identify students at risk for listening problems, it has proven to be useful in establishing efficacy of intervention in the classroom. When SIFTER is used in a pretest/posttest paradigm, any change in the child's classroom performance as a result of the FM intervention can be noted and documented.

LIFE-R (Listening Inventories for Education—Revised)

Using the LIFE-R (Anderson, Smaldino, & Spangler, 2011), the student self-rates his or her ability to hear and understand in each of 15 listening situations. A separate form allows the teacher to evaluate the student's listening difficulty. Sections include classroom listening situations, situations outside the classroom, and self-advocacy. The addition of students' input about their personal classroom listening difficulties improves the overall validity of this subjective approach to efficacy. A new online interactive version makes using this tool easier than ever.

CHILD (Children's Home Inventory of Listening Difficulties)

The CHILD (Anderson & Smaldino, 2001) is a further extension of the LIFE, wherein teachers in the classroom environment, and parents and children in the home environment, can assess the adequacy of the environment for listening and observe changes as a result of intervention both at school and in the home.

CHAPS (Children's Auditory Performance Scale)

This questionnaire, appropriate for children age 7 and older, consists of six subsections that were selected to represent the most often reported auditory difficulties experienced by children diagnosed as having

CAPD (Smoski, Brunt, & Tannahill, 1998). The 36-item scale concerns six listening conditions: quiet, ideal, multiple inputs, noise, auditory memory/sequencing, and auditory attention span. Parents or teachers are asked to judge the amount of listening difficulty experienced by the child in question compared with that of a typical child of similar background and age.

Equipment Efficacy for the School System

The key to securing technology from the school system is to obtain data documenting need (Ackerhalt & Wright, 2003). A multifactored comprehensive evaluation, which is a thorough evaluation by a multidisciplinary team, is necessary to document the need for a child to receive special services (see Chapter 30 for more information about laws). The last category on most multifactored comprehensive evaluation forms is Assistive Technology Needs. In order for assistive technology to be recommended within any legislative framework, some type of evaluation must be conducted. It must be documented that the child in question cannot obtain an appropriate education unless a personal FM system or an FM or IR CADS is used. Can the child's access to and performance in the general education environment be linked to hearing difficulties in the classroom? What tests can be administered to document acoustic access and listening difficulties in the classroom?

◆ Conclusion

Improving listening and learning environments is a primary focus of pediatric and educational audiologists. This focus should include home, day care, and classroom environments.

The ANSI classroom acoustic stipulations are an important goal for every classroom. Acoustical modifications in the form of personal FM or CADS (FM or IR) SNR-enhancing technologies are viable and cost-effective means for ensuring signal saliency and auditory focus for children, whether or not they have diagnosed hearing problems. Numerous studies suggest that every classroom ought to have well-installed and used CADS as a necessary learning condition for all children.

Discussion Questions

1. Why do efficacy measures need to be conducted after acoustic interventions like personal FM or CADS are implemented?

2. What common-sense questions should the audiologist consider when deciding on the use of SNR-enhancement technology?

3. Compliance with ANSI classroom acoustics standard is currently voluntary. Why should the standard be compulsory for all classrooms?

4. What are the possible advantages of using SNR-enhancing technology in the home environment?

5. Why are certain populations, who do not exhibit hearing loss per se, candidates for SNR-enhancing technologies?

◆ Sampling of Manufacturer Web Sites

- http://www.audioenhancement.com (personal FM, FM and IR CADS)
- http://www.comtek.com (personal FM and CADS)
- http://gofrontrow.com/en/classroom?gclid=CObb93uyqrLICFac7MgodQVQA_w Front Row to Go (CADS)
- http://oticon.com/products/wireless-accessories/amigo-fm/about-amigo.aspx (Oticon Amigo Personnel FM)
- http://www.lifelineamp.com (personal FM, FM and IR CADS)
- http://www.lightspeed-tek.com (personal FM, FM and IR CADS)
- http://www.ovalwindowaudio.com (loop systems, CADS)
- http://www.phonak.com/com/b2c/en/products/pediatric_solutions/solutions.html (personal FM systems and CADS)
- http://www.sennheiserusa.com (personal FM, FM and IR classroom amplification)

◆ Dedication

Carl Crandell was a dear friend and colleague to both of us. Although he did not physically contribute to this chapter, his thoughts and spirit run through every word. Carl was a passionate proponent of the use of SNR-enhancing technologies to improve listening and learning for all children. His wish was for others to become advocates for children, and we hope that by reading this chapter you will understand that that is our wish too.

References

Access Board (United States). (2013). Classroom acoustics. Retrieved from http://www.access-board.gov/acoustic

Ackerhalt, A. H., & Wright, E. R. (2003). Do you know your child's special education rights? Volta Voices, 10, 4–6.

American Academy of Audiology. (2008). Clinical Practice Guidelines for Remote Microphone Hearing Assistance Technologies for Children and Youth Birth–21 Years. Retrieved from http://www.audiology.org/resources/documentlibrary/Documents/HATGuideline.pdf

American National Standards Institute. (2002). American National Standard Acoustical Performance Criteria, Design Requirements, and Guidelines for Schools (ANSI/ASA S 12.60–2002). New York, NY: American National Standards Institute.

American National Standards Institute. (2009). American National Standard Acoustical Performance Criteria, Design Requirements, and Guidelines for Schools, Part 2: Relocatable Classroom Factors (ANSI/ASA S12.60–2009). New York, NY: American National Standards Institute.

American National Standards Institute. (2010). American National Standard Acoustical Performance Criteria, Design Requirements, and Guidelines for Schools, Part 1: Permanent Schools (ANSI/ASA S12.60–2010). New York, NY: American National Standards Institute.

American Speech-Language-Hearing Association. (1995). Guidelines for acoustics in educational environments. ASHA, Supplement, 37, 15–19.

American Speech-Language-Hearing Association. (2005). Acoustics in educational settings: position statement. Retrieved from http://www.asha.org/policy/PS2005-00028.htm

Anderson, K. L. (1989). Screening instrument for targeting educational risk (SIFTER). Tampa, FL: Educational Audiology Association. Retrieved from http://www.hear2learn.com

Anderson, K. L. (2001). Voicing concern about noisy classrooms. Educational Leadership, 58, 77–79.

Anderson, K. (2004). The problem of classroom acoustics: the typical classroom soundscape is a barrier to learning. Seminars in Hearing, 25, 117–129.

Anderson, K., & Arnoldi, K. A. (2011). Building skills for success in the fast-paced classroom. Hillsboro, OR: Butte.

Anderson, K., & Smaldino, J. (2001). Children's home inventory for listening difficulties (CHILD). Retrieved from http://www.hear2learn.com

Anderson, K. L., Goldstein, H., Colodzin, L., & Inglehart, F. (2005). Benefit of S/N enhancing devices to speech perception of children listening in a typical classroom with hearing aids or a cochlear implant. Journal of Educational Audiology, 12, 14–28.

Anderson, K., Smaldino, J., & Spangler, C. (2011). Listening Inventory for Education—Revised (LIFE-R). Retrieved from http://successforkidswithhearingloss.com/wp-content/uploads/2011/08/Teacher-LIFE-R.pdf

Blair, J. C. (2006). Teachers' impressions of classroom amplification. Educational Audiology Review, 23, 12–13.

Boothroyd, A. (2002). Optimizing FM and sound-field amplification in the classroom. Paper presented at the American Academy of Audiology National Convention, Philadelphia.

Boothroyd, A. (2004). Room acoustics and speech perception. Seminars in Hearing, 2, 155–166.

Bradley, J. S. (1986). Speech intelligibility studies in classrooms. The Journal of the Acoustical Society of America, 80(3), 846–854.

Cole, E., & Flexer, C. (2011). Children with hearing loss: developing listening and talking, birth to six (2nd ed.). San Diego, CA: Plural.

Crandell, C., & Smaldino, J. (1995). An update of classroom acoustics for children with hearing impairment. The Volta Review, 1, 4–12.

Crandell, C. C., Smaldino, J. J., & Flexer, C. (2005). Sound-field amplification: applications to speech perception and classroom acoustics (2nd ed.) New York, NY: Thomson Delmar Learning.

Dillon, H. (2012). Hearing aids (2nd ed.). New York, NY: Thieme.

Edwards, D., & Feun, L. (2005). A formative evaluation of sound-field amplification system across several grade levels in four schools. Journal of Educational Audiology, 12, 57–64.

Estabrooks, W. (2006). Auditory-verbal therapy and practice. Washington, DC: Alexander Graham Bell Association for the Deaf and Hard of Hearing.

Finitzo-Hieber, T., & Tillman, T. W. (1978). Room acoustics effects on monosyllabic word discrimination ability for normal and hearing-impaired children. Journal of Speech and Hearing Research, 21(3), 440–458.

Flexer, C. (2004). The impact of classroom acoustics: listening, learning, and literacy. Seminars in Hearing, 25, 131–140.

Flexer, C., & Long, S. (2003). Sound-field amplification: preliminary information regarding special education referrals. Communication Disorders Quarterly, 25, 29–34.

Flynn, T. S., Flynn, M. C., & Gregory, M. (2005). The FM advantage in the real classroom. Journal of Educational Audiology, 12, 35–42.

French, N., & Steinberg, J. (1947). Factors governing the intelligibility of speech sounds. The Journal of the Acoustical Society of America, 19, 90–119.

Gabbard, S. A. (2003). The use of FM technology for infants and young children. Paper presented at ACCESS Conference, Chicago, IL.

Gargiulo, R. M., & Metcalf, D. (2013). Teaching in today's inclusive classrooms: a universal design for learning approach (2nd ed.). Belmont, CA: Cengage Learning.

Hall, J. W. (2011). Auditory processing disorder: application of FM technology. In J. R. Madell & C. Flexer (Eds.), Pediatric audiology casebook (pp. 32–36). New York, NY: Thieme.

Hawkins, D. B., & Yacullo, W. S. (1984). Signal-to-noise ratio advantage of binaural hearing aids and directional microphones under different levels of reverberation. The Journal of Speech and Hearing Disorders, 49(3), 278–286.

Hornickel, J., Zecker, S. G., Bradlow, A. R., & Kraus, N. (2012). Assistive listening devices drive neuroplasticity in children with dyslexia. Proc. Natl. Acad. Sci. USA, 109(41), 16731–16736.

International Electrotechnical Commission. (2006). 60118–4: Inductance Loop Standard. Geneva, Switzerland: International Electrotechnical Commission.

John, A., & Kreisman, B. (2012). Classroom audio distribution systems: literature review 2003–2011. In J. J. Smaldino & C. Flexer, (Eds.), Handbook of acoustic accessibility: best practices for listening, learning and literacy in the classroom (pp. 55–71). New York, NY: Thieme.

Johnston, K. N., John, A. B., Kreisman, N. V., Hall, J. W., III, & Crandell, C. C. (2009). Multiple benefits of personal FM system use by children with auditory processing disorder (APD). International Journal of Audiology, 48(6), 371–383.

Killion, M. (1997). SNR loss: I can hear what people say, but I can't understand them. Hearing Review, 4(12), 8–14.

Knecht, H. A., Nelson, P. B., Whitelaw, G. M., & Feth, L. L. (2002). Background noise levels and reverberation times in unoccupied classrooms: predictions and measurements. American Journal of Audiology, 11(2), 65–71.

Knittel, M. A. L., Myott, B., & McClain, H. (2002). Update from Oakland schools sound field team: IR vs FM. Educational Audiology Review, 19, 10–11.

Launer, S. (2003). Wireless solutions: the state of the art and future of FM technology for the hearing impaired consumer. Paper presented at ACCESS Conference, Chicago, IL.

Leavitt, R., & Flexer, C. (1991). Speech degradation as measured by the rapid speech transmission index (RASTI). Ear and Hearing, 12(2), 115–118.

Ling, D. (2002). Speech and the hearing impaired child (2nd ed.). Washington, DC: Alexander Graham Bell Association of the Deaf and Hard of Hearing.

Mendel, L. L., Roberts, R. A., & Walton, J. H. (2003). Speech perception benefits from sound field FM amplification. American Journal of Audiology, 12(2), 114–124.

Moeller, M. P., Donaghy, K. F., Beauchaine, K. L., Lewis, D. E., & Stelmachowicz, P. G. (1996). Longitudinal study of FM system use in nonacademic settings: effects on language development. Ear and Hearing, 17(1), 28–41.

Morrow, S. L., & Connor, N. P. (2011). Voice amplification as a means of reducing vocal load for elementary music teachers. Journal of Voice, 25(4), 441–446.

Nelson, E., Smaldino, J., Erler, S., & Garstecki, D. (2008). Background noise levels and reverberation times in old and new elementary school classrooms. Journal of the Educational Audiology Association, 14, 16–22.

Rosenberg, G. (2005). Sound field amplification: a comprehensive literature review. In C. C. Crandell, J. J. Smaldino, & C. Flexer. (Eds.), Sound-field amplification: applications to speech perception and classroom acoustics (2nd ed., pp. 72–111). New York, NY: Thomson Delmar Learning.

Rosenberg, G. G., & Blake-Rahter, P. (1999). Improving classroom acoustics (ICA): a three-year FM sound field classroom amplification study. Journal of Educational Audiology, 7, 8–28.

Sapienza, C. M., Crandell, C., & Curtis, B. (1999). Effect of sound field FM amplification on vocal intensity in teachers. Journal of Voice, 13, 375–381.

Sexton, J. (2003). FM as a component of primary amplification. Educational Audiology Review, 20, 4–5, 43.

Shannon, C. (1948). A mathematical theory of communication. The Bell System Technical Journal, 27, 379–423, 623–656.

Smaldino, J. J., & Crandell, C. C. (2004). Classroom acoustics. Seminars in Hearing, 25, 113–206.

Smaldino, J., & Flexer, C. (2012). Handbook of acoustic accessibility: best practices for listening, learning and literacy in the classroom. New York, NY: Thieme.

Smoski, W. J., Brunt, M. A., & Tannahill, J. C. (1998). Children's auditory performance scale (CHAPS). Tampa, FL: Educational Audiology Association.

Tharpe, A. M. (2004). Who has time for functional auditory assessments? We all do! Volta Voices, 11, 10–12.

Valente, D. L., Plevinsky, H. M., Franco, J. M., Heinrichs-Graham, E. C., & Lewis, D. E. (2012). Experimental investigation of the effects of the acoustical conditions in a simulated classroom on speech recognition and learning in children. The Journal of the Acoustical Society of America, 131(1), 232–246.

Wilson, W. J., Marinac, J., Pitty, K., & Burrows, C. (2011). The use of sound-field amplification devices in different types of classrooms. Language, Speech, and Hearing Services in Schools, 42(4), 395–407.

Wróblewski, M., Lewis, D. E., Valente, D. L., & Stelmachowicz, P. G. (2012). Effects of reverberation on speech recognition in stationary and modulated noise by school-aged children and young adults. Ear and Hearing, 33(6), 731–744.

Chapter 24

Red Flags: Identifying and Managing Barriers to the Child's Optimal Auditory Development

Jane R. Madell, Joan G. Hewitt, and Sylvia Rotfleisch

Key Points

- The audiologist's responsibility is greater than simply fitting and evaluating hearing aid technology; audiologists also have the responsibility of studying the whole child and making appropriate recommendations.

- All professionals are responsible for fully understanding the child's abilities within their areas of specialization and for collaborating with other professionals to provide a comprehensive picture of the child and his abilities.

- If an audiological evaluation does not include assessment of aided speech perception at normal and soft conversational levels in quiet and with competing noise using age-appropriate testing materials, professionals and parents will have an incomplete picture of the child's auditory access to spoken language, which will limit their ability to plan appropriately for the child.

- When a child has appropriate parental and interventional support, red flags point to the type of technology or the technology settings as the source of the child's lack of progress.

- A child's phoneme perception and production, voice quality, and language development can provide significant data concerning the child's auditory access and the appropriateness of technology settings.

- Variability or delay in a child's progress should merit investigation into all aspects of the child's intervention.

Many children with hearing loss attain the listening and spoken language outcomes expected by family and professionals. Many children are fitted with technology and do well. They appear to hear sufficiently well to develop speech and language and learn. However, not every child with hearing loss is a superstar. Why is there a huge variation in performance among children who seem to be equal? We know that not all children achieve the same level of listening, spoken language, literacy, and academic proficiency, but why?

Certain things are clearly a problem that will explain some differences in performance. For example, some children do not hear well with technology, some are not receiving appropriate therapy, some have parents and family who are not involved and not providing speech and language stimulation, and some have other developmental issues that interfere with progress. However, sometimes all variables seem to be managed in a positive fashion, yet the child still does not make the expected progress.

◆ The Audiologist's Responsibility When a Child is Not Attaining Expected Outcomes

The audiologist has a larger responsibility than evaluating hearing and fitting hearing aid (HA) and cochlear implant (CI) technology. As audiologists, we have the responsibility to study the whole child. All professionals are responsible for fully understanding the child's abilities within their areas of specialization. Each professional who works with a child with hearing loss needs to evaluate the child's use of auditory information. Audiologists need to obtain threshold information and assess speech perception with technology, while speech-language pathologists and listening and spoken language specialists (LSLS) need to monitor how well the child functions daily while wearing and using auditory technologies in all environments. Teachers of the deaf (TOD) need to monitor the child's use of hearing in the classroom, and parents are responsible for monitoring the child's performance at home and in social settings. The audiologist may need to teach parents and other professionals how to monitor the child's hearing and the child's use of technology accurately.

We must accept and understand that a child's ability to hear is the fundamental basis for all speech and language development and that the success of our audiological intervention is reflected in the success of the child. "Success" should be defined as reaching the family's desired outcomes so that the child's spoken language, literacy, and academic skills are consistent with hearing peers. The audiologist has the responsibility to understand not only the audiological data as it pertains to the child, but also the child's development in the critical areas of speech, language, and functional listening skills. We need to obtain relevant information from evaluations administered by other team members to make a determination about the child's progress. If a child is not making one year's progress in one year's time, all team members should be concerned. Clinicians must look at the overall progress of the child, beyond their own area of specialization (see Chapter 25 about collaborative team management). If clinicians look only to their own area of specialization and report that the problem is not in their area, then the child's development is compartmentalized and the ability of one area of the child's development to positively or adversely affect others is ignored. All professionals must make the commitment to hold themselves accountable and take responsibility to recognize and examine issues in their own areas. To address red flags and improve the child's progress, we must each collaborate with other team members, understand the significance of the measures collected by colleagues in their areas of expertise, and evaluate how these data can contribute to analyzing test results in our own area of expertise. It is critical that the child's lack of progress be discussed with the entire team: all the professionals who work with the child and the family. Only by evaluating all aspects of the child's performance, and being willing to accept that some of the responsibility might be ours, can we determine what needs to be done to improve a child's outcomes. The child's lack of progress may be the result of audiological, speech-language, educational, auditory enrichment, or developmental issues. Regardless of the cause, all clinicians involved must participate in working together to problem solve the child's lack of progress.

> **Pearl**
>
> • All clinicians must look at the overall progress of the child, beyond their own area of specialization.

◆ Red Flags That Might Signal a Barrier to the Child's Optimal Auditory/Neural Development

Red Flag: Basic Behavioral Observations

Children Not Wanting to Wear Technology

If children hear well with their technology, they should want to wear their technology all day, every day. A child who does not want to wear technology is demonstrating the most basic red flag. A child may not tolerate technology because it is too loud and uncomfortable or because it is too soft and he cannot hear with it.

Hypersensitivity

A red flag that should raise immediate concern is hypersensitivity to auditory stimuli. A child demonstrating eye blinks or facial sensation to auditory stimulation should provoke serious concern and prompt immediate professional action.

Behavioral Control Issues

Occasionally, children refuse to wear technology because of their behavioral control issues; however, in the authors' experience, this is unusual. Other factors should be eliminated before reaching the conclusion that the child's own behavior is the source of the problem.

Poor Responses to Auditory Stimuli

Poor responses to auditory stimuli are a red flag. A child who has no responses or poor responses to sound (even as an infant) is a focus of serious concern.

Failure to Make One Year's Progress in One Year's Time

In addition, children who are not making one year's progress toward desired outcomes in one year's time are demonstrating another significant red flag. Audiologists need to inquire about speech-language and academic progress. Speech-language pathologists, auditory verbal therapists, and TODs need to ask about technology thresholds and speech perception in quiet and in noise to be sure the child is performing as well as possible.

Red Flag: Ineffective Audiological Intervention

All professionals need to ensure that they are providing effective intervention, while parents need to ensure that their children are receiving effective intervention. Audiology services are ineffective if they fail to evaluate regularly how a child hears and understands speech with each piece of technology. Testing should include unaided thresholds and aided thresholds with the right and left ear technology individually and with the technology worn binaurally. Speech perception testing should be performed at normal and soft conversational levels in quiet and in competing noise (see Chapter 11 for more detail on performing speech perception testing and selecting appropriate tests).

Audiological red flags are indicated when audiologists obtain aided thresholds that are too soft (0–15 dB hearing level [HL]), aided thresholds that are not loud enough (35 dB HL or poorer), poor speech perception scores in any of the test conditions (50 dB HL and 35 dB HL in quiet, and 50 dB HL +5 SNR), or speech perception results completed with inappropriate test materials (such as using a picture-pointing test for a mainstreamed child in third grade) (see Chapters 11 and 18). Audiologists can support effective intervention by doing the following:

- Understanding normal auditory skill development and the effect of hearing loss on auditory skills development
- Ensuring that technology is appropriately fitted through regular audiologic evaluations and programming visits
- Recognizing that only appropriately fitted technology can provide optimal auditory access to the brain
- Collecting data from other professionals who work with the child and from parents
- Evaluating comprehensively any signs of difficulty noted by any of the professionals or parents

Red Flag: Ineffective Speech, Language, and Listening Intervention

In addition to the audiology and the technology aspects, audiologists must examine the speech-language and listening intervention being provided to the child. Red flags indicative of ineffective intervention would be noted in the delay of initial and basic auditory skill development. The clinician would primarily note a lack of clinical behaviors expected early in the auditory hierarchy (Rotfleisch, Madell, & Hewitt, 2012; **Table 24.1**). All interventionists should be concerned when a child responds to fewer sounds with his HAs on than with them off, responds to fewer sounds with his CI than previously with his HAs, or when skills acquired with his HAs do not transfer to his CI.

Red flags include, but are not be limited to, no response to a child's name; a lack of "listening attitude"; a poor voice quality; no evidence of improvement in speech production; an inability to discriminate and/or identify suprasegmentals, vowels, and consonant features; and limited comprehension of familiar phrases based only on suprasegmentals and/or key words.

Red Flag: Vision as Primary Modality

When a child's intervention does not primarily focus on audition and instead uses vision as the primary input modality for receiving spoken language, problems in the child's speech production often are observed. These speech errors are a consequence of the limited visual availability of acoustic speech features. Ling (2002) states that "because audition (auditory brain development) is the only sense capable of appreciating all aspects of speech . . . it is emphasized that whatever residual hearing a child may possess should be exploited."

Indications of speech acquisition through vision and the resulting error patterns would include confusions of phonemes produced in the same place, voicing errors for cognate pairs, pitch-dependent vowels, and poor control of suprasegmentals. Utilizing even minimal auditory cues would typically prevent most of these error patterns. To address and/or prevent visual speech errors, the intervention must focus on the child's use of audition and eliminate the child's reliance on vision for the reception of spoken communication.

The child with hearing loss who is provided with optimal hearing technology and appropriate intervention should develop auditory, speech, and language skills in the typical sequence and at an appropriate rate in a given time interval (Connor, Craig, Raudenbush, Heavner, & Zwolan, 2006; Geers, Nicholas, & Sedey, 2003; May-Mederake, 2012; Tait, De Raeve, & Nikolopoulos, 2007).

Red Flag: Child Making Insufficient Progress toward Attaining Desired Outcomes

When a child is not developing skills at the appropriate rate, weak areas of development and the rate of progress must be examined to detect the red flags revealing issues possibly affecting the child. When assessing for an appropriate rate of change over time, interventionists should be alert to any signs of deterioration of skills in the areas being monitored. A deterioration of skills (e.g., loss of ability in speech discrimination, identification, or production) can be

Table 24.1 Professional expectations for a baby aided by 3 months or implanted by 12 months

Preliminary-level skills	Hearing Age (months)					
Skill	1	3	6	9	12	> 12
Responds to Ling sounds		HA, CI				
Responds to name		HA, CI				
Discriminates suprasegmentals		CI	HA			
Babbles 5 vowels			HA, CI			
Discriminates nasal from plosive			HA, CI			
Produces nasal			HA, CI			
Produces plosive			HA, CI			
Discriminates fricative			CI	HA		
Comprehends 5 words			CI	HA		
Produces fricative				HA, CI		
Babbles 4 consonants				HA, CI		
Comprehends 2–3 stereotypic phrases				HA, CI		
Expressive vocabulary of 5–10 words					HA, CI	
Babbles 5 voiceless consonants					HA, CI	
Higher-level skills	**Hearing Age (months)**					
Skill	12	18	24	30		
Comprehends 50 words	HA, CI					
Comprehends 100 words		HA, CI				
Comprehends simple sentences		HA, CI				
Produces 10 words		HA, CI				
Produces 50 words			HA, CI			
Produces 2-word phrases			HA, CI			
Produces 2-word combinations			HA, CI			
KEY:						

Abbreviations: HA, hearing aid; CI, cochlear implant.

Note: This table shows the results of a survey of professionals who work with infants and children with hearing loss (Rotfleisch et al, 2012).

evidenced by the child's inability to demonstrate a previously emerging or mastered skill. A negative change in the child's abilities merits troubleshooting for any possible cause. Deterioration of speech production might be shown by an inability to produce a phoneme previously mastered. In the areas of comprehension, vocabulary, and language development, evidence data from testing might indicate a plateau or regression. Additionally, observations in therapy of the child not demonstrating comprehension abilities previously mastered could be a red flag.

Red Flag: Speech Production

Listening to the child's speech will indicate what he is hearing. Children speak what and how they hear. If a child is not producing a particular phoneme, it is as likely as not the child is not hearing that speech sound well enough or often enough to cement appropriate connections in the auditory centers of the brain. A red flag is indicated by children exhibiting poor voice quality, such as a gravelly quality or glottal fry. Another red flag is evidenced by the inappropriate use of intensity demonstrated by the child who always whispers, is always too loud, or is unable to simulate whisper in his productions. Additional red flags are noted in speech production with issues of oral/nasal balance, lack of pitch control, and vocalizations that occur on inhalation rather than on exhalation of the breath stream.

Red flags are indicated when development of phonemes is atypical or does not follow the normal rate or sequence. The most typical speech error patterns noted are: poor syllabification; poor vowel variety and productions; vowel development but no consonant development; inappropriate and/or atypical consonant development, primarily in limited frequency areas; nasal emissions; and lateral fricatives. When monitoring speech production, interventionists must be aware if the variety of manners of production or place of production is too limited. An inappropriate developmental sequence would be indicated when the child utilizes more advanced phonemes but demonstrates gaps in phoneme repertoire for earlier acquired phonemes. Another red flag would appear when a child is unable to produce phonemes with particular speech features, such as unvoiced consonants or bilabials.

Red Flag: Language Development

Interventionists must monitor the child for indications of appropriate emergence of language skills even prior to the initial expressive use of words. An overall lack of development of "conversational" babbling/jargoning is a concern. A child without intelligible vocabulary or language development who produces only canonical babbling and jargoning is not developing the next level of language abilities. Interventionists must be concerned when they observe receptive language development, but no parallel development of expressive language or speech production abilities by the child.

◆ Recognizing Effective Auditory Intervention

To ensure effective intervention, the child's use of audition must be the fundamental component. For a child with a hearing loss, the hearing loss itself can significantly limit access to speech and language, thus creating the delayed speech and language skills. To address this problem, intervention requires a defined auditory component such that the focus of therapy is auditory skill development in the appropriate sequence through the auditory modality (Estabrooks, 2006; Ling, 1989). In this auditory model, a sequence of auditory goals determined through the knowledge of the normal progression of audition is established. The auditory-verbal therapist or speech-language pathologist must assess the child to determine baseline auditory abilities and then begin at the appropriate level of difficulty. Intervention then moves through the sequence by incorporating auditory goals in every activity in every session. Effective intervention provides guidance and coaching to parents, enabling auditory goals to be incorporated throughout the child's daily life and in all settings (**Table 24.1**).

◆ Supporting Intervention through Auditory Demand

Auditory Support

All clinicians working with a child must determine whether the demand for the child to use audition extends across all environments—therapy, home, and school. Is the child wearing technology during all waking hours in every setting? Is there a determined way to respond if the child removes her technology? Is the child expected to report age-appropriate issues with her equipment? The adults interacting with the child must have an expectation that the child will respond to sound, and adults should have a clear understanding of what the child can and cannot hear in each specific environment. Then, adults interacting with the child will have an appropriate auditory expectation for each particular situation.

Checking Technology

Everyone on the child's team must support effective intervention. The bottom line remains that effective intervention is impossible without appropriately functional technology. Technology must be aggressively monitored and checked correctly and thoroughly on a daily basis by the adults who have appropriate listening technology (HA stethoscope, CI earbuds, CI listening check). Adults across the environments must know how to use the technology with ease. The parent or teachers/school professionals must be able to determine whether the child's technology is not functioning and troubleshoot for issues such as a dead battery, a broken device, and/or intermittent use. All professionals must be sensitive to situations where a child is not using technology fully—for example, if the child arrives at the clinic or school with the the technology in the mother's purse or the child's backpack. Listening and hearing (auditory brain access, exposure, and enrichment) are the critical components of all activities in therapy and everyday life across environments and cannot be achieved without full use of appropriately functioning technology.

Pearl

- All clinicians working with a child need to be able to monitor performance with technology daily and immediately refer to the audiologist if the child is not hearing well.

Parental Support for Effective Intervention

Parents support effective intervention by finding knowledgeable, experienced professionals and actively participating in all intervention. Full participation in their child's intervention allows parents to reinforce all goals and objectives at home as well as ensure that all family members and caregivers are also able to do so. Parents must document observations about the child's auditory, speech, and language development so that they can provide feedback to all professionals. Parents do need to "trust their gut." If the intervention and progress do not seem optimal, then they probably are not. Seeking out additional professional resources or obtaining a second opinion may be necessary. Parents should be supported so that they can become strong advocates for their child and competent medical consumers. Professionals need to support parents in seeking a second opinion and not feel insulted when parents do so.

Pearl

- Parents should be supported so that they can become strong advocates for their child and competent medical consumers. Professionals need to support parents in seeking a second opinion and not feel insulted when parents do so.

Interventionist Support for Effective Intervention

An auditory focus in therapy or intervention would ensure that input through sensory modalities other than audition is minimized; thus, professionals must model and coach strategies to maximize use of auditory input for parents. Interventionists must fully involve parents in the intervention. Expectations in therapy should be clear to the parents and the child. The therapist's role is to teach carryover of these expectations into the child's daily life, allowing parents to have appropriate and consistent auditory expectations and knowledge of therapy targets and outcome goals. Through support and involvement of the par-

ents or caregivers, interventionists enable consistency and the needed carry-through beyond the therapy sessions.

◆ Why is Careful Monitoring of Red Flags Important?

Developmental expectations are based on normal development. Expectations for children with hearing loss should follow normal developmental patterns. If a child is fitted with appropriate technology early and receives appropriate therapy, we should expect one year's development in one year's time. However, if a child receives technology late, or if therapy intervention is not optimal, development will be impacted. Listening age (Patton, Hackett, & Rodriguez, 2004), which is the length of time a child has been appropriately fitted with technology, may be a matter of concern when compared with chronological age. Any deviations from normal development are a matter for concern.

Parents are novices and rely on professionals for guidance. Parents report that they do not feel professionals from different disciplines have the same expectations for development. For example, audiologists may not always recognize a concern when auditory therapists report that a child cannot hear high frequencies at a distance. When members of different disciplines disagree, parents are put in a difficult position. They become confused, frustrated, and anxious when different disciplines have conflicting expectations and levels of concern.

Table 24.1 shows the results of a survey of professionals who work with infants and children with hearing loss (Rotfleisch et al, 2012). The survey outlines expectations for a baby aided by 3 months or implanted by 12 months of age. Auditory therapists, who work on development of auditory skills, are in an excellent position to determine appropriate expectations. If all clinicians applied this kind of information as a guideline, then they would all be using the same criteria for performance, which would lead to more cohesive expectations from all interventionists working with the child.

Pearl

- If all clinicians applied information about developmental milestones as a guideline, then they would all be using the same criteria for performance, leading to more cohesive expectations from all interventionists working with the child.

◆ When Red Flags Point to Technology as the Source of the Problem

Speech-language perception issues result from one or more of four conditions experienced by the child with hearing loss:

- I did not understand because the sound was too quiet.
- I did not understand because the sound was too loud.
- I did not understand because the sound was not clear.
- I did not understand because I do not have sufficient language development.

Real-ear measures and CI programming do not tell us what a child is hearing. Real-ear measures report the sound that is reaching the eardrum, not the sound that is processed by the auditory brain. Cochlear implant programming and neural response telemetry (NRT) values tell us how much electrical stimulation is being provided but, again, not what is being received by the auditory brain. Children provide us with accurate and reliable information about what they hear when we observe and understand their behavior, when we document their auditory skill development, when we listen carefully to their speech-language production, and when we verify their speech perception through audiological testing.

Pearl

- If a child does not clearly understand spoken language while wearing technology, something is wrong. The audiologist must act quickly to modify the technology to enable the child to comprehend speech.

◆ Evaluating Audiology Test Results

Red Flags That Indicate Speech Is Too Soft

When HAs are not providing sufficient amplification or CIs are not providing sufficient stimulation, children will exhibit a variety of behaviors that should indicate to the professionals and parents that speech is too soft. **Table 24.2** provides a list of specific behaviors children may exhibit that indicate that speech is too soft. A lack of response to sound and a reliance on visual input are obvious indicators that speech may not be audible, but other behaviors are often present that provide further evidence that sound is too soft.

Inadequate access to speech and language must be considered for children who are making slow or nonexistent progress in their language development. In addition, while some professionals insist that children must learn to "wear" their devices, in our experience children who are receiving little benefit from their amplification will often remove the HAs or CIs because they serve little purpose. Older children may try to increase the volume or sensitivity of their devices to make speech louder, but if they are unsuccessful, even they will develop a lax attitude toward wearing their technology. Formal speech perception testing can also provide strong evidence that sound is too soft. If a child's speech perception improves by 12% or more when the intensity level is increased from 50 dB HL to 70 dB HL, then this indicates that conversational speech is too quiet and an increase in amplification or stimulation is needed.

While most behaviors that indicate speech is too soft are consistent between HA and CI users, the authors have observed the vocal intensity of the users may differ. Children with HAs who are underamplified will often speak loudly, since increasing their vocal intensity provides them with an amplified signal. However, children whose CIs are not providing sufficient stimulation will often speak in a quiet or

---

Table 24.2 When speech is too soft: Signs of underamplification or understimulation

Hearing aids	Cochlear implants
Child consistently removes technology	Child consistently removes technology
Turns up volume	Turns up volume and/or sensitivity
Relies on visual input	Relies on visual input
Does not turn or respond to name	Does not turn or respond to name
Vocalizations do not change with technology	Vocalizations do not change with technology
Voice is loud	Voice is whispered
Listening/speech/language development is slow or nonexistent	Listening/speech/language development is slow or nonexistent
Speech perception at 70 dB HL is better (> 12%) than at 50 dB HL	Speech perception at 70 dB HL is better (> 12%) than at 50 dB HL

even whispered voice. For these children, sound does not appear to grow appreciably in loudness, so their voice is often soft and reflects their perception of the quietness of others' voices and the environment around them.

If the audiologist suspects that speech is too soft, she must first perform informal listening checks and also a formal analysis of the technology to ensure that it is functioning properly. If the technology is working appropriately, then aided speech perception testing should be completed at 35 dB HL, 50 dB HL, and 70 dB HL to ensure that the patient has optimal access to soft, conversational, and loud speech. Unaided pure tone testing may also be necessary if threshold changes are suspected. Phoneme perception can provide additional information about the area or areas of speech that are not clearly audible. Once audiologic assessments are completed and the results analyzed, reprogramming of the HAs or CIs may be necessary to improve access to soft speech, normal conversational speech, and possibly even loud speech. Finally, if a child's current HAs cannot provide sufficient access to all speech inputs, then a trial with new amplification or an evaluation for cochlear implantation is warranted.

Red Flags That Indicate Speech Is Too Loud

From the authors' clinical experiences and from the reports of parents and educational professionals, overamplification and, especially, overstimulation are a growing concern with children. Moreover, the consequences of overstimulation and overamplification can be extremely detrimental to speech and language development.

Table 24.3 provides a list of specific behaviors children may exhibit when speech is too loud.

As stated above, children should want to wear their technology during all their waking hours. Thus, if a child resists or flinches or grimaces or cries when the technology is applied, parents and professionals should be concerned. In addition, any time a child removes his technology or has a marked startle and/or involuntary eye blink in response to loud sounds, we should again be very concerned. We should also be suspicious when children exhibit obvious responses to distant environmental sounds or to very soft sounds, such as a door moving on carpet or a pen on paper. Formally, speech should be considered to be too loud when a child cannot tolerate speech presented in the sound booth at 70 dB HL or when his speech perception scores decrease significantly as the intensity increases from 35 dB HL to 50 dB HL or from 50 dB HL to 70 dB HL. Berger et al (2011) reported that many of these children also appear to have a shortened attention span, or agitated behavior, or both.

Overamplification and overstimulation can have deleterious effects on speech and language development. First, the vocal quality of these children is often affected, but, as previously discussed, differences in this area are noted between HA and CI recipients. Children with HAs will often use a quiet voice in an attempt to reduce the intensity of the speech signal. However, children with implants who are overstimulated appear to perceive sound, including speech, as being louder than it actually is. Parents of these children often complain that their children speak in unusually loud voices and are unable to imitate a whisper. Speech-language pathologists and TODs often remark that these children have a gravelly feature to their voices that does not improve with

Table 24.3 When speech is too loud: Signs of overamplification or overstimulation

Hearing aids	Cochlear implants
Consistently resists or removes technology	Consistently resists or removes technology
Turns down volume	Turns down volume or sensitivity
Startles, cries, or blinks to loud sounds	Startles, cries, or blinks to loud sounds
Has robust responses to very soft sounds	Has robust responses to very soft sounds
Is very quiet or withdrawn	Is very quiet or withdrawn
Voice is quiet	Voice is loud and/or gravelly; voices when whispering
Poor or deviant consonant development	Poor or deviant consonant development; Produces only vowels and voiced consonants
Receptive language development without expressive language development	Receptive language development without expressive language development
Speech perception at 70 dB HL is poorer (> 12%) than at 50 dB HL	Speech perception at 70 dB HL is poorer (> 12%) than at 50 dB HL

therapy. In some cases, children who are overstimulated have been observed to babble very little or to be completely silent; the sound of their own voices may be too loud to be tolerated.

Moreover, when sound is too loud, significant distortion or masking can occur. Since audition is the basis for speech development, overamplification and overstimulation can cause consonants to be indistinct or intense, leading to poor consonant development, and even to the production of only vowels and voiced consonants, since even voiceless consonants will have significant intensity. Berger et al (2011) reported that, in addition to refusal to wear the implant and an unusually loud voice, children who are overstimulated can also exhibit poorly defined borders between their words and poor voice modulation with high-pitched sounds. Moreover, for these children, no improvement in their vocal quality or articulation was noted despite intensive and appropriate auditory and speech therapy. Finally, the authors have noted several children in this category whose receptive language appeared to be developing appropriately, but whose expressive language was not developing. Receptive language development without concurrent expressive language development should always be considered a red flag.

Again, if the audiologist suspects that speech is too loud, she should informally and formally ensure that all technology is functioning appropriately. Unilateral and bilateral assessment of aided speech perception of soft, conversational, and loud speech will provide information about the intensity levels at which speech is distorting or even becoming painful. For hearing aid patients, real-ear measurements performed at high intensity levels may provide information about frequencies that are being overamplified. While loudness scaling has long been a part of cochlear implant programming, its use with children should be carefully reviewed. Since hearing adults have been shown to be poor raters of loudness (Madell and Goldstein, 1972), it is imprudent and even unrealistic to assume that children who are profoundly deaf are able to complete this highly subjective task accurately. On the other hand, the use of neural response assessment (NRT, neural response imaging [NRI], and auditory response telemetry [ART]) can provide objective information for determining stimulation levels. Berger et al (2011) found that for patients with the cochlear device, reducing the comfort level stimulation to tNRT levels led to spontaneous resolution of the behavioral and interventional problems previously noted.

Pearl

- Overamplification and overstimulation can have deleterious effects on wearing compliance, speech and language development, attention, and behavior.

Red Flags That Indicate Speech is Not Clear

First, as with other speech perception problems, interventionists must always consider that the technology may be affecting the clarity of speech. HAs and CI processors should undergo a daily listening check to ensure that the microphones and other components are not the source of distortion. If parents or professionals are unsure whether a hearing aid or processor is functioning appropriately, it should be analyzed and replaced. The motto should be, "When in doubt, swap it out!" Especially with CIs, if the processor is functioning appropriately, but a child has poor speech perception, parents and sometimes professionals may begin to have concerns about an internal device failure. Although device failures do occur, failure rates are very low (Eskander et al, 2011). If the child can hear, detailed documentation of speech perception and production errors, a complete audiological assessment, and careful reprogramming should always occur prior to considering an internal device failure.

When speech is audible, but not clear, children will exhibit behaviors like those listed in **Table 24.4**. Children speak what they hear, which means articulation errors may be "hearing" errors. Thus, since a child's speech production should be the most accurate reflection of his speech perception, professionals and parents should make careful and accurate observations and note the consistent production, omissions, and substitutions a child makes. After consideration is given for normal developmental patterns, the remaining errors provide us with significant information about the child's speech perception.

For children with hearing loss to acquire good speech production and morphemic functions in spoken English, they must be able to clearly perceive all of the ~44 phonemes of the language. However, many clinicians and parents utilize the Ling six-sound test, with the assumption that this test is indicative of accurate phoneme perception. Although the Ling six-sound test is helpful in determining whether a child has access across the speech spectrum, it provides us with a very limited understanding of a child's phoneme perception. In a retrospective review of more than 230 cochlear implant mappings, Hewitt, Hewitt, Owen, and Madell (2012) found that the most common speech perception errors were not identified by the six phonemes of the Ling test. In addition, this review indicated that, when a child has widespread vowel errors as identified by the Ling six-sound test or an expanded vowel perception test, significant global programming issues may exist. Nevertheless, to ensure that a child is able to perceive every phoneme in English clearly, identification, not detection, should be regularly assessed for all phonemes, with emphasis on consonant perception for speech from distances of 3 feet and 10 feet. The Iowa Medial Consonant Test is an example of a format that can

Table 24.4 When speech is not clear: Signs of poor clarity

Hearing aids	Cochlear implants
Relies on visual input	Relies on visual input
Poor or unusual voice quality	Poor or unusual voice quality
Inappropriate/unusual consonant development	Inappropriate/unusual vowel and/or consonant development
Consistent omission/substitution of specific consonants	Consistent omission/substitution of specific consonants
Speech production not improving	Speech production not improving
Hearing aid program is completely flat or heavily weighted to lows and highs	CI map is completely flat or heavily weighted to lows and highs
Very small or very large difference between gain for soft and normal conversation	Very small or large difference between T levels and C/M levels
Speech perception is poor at 35 dB HL, at 50 dB HL, and/or in noise	Speech perception is poor at 35 dB HL, at 50 dB HL, and/or in noise

be used by parents and professionals to assess perception of all consonants. Analysis of formal speech perception tests presented at 35 dB HL and 50 dB HL in quiet and in noise can provide additional information about the clarity of speech and perception of specific phonemes.

Since audiologists have contact with children for only a small number of hours every few months or once a year, the majority of information concerning a child's speech perception will be documented by listening and spoken language specialists, speech-language pathologists, TODs, and parents working with the child. Audiologists must be considerate of and receptive to the accumulated speech perception data that parents and interventionists provide. Responses to normal conversational speech, assessed informally at 3 feet and/or formally at 50 dB HL, and to soft speech, assessed informally at 10 feet and/or formally at 35 dB HL, should be carefully reviewed to determine whether changes need to occur in the soft speech/threshold settings and/or the normal conversational/comfort level settings. Analysis of the errors on informal and formal measures and review of a frequency allocation chart for speech phonemes can identify specific frequency bands that need to be adjusted. Making needed changes in specific frequency bands, rather than globally increasing or decreasing all bands, can improve speech perception for those sounds that are not clear to the patient without jeopardizing information that is already clear. In further analyzing the data, audiologists must remember to apply their knowledge of basic principles of sound. For instance, if a child is unable to hear high-frequency sounds, not only should high-frequency settings be checked, but low-frequency settings should be reviewed to determine whether upward spread of masking is occurring. In the authors' experience,

careful analysis of phoneme perception errors and specific programming changes targeted to improve perception can have an immediate impact on a child's speech perception and production.

> **Pearl**
>
> - Careful analysis of phoneme perception errors and specific programming changes targeted to improve perception can have an immediate impact on a child's speech perception and production.

Red Flags That Indicate Speech Is Not Balanced

The benefits of binaural hearing are well documented (Litovsky et al, 2012; Litovsky, 2011; Peters, 2006). As a result of binaural summation, the auditory input from two ears will be louder and clearer than a monaural input. Furthermore, the auditory input to both ears should appear balanced to prevent binaural interference, in which the acoustic input from one device interferes with the ability to receive clear auditory input from the other device. A correlation to this is the Stenger principle, where if the same auditory input is provided to both ears at different intensity levels, only the louder input will be perceived (Stenger, 1907).

Although audiologists are well versed in the benefits of binaural hearing, in practice some fail to apply these basic principles to binaural technology. While audiologists work to ensure that each ear individually is fitted with appropriately programmed technology, they must also determine whether the two devices together provide optimal binaural benefit. When a patient has been utilizing only one device, the programming and/or volume of that device will often be elevated to compensate for the lack of binaural summation. Often, HA programming algorithms automatically provide additional gain if a fitting is monaural only. However, when the patient receives a second device, the ability to fit the second device optimally will be compromised if the output of the first device is not readjusted and often reduced. Blamey, Dooley, James, and Parisi (2000) found that standard programming methods for fitting HAs and/or CIs were not likely to accomplish a balanced binaural fitting and that the output of devices fitted monaurally would most likely need to be reduced to compensate for the occurrence of binaural summation. Moreover, when their technology is not balanced or when binaural summation has created an overly loud input, children will often go to great lengths, such as removing the battery or turning off the loud or interfering device, to make the sound more tolerable. Children, and parents, generally do not realize that binaural summation is occurring and will assume that the new device is creating the excessive loudness or interference, since the problem did not exist prior to the introduction of the second device. **Table 24.5** provides examples of behaviors noted in children when their technology is not binaurally balanced.

With the introduction of a new implant or HA, children should immediately begin receiving some of the benefits of binaural hearing, even if the listening abilities in the ear with the new device are just developing. If both devices are reprogrammed and balanced, the sound quality of both, when worn together, should be good. However, failure to review and adjust the programming of the first device fully when a second device is added is a red flag. If the loudness is not balanced between the two devices, only the louder device may be audible, potentially causing auditory progress in the ear with the new device to be limited and/or rejection of the new device to occur.

Table 24.5 When sound is not balanced: Signs of unbalanced binaural technology

HA + HA / HA + CI / CI + CI Unbalanced
Consistently localizes to one direction
Consistently turns one ear to speaker/music/TV
Does not replace one device when it falls off
Startles, blinks, or asks for quiet when putting on 2nd device
Does not indicate when one battery dies
Original HA or CI is not reprogrammed when 2nd is added
Can tell that one device is louder than the other

Assessing binaural balance is generally quite easy. One of the simplest ways to determine whether a child's technology is balanced is to ask "Which ear is louder, this one or that one?" The correct answer is, "None" or "I don't know." Even preschoolers are often able to identify when one device is louder than the other. By asking the child, "Does this ear need to be louder or this ear need to be quieter?" the audiologist can obtain information to help guide programming changes. Formal aided speech perception measures can also be completed in the monaural and binaural conditions to determine whether binaural summation is improving the ability to hear soft sounds or creating a signal that is too loud. Furthermore, while parents or children may report that one device appears to be bothersome, clear evidence of interference may be documented only when testing with speech in noise. If the technology is programmed and balanced appropriately, speech perception scores should improve in the binaurally aided condition when compared with the monaurally aided condition, especially in the presence of noise.

Pearl

- With the introduction of a new implant or hearing aid, children should immediately begin receiving some of the benefits of binaural hearing, even if the listening abilities in the ear with the new device are just developing. If both devices are reprogrammed and balanced, the sound quality of both, when worn together, should be good.

◆ Summary and Conclusions

Different professionals can have conflicting viewpoints about a child's developmental expectations and outcomes. If one professional has lower expectations, he may discount the input of others and fail to assess objectively in his area of expertise, causing collaboration to be adversely affected. Resolution of legitimate concerns, and ultimately a child's progress, can be affected by professionals who have different viewpoints and are not willing to listen openly to colleagues. It is critical that all clinicians working with children listen with an open ear to colleagues and to parents. Listening to the children also is essential; their speech production is a reflection of how well they are hearing.

In the authors' recent survey of experienced professionals working with children with hearing loss to determine what issues contributed to a child's poor progress, the vast majority of interventionists (> 94%) were "very" or "quite" willing to consider technology as a factor in the child's poor outcomes (Rotfleisch et al, 2012). The greatest percentage of respondents ranked inappropriate technology (63.9%) and inappropriate technology settings (64.3%) as most frequently causing problems with the child's performance, with resolution of these problems most frequently leading to improvement in the child's progress. If technology is so frequently considered a likely factor in a child's poor progress, audiologists must be prepared to listen to their colleagues when such concerns are expressed and accept responsibility to carefully assess technology and modify it as needed.

It is essential that data are collected before making assumptions about performance. Returning to basic audiological principles, audiologists need to test to be certain a child is hearing what we think she is hearing. Real-ear measures, NRT, and electrical stapedial reflex threshold (ESRT) are important tools, but they do not tell us what is reaching the brain. Only behavioral testing of thresholds with technology and speech perception testing in multiple conditions will validate how a child is performing.

Audiologists who have appropriate developmental expectations, collaborate fully with other interventionists, consistently assess a child's ability to clearly perceive speech and language, and actively pursue appropriate technology fittings and programming can and will positively impact the development of their young patients. Inappropriate technology or inappropriate technology settings are solvable problems. Audiologists can solve them, and the children we serve deserve to have them solved.

Pearl

- Audiologists who have appropriate developmental expectations, collaborate fully with other interventionists, consistently assess a child's ability to clearly perceive speech and language, and actively pursue appropriate technology fittings and programming can and will positively impact the development of their young patients.

Discussion Questions

1. What red flags may be present for children who are not making optimal progress?

2. Why is carefully monitoring a child's speech perception and speech production essential in evaluating a child's benefit from hearing technology?

3. Why is the monitoring of red flags important for all professionals?

4. What information can be gleaned from collaboration with parents and other professionals about the child's overall progress?

5. What red flags indicate that the perception of speech through the child's technology is: (1) too soft? (2) too loud? (3) unclear? (4) unbalanced?

6. What speech production issues would merit cross-disciplinary assessment to determine the cause of the child's errors?

References

Berger., et al. (2011). Overstimulation in children with cochlear implants. Presented at Cochlear Implant Symposium 2011, Chicago, IL. July 14–16, 2011.

Blamey, P. J., Dooley, G. J., James, C. J., & Parisi, E. S. (2000). Monaural and binaural loudness measures in cochlear implant users with contralateral residual hearing. Ear and Hearing, 21(1), 6–17.

Connor, C. M., Craig, H. K., Raudenbush, S. W., Heavner, K., & Zwolan, T. A. (2006). The age at which young deaf children receive cochlear implants and their vocabulary and speech-production growth: is there an added value for early implantation? Ear and Hearing, 27(6), 628–644.

Eskander, A., Gordon, K. A., Kadhim, L., Papaioannou, V., Cushing, S. L., James, A. L., & Papsin, B. C. (2011). Low pediatric cochlear implant failure rate: contributing factors in large-volume practice. Archives of Otolaryngology–Head & Neck Surgery, 137(12), 1190–1196.

Estabrooks, W. (2006). Auditory-verbal therapy and practice. Washington, DC: Alexander Graham Bell Association for the Deaf and Hard of Hearing.

Geers, A. E., Nicholas, J. G., & Sedey, A. L. (2003). Language skills of children with early cochlear implantation. Ear and Hearing, 24(1, Suppl), 46S–58S.

Hewitt, L., Hewitt, J., Owen, L., & Madell, J. (2012). Analysis of common speech perception errors prior to cochlear implant MAPping and successful, remedial programming changes.

Ling, D. (1989). Foundations of spoken language. Washington, DC: Alexander Graham Bell Association for the Deaf and Hard of Hearing.

Ling, D. (2002). Speech and the hearing-impaired child: theory and practice (2nd ed.). Washington, D.C.: The Alexander Graham Bell Association for the Deaf and Hard of Hearing.

Litovsky, R. (2011). Review of recent work on spatial hearing skills in children with bilateral cochlear implants. Cochlear Implants International, 12, 30–33.

Litovsky, R. Y., Goupell, M. J., Godar, S., Grieco-Calub, T., Jones, G. L., Garadat, S. N., . . . Misurelli, S. (2012). Studies on bilateral cochlear implants at the University of Wisconsin's Binaural Hearing and Speech Laboratory. Journal of the American Academy of Audiology, 23(6), 476–494.

Madell, J. R., & Goldstein, R. (1972). Relation between loudness and the amplitude of the early components of the averaged electroencephalic response. Journal of Speech and Hearing Research, 15(1), 134–141.

May-Mederake, B. (2012). Early intervention and assessment of speech and language development in young children with cochlear implants. International Journal of Pediatric Otorhinolaryngology, 76(7), 939–946.

Patton, J. B., Hackett, L., & Rodriguez, L. (2004). The listening age formula. San Antonio, TX: Sunshine Cottage School for the Deaf.

Peters, B. R. (2006). Rationale for bilateral cochlear implantation in children and adults. Sydney, Australia: Cochlear Corporation.

Rotfleisch, S., Madell, J., & Hewitt, J. (2012). Developmental expectations with early amplification and/or implantation. Presented at the annual convention of the American Academy of Audiology, Boston.

Stenger, P. (1907). Simulation and dissimilation of ear diseases and their identification [in German]. Deutsch Medizinsche Wochenschrift, 33(24), 970–973.

Tait, M., De Raeve, L., & Nikolopoulos, T. P. (2007). Deaf children with cochlear implants before the age of 1 year: comparison of preverbal communication with normally hearing children. International Journal of Pediatric Otorhinolaryngology, 71(10), 1605–1611.

Part IV

Educational and Clinical Management of Hearing Loss in Children

Chapter 25

Collaborative Team Management of Children with Hearing Loss

Jane R. Madell and Carol Flexer

Key Points

- The goal of team management is to have all involved professionals provide services in a coordinated way and with a unified philosophy to a child with hearing loss and his family.
- The child and family are always at the center of the team.
- A system of communication, shared among clinicians and the family, needs to be formulated that will provide information about how a child is performing. Some families have found a communication notebook, e-mails, or blogs to be useful tools for sharing information among team members in multiple settings.
- For team coordination to work well, someone must be assigned to be the case manager; as the child's needs change over time, the case manager may change.
- Disagreements among clinicians need to be handled in a way that does not involve families in interprofessional disputes.

◆ The Goal of Team Management

Multiple professionals are involved in providing services to children with hearing loss and their families. Even though the professionals may do their best individually, they do not always work together as a coordinated team or communicate with each other when planning and implementing services. As a result, the totality of services that the child actually receives can be far from optimal (Madell et al, 2003; Yoshinaga-Itano, 2011).

The goal of team management is to have all involved professionals provide services in a coordinated way to a child with hearing loss and his family. Sometimes all services are provided by a single program in one location. In other instances, services are

provided by clinicians working out of different programs, including clinicians working in hospital-based audiology programs, in schools, and in private practices. Whether at one or at multiple centers, services should be delivered with a unified philosophy and by clinicians who communicate regularly with each other (Madell et al, 2003; McNamara & Richard, 2012).

Teaming can be a very positive experience for professionals and families, in the following ways:

- Observations made by one clinician are helpful to other clinicians in understanding the child's overall performance and behaviors and can help clinicians rethink and improve their individual recommendations.
- Collaborating with service providers from other specialties helps clinicians expand their knowledge base and helps them better understand all children they serve.
- Collaboration with a team provides each professional with a broader view of the effects of hearing loss on the child and the family.

This chapter will discuss the composition of a team and the roles of team members. The critical position of the team manager will be detailed. The chapter will end with four case studies that illustrate the value of a coordinated team and the recognition that the role of team manager shifts as the child's primary needs change over time.

◆ Who Is on the Team?

The composition of the team will be different for every child and will depend on the child's individual needs (**Fig. 25.1**). The child is always at the center of the team. All team efforts focus on the child, the family, and their needs. In some cases, the family includes only the parents. In other cases, extended family members (grandparents, aunts, uncles, siblings, and other caregivers) are included as well.

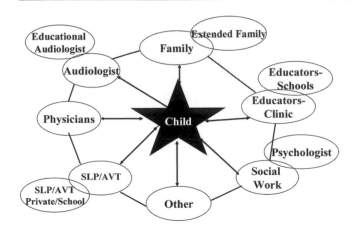

Fig. 25.1 The team. AVT, auditory-verbal therapist; SLP, speech-language pathologist.

Audiologist

For every child with hearing loss or central auditory processing disorder (CAPD), a pediatric audiologist is a key member of the team. The audiologist is responsible for:

- Identifying hearing loss
- Monitoring hearing loss over time
- Evaluating auditory behaviors
- Evaluating speech perception capabilities
- Selecting and fitting amplification technologies (hearing aids, cochlear implants, frequency modulation [FM] systems)
- Monitoring use of technologies to be certain that they are providing the necessary benefit
- Evaluating the need for and selection of assistive technologies, including personal FM and classroom listening systems
- Counseling parents and other team members about hearing loss and technology
- Identifying other auditory problems, such as CAPDs
- Educating parents, teachers, and others about hearing loss, the effect of hearing loss on learning, and about ways to maximize auditory skills in children with hearing loss and other auditory disorders

Because the audiologist sees the child less frequently than some of the other team members, she can and should observe the child's progress over time, including the child's speech, language, and auditory development. If the child is not making appropriate progress, the audiologist needs to discuss concerns with other team members and encourage them to reevaluate the child's developmental, listening, and linguistic status.

Once a child enters school, an educational audiologist frequently joins the team. The educational audiologist will be responsible for monitoring personal technology in school, selecting and monitoring assistive technology (including frequency modulation [FM] systems), and teaching school staff how to use the systems appropriately. In some schools, the educational audiologist is responsible for educating classroom teachers about hearing loss and maximizing learning in the classroom for children with hearing loss. In other schools, training school personnel is the responsibility of the teacher of the deaf (TOD). In some cases, the educational audiologist may provide all the audiology services a child requires, and the child may not receive audiologic services from an outside clinic or hospital. In other cases, the school audiologist will not deal with personal technology and will deal only with school equipment. A few audiology centers employ an educational audiologist in-house who may provide both clinical and educational audiologic services. If an educational audiologist is not employed by the school district, it may fall to the clinical audiologist to provide the services that are the responsibility of the educational audiologist in other districts (Madell, 2011).

Medical Professionals

Every child with hearing loss will receive medical services from at least two physicians: a pediatrician and an otolaryngologist. The pediatrician will manage routine medical issues, and the otolaryngologist will be responsible for ear issues.

Infants with hearing loss ought to have the benefit of a medical home (American Academy of Pediatrics [AAP], 2002), which the AAP defines as an approach to providing health care services where care is "accessible, family-centered, continuous, comprehensive, coordinated, compassionate, and culturally competent." For most children, the medical home will reside with the pediatrician; however, this may not be the case for every child.

All children with hearing loss should see an otolaryngologist at least annually. Obviously, it is necessary for pediatricians and otolaryngologists to work well together so that medical issues can be treated in a timely fashion. These key physicians will be responsible for making referrals to other medical personnel as needed, including referrals for genetics evaluations, neurology, and ophthalmology consultation. (See Chapter 4 for a complete discussion of medical management of the child with hearing loss.)

Speech-Language-Auditory Therapist

A speech-language pathologist (SLP) with specific training in the provision of auditory therapy for children with hearing loss, or an auditory-verbal therapist, needs to be involved in the evaluation and management of all children with hearing loss (see Chapter 28). As soon as the hearing loss is identified and at least annually thereafter, the child's speech-language skills and functional listening skills should be assessed. This evaluation will include assessing and monitoring the child's performance with his technology, and participating in determining the need to change technology (e.g., to new or more powerful hearing aids or to shift from hearing aids to cochlear implants). After speech-language and auditory assessments are conducted, recommendations are made for appropriate therapies and for providing training and coaching to parents to enable them to carry therapy over at home. When a child reaches school age, services may move from the clinic to the school. However, if the school SLP does not have the skills to work with children with hearing loss, it may be necessary for the child to continue to receive services outside the school environment or to train school personnel to work with children with hearing loss.

Educational Personnel

A TOD typically is involved in the management of all school-aged children with hearing loss. (The title of this teacher may vary; forms include "teacher of the deaf," "teacher of the hearing-impaired," and "teacher of the deaf or hard of hearing.") In some areas of the country, a TOD will be involved with preschool children also (see Chapter 29). For children enrolled in self-contained classes for children with hearing loss, the TOD will be the primary provider of educational services. For children who are mainstreamed, a general education teacher will be responsible for providing academic instruction. As a support, the TOD may provide individual or resource room instruction on a daily basis or several times per week to preview material that will be covered in the mainstream class and to review material previously covered. The TOD, in some schools, will also be responsible for monitoring the FM equipment and for teaching the regular school staff about hearing aids, cochlear implants, and FM systems.

Social Worker

Social workers meet with newly diagnosed families to help them deal with their feelings about having a child with hearing loss and to help them work through the paperwork involved in procuring services and technology for their children. Social workers can help families enroll in early intervention, obtain Medicaid funding as appropriate, and navigate insurance issues. In some centers, they work with families who are trying to decide the value of shifting from hearing aids to cochlear implants. They provide crisis intervention for families: when a hearing loss is identified, when a child has a decrease in hearing or a cochlear implant device failure, or when family issues occur that are not related to hearing loss. In some centers, the social worker may run support groups for teenagers and for parents. Support groups could be run by the social worker alone or collaboratively with other staff members.

Psychologist

School systems and other clinics may have an educational psychologist who evaluates children on a regular basis (usually every 3 years) to assess learning strengths and weaknesses and to make recommendations for educational placement and special service needs. Psychologists also may offer the support services provided by social workers as described in the preceding paragraph, including counseling for newly diagnosed hearing loss, managing support groups, and providing assistance in crisis intervention.

Family

Families play a critical role in a child's success. The word *family* is used here in its broadest definition. *Family* certainly implies parents, but also can include grandparents, siblings, and other relatives or caregivers (nannies, etc.) who are involved in a child's day-to-day care. Even the most talented group of clinicians will not be successful in educating a child if the family is not involved (Boons et al, 2012). Language learning must take place all day long. Infants and young children are at home many hours each day. If the family is not working with the child for many hours every day, the child will not reach the outcomes desired by the family.

A family who has selected an auditory-oral (now called Listening and Spoken Language [LSL]) or auditory-verbal program for their child needs to be responsible for making sure that the child's technology is always working optimally. In addition, they need to know how to talk, talk, talk to the child to build language and communication (Cole & Flexer, 2011). Families who have selected sign language as a communication mode for their child need to learn sign language way above the level of baby and preschool signs. They need to communicate with the child using sign language in the same way and at the same level of language complexity used to communicate with their hearing children in order for the child's language to develop to age-appropriate levels.

In addition to working with their child at home, a family needs to transport their children to and from therapy. Once the child is in school, the family must be sure that the child goes to sleep early enough to be bright and alert and ready to learn when at school. Further, the family needs to check and assist with homework. The family needs to know what is happening at school and in therapy to be sure the child is receiving the services he needs. In addition, the family needs to verify that professionals working with the child have high enough expectations, and that the child is doing the best that he can do.

Providing support even for normally developing children is very often stressful for parents. Children with special needs, including children with hearing loss, require even more effort on the part of the family (see Chapter 34). Even though parents are primarily responsible, grandparents and others can be very helpful in providing the necessary assistance.

Occupational and Physical Therapists

Many children who are deaf or hard of hearing, especially in the preschool years, need the services of physical or occupational therapists. Services include strengthening fine and gross muscle development as well as vestibular development and sensory integration. These services may be provided in schools or may be obtained from clinicians outside of school. If the clinicians providing these services are not familiar with hearing loss, the audiologist or another member of the team should work with the clinicians to help them understand about hearing loss and about how they can work to improve the child's listening skills during their therapy sessions.

Professionals in the Community

When children receive services from clinicians in more than one center or from individual providers, everyone on the team must make a commitment to open communication. A child may receive speech-language services from a provider at one center and audiology services from a provider at another. The audiologist can deliver the best possible audiology services only when she knows how the child is performing with hearing aids at home and at school. For example, the speech-language pathologist, auditory therapist, and classroom teacher should be able to tell the audiologist what specific phonemes the child is not hearing or that the child is having difficulty hearing soft speech. With this information, the audiologist can adjust technology to improve functioning.

A system of communication, shared among clinicians, needs to be formulated that will provide ongoing information about how a child is performing. Certainly everyone working with a child should send diagnostic and evaluation reports to others on the team. However, evaluations usually do not occur frequently, so any problems that develop between evaluations may not be reported to team members in a timely fashion.

Some families have found a communication notebook to be a useful tool for sharing information among team members. The notebook travels with the child to every setting and team member. Then, everyone who works with the child writes down what is happening during each contact, including concerns about performance, homework, and questions for others on the team. Some families have developed a Web site or blog where everyone involved with the child can share information. Paper or electronic notebooks are effective only if everyone, including parents, is committed to both writing a summary of contact with the child and reading other clinicians' entries.

Fig. 25.2 is an example of another communication tool that can be useful. It is an information sheet that can be shared between the audiologist and SLP. Because the SLP or auditory verbal therapist sees the child frequently, she is in a good position to identify the child's auditory problems specifically. Sharing this information with the audiologist in a clear and concise way places the audiologist in a good position to make changes in equipment to improve listening skills.

OBSERVATIONS OF AUDITORY PERCEPTION

Child's Name_____   Date: _____

Observed by: _____   Title: _____

Cochlear Implant: ____Cochlear Corp.   ____Advanced Bionics   ____MED-EL

Speech Processor: _____

Program #_____   Volume #_____   Sensitivity #_____

Program #_____   Volume #_____   Sensitivity #_____

Program #_____   Volume #_____   Sensitivity #_____

Program #_____   Volume #_____   Sensitivity #_____

Hearing Aid Type: Right Ear_____   Left Ear _____

Volume: Right Ear_____   Left Ear_____

Program Information: _____

Changes in Perception since last MAP or Hearing Aid Adjustment

Date(s) of Observation:_____

Has the child demonstrated misperceptions since the last MAP/Hearing Aid adjustment?_____

_____

Has the child demonstrated phonemic confusion since the last MAP/Hearing Aid adjustment?_____

_____

Have there been changes in voice quality?_____

Have there been changes in resonance? _____

Has the child asked for more repetitions of information?_____

Has the child been clipping syllables or lengthening vowel?_____

Has the child had difficulty adhering to word boundaries? _____

Has there been changes in FM usage? _____

Additional Comments or Observations:

Fig. 25.2 Communication between the speech-language-auditory therapist and audiologist: Observation of auditory perception.

◆ The Case Manager

For team coordination to work well, someone must be designated to be the case manager. There must be a go-to person, or critical problems may remain unsolved.

How Is It Decided Who the Case Manager Will Be?

Interesting issues evolve around the selection of the case manager. For example:

- Is there thoughtful discussion between team members about the child's needs at this point in time and who is best suited to manage them?
- Does the case management decision happen by accident?
- Does the case management decision happen by default?
- Is the case manager the practitioner who sees the child most often?
- Who has input into selecting the manager?
- What is the role of the parent in selecting the manager?
- Do all team members recognize who is the team manager?

Because the case manager must assume a critical leadership role, these questions should be thoughtfully answered in order for the team to work together effectively to attain the family's desired outcome.

The case manager is responsible for:

- Collecting information from everyone working with the child
- Being sure that the information is distributed to all team members
- Determining the services that are needed
- Addressing problems as they arise
- Ensuring that the child actually is receiving all the necessary services
- Being available to provide support to the family
- Communicating with all clinicians, either at case conferences or by phone, mail, or email

If a child is receiving services from many facilities, the parents will often be responsible for coordinating services. Although the parents are certainly ultimately responsible for their child, it can be difficult for them to negotiate differences of opinion between clinicians. Therefore, it is often useful if one of the clinicians involved in the case acts as the coordinator. As the child's needs change over time, the coordinator may change.

When audiologic issues are paramount, such as when a child is initially diagnosed or when hearing loss is fluctuating, the audiologist usually assumes the case manager role. On the other hand, when patients are receiving ongoing habilitation services, especially in preschool years, the SLP or auditory therapist is usually the case manager. When a child requires integrated educational planning, a TOD typically becomes the case manager. When there are complex otologic medical issues, the otologist will be the case manager.

Team Meetings

The optimal way for all players to communicate is to have periodic interdisciplinary team meetings. If many children are seen by the same group of clinicians in one location, or in different locations, it will be beneficial for the team members to meet monthly or bimonthly to discuss all children as needed. However, if clinicians from different facilities are involved in providing services, it can be difficult for them to meet in one room at the same time. A conference call using telephone or Skype may be useful for discussing specific issues as they arise and in planning for joint recommendations. For children who are in school, the annual individual education plan (IEP) meeting is frequently a good time to have a team meeting. Clinicians from the community center can go to the school or can participate by phone or Skype. When there are multiple clinicians from one facility, they can meet to discuss the case and have one representative participate at the IEP meeting.

Dealing with Disagreements among Team Members

The child and family will benefit most from receiving a consistent message from all clinicians about goals for the child and ways of achieving the goals. If, for example, one clinician works with the child using American Sign Language (ASL) and another uses auditory-based therapy, the child is not receiving consistent intervention. Moreover, the family is put under a great deal of stress as they attempt to determine what is best for their child while managing very divergent treatments that have different desired outcomes.

Even though clinicians may have legitimate disagreements about recommendations for the child, they should try to work out differences with each other before discussing recommendations with families. Disagreements among clinicians need to be handled in a way that does not involve families in interprofessional disputes. When there is a serious disagreement, such as whether a child should receive a cochlear implant, or whether one educational placement is better than another for a child, parents should be advised of the different opinions, should be presented with complete information, and should be given assistance in making their decision. Clinicians are experts in their own areas; however, the family is always the final arbiter about what is best for their child. Professionals must behave professionally and respectfully toward parents and other professionals, regardless of the decisions made by the family.

◆ Case Examples and Discussion of Case Management Issues

Case 1

"Vic" (not his real name) is a preschooler who is ready to transition to his local school district. Vic has hearing loss that was identified at 12 months of age; he was fitted with hearing aids and an FM system at that time. He received in-home early intervention that included services provided by an SLP and a TOD. The speech-language pathologist was the initial case manager.

Before Vic reached 2 years of age, the audiologist, SLP, and TOD met to discuss the case. It was determined that Vic was not receiving sufficient benefit from his hearing aids. When wearing his hearing aids, he was detecting sounds in the moderate hearing loss range, an insufficient loudness to provide access to the speech spectrum at average and soft conversational levels. Everyone working with Vic recognized that he could function well only when it was quiet or when he was listening through the FM system. He was not able to hear well at a distance or when there was competing noise. A cochlear implant was recommended, and Vic received the implant at 2 years of age. Three months later, he started wearing a hearing aid on the unimplanted ear.

At age 3, Vic entered an auditory-oral (listening and spoken language) preschool program at a school for the deaf. In addition, he attended a mainstream preschool two afternoons per week. The TOD from the Hearing and Speech Center became the case manager and coordinated services between the center, the school for the deaf program, and the mainstream preschool. Even though Vic was doing very well with his cochlear implant, he continued to detect sound at only moderate hearing loss levels with the hearing aid worn in his unimplanted ear. So, at 4 years of age, he received a second cochlear implant. Testing with two cochlear implants indicated that Vic could now detect sound at borderline normal hearing levels. Word recognition scores, obtained during an audiologic evaluation using the Northwestern University Children's Hearing in Pictures (NU-CHIPS) test (Elliot & Katz, 1980), were 84% at a normal conversational level of loudness (50 dB hearing level [HL]), and 60% at a soft conversational level (35 dB HL). In his speech-language-listening evaluation (Kirk, Pisoni, & Osberger, 1995), Vic obtained listening scores of 80 to 100% on the Lexical Neighborhood Test (LNT) and Common Phrases (Osberger et al, 1991) test. Language testing indicated an age equivalent of 5.5 years on the Peabody Picture Vocabulary Test (PPVT)-III (Dunn & Dunn, 2007), and he was in the 75th percentile on the Clinical Evaluation of Language Fundamentals—Preschool (CELF-P) (Wigg, Secord, & Semel, 1992).

The team, consisting of the audiologist and TOD consultant from the Hearing and Speech Center, the speech-language-listening therapist, and the teachers from both the mainstream preschool and the preschool deaf infant program, met again and determined that Vic was ready to be transitioned back to his local school district. The TOD attended the IEP team meeting at the school district and discussed the services that Vic would require to be successfully mainstreamed.

When Vic started school, the TOD visited the mainstream class and met with the staff to provide training about hearing loss and ways to maximize Vic's auditory performance. The TOD from the Hearing and Speech Center remained in touch with both the school and clinic staffs to make sure that Vic was performing well in school.

Case 2

"Gail" (not her real name) is an example of a child with auditory neuropathy spectrum disorder (ANSD). Gail passed otoacoustic emissions (OAE) screening at birth, but as time went on, she demonstrated delayed speech and language development. The parents reported their concern to the pediatrician on several occasions, and finally, at age 18 months, Gail was referred for an audiologic evaluation. At that time, she was identified with a moderate, bilateral sensorineural hearing loss (SNHL). At 19 months, a click auditory brainstem response (ABR) confirmed moderate, bilateral hearing loss; however, ABR testing at that time did not include tonal air and bone thresholds and did not test reversed polarity to check for ANSD. (See Chapter 32.)

Although Gail wore her hearing aids consistently, participated in a good preschool therapy program, and had parents who worked consistently with her, she was not making good progress. Her speech and language skills were slow to develop, and she was not able to use hearing to understand speech. The school suggested that the family consider moving Gail to a program using ASL because of her lack of progress developing auditory skills. At 2.5 years of age, the family sought a second opinion about her diagnosis. The audiologist at the second opinion center was concerned about Gail's performance and poor auditory skills. With her hearing aids, Gail was detecting sound at borderline normal levels, and she was involved in a good auditory therapy program, but she was not making the expected progress. Consequently, the ABR was repeated, including testing with reversed polarity. This time, testing suggested ANSD.

Gail's case was reviewed at a team meeting. The audiologist became the case manager. Bilateral cochlear implants were recommended. Gail received the implants at 38 months of age. She remained in the auditory-oral (listening and spoken language) preschool and made excellent progress. At the 6 month cochlear implant evaluation, word recognition tests indicated the NU-CHIPS test (Elliot & Katz, 1980) scores of 93% at 50 dB HL, 87% at 35 dB HL, and 80% at 50 dB HL +5 dB SNR. Speech and language evaluation at 4.5 years of age indicated delayed language (PPVT) with performance at a 3 year, 7 month age level. Expressive language scores were at 3.7 years. Speech production was excellent at 5.5 years.

Gail's case management then shifted from the audiologist to the TOD as education issues became paramount. The team met again and decided to return Gail to her local school district in an integrated kindergarten class because her language scores were not sufficient for her to be in a mainstream class. Services now included speech-language-auditory services and TOD services, each delivered five times weekly. A personal FM system was recommended for school use. The TOD from the Hearing and Speech Center met with the school to confirm that Gail was going to receive all necessary services. She visited the school, observed the class, and met with the staff to provide training about hearing loss and ways to maximize Gail's auditory performance. She continued to be in touch with the school and clinic staff to ensure that Gail was making good progress.

Case 3

"Suzy" (not her real name) is an example of shifting case management over time. Suzy is a college student who had profound hearing loss identified as a toddler. As a toddler, Suzy was fitted with hearing aids and an FM system; however, her hearing aids enabled her to detect sound only at moderate hearing loss levels. Early psychological testing indicated normal intelligence, and Suzy was enrolled in an auditory-verbal therapy program. The SLP was the first case manager.

Suzy did not make the progress that was expected. She was clearly intelligent but could not seem to learn auditorally, and her speech and language skills were delayed. Because Suzy was not making sufficient progress, when the team met, they felt that they could not recommend a mainstream kindergarten placement. The team discussed Suzy's lack of progress with the family and recommended an alternate therapy program, such as cued speech or ASL. Because

the family was anxious to attempt mainstreaming Suzy, they decided to try cued speech. Consequently, Suzy entered kindergarten with a cued speech interpreter. The cued speech interpreter then became the next case manager.

Suzy continued to receive speech-language-auditory therapy. With the use of the cued speech interpreter, Suzy was able to improve her speech and language skills, but her auditory skills remained poor.

At 7 years of age, the family decided to consider a cochlear implant. Following implantation, Suzy's auditory skills improved dramatically. Within a year, Suzy felt that she no longer required the cued speech interpreter. Her mother and the other clinicians involved in Suzy's management were skeptical about Suzy's attending school without an interpreter. As a result, the interpreter remained in the class for another 6 months; however, she provided less and less assistance. Finally, everyone was comfortable having Suzy in the classroom without that support.

Responsibility for case management shifted again and returned to the speech-language-auditory therapist, who continued to provide services. By fourth grade, Suzy began using a note-taker, and when she entered high school, she stopped receiving speech-language services.

Suzy's mother now became the case manager. Suzy received Communication Access Real-time Translation (CART) services in high school for academic subjects. At the time she entered high school, she also decided to receive a cochlear implant for her second ear. Suzy then returned to auditory therapy for 1 year after receiving the second cochlear implant. She is now a freshman in college, majoring in psychology. She receives CART services in the classroom and extended time for tests. Her grades are good. She is now her own case manager.

Case 4

"Lenny" (not his real name) has Down syndrome. Lenny's auditory management began when he was 5 months old. Lenny failed his newborn hearing screening. Follow-up behavioral and ABR testing indicated moderate hearing loss by air conduction, but bone conduction thresholds were within normal limits. He had flat tympanograms, consistent with middle ear pathology. Lenny was referred to an ear, nose, and throat specialist. Otologic evaluations revealed very narrow external auditory canals and bilateral serous otitis media.

Management issues were discussed. Should Lenny receive myringotomy tubes? Should he receive hearing aids? In either case, he needed speech-language-auditory therapy. Management became the responsibility of the otologist because medical issues were paramount. The decision was made by the team to not use myringotomy tubes because of the narrowness of the ear canals. In addition, since it was now spring, it was hoped that Lenny's health would improve and his ears would clear of fluid.

Subsequently, Lenny was fitted with amplification and was doing well, even though fluid was still present in his middle ears. He was closely monitored otologically and received several courses of antibiotics. Middle ear disease cleared up for short periods of time but returned, with associated hearing loss that negatively affected his speech and language development.

Responsibility for case management moved to the audiologist to deal with amplification issues. Lenny received speech-language-auditory therapy and was enrolled in a special education preschool. At 3 years of age, hearing testing continued to indicate a primarily mild hearing loss with moderate thresholds in the low frequencies. Unaided word recognition testing using a test appropriate for Lenny's receptive language level indicated poor word recognition scores (48%) at a normal conversational level (50 dB HL), 0% at soft conversational levels (35 dB HL), and very poor word recognition (24%) at a normal conversational level with competing noise added. Fortunately, testing with hearing aids revealed excellent word recognition scores (86 to 94%) in all three conditions.

The case was discussed again with the team. The otologist felt that the situation in Lenny's ears had changed sufficiently so that myringotomy tubes could be inserted. Surgery was performed and hearing improved slightly, but hearing aids were still necessary.

Case management then moved to the speech-language-auditory therapist, who was now the primary provider. When Lenny entered kindergarten in a special education class, management was shared between the classroom teacher and the speech-language-auditory therapist, who continued to provide services to Lenny.

◆ Summary

Although providing collaborative services requires increased effort on the part of all involved, the extra work is more than worth the effort because collaboration is essential for the provision of quality services to infants and children. In some ways, teaming makes the jobs of all professionals easier, because collaboration enables each to work in designated areas of expertise and allows other team members to contribute their unique knowledge. Each team member values his place on the team and respects and appreciates the roles of the others. Furthermore, having multiple clinicians provides more support to families.

The case manager typically changes over time (Madell & Flexer, 2012), and eventually the family usually takes over that responsibility. When children reach college age, many are capable of taking over responsibility for their own services. Self-advocacy is, of course, the ultimate goal.

Discussion Questions

1. What factors should be considered when determining which professional should be the team manager for a child with hearing loss at any point in time?

2. How are members of the team selected?

3. What are some ways that team disagreements might be resolved?

4. What strategies and techniques will allow all team members to stay in communication with one another?

References

American Academy of Pediatrics. (2002). The medical home. Pediatrics, 110(1 Pt 1), 184–186.

Boons, T., Brokx, J. P., Dhooge, I., Frijns, J. H., Peeraer, L., Vermeulen, A., . . . van Wieringen, A. (2012). Predictors of spoken language development following pediatric cochlear implantation. Ear and Hearing, 33(5), 617–639.

Cole, E., & Flexer, C. (2011). Children with hearing loss: developing listening and talking, birth to six (2nd ed.). San Diego, CA: Plural.

Dunn, L. M., & Dunn, L. M. (2007). Peabody Picture Vocabulary Test, 4th Edition, (PPVT-4 Scale). New York, NY: Pearson Assessments.

Elliot, L., & Katz, D. (1980). Development of a new children's test of speech discrimination. St Louis, MO: Auditec.

Kirk, K. I., Pisoni, D. B., & Osberger, M. J. (1995, Oct). Lexical effects on spoken word recognition by pediatric cochlear implant users. Ear and Hearing, 16(5), 470–481.

Madell, J. R. (2011). Acoustic accessibility: the role of the clinical audiologist. In J. Smaldino, & C. Flexer (Eds.), Handbook of acoustic accessibility: best practices for listening, learning, and literacy in the classroom (pp. 128–142). New York, NY: Thieme.

Madell, J., & Flexer, C. (2012). Who is in charge? Case management of children with hearing loss. AudiologyOnline, Recorded Course #21112. Retrieved from http://www.audiologyonline.com/audiology-ceus/course/early-intervention-aural-habilitation-children-who-in-charge-case-management-21112

Madell, J. R., Hoffman, R. A., Kooper, R., Cheffo, S., Heymann, L., Rothschild, P., . . . Houston, K. R. (2003). Coordination of cochlear implant services. Audiology Today (Special Issue), FT1–FT20.

McNamara, T., & Richard, G. (2012). Better together. The ASHA Leader, 17(3), 12–14.

Osberger, M. J., Miyamoto, R. T., Zimmerman-Phillips, S., Kemink, J. L., Stroer, B. S., Firszt, J. B., & Novak, M. A. (1991). Independent evaluation of the speech perception abilities of children with the Nucleus 22-channel cochlear implant system. Ear and Hearing, 12(4, Suppl), 66S–80S.

Wigg, E., Secord, W., & Semel, E. (1992). Clinical Evaluation of Language Fundamentals—Preschool (CELF-P). New York, NY: The Psychological Corporation.

Yoshinaga-Itano, C. (2011). Achieving optimal outcomes from EHDI. The ASHA Leader, 16(11), 14–17.

Chapter 26

Communication Approaches for Managing Hearing Loss in Infants and Children

Carol Flexer

Key Points

- The main communication approaches first discussed with families typically include: those that focus on listening and spoken language (LSL), including auditory-oral (A-O)—now called auditory-verbal education (AVEd)—and auditory-verbal therapy (AVT); cued speech; sign language (BiBi); and total communication (TC).

- Families need to be provided with full information about each approach; one way to begin the communication options conversation is to ask families about their desired outcome for their baby or child.

- The professional must recognize that ~95% of children with hearing loss are born to hearing and speaking families; these families are very interested in having their child learn to listen and talk.

- Some communication approaches are primarily auditory in orientation, and some are primarily visual.

- Not every child will do well with every approach, for a multiplicity of reasons.

A variety of communication approaches are available for managing hearing loss in infants and children (Schwartz, 2007). The decision about selecting the best approach for a particular child and her family is usually overwhelming because parents are asked to make this important decision at a time when they have just learned they have a baby or child who is deaf or hard of hearing, and when they have had little or no experience with hearing loss, hearing aids, or cochlear implants.

The purpose of this chapter is to present a summary overview of the various communication approaches and to provide a list of resources and Web sites that offer additional and detailed information about each approach.

◆ What Are the Communication Approaches?

Multiple approaches are available for teaching babies and children who are deaf or hard of hearing to communicate. Some approaches are primarily auditory, and some are primarily visual; these different orientations likely will lead to different outcomes.

Auditory Approaches

An auditory approach is based on the assumption that a baby or child with hearing loss can have primary access to auditory information through the use of hearing aids or cochlear implants (Cole & Flexer, 2011; Estabrooks, 2006; Ling, 2002; Nicholas & Geers, 2006). The goal of an auditory approach is to develop spoken language and communication through listening, leading to full and independent integration of the child into the general hearing community (Cole & Flexer, 2011; Fitzpatrick, Crawford, Ni, & Durieux-Smith, 2011; Pollack, Goldberg, & Caleffe-Schenck, 1997). The main auditory approaches historically have been A-O and AVT. Recently, a new certification program has been developed called the LSLS (Listening and Spoken Language Specialist) that recognizes the unity and similarities in both listening and spoken-language approaches. There are two branches of the LSLS program: LSLS Cert. AVEd (Auditory-Verbal Educator) and LSLS Cert. AVT (Auditory-Verbal Therapist). For more information about the LSLS program, please refer to AG Bell Academy for Listening and Spoken Language (n.d.).

Pearl

- If spoken communication is the family's desired outcome for their baby, auditory brain access through the use of technology followed by extensive, parent-centered auditory language enrichment is essential.

Cued speech may be placed in the spoken-language category, because even though it uses a visual system of hand shapes and signals that the family must learn, the goal of cued speech is to facilitate programming, mainstreaming, and spoken communication, not to develop a sign language system.

Visual Approaches

Visual approaches, on the other hand, focus on looking, not on listening. They are based on the assumption that a baby or child who experiences hearing loss cannot access her auditory environment in a foremost way and cannot become proficient in spoken communication, even with amplification (Marschark & Spencer, 2010). The goal of a visual approach is to use sign language as the primary communication, and to be part of the deaf community (Schwartz, 2007). Families must become proficient in sign language to communicate with their children beyond the preschool level. Examples of visual approaches are BiBi, American Sign Language (ASL),

Manually Coded English (MCE), and Conceptually Accurate Signed English (CASE) (**Table 26.1**).

Some approaches attempt to teach both spoken and sign language communication (Watkins, Taylor, & Pittman, 2004). Examples are Simultaneous Communication, Sign-Supported Speech and Language, and Total Communication (TC). The terms *simultaneous communication* and *total communication* often are used interchangeably.

Approach Issues

There are advantages and disadvantages to each approach (Kretschmer & Kretschmer 2001) depending in part on:

- The nature and needs of the child and family
- The ability of the family to do what it takes to implement a particular approach
- The presence of qualified providers to work with and support the family

In addition, reports vary about how successful or unsuccessful a particular approach might be (Moog & Geers, 2003).

Pearl

- Success can be defined as reaching the desired outcome expressed by the family through the implementation of the chosen communication approach.

Table 26.1 Visual languages, systems, and strategies

Communication approach	Characteristics of communication
ASL	ASL is a visual-gestural language that is used by some deaf people in the United States and Canada. It has its own set of language rules that are separate from spoken or written English. It is not possible to speak English and sign ASL at the same time. Speech is not used, and the goal is to communicate using sign language, not spoken language. Different sign language systems are used in different countries.
CASE or PSE	Signs from ASL are used in English word order. The focus is on conceptual accuracy to augment understanding, and no attempt is made to provide a one-to-one relationship with spoken English. Specific features of ASL, such as facial expression and use of space, may be used. Both CASE and PSE rely on context and mechanisms such as initialization to support meaning.
MCE	These systems, including Seeing Essential English (SEE1) and Signing Exact English (SEE2), were constructed by educators to teach English. The sign systems attempt to represent English by combining ASL signs, English word order, and some invented signs to represent grammatical markers (plurals, possessives, tenses) in English. Each word, including each morpheme, is signed. An example would be to sign the word "*working*" by signing the word "*work*" and then signing the ending "*ing*." All structure words, such as "*the*" and "*to*," are signed in this system.

Abbreviations: ASL, American Sign Language; CASE, Conceptually Accurate Signed English; MCE, Manually Coded English; PSE, Pidgin Signed English.

Note: Teachers or interpreters with special skills in each of these visual modes will be required to implement the communication approach. In addition, family members will need to become proficient in these visual approaches to communicate with their children beyond a preschool level.

Not every child will do well in every approach, for many reasons. It is not unusual for a family to select one approach or even to combine approaches, and then change their mind as they acquire more information and experience (Luterman and Maxon, 2002). The selection of a particular communication approach at any point in the habilitative process is influenced by many variables, including:

- The child's age at the time of diagnosis of hearing loss
- Other problems, disabilities, or challenges not related to hearing loss that the child may have or that may surface as the child ages
- The family's ability to help instruct the child over time
- The quality of intervention programs that are available for infants and school-aged children in the family's geographic area

Summary of Approaches

Many Web sites and books explain each approach in detail; some of these resources are included at the end of this chapter. **Table 26.1** and **Table 26.2** summarize these approaches.

Families need to be provided with full information about each approach (Joint Committee on Infant Hearing, 2007). One way to begin the communication options conversation is to ask the family about their desired outcome for their baby or child. That is, how do they want their child to communicate in the family constellation, in school, and in the community? The professional must recognize that ~ 95% of children with hearing loss are born to hearing and speaking families (Mitchell & Karchmer, 2004); these families are very interested in having their child learn to listen and talk. The conversation then needs to focus on what it takes from both the family and a qualified interventionist to implement each approach, because every approach requires family involvement (Watkins et al, 2004).

Factors to Consider

A family might consider many factors when choosing how to communicate with their child (Cole & Flexer, 2011; Fitzpatrick et al, 2011; Ling, 2002; Luterman & Maxon, 2002; Madell & Flexer, 2011; Watkins et al, 2004):

- Is the communication approach in the best interest of the child and family?
- Does the communication approach enable the child to have control and influence over the environment, to converse about needs, and to take part in the world of abstract thought?

- Does the communication approach enable all family members to communicate deeply—not only on the surface—with the child?
- Does the communication approach permit the child to feel part of the family unit through pleasurable and significant interaction?
- How will the child communicate with peers, with extended family, and with the community as a whole?
- Is the family ready to take on the commitment that the communication approach requires?
- Will the child be equipped by school age with the necessary language, thinking, and learning skills?

Programming decisions are very difficult and can be made only after a great deal of thought. Before a family makes a communication approach decision, they are advised to do the following (Watkins et al, 2004):

- Visit the various programs and individual therapists in the community
- Meet and speak with parents of other children with hearing loss who are enrolled in different programs
- Meet and speak with older teens and adults with hearing loss who have been taught using the various approaches, keeping in mind that they were born at a time that did not have newborn hearing screening, early intervention, cochlear implants, or digital hearing aids

◆ Summary

Every communication approach decision should be reviewed regularly. Not every program is right for every child, and families may change approaches over time. As the child grows and learns, the family and therapists will discover more about what is best for the child.

Pearl

- A key issue is expectations. In this time of early identification and multiple technologies, parents and family ought to have high expectations for outcomes, if all parties do what it takes.

During the beginning stages of therapy, the child's progress should be reviewed often, and diagnostics should be a part of therapy sessions. If the selected approach does not seem to be a match for the child or family, or if the child is not progressing as originally expected, an approach change could be investigated. (See Chapter 24 of this book for "red flags" that might interfere with progress.)

Table 26.2 Summary of communication approaches and philosophies

Communication approaches and philosophies	Definition
A-O Approach (now called AVEd by many professionals)	This approach has spoken language as a desired outcome. Active listening, enhanced by the use of hearing aids or cochlear implants, is accompanied by speech reading to receive instructional and conversational information (Clark, 2006). The use of natural gestures is acceptable; sign language is not used. Children with hearing loss may be grouped together in auditory-oral classrooms for specialized oral instruction, at least in preschool and kindergarten, with mainstreaming being a goal. Family members will need to learn how to manage auditory technology and how to provide an enriched spoken language environment for their child.
AVT Approach (AVT has also been called "unisensory" and "acoupedic")	This is primarily an early intervention therapeutic approach in which technology (hearing aids or cochlear implants) is paired with specific techniques and strategies that teach children to listen and understand spoken language. The 10 Principles of Auditory-Verbal Practice focus on parent coaching to foster cognition, speaking, reading, and learning through the auditory modality. Visual cues (lip reading and sign language) are not used or taught during therapy, so that the child can develop the auditory system through directed listening practice. The foremost goals of A-V therapy are to guide parents and caregivers as the primary facilitators for helping their children develop intelligible spoken language through listening and to advocate for their children's inclusion in regular schools. AVT uses one-on-one teaching of parent or caregiver and child, focusing on strong family involvement; children are mainstreamed from the beginning (Estabrooks, 2006). However, some children will require additional auditory support after entering the mainstream. Parents are key partners in AVT.
BiBi	A person who achieves fluency in ASL and English (or another language) is bilingual. Using this approach, ASL is often taught as the first language and English is taught as a second language to develop literacy skills. English may be taught by using a sign system or through print—spoken English is not featured. The child will need to be in an ASL self-contained classroom or will require an ASL interpreter if placed in a general education classroom. Family members will also need to learn ASL and the English-based sign system to communicate with their child.
Cued Speech	A supplement to spoken English, Cued Speech is intended to make important features of spoken language fully visible, since ~ 60% of the phonemes are not visible through speech reading. This system enhances speech reading by employing phonemically based gestures to distinguish between similar visual speech patterns. The goal of Cued Speech is the reception and expression of spoken communication. Family members will need to learn Cued Speech to communicate with their child. Children are expected to be able to drop the use of cues once their oral language skills are firmly established.
Sign-Supported Speech	Signs are used occasionally to support spoken language development. Signs function as a bridge and language to enhance the meaning of oral communication. The signs also can serve to enhance understanding in certain challenging situations, such as noisy environments or when a hearing device is not in use. Family members will need to learn sign language in addition to oral communication techniques to communicate with their child.
Simultaneous Communication	This is the concurrent use of signs and speech. To provide language using two modalities simultaneously, a sign system, rather than a signed language, is used. This visual representation of the oral language is accomplished using manual symbols and signs. If not in a self-contained classroom that uses sign language, the child will require a sign language interpreter. Family members will need to learn both sign language and oral communication techniques to communicate with their child.
TC	Introduced in the 1960s, this philosophy aims to make use of several strategies or modes of communication, including sign, speech, auditory, written, and other visual aids. First developed by Roy Holcomb, the choice of modalities depends on the particular needs and abilities of the child and professes to provide whatever is needed to foster communicative success. Children will need to be placed in a TC classroom or have an interpreter if in general education classrooms. Family members also will need to learn sign language and other prescribed techniques to communicate with their child.

Abbreviations: AVEd, Auditory–Verbal Education; A-O, Auditory-Oral; ASL, American Sign Language; AVT, Auditory-Verbal Therapy; BiBi, Bilingual Bimodal; TC, Total Communication
(Developed with Arlene Stredler Brown; see Chapter 24 for more information about early intervention practices.)

Discussion Questions

1. How might the pediatric audiologist initiate a communication approach conversation with a family?

2. What is the role of a pediatric audiologist relative to a family's choice and implementation of a communication approach?

3. Does the management of hearing loss play a role in every communication approach? Why or why not?

4. Does the recommendation of amplification technology play a role in visual approaches as well as in auditory approaches?

◆ Web-Based Resources

General Information

- http://www.ncbegin.org
- http://www.handsandvoices.org
- http://www.babyhearing.org
- http://www.successforkidswithhearingloss.com

Information about Listening and Spoken Language (LSL) Approaches

- http://www.agbell.org
- http://www.oraldeafed.org
- http://www.listen-up.org
- http://www.johntracyclinic.org

Information about Cued Speech

- http://www.cuedspeech.org
- http://www.dailycues.com
- http://www.tecunit.org
- http://www.language-matters.com

Information about ASL and Visual Approaches

- http://www.deafchildren.org
- http://www.nad.org
- http://deafness.about.com/cs/communication/a/totalcomm.htm
- http://clerccenter.gallaudet.edu
- http://www.seecenter.org

References

AG Bell Academy for Listening and Spoken Language. (n.d.). AG Bell Academy. Retrieved from http://www.listeningandspokenlanguage.org/AGBellAcademy/

Clark, M. (2006). A practical guide to quality interaction with children who have a hearing loss. San Diego, CA: Plural.

Cole, E., & Flexer, C. (2011). Children with hearing loss: developing listening and talking, birth to six (2nd ed.). San Diego, CA: Plural.

Estabrooks, W. (2006). Auditory-verbal therapy and practice. Washington, DC: Alexander Graham Bell Association for the Deaf and Hard of Hearing.

Fitzpatrick, E. M., Crawford, L., Ni, A., & Durieux-Smith, A. (2011). A descriptive analysis of language and speech skills in 4- to 5-yr-old children with hearing loss. Ear and Hearing, 32(5), 605–616.

Joint Committee on Infant Hearing. (2007). Year 2007 position statement: principles and guidelines for early hearing detection and intervention programs. Pediatrics, 102(4), 893–921.

Kretschmer, L., & Kretschmer, R. (2001). Children with hearing impairment. In T. Layton, E. Crais, & L. Watson (Eds.), Handbook of early language impairment in children: nature (pp. 560–584). Albany, NY: Delmar.

Ling, D. (2002). Speech and the hearing impaired child (2nd ed.). Washington, DC: Alexander Graham Bell Association for the Deaf and Hard of Hearing.

Luterman, D. M., & Maxon, A. (2002). When your child is deaf: a guide for parents (2nd ed.). Austin: Pro-Ed.

Madell, J., & Flexer, C.(2011). Pediatric audiology casebook. New York: Thieme Medical Publishers, Inc.

Marschark, M., & Spencer, P. A. (2010). The Oxford handbook of deaf studies, language, and education, Vol. 2. New York, NY: Oxford.

Mitchell, R. E., & Karchmer, M. A. (2004). Chasing the mythical ten percent: parental hearing status of deaf and hard of hearing students in the United States. Sign Language Studies, 4, 138–163.

Moog, J. S., & Geers, A. E. (2003). Epilogue: major findings, conclusions and implications for deaf education. Ear and Hearing, 24(1, Suppl), 121S–125S.

Nicholas, J. G., & Geers, A. E. (2006). Effects of early auditory experience on the spoken language of deaf children at 3 years of age. Ear and Hearing, 27(3), 286–298.

Pollack, D., Goldberg, D., & Caleffe-Schenck, N. (1997). Educational audiology for the limited-hearing infant and preschooler: an auditory-verbal program. Springfield, IL: Charles C. Thomas.

Schwartz, S. (2007). Choices in deafness: a parent's guide to communication options (3rd ed.). Bethesda, MD: Woodbine House.

Watkins, S., Taylor, D. J., & Pittman, P. (2004). SKI-HI curriculum: family-centered programming for infants and young children with hearing loss. Logan, UT: HOPE, Inc.

Chapter 27

The Importance of Early Intervention for Infants and Children with Hearing Loss

Arlene Stredler-Brown

Key Points

- Several federal initiatives support early intervention for infants and toddlers with hearing loss. The Individuals with Disabilities Education Act (IDEA), Part C, mandates services for children younger than 36 months. The Early Hearing Detection & Intervention initiative has been supported legislatively; most recently, the Early Hearing Detection and Intervention (EHDI) Act of 2010 was signed into law. The EHDI initiative provides funding to states to develop screening, audiologic diagnostic, and early intervention programs.

- Early intervention for children with hearing loss is a relatively new profession. Providers continue to rely on in-service training to meet quality standards.

- Very young children practice communication in their daily routines. In family-centered intervention, parents and other family members are the primary recipients of the care. Family-centered intervention is a three-pronged approach that provides information and support for parents, facilitates child development, and provides instruction on optimal characteristics of parent–child interaction. There are specific curriculums for each of these domains.

- The goal for infants and toddlers with hearing loss is to achieve communication and language skills commensurate with their hearing peers. It is valuable to rely on objective assessment information to guide the intervention; evidence is key.

- Many children live in remote or rural communities where access to well-qualified interventionists may be limited. Telepractice, the delivery of early intervention from a distance, can provide access to family-centered services that are delivered remotely by experts in hearing loss.

Case studies have been used to illustrate the key points in this chapter. These vignettes are based on events in families' lives. Each anecdote encourages the reader to think about the way she delivers information to families.

◆ Case One

An 8-week-old child failed her newborn hearing screening test. The audiologist has just used state-of-the-art diagnostic tests to confirm hearing loss. The family has much to learn about the early intervention system in their community.

Part C of the Individuals with Disabilities Education Act

The Individuals with Disabilities Education Act (IDEA) ensures that children with disabilities have access to services. Part C of IDEA addresses the needs of children from birth to 36 months of age. This federal law establishes minimum guidelines, and each state develops its unique state plan. In most states, a child younger than 36 months with bilateral hearing loss is eligible for early intervention services. However, children with minimal hearing loss may not meet a state's eligibility criteria. A survey conducted by the National Center for Hearing Assessment and Management (NCHAM) (2006) reviewed eligibility criteria in each state. Some states provide services to children with all degrees and types of hearing loss. Other states require a child to have a moderate to severe degree of hearing loss to qualify for services. Some states exclude children with mild, unilateral, or other minimal degrees of hearing loss, even though these degrees of hearing loss may have a negative effect on a child's development (Stredler-Brown, Hulstrom, & Ringwalt, 2008). If a child is denied services, the decision can be appealed.

Pitfall

- A state's eligibility criteria can change over time, so it is important for the audiologist to verify criteria and stay current.

The law entitles infants and toddlers with disabilities, and their families, to receive several different services. First, each family has the right to have a service coordinator. The Part C service coordinator is the designated point of entry into early intervention. For a child with hearing loss, the service coordinator serves as a conduit between the diagnosing audiologist and the early intervention provider. The service coordinator helps parents obtain the services they need, facilitates timely delivery of these services, and helps the family to coordinate the services that are provided by different professionals from various agencies.

The law states that it is appropriate for the service coordinator to be from the profession most immediately relevant to the infant's or toddler's or family's needs (EHDI Act, 2010). Since most families are unfamiliar with audiology, early intervention, and therapy, they may want to know whether the service coordinator is familiar with the type and degree of hearing loss of their child. Families typically want to know the impact hearing loss can have on the development of speech and language. Most families want the different communication approaches that are used with children who are deaf or hard of hearing (DHH) to be explained and demonstrated. Hopefully, the service coordinator can answer these questions and provide this information. Each state is responsible for developing a system of service coordination to meet the needs of families.

A few states have augmented the Part C service coordination system by offering expertise specifically about hearing loss. In some of these states, a professional who is an expert on hearing loss in young children has contact with the family shortly after diagnosis. At one time, in the state of Colorado, a group of specially trained professionals were strategically placed in 10 geographic regions. These hearing resource coordinators worked, in tandem, with the local Part C service coordinators. The primary responsibilities of the hearing resource coordinators were to provide information and emotional support to family members as they handled their child's diagnosis. The average age of entry into early intervention in Colorado was less than 4 months in 2004 (Clinical Health Information Records of Patients [CHIRP], 2005). The network of hearing resource coordinators was credited, at least in part, with this early start of services. Another model supporting Part C service

coordinators is the Guide By Your Side (GBYS) program, which currently operates in 19 states. GBYS is sponsored by Hands and Voices, which is a parent organization specifically for families who have children who are DHH. The majority of the GBYS affiliates have a component in their curriculum that addresses questions families typically ask when their child's hearing loss has just been diagnosed.

A second entitlement in the law ensures access to funding. Each state plan identifies specific eligibility criteria for Part C services. If a child with hearing loss meets eligibility criteria, the state system is responsible for funding early intervention services.

When a child is eligible for services, a meeting is conducted. One outcome of this meeting is the creation of an Individual Family Service Plan (IFSP), which must include specific information. The components of the IFSP are identified in **Table 27.1**. The law is clear about the importance of this plan; the IFSP identifies specific services, identifies who will provide each service, and guides the intervention. The IFSP also identifies the agency or individual who will pay for each service.

Implicit in the IFSP is the need to collect data to monitor progress. A measurement of the child's development is conducted and reported in the IFSP. The IFSP is reviewed at 6-month intervals, and a new plan is created annually. Each time a new IFSP is created, a new measurement of the child's development is to be obtained and reported.

Table 27.1 The Individual Family Service Plan (IFSP)

1. A statement of the child's present level of development

2. A statement of the family's resources

3. A statement of the family's priorities and concerns

4. A statement of the major outcomes expected

5. The criteria, procedures, and timelines used to measure outcomes

6. A statement of necessary early intervention services

7. A statement of the natural environments, to the maximum extent appropriate, in which services will be provided (or a justification when services should not be provided in a natural environment)

8. The projected dates for the start of services and the anticipated duration of services

9. Identification of the service coordinator

10. The steps to be taken to support the transition of the child to preschool services when the child is 2½ years of age

Pearl

- The collection of developmental information over time is crucial because this is how parents know the early intervention program is effective for their child.

Pearl

- The goal is to develop the child's communication and language so that these skills remain on track with their hearing peers.

◆ Case Two

A family has just met with their service coordinator and knows that at least one early intervention program is available in their community. The family needs to select the program that provides what they want. The parents look to one another. How will they make a choice?

Early Intervention Providers and Their Qualifications

An early attempt to develop consensus on the competencies needed by early interventionists was initiated by Compton, Niemeyer, and Shroyer (2001). Since that time, the need has been reinforced by another consensus document encouraging personnel providing early intervention to be thoroughly knowledgeable about issues related to the unique language and communication abilities and needs of this population (Marge & Marge, 2005). Marge and Marge (2005) stated that "the specialized and technological needs of infants and children with hearing loss are unique and require a professional with specific training in providing services for these children" (p. 24). Another commitment to the provision of high-quality services is in the 2007 Position Statement issued by the Joint Committee on Infant Hearing (JCIH) (2007). This position statement focuses on these benchmarks for early intervention: (1) Families should have access to information describing all intervention and treatment options, including counseling, regarding hearing loss; and (2) appropriate interdisciplinary intervention programs for infants with hearing loss and their families should be provided by professionals who are knowledgeable about childhood hearing loss. EHDI (EHDI Act, 2010) programs, operating in each state, can also encourage early intervention programs to address the unique needs of infants and toddlers who are DHH. Each state's EHDI program is unique.

When selecting an early intervention program, the family can consider the delivery model. Services can be family-centered or child-centered. Both are reasonable options. However, Part C strongly endorses family-centered practices for children younger than 36 months.

In family-centered intervention, all family members are the clients (Dunst, Boyd, Trivette, & Hamby, 2002). A family-centered approach establishes a partnership between the therapist and the parents. The therapist provides access to information about the child's disability and its potential impact on development. In addition, family members are encouraged to communicate their opinions, their expectations, and their feelings. The therapist, with appropriate training, provides emotional support to family members and caregivers. The family-centered therapist is also responsible for parent education or parent-mediated intervention–a process of teaching parents specific skills (Hanft, Rush, & Shelden, 2004; Klass, 2003; Mahoney et al, 1999; Muma, 1998; Wasik & Bryant, 2001). Guidelines for parent-mediated intervention have been defined explicitly for children who are DHH (AG Bell Academy for Listening and Spoken Language, 2012). According to this document, when delivering parent-centered intervention to a child with hearing loss, an interventionist is expected to demonstrate these competencies: (1) having conceptual knowledge of the intervention strategy to be taught to the parents; (2) having the skill to implement the strategy with the child; (3) having the ability to provide the parents with clear information about the strategy and concrete examples to demonstrate it; (4) having knowledge of coaching skills and the ability to use them; and (5) having the ability to provide specific feedback to the parents.

Child-centered therapy continues to be a viable option, even though it is not encouraged by Part C. In this paradigm, the professional works directly with the child to investigate, identify, and implement specific communication strategies. Parents may observe these therapy sessions, but the intent is for the professional to provide direct one-on-one instruction to the child.

The Natural Environment

Another consideration is the environment in which intervention occurs. Part C of the IDEA Act strongly endorses treatment in natural environments (34 CFR §303.26). Each state's Part C lead agency is obliged to include policies and procedures to ensure that, to the maximum extent appropriate, early intervention services are provided in natural environments, which are defined as settings that are natural or typical for an infant or toddler without a disability, such as the home. There are also a variety of community settings that are considered natural environments. The regulations do include allowances for the provision of early intervention services in a setting other than the natural environment; this is a determination made by the parents and the IFSP team, and it must be based on the unique needs of the child, family routines, and developmental outcomes. The language in the newest Part C regulations makes it clear that a justification is always required when early intervention services are not provided in a natural environment, and the reason must be based on the fact that early intervention cannot be achieved satisfactorily in the natural environment. The increasing popularity of telepractice, discussed later in this chapter, offers "virtual home visits" (Olsen, Fiechtl, & Rule, 2012) delivered through interactive video. This service delivery platform seems to meet the definition of a natural environment because services are provided, virtually, in the family's home.

Provider Competencies

Next, consider the qualifications of the early interventionist. Historically, interventionists have been a hybrid group, as they come from a variety of preservice training programs. A survey of 16 states (Arehart, Yoshinaga-Itano, Thomson, Gabbard, & Stredler-Brown, 1998) reported that most professionals received preservice training in three types of programs: teacher education for the deaf and hard of hearing, speech-language pathology, and audiology. A small number of providers received preservice training in early childhood education or early childhood special education. Unfortunately, a graduate degree in any one of these training programs does not guarantee that the professional has the requisite competencies to work with children with hearing loss and their families. Families, then, have the responsibility to determine whether the early interventionists have the skills, competencies, knowledge, and experience to effectively teach their child. Recently, leaders in the fields of early intervention and hearing loss provided resounding support for the development of a consensus statement listing the core knowledge and skills required to work effectively with infants and toddlers under 3 years of age who are DHH. A set of competencies, knowledge statements, and skills was developed based on a review of eight published documents (Sass-Lehrer, Stredler-Brown, Moeller, Clark, & Hutchinson, 2011). These competencies, appended to a larger document on early intervention, have been published in the most recent position statement of the Joint Committee on Infant

Hearing (Muse et al, 2013). The competencies could be used to create a systematic approach to training in preservice programs. The competencies can also be used to develop a prescriptive in-service training for working professionals. An overview of these competencies and skills is presented in **Table 27.2**.

◆ Case Three

At our IFSP, we scheduled sessions with an early interventionist six times each month. We identified many outcomes and procedures. What exactly can we expect our early interventionist to teach us?

Curriculums

Family-centered early intervention is a three-pronged approach. The content that is taught falls into three categories: (1) services to the family; (2) strategies to foster the child's development; and (3) techniques that influence the quality of parent–child interaction.

Table 27.2 Competencies for an early interventionist providing family-centered intervention

- Family-centered practice: Family-professional partnerships, decision making, & family support
- Socially, culturally, and linguistically responsive practices, including deaf/hard-of-hearing cultures and communities; sensitivity to and respect for an individual family's characteristics
- Language acquisition and communication development: typical development, communication approaches available to children with hearing loss, and impact of hearing loss on access to communication
- Factors influencing infant and toddler development
- Screening, evaluation, and assessment: Interpretation of hearing screening and audiologic diagnostic information, ongoing developmental assessment, and use of developmental assessment tools to monitor progress
- Technology: Supporting development by using technology to access auditory, visual, and tactile information
- Planning and implementation of services: Creating a lesson plan, conducting a home visit, developing the IFSP, and using appropriate curriculums, methods, and resources
- Collaboration and interdisciplinary models and practices
- Professional and ethical behavior: Fundamentals of early intervention practice, legislation, policies, and research

Source: Stredler-Brown, Sass-Lehrer, Clark, & Moeller (2012).

Services to the Family

In a family-centered approach, the parents are the clients. Parents and other caregivers learn to understand hearing loss and its potential impact on development. Most parents, especially those who do not have experience with hearing loss, have an emotional reaction to the diagnosis of hearing loss in their child (Moses, 1985). The intervention process can support family members emotionally. Because hearing loss has a significant impact on communication and language, parents are taught specific techniques to foster their child's communication and language. The early interventionist teaches these strategies to the parents and other caregivers.

Strategies to Foster Child Development

Many developmental domains need to be considered, and all affect the child's learning. The first consideration is cognitive development. For a young child, cognition is exhibited and measured through play. In addition, motor skills, personal-social skills, and self-help skills all contribute to development. A child's growth in each of these domains needs to be observed carefully over time because a disability in any of these developmental areas can have a negative impact on communication and language. If problems occur, techniques to support the child's progress need to be taught. When development in these domains is age appropriate, the child's inherent skills can be harnessed to enhance communication and language.

The traditional focus of the early interventionist promotes the development of the child's communication. Communication includes any and all of the following domains: auditory skill development, speech, preverbal communication (e.g., vocalizations and gestures), and verbal communication (starting with first words). Verbal communication, or language, includes four specific domains, listed in **Table 27.3**.

With guidance from the professionals, a family selects a communication approach. See Chapter 26 for an overview of communication approaches.

Techniques That Affect the Quality of Parent–Child Interaction

Communication is reciprocal; it is a dynamic process that happens between two or more people. Therefore, the interventionist must consider the attributes of the communicative dyad. Mahoney and Powell (1986) stated that "interventions impact child development to the extent that parents are supported and encouraged to engage in responsive interactions with the child." A goal is to have an optimal interactive match (Bailey & Simeonsson, 1988). The premise here is to allow the child's

mode of communication to influence the modality used by the parents. The parent is encouraged to recognize and imitate the mode used by the child. Children learn language best when they are exposed to a complete language model. Professionals, in partnership with parents, can conduct informal and formal observations of the parent-child communication and strive to provide full access to a complete language model (Stredler-Brown, 2010). Parents are taught to provide a language-rich environment; one in which language is complete, expanded, and reinforced to provide appropriate repetition (DesGeorges, Johnson, & Stredler-Brown, 2006). When a child who is deaf or hard of hearing is immersed in a language-rich environment, there is potential to override the potential influences of hearing loss.

Parents have a lot to learn. Many state EHDI programs have created a resource guide specifically for parents of children who are deaf or hard of hearing. There are many topics in these resource guides, including a description of hearing loss; the potential effects of hearing loss; information about amplification, cochlear implants, and assistive listening technology; access to early intervention in one's community; intervention programs with expertise in hearing loss; communication approaches; support for evidence-based practices; funding for amplification and intervention; and lists of organizations in the state and country that focus on hearing loss.

◆ Case Four

Our early interventionist meets with our family regularly. She works with the adults for most of the session. Only some of her time is spent with our child. I am confused about the purpose of intervention. Who is the client? Is the intervention for the adults or is it for our child?

Table 27.3

Components of language learning	Description
Semantics	The study of word meanings and word relations
Syntax	The aspect of language that governs the rules for how words are arranged in sentences
Morphology	The study of the minimal units of language that are meaningful, such as –s for plural nouns or third-person verb tenses, –ing for present progressive, and –ed for past tense
Pragmatics	The functional use of language

Source: Schow and Nerbonne (2002).

Family-Centered Intervention

Parents have many questions about hearing loss and its impact on communication. When intervention starts, information is provided to the family. There is an endless list of issues, and the interventionist needs to answer the parents' questions first.

Pearl

- Parents know what they want to learn. The interventionist must respect the rate at which different parents acquire information.

Next, communication and intervention techniques are taught to the adults. The characteristics of the parent–child interaction can be judiciously appraised. The techniques that are taught are based on informal assessments, prescriptive analyses, and parent priorities. These techniques may focus on preverbal communication, receptive language, expressive language, listening skills, speech skills, play skills, and others. The goal is for each adult in the child's life to use these techniques and to use them daily. The venues that support responsive interactions include frequent play, matching a child's interests, having parent and child take an equal number of turns, and increasing responsive comments (Cole & Flexer, 2011). Daily practice of these strategies is recommended. By working with typically occurring routines, parents have more opportunities to practice strategies. For instance, communication occurs during typical child routines, such as eating, dressing, bathing, or getting into the car. Typical parent routines include vacuuming, dusting, cooking, marketing, and laundry, just to name a few. In family-centered intervention, the provider can teach specific skills while engaging in these familiar and frequently occurring routines.

A rubric for a home visit is illustrated in **Fig. 27.1** (Stredler-Brown, Moeller, Gallegos, Corwin, & Pittman, 2004). It is explained here. At a home visit, the interventionist first reconnects with family members and reviews the events since the last visit. The early interventionist learns about the experiences of each family member. The interventionist often needs to set aside her agenda to address the current events in the family's life.

Next, family members identify their priorities. Of course, the interventionist has a well-developed plan for each session. However, the family's questions, concerns, and accomplishments are of paramount importance, because the specific strategies that will be taught during the session must be appropriate for the child *and* for the family.

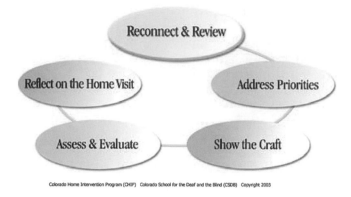

Fig. 27.1   Rubric for a home visit *(Contributors: A. Stredler-Brown, M.P. Moeller, R. Gallegos, P. Pittman, J. Corwin, M. Condon). Source:* Stredler-Brown et al (2004).

The next step in the rubric is a familiar one for the interventionist. A brief explanation of a strategy or technique is offered. Then the play begins. The interventionist shows the craft underlying communication. The family members are active and engaged in this process. The interventionist uses coaching strategies to explore, with the family, the techniques that work. Several strategies can be explored during one session. This process helps parents feel competent and confident.

Each session includes assessment and evaluation of the family's and child's progress. The early interventionist and the parents discuss the child's skills before, during, and after each technique is taught. The purpose is to identify the effectiveness of the communication strategy. Did the child's behavior change because of it? If so, how did it change? If not, why not? In a family-centered program, evaluation also includes consideration of the family members. The interventionist helps each family member to comment on his comfort with the new strategies. Parents are expected to integrate these strategies into their daily routines, and to do so, they must be comfortable using the technique.

As the family-centered session draws to an end, the family members reflect on the session. The interventionist is looking for input from the parents. Were particular strategies or techniques successful? Were the questions from family members answered? Were family members satisfied with the information they received? Are they ready to use the new information and novel strategies in their daily routines?

Experienced professionals working with infants and toddlers with hearing loss assert there is an art and a science to family-centered early intervention (Stredler-Brown, 2005; Stredler-Brown et al, 2004). These relationship-based techniques provide information and emotional support to parents. These techniques, called tools of the trade, are described in **Table 27.4**.

Table 27.4 Tools of the trade

Information resource: The early interventionist has an exhaustive amount of information about hearing loss. Specific information can be gathered in response to the questions from family members.

Coach and partner: The interventionist is an observer and provides reinforcement. The interventionist points out desirable behaviors. As the early intervention process unfolds, parents begin to recognize what is important. Family members learn to identify what is working for them and for their child.

Sounding board: The interventionist uses active listening (Rogers, 1961) and reflects what is heard back to the family. The interventionist can notice the content of the message. Of equal importance, the interventionist can listen for the emotions the family members reveal.

News commentator (Moeller & Condon, 1994): The early interventionist provides an on-the-spot commentary. This gives immediate feedback to the family. This technique is used as parents discover the effectiveness of a specific strategy.

◆ Case Five

Our early interventionist says our 24-month-old child is making progress. We're happy to hear this. But our child's communication is not like that of her hearing peers. Is there a way to measure her progress?

Formal and Informal Assessment Practices

Children are identified with hearing loss, in increasing numbers, at a very young age. There is a call to action to measure the developmental outcomes of all of these children who are receiving early intervention (Dunst et al, 2002). How can outcomes be quantified? Do we have the appropriate tests to do this? Do we know who will administer the tests? The answers are a resounding "yes" to each of these questions.

Now that systems support children entering early intervention by 6 months of age, it is appropriate to raise our expectations. No longer should one hear, "He is doing well for a deaf child." Rather, the expectation is for a child with hearing loss of any degree who has received early intervention by 6 months of age to be doing well. The communication and language skills of a child with hearing loss can be commensurate with their hearing peers. For children with cognitive disabilities, the standard will be their developmental age, rather than their chronological age. A key activity when providing intervention is to document the effectiveness of what is done. Several studies have documented the effectiveness of early identification and an early start of intervention (Kennedy, McCann, Campbell, Kimm, & Thornton, 2005;

Moeller, 2000; Yoshinaga-Itano, Sedey, Coulter, & Mehl, 1998).

Data are compelling. Each interventionist can collect assessment data to document the progress made by each child. Informal assessment is an integral part of each session. Formal testing is completed at 6-month intervals and documented on the IFSP. Each program, subsequently, can take the individual child data and analyze it to identify program trends. The areas of development that merit assessment are identified in **Table 27.5** (Clark, Abraham, Lambourne, Madsen, & Welch, 2004).

Assessment serves several purposes. First, the data provide an ongoing record of progress. Is the one-for-one rule being met (Johnson, 2006)? The one-for-one rule expects a child to make 1 year's growth in 1 year's time. For the infants and toddlers, progress is measured more frequently. The expectation for these very young children is 1 month of progress in 1 month's time or 3 months of progress in 3 months' time. Outcome data are used to acknowledge the efficacy of the individualized intervention program. The number of sessions, the communication approach, and the skills of the interventionist and parents all contribute to the child's development. If the requisite amount of progress is being made, the program, including the selected communication approach, must be a good fit. Conversely, if progress is not being made, there is due cause to review the strategies being used. Not to be mistaken for research, assessment is a relevant, indeed integral, aspect of intervention (Kamhi, 2006; Ratner, 2006).

Assessment also benefits the administrative unit. Collecting and analyzing data are powerful ways for a program to measure outcomes. The program can identify its achievements, prioritize present and future initiatives, and designate funding appropriately.

Table 27.5 Developmental domains for assessment

- Communication and language
- Functional auditory skills
- Speech
- Play and cognition
- Parent–child interaction
- Social-emotional development
- Physical development
- Vision
- Family needs and environment

Source: Clark et al (2004).

Transition to Preschool

The transition from early intervention to preschool services starts when a child is 2½ years old. The early interventionist can support parents as they learn about preschool placements. Parents are encouraged to visit preschool programs; parents usually appreciate having the early intervention provider accompany them on these site visits. A checklist to guide these observations was developed by Johnson, Beams, and Stredler-Brown (2005). The considerations are listed in **Table 27.6**.

There are several types of preschool programs. The least restrictive option places the child with hearing loss in a program with hearing children. This could be a publicly funded preschool program or a private preschool. Another option enrolls the child with hearing loss in a noncategorical preschool program, which has children with different types of disabilities in the same classroom. A third option, often found in larger metropolitan areas, is a center-based program, which enrolls as many children with hearing loss as possible in one classroom. To have this critical mass of children, students may be transported to one school from different catchment areas. All these options, to varying degrees, can enroll peers who do not have disabilities. These peers serve as models for typical development.

Table 27.6 Criteria for selecting a preschool program

- Total number of students in the classroom
- Number of students with hearing loss in the classroom
- Adult-to-child ratio
- Communication approach used by each child in the classroom
- Accommodations for amplification
- Related services (e.g., speech-language pathologist, educational audiologist, occupational therapist, physical therapist, psychologist)
- Parent support
- Physical environment
- Acoustic accommodations
- Curriculums
- Communication between school and home
- Family involvement in day-to-day preschool activities
- Role models who are deaf or hard of hearing
- Assessment

Source: Johnson, Beams, and Stredler-Brown (2005).

◆ Case Six

Our family has met with the audiologist and our service coordinator. We have carefully chosen the communication approach we want to use with our child. The early interventionist in our community has not had training, nor does she have experience using this approach. The nearest interventionist with this expertise is 220 miles away. We are unable to move at this time. Is there a way for us to access the therapy we want?

Equal Access to Services

Families living in remote or rural areas often have limited access to services. Limitations can be due to the training, expertise, and experience of the providers in the community. There can be geographic barriers that limit access to or frequency of services as well. And yet, the goal is for young children with hearing loss, and their families, to receive appropriate and high-quality services irrespective of where they live.

Telepractice Defined

Telepractice is the use of information and telecommunications technologies to provide health services to persons who are located at some distance from a provider. Modern video conferencing technology allows practitioners to have audio and video interactions in real-time on a range of devices. The American Speech, Language, Hearing Association (ASHA) officially adopted the term telepractice to describe the use of a remote service delivery model by speech-language pathologists and audiologists (ASHA, 2005). ASHA (2012) defines telepractice as "the application of telecommunications technology to delivery of professional services at a distance by linking clinician to client, or clinician to clinician, for assessment, intervention, and/or consultation" (paragraph 1).

Telepractice Technology

When using telepractice, one must consider the type of equipment that is used to deliver services remotely. The audio and video components of the technology, as well as the synchronicity of the two signals, need to be addressed (Puskin, Cohen, Ferguson, Krupinski, & Spaulding, 2010). The standards for delivering this service to children with hearing loss may need to be higher than those standards adopted by other professions. For instance, a higher speed for video transmission may be needed to enable the transmission of visual communication supports (e.g., sign language and speechreading) in real time. When treatment focuses on the development of listening and spoken language, enhanced audio is important.

Another consideration is the type of Internet connection available in the remote community and at the professional's site. The speed of the Internet connection is a critical component for a successful interaction.

Evidence Supporting Telepractice

Telepractice has been associated with positive outcomes for infants and toddlers who are deaf or hard of hearing (Houston, 2011; McCarthy, Muñoz, & White, 2010). Practitioners and parents of children with hearing loss are overwhelmingly satisfied with this service (Blaiser, Edwards, Behl, & Munoz, 2012; Broekelmann, 2012; Peters-Lalios, 2012; Simmons, in press). Colleagues in Australia have been pioneers in delivering early intervention through telepractice to children who are DHH (Davis, Phil, Hopkins, & Abrahams, 2012; McCarthy, 2012). The work in Australia has shown that telepractice has the potential to span time zones and continents (McCarthy, Duncan, & Leigh, 2012). In the United States, administrators and practitioners, coast to coast, are starting to initiate services using telepractice to provide early intervention to infants and toddlers who are DHH (Blaiser et al, 2012; Broekelmann, in press; Hamren & Quigley, 2012; Hopkins, Keefe, & Bruno, 2012; Peters-Lalios, 2012).

Professional Issues

As with any new service, many practical, ethical, and legal considerations must be studied. It seems fair to say that technology is advancing faster than the documents that will guide ethical, privacy, and policy issues. Policies related to speech-language pathologists are cited in ASHA documents (ASHA, 2005; 2010). Policies for teachers of the deaf or hard of hearing are only now being considered. At this time, different insurers reimburse telepractice services in various ways. Medicaid reimbursement is governed by each individual state's program. State licensure is very clear for speech-language pathologists; there is currently no interstate licensure portability for services to youth (ASHA, 2005, 2010). The professional

must be certified to provide services in the state in which the child resides.

Pearl

- Where a child lives need not dictate access to services, nor should one's geographic location dictate the type of services.

◆ Summary

Early intervention is complex. It must start early—within weeks of the diagnosis of hearing loss. It must be provided by well-trained providers. An individualized curriculum must be created. The infant/child's progress must be monitored by assessing evidence of outcomes. More and more often, young children with hearing loss, birth to three years of age, exhibit communication and language skills at age level (Yoshinaga-Itano, 2004). In the not-too-distant future, this benchmark can become a standard for children with hearing loss.

There is an art and a science to early intervention. Technological advances contribute to the science, and the skills of the providers and the prescriptive nature of intervention represent the art.

Discussion Questions

1. How does a family learn about the early intervention programs in their community?

2. What are the criteria for selecting a program that meets the family's and the child's needs?

3. What are the qualifications for an early interventionist working with children with hearing loss?

4. What is included in a curriculum for an infant or toddler with hearing loss?

5. Why is family-centered programming valued?

6. How does information collected from ongoing assessment benefit a child and the child's family?

7. How can I find out if telepractice is offered in my state?

References

AG Bell Academy for Listening and Spoken Language. (2012). How to apply. Retrieved from http://www.listeningand spokenlanguage.org/AcademyDocument.aspx?id=628

American Speech-Language-Hearing Association. (2005). Audiologists providing clinical services via telepractice: Position statement [Position Statement]. doi:10.1044/policy.PS2005-00029. Retrieved from http://www.asha.org/policy

American Speech-Language-Hearing Association. (2010). Professional issues in telepractice for speech-language pathologists (professional issues statement). Retrieved from http://www.asha.org/policy

American Speech-Language-Hearing Association. (2012). Telepractice for SLPs and audiologists. Retrieved from http://www.asha.org/practice/telepractice

Arehart, K., Yoshinaga-Itano, C., Thomson, V., Gabbard, S., & Stredler-Brown, A. (1998). State of the states: The status of universal newborn hearing screening, assessment & intervention systems in 16 states. American Journal of Audiology, 7, 101–114.

Bailey, D., & Simeonsson, R. (1988). Family assessment in early intervention. Columbus, OH: Merrill.

Blaiser, K. M., Edwards, M., Behl, D., & Munoz, K. F. (2012). Telepractice services at Sound Beginnings at Utah State University. The Volta Review, 112(3), 365–372.

Broekelmann, C. (2012). Ihear internet therapy program: a program by St. Joseph Institute for the Deaf. The Volta Review, 112(3), 417–422.

Clark, K., Abraham, H., Lambourne, M., Madsen, M., & Welch, P. (2004). Assessment. In S. Watson, D. J. Taylor, & P. Pittman, (Eds.). SKI-HI curriculum: Family-centered programming for infants and young children with hearing loss (pp. 55–166). Logan, UT: HOPE, Inc.

Clinical Health Information Records of Patients. (2005). [Electronic data]. Denver, CO: Colorado Department of Public Health and Environment.

Cole, E., & Flexer, C. (2011). Children with hearing loss: Developing listening and talking, birth to six (2nd ed.). San Diego: Plural Publishing

Compton, M. V., Niemeyer, J. A., & Shroyer, E. (2001). CENTe-R: Collaborative early intervention national training e-resource needs assessment. Unpublished manuscript, University of North Carolina at Greensboro, Greensboro, NC.

Davis, A., Phil, M., Hopkins, T., & Abrahams, Y. (2012). Maximizing the impact of telepractice through a multifaceted service delivery model at The Shepherd Centre, Australia. The Volta Review, 112(3), 383–391.

DesGeorges, J., Johnson, C. D., & Stredler-Brown, A. (2006). Natural environments: A call for policy guidance for infants and toddlers (0–3) who are deaf/hard of hearing. Unpublished manuscript.

Dunst, C. J., Boyd, K., Trivette, C. M., & Hamby, D. W. (2002). Family-oriented program models and professional helpgiving practices. Family Relations, 51(3), 221–229.

Early Hearing Detection and Intervention Act (2010). Pub. L, No. 111-337.

Hamren, K., & Quigley, S. (2012). Implementing coaching in a natural environment through distance technologies. The Volta Review, 112(3), 403–407.

Hanft, B. E., Rush, D. D., & Shelden, M. L. (2004). Coaching families and colleagues in early childhood. Baltimore, MD: Brookes.

Hopkins, K., Keefe, B., & Bruno, A. (2012). Telepractice: creating a statewide network of support in rural Maine. The Volta Review, 112(3), 409–416.

Houston, K. T. (2011). TeleIntervention: improving service delivery to young children with hearing loss and their families through telepractice. Perspectives on Hearing and Hearing Disorders in Childhood, 21(2), 66–72.

Johnson, C. D. (2006). One year's growth in one year, expect no less. Hands & Voices Communicator, 9, 3.

Johnson, C. D., Beams, D., & Stredler-Brown, A. (2005). Preschool-kindergarten placement checklist for children who are deaf and hard of hearing. Retrieved from http://www.cde.state.co.us/cdesped/download/pdf/dhh-PS-KPlcmntCklst.pdf

Joint Committee on Infant Hearing. (2007). Year 2007 position statement: Principles and guidelines for early hearing detection and intervention programs. Pediatrics, 102(4), 893–921.

Kamhi, A. G. (2006). Epilogue: some final thoughts on EBP. Language, Speech, and Hearing Services in Schools, 37(4), 320–322.

Kennedy, C., McCann, D., Campbell, M. J., Kimm, L., & Thornton, R. (2005). Universal newborn screening for permanent childhood hearing impairment: an 8-year follow-up of a controlled trial. Lancet, 366(9486), 660–662.

Klass, C. S. (2003). The home visitor's guidebook. Baltimore, MD: Brookes.

Mahoney, C., & Powell, A. (1986). Transactional intervention program. Farmington, CT: University of Connecticut School of Medicine.

Mahoney, G., Kaiser, A., Girolametto, L., MacDonald, J., Robinson, C., Safford, P., & Spiker, D. (1999). Parent education in early intervention: A call for a renewed focus. Topics in Early Childhood Special Education, 19(3), 131–140. DOI:10.1177/027112149901900301

Marge, D. K., & Marge, M. (2005). Beyond newborn hearing screening: Meeting the educational and health care needs of infants and young children with hearing loss in America. Report of the National Consensus Conference on Effective Educational and Health Care Interventions for Infants and Young Children with Hearing Loss, September 10–12, 2004. Syracuse, NY: SUNY Upstate Medical University.

McCarthy, M. (2012). RIDBC Teleschool: A hub of expertise. The Volta Review, 112(3), 373–381.

McCarthy, M., Duncan, J., & Leigh, G. (2012). Telepractice: The Australian experience in an international context. In A. Stredler-Brown (Ed.), The Volta Review, 112(3), 297–312.

McCarthy, M., Muñoz, K., & White, K. R. (2010). Teleintervention for infants and young children who are deaf or hard-of-hearing. Pediatrics, 126(Suppl 1), S52–S58.

Moeller, M. P. (2000). Early intervention and language development in children who are deaf and hard of hearing. Pediatrics, 106(3), 1–9.

Moeller, M. P., & Condon, M. C. (1994). A collaborative problem-solving approach to early intervention. In J. Roush & N. D. Matkin (Eds.), Infants and toddlers with hearing loss (pp. 163–194). Baltimore, MD: York Press.

Moses, K. (1985). Infant deafness and parental grief: Psychosocial early intervention. In F. Powell, T. Finitzo-Hieber, S. Friel-Patti, & D. Henderson (Eds.), Education of the hearing impaired child. San Diego, CA: College-Hill.

Muma, J. (1998). Effective speech-language pathology: A cognitive socialization approach. Mahwah, NJ: Erlbaum.

Muse, C., Harrison, J., Yoshinaga-Itano, C., Grimes, A., Brookhouser, P. E., Epstein, S., . . . Martin, B. (2013). Supplement to the JCIH 2007 position statement: Principles and guidelines for early intervention after confirmation that a child is deaf or hard of hearing. Pediatrics, 131(4), e1324–e1349. doi: 10.1542/peds.2013-0008

National Center for Hearing Assessment and Management. (2006). Criteria for infants and toddlers with hearing loss to be eligible for early intervention services under IDEA. Retrieved from http://www.infanthearing.org/early intervention/eligibility.pdf

Olsen, S., Fiechtl, B., & Rule, S. (2012). An evaluation of virtual home visits in early intervention: feasibility of "virtual intervention." The Volta Review, 112(3), 267–281.

Peters-Lalios, A. (2012). ConnectHear teleintervention program. The Volta Review, 112(3), 357–364.

Puskin, D. S., Cohen, Z., Ferguson, A. S., Krupinski, E., & Spaulding, R. (2010). Implementation and evaluation of telehealth tools and technologies. Telemedicine and e-Health, 16(1), 96–102.

Ratner, N. B. (2006). Evidence-based practice: an examination of its ramifications for the practice of speech-language pathology. Language, Speech, and Hearing Services in Schools, 37(4), 257–267.

Rogers, C. R. (1961). On becoming a person: A therapist's view of psychotherapy. Boston, MA: Houghton Mifflin Company.

Sass-Lehrer, M., Stredler-Brown, A., Moeller, M. P., Clark, K., & Hutchinson, N. (2011). Defining core competencies: A three year investigation. Paper presented at the National Conference for Early Hearing Detection and Intervention (EHDI), Atlanta, GA.

Schow, R. L., & Nerbonne, M. A. (2002). Overview of audiologic rehabilitation. In R. L. Schow & M. A. Nerbonne (Eds.), Introduction to audiologic rehabilitation. Boston, MA: Allyn and Bacon.

Simmons, N. R. (2012). Virtual hearing resource services for children who are deaf and hard of hearing. In A. Stredler-Brown (Ed.), The Volta Review, 112(3), 423–427.

Stredler-Brown, A. (2005). The art and science of home visits. ASHA Leader, 6–7, 15.

Stredler-Brown, A. (2010). Communication choices and outcomes during the early years: An assessment and evidence-based approach. In M. Marschark & P. E. Spencer (Eds.), Oxford handbook of deaf studies, language, and education (pp. 292–315). New York, NY: Oxford University Press.

Stredler-Brown, A., Hulstrom, W. J., & Ringwalt, S. S. (2008). The need for early intervention. Seminars in Hearing, 29(2), 178–195.

Stredler-Brown, A., Moeller, M. P., Gallegos, R., Corwin, J., & Pittman, P. (2004). The art and science of home visits (DVD). Omaha, NE: Boys Town Press.

Stredler-Brown, A., Sass-Lehrer, M., Clark, K., & Moeller, M. P. (2012, March). Competency-based professional development: strategies for early interventionists. Paper presented at the meeting of the National Early Hearing Detection and Intervention (EHDI) Conference, St. Louis, MO.

Wasik, B. H., & Bryant, D. M. (2001). Home visiting: procedures for helping families (2nd ed.). Thousand Oaks, CA: Sage.

Yoshinaga-Itano, C., Sedey, A. L., Coulter, D. K., & Mehl, A. L. (1998). Language of early- and later-identified children with hearing loss. Pediatrics, 102(5), 1161–1171.

Yoshinaga-Itano, C. (2004). The impact of early access to language and communication for children with hearing loss (pp. 69–84). In D. Powers & G. R. Leigh (Eds.), Education of deaf children: Global perspectives. Washington DC: Gallaudet University Press.

Chapter 28

Speech/Language/Auditory Management of Infants and Children with Hearing Loss

Elizabeth Ying

Key Points

- The role of a speech-language pathologist (SLP) encompasses diagnostic and therapeutic responsibilities for a child who is deaf or hard of hearing.

- The need to assess functional listening distinguishes the communication evaluation of a child with hearing loss from the communication evaluation of a child with normal hearing.

- Audition is the most effective and efficient modality for acquiring and monitoring spoken language skills.

- The primary objective of aural habilitation and rehabilitation training is to develop functional listening skills for continued language learning and enhanced communicative interactions.

- Advances in amplification technology and early identification and intervention have helped more children with hearing loss to acquire functionally adequate listening and age-appropriate spoken language skills.

Since passage of the Walsh Act in 1997, most states now implement programs of universal newborn hearing screening. As a result, hearing loss is being identified at earlier ages than they were even a decade ago, and more families and their infants or toddlers are seeking assessment and treatment of the communication deficits accompanying hearing loss by the time the child is 1 to 3 months of age (Moeller, 2000). Advances in technology options (including digital hearing aids and cochlear implants), as well as the increased availability of parent-child-focused early intervention programs that emphasize auditory skill development and the comprehension and use of spoken language, have significantly altered what are considered functionally adequate progress and performance. Whereas in the recent past it was considered exceptional for a child with significant hearing loss to achieve age-level communication skills by any age, it is now commonly expected that children whose hearing loss was identified early will function receptively and expressively on par with their typically hearing peers by preschool or kindergarten. This evolution of the student with severe to profound hearing loss from a functionally deaf to a functionally hard of hearing student places unique social and educational management challenges on professionals and school systems alike.

◆ Role of the Speech-Language Pathologist (SLP)

It is widely accepted that a speech-language pathologist (SLP) is an integral member of the interdisciplinary diagnostic team that serves children with hearing loss. Traditionally, findings from an initial speech-language evaluation yield the following baseline information about a child who is deaf or hard of hearing: vocabulary and receptive-expressive language functioning, and speech production stimulability and capability. These important findings will determine initial training needs and serve as comparative data for the measurement of therapy benefit and progress.

The communication profiles of children with any degree of hearing loss are characterized by a wide variability in functional listening skills and linguistic competency. Therefore, for any child with hearing loss, the communication evaluation should encompass a functional listening assessment. This component is needed to obtain critical information about speech perception abilities (e.g., the nature and extent of a hearing aid or implant on the user's reliance on auditory input for continued language learning, literacy development, and enhanced communicative interactions). This functional listening assessment requirement distinguishes the speech-language assessment of a child with hearing loss from the communication assessment of his normal-hearing peers, because formulating and implementing aural habilitation/rehabilitation training also fall within the professional domain of the SLP.

Pitfall

- Few graduate training programs offer the coursework or practical experiences that are necessary to prepare the average SLP with skills to work with children with hearing loss. The academic preparation of an SLP should prepare clinicians to conduct the evaluation and treatment programs for pediatric patients with hearing loss. Furthermore, SLPs must be prepared to assume additional responsibilities for the student with hearing loss who is enrolled in general education settings (e.g., monitoring amplification, serving as a resource to the classroom teacher, providing preteaching of classroom vocabulary and content, and facilitating social interactions).

◆ Diagnostic Evaluations

There are two major purposes for conducting speech-language evaluations and functional listening assessments: (1) to identify communicative strengths and weaknesses (during the initial assessment); and (2) to monitor progress over time (during progress assessments). Identifying the purpose of the assessment is essential to determining the scope of the assessment and in selecting the most appropriate assessment tools.

Upon receiving a referral for evaluation, it is first absolutely critical to review the audiologic findings and general case history. The SLP must understand the child's hearing loss, including aided and unaided hearing. In addition, the SLP must perform a listening check of the child's technology to ensure it is working and the child has auditory access to the information presented during the SLP assessments.

Initial Assessment

Findings from an initial speech-language evaluation/functional listening assessment identify areas of strength and weakness in several skill domains, including

- Phonemic awareness (encompasses assessment of detection, discrimination, and identification of vowel elements and consonants as they occur in isolation or in different positions within words)

- Word recognition (encompasses comparison of open-set word identification under separate ear and binaural listening conditions, in both quiet and noise)
- Vocabulary (encompasses the assessment of the understanding or expressive use of real words or sound associations representing real words, e.g., *woof-woof* for *dog*)
- Language comprehension (encompasses the assessment of the understanding and contingent response to spoken language, including acting on directions and questions by performing actions, manipulating objects, pointing to pictures, or verbally responding)
- Expressive language (encompasses the assessment of nonverbal and verbal behaviors produced to intentionally convey meaning)
- Speech production (encompasses the assessment of the articulation of speech sounds in isolation, repeated and alternated syllables, words, and word combinations, as well as overall voice quality, prosody, and intonational characteristics)
- Pragmatic functioning (encompasses the assessment of how spoken language is used for various communicative purposes, such as labeling, commenting, requesting, directing, and questioning)

Performance data yield critically needed information to determine future habilitation and rehabilitation management as well as educational placement and related services needs.

During the communication assessment, additional information is also gathered about factors (listed below) that account for much of the variability in the performance of pediatric hearing aid or cochlear implant users. Through formal and informal measures, the SLP obtains information about: (1) age of identification (Sininger, Grimes, & Christensen, 2010; Yoshinaga-Itano, Sedey, Colter, & Mehl, 1998); (2) previous communication modality (Geers, Strube, Tobey, Pisoni, & Moog, 2011); (3) cognitive factors (such as attention span and memory) (Geers et al, 2011; Pisoni & Geers, 2000); (4) environmental considerations, such as everyday communicative demands and expectations (Anderson & Arnoldi, 2011; Quittner, Leibach, & Marciel, 2004); and (5) parental input/language proficiency (Cole & Flexer, 2011; Stallings, Kirk, Chin, & Gao, 2004).

Testing may also reveal areas that should be addressed to ensure there is sufficient and appropriate support for the child with hearing loss, both at home and in school. Considerations such as consistency of present technology use, realistic understanding of the impact of hearing loss on language learning, and availability of aural habilitation and rehabilitation training, should be identified during the initial diagnostic assessment. Most important, it should be possible to formulate aural habilitation training objectives and strategies based on the results of a comprehensive communication evaluation.

Progress Assessments

In contrast, subsequent assessments (routinely occurring at 6-month intervals or annually) provide all of the foregoing, but also slightly different, information. Comparative analysis of performance on criterion-referenced or standardized measures affords an objective means of monitoring progress and benefit (of both therapy and technology) for the child who is deaf or hard of hearing. Subsequent assessments also present the necessary information for making changes in the child's aural habilitation/rehabilitation training.

◆ Determining the Focus of Therapy

Children entering the aural habilitation and rehabilitation process fall within four major age groupings: infants, preschool-aged, school-aged, and teenagers. Each of these developmental groups has distinctly differing diagnostic and training requirements. Recognizing the unique needs of each group is critical both in selecting the appropriate diagnostic tools and in interpreting the test findings and formulating appropriate training programs.

Infants

It is increasingly more common to be asked to conduct a speech-language evaluation and functional listening assessment on an infant who has only recently been diagnosed with hearing loss or who is just beginning a hearing aid trial process. Because of their young ages, infants exhibit few skills that can be assessed using standard testing protocols. Therefore, a large part of the evaluation process involves parent questionnaires of observed auditory and basic communication behaviors. Parental responses on such questionnaires provide important information about parental understanding of the impact of hearing loss on future language learning and social-communicative interactions as well as parental understanding of amplification use and aural habilitation training on the development of desired skills (Anderson & Arnoldi, 2011).

Frequently, the infant or toddler has already undergone some type of global early intervention (EI) eligibility assessment. Rarely, however, has there been a systematic attempt during such assessments to observe or document the auditory responsiveness and stimulability of the infant-toddler with hearing loss. Generic early intervention providers may have limited experience with hearing loss (and even

less experience in determining potential candidates for more advanced technologies, such as frequency modulation [FM] devices or cochlear implants, as the child's primary amplification at home).

Early intervention providers or speech-language pathologists often lack the special training or experience to support the necessary preimplant training or to assist in the infant's or toddler's initial acclimation to either hearing aids or cochlear implants. In addition, the concept of fast-tracking an infant or toddler for cochlear implantation is often misinterpreted as affording minimal services to the child and family until an implant is fitted, when, in fact, the early interventionist should be an active participant in preparing the baby and parents for the implant procedure.

During the hearing aid trial, it is valuable to attempt to establish some prerequisite communication behaviors while establishing an awareness of speech and environmental sounds, such as developing visual attending skills, sustained attention to sound-making toys, and exposure to a variety of low-frequency listening and vibrotactile experiences.

Preschoolers

The primary component of the evaluation process for the preschool-aged child is to assess the present level of functioning in light of the child's amplification history and previously delivered aural habilitation training. If the preschooler with hearing loss has been fortunate enough to have had some auditory-verbal training but had achieved minimal gains, the evaluator might assume that (1) the child has limited potential to use auditory input from hearing aids or implants that are currently being used, or (2) the technology has not been providing sufficient acoustic access to the child's brain. In contrast, if previous early intervention programming has been more visually based or used sign support, one must question whether there has been sufficient focus on auditory skill emergence to determine ultimate benefit from the hearing aid trial or implant program (e.g., perhaps the lack of auditory progress is an artifact of training as opposed to either a subject-specific or device-related issue). This communication modality issue becomes particularly important in borderline cases for cochlear implantation (e.g., for children whose audiograms suggest they should be hearing better with hearing aids). At times, potential implant recipients might exhibit behaviors during formal testing that suggest they are more stimulable (e.g., have greater auditory potential) than reported by the parents or their ongoing speech-language clinicians. This finding would, in turn, suggest that changes are needed in the preschooler's aural habilitation objectives and strategies.

Depending on the child's age, exploration of present or future school-based aural habilitation services might also be a component of the evaluation process. When the child with hearing loss continues to exhibit limited functional listening or oral communication skills, the most appropriate evaluation measures may be largely parent-report inventories or criterion-referenced assessment tools; keeping in mind that it is critical to include some tool to assess the nature and consistency of the preschooler's auditory and communicative demands (Anderson & Arnoldi, 2011).

The recommended protocol for direct observation of the auditory skill emergence of an infant, toddler, or preschooler who is not yet talking or able to respond on formal diagnostic measures encompasses exposing the child to a range of noisemakers and speech, spanning the speech frequency range within interactive play routines. After a period of exposure, the child's visual attention should be engaged in play with an alternative manipulative toy. Then, while his visual attention is averted from the examiner, these now "familiar" noisemakers or speech stimuli are presented, and the child's response is observed. Specific responses could range from stopping an ongoing action, looking up, moving rhythmically in response to the sound stimuli, visually scanning the environment to locate the sound source, or attempting to imitate what was heard. Having knowledge of both the acoustic features of the sounds presented as well as the normal progression for auditory skill development will permit the examiner to assess the appropriateness of the child's observed behaviors.

School-Aged Children

For school-aged children, communication mode (total communication versus listening and spoken language/auditory-verbal) and current communication skills have impact on both the diagnostic and therapeutic management of a child with hearing loss. Potential first-time cochlear implant candidates in this age group are assumed to have missed the window of opportunity for optimal verbal language learning (unless the referral for implantation is being made because of a change in hearing). This may create a need to assess the child's level of linguistic competency in her first language (e.g., a manual communication system). In addition, when the school-aged child is being evaluated for implant candidacy, assessment measures should also be used to determine whether parents and professionals (who have often initiated the implant process) have realistic expectations of the ultimate benefit for the particular implant candidate.

It is expected that the school-aged hearing aid user or implant recipient can take formal standardized testing, preferably administered in the child's primary mode of communication. In addition, if the present or future educational placement for this child is a regular classroom setting, it is strongly recommended that tests standardized on children with normal hearing, rather than on children with impaired hearing, be used. This will provide a more representative sample of how the skills of the school-aged student with hearing loss compare with those of her classroom peers. The results of this evaluation are used to determine the child's areas of strengths and weaknesses, to serve as a baseline from which to measure future progress, and to identify specific modifications needed in his ongoing aural habilitation and rehabilitation management.

Teenagers

Teens and parents who enter the evaluation or rehabilitation process often do so in response to having experienced a change in hearing status or a failure in some aspect of their social-communicative interactions. If considering cochlear implantation, the device may be viewed as a potential cure for deafness. Other precipitating variables for pursuing a cochlear implant in this age group, however, include obtaining a second cochlear implant or simply the relaxing criteria for implant candidacy.

The requirements of the communication evaluation for a teenager are the same as those for the school-aged child. However, it is also critical to involve the teen actively in the decision-making process regarding future amplification devices (including trying a digital hearing aid, using an FM system, or obtaining a cochlear implant). Similarly, it is unrealistic to expect that any progress will be made in the recommended therapy programming without the teen's motivation and commitment to such training. If the teen has restricted language skills, it is difficult to determine whether her limited understanding of the issues will allow her to offer an informed consent.

Professionals who are actively involved in the diagnostic and therapy processes with teenagers recognize that teens who have adjusted to compromised auditory input over many years may perceive increased or continuous sound from present technology as bothersome and aversive. The use of social-communicative questionnaires, such as the Listening Inventory for Education (LIFE) (Anderson & Smaldino, 1998) or the Secondary Screening Instrument for Targeting Educational Risk (Secondary SIFTER) (Anderson, 2004), has been found to be extremely useful in assessing whether the teen and parents have realistic expectations of an amplification device, the listening environment, or present level of functioning. Similarly, sharing test results and training strategies throughout the habilitation and rehabilitation process is motivating but also ensures that the teen maintains realistic expectations about her course of management and develops a better understanding of what is needed for her own self-advocacy.

In recent years, there has been a growing group of children from all developmental groups who reenter the evaluation and hearing habilitation process to receive a second cochlear implant. (Special note should be made that, ideally, a hearing aid trial has already been completed as part of the evaluation process for the second cochlear implant, involving the full-time use of a hearing aid in the unimplanted ear.) Particularly if the teen received an initial implant at a young age, she likely has few memories of the time commitment or training required to achieve benefit from the first device. Determining whether the teen and family have realistic expectations for the second device (compared with the dramatic gains received from the first) is a critical component of the evaluation procedure for this group. The second implant can be expected to improve hearing in competing noise, extend distance hearing, and assist in localization. Some children may derive little increased benefit in overall speech reception in quiet. Therapeutically, the challenge lies in devising a motivating and effective protocol for integrating the likely different signals the user initially receives from each implant.

◆ Selection of Test Protocols

The need to ensure accurate reception/perception of verbal test stimuli distinguishes the test administration for a child with hearing loss from that of her normal-hearing peers. Accordingly, all technology must be carefully checked to determine that it is functioning as intended before any speech-language-listening assessments are conducted. Furthermore, as previously cited in this chapter, assessing functional listening at the suprasegmental, phoneme, word, and sentence levels is also a necessary component of a comprehensive speech-language assessment for this population. Depending on the child's age, selected diagnostic protocols may encompass informal and formal measures. These measures, in turn, might involve criterion-referenced or norm-referenced tools. The advantage of norm-referenced diagnostic measures is that they permit comparison of the child's performance data to those of typically developing peers.

The components of a comprehensive communication evaluation should consist of three distinct skill domains: (1) auditory perception measures in contrasting listening environments; (2) receptive and expressive language functioning: and (3) speech production measures in contrasting listening environments. **Table 28.1** provides an organizational framework for conducting such an assessment. Given the wealth of available diagnostic tools, it is clearly evident that no single test can appropriately

meet the requirements of all of the necessary skill domains. A suggested protocol of tests has been included in the Appendix at the end of this chapter to offer a model for designing an appropriate diagnostic protocol.

Pearl

- Supplementary information may be obtained by using an assortment of subtests from various tests to obtain a more representative sample of the child's level of functioning and management needs, rather than using one prescribed test completely. Using tests normed on children with hearing loss often yields ceiling-effect scores and an inflated view of the child's present level of functioning.

◆ Service Delivery

The SLP or auditory-verbal practitioner provides direct instructional services to a child with hearing loss, either individually or within a group setting. The mandate for an early interventionist to provide services within the child's natural environment (Disability Education Act, 1991) has substantially altered the delivery of services to children under the age of 3 years. The focus of such services has been modified to address the social-communicative interactions of the child within family dynamics and daily home routines. Previously, it was not uncommon for an infant or toddler to be taken to a hospital or clinic setting, where frequently the parents were either not present in the session or they passively observed the therapy session. The expectation of naturalistic early intervention programming is that the parent or caregivers are actively involved in the training sessions, taking conversational turns and using the clinician's modeled techniques for stimulating functional listening and speech-language skills (Cole & Flexer, 2011).

This commitment to active parental involvement is not unique to early intervention. Quite the contrary, one of the primary tenets of the auditory-verbal and Listening and Spoken Language approaches from their inception has been the importance of active parental involvement (see Chapters 26 and 27). Skilled clinicians within clinical settings have been able to implement naturalistic training tasks effectively to facilitate the child's acquisition of a target skill (in a less distracting environment), with active parent involvement. The expectation is that because the parents have been actively involved, they will be able to reinforce the skills within naturally occurring situations at home.

Table 28.1 Functional listening assessment

Functional Listening Assessment						
Background Information						
Name:			Device: (RE) (LE)			
Date:			Settings: (RE) (LE)			
	Listen Alone (Quiet)			**Listen Alone (Noise)**		
Linguistic Level	RE	LE	Bin.	RE	LE	Bin.
Suprasegmentals						
Phonemes						
Words						
Sentences						
Connected Speech						
	Listen & Listen (Quiet)			**Listen & Listen (Noise)**		
Linguistic Level	RE	LE	Bin.	RE	LE	Bin.
Suprasegmentals						
Phonemes						
Words						
Sentences						
Connected Speech						
Speech Production	Standard Score Percentile Rank Age Equivalent		Intelligibility			
			Voice Quality			
			Resonance			
			Prosody			
			Vowels			
			Consonants			
			Syllables			
Verbal Comprehension	Standard Score Percentile Rank Age Equivalent		Expressive Language			
Pragmatic Functioning						

Abbreviations: LE, left ear; RE, right ear.
Source: Ying, 1990.

Similarly, the education initiatives of the 1980s and early 1990s, which require that general education classroom must change to accommodate the individual learning needs of all students, has most influenced the delivery of support services to the student with hearing loss, from the preschool years throughout the college experience (National Council on Disability, 1989). Ideally, instructional flexibility should be written into the child's individualized educational plan (IEP), allowing for push-in and pull-out services as needed. In a push-in delivery model, the student's auditory and speech and language training objectives are provided within the classroom setting; a pull-out model affords training outside the classroom.

During pull-out therapy sessions, the SLP or auditory-verbal practitioner can work in a less distracting environment on areas of weakness that are difficult to address in a classroom setting (e.g., resolving specific phonemic confusions or addressing the child's preteaching needs). On the other hand, by going into the classroom environment, the clinician has the valuable opportunity to observe the imposed communicative demands and teacher-talk used by the classroom teacher to navigate the behavior of her students, and to engineer social-communicative interactions between peers and adults while concomitantly addressing the child's individual training objectives.

Pitfall

- In all service delivery models, care needs to be taken to avoid having the student become overly dependent upon the service provider, and therein fostering less independent functioning in the classroom than the student is capable of demonstrating.

◆ Components of Hearing Habilitation/ Rehabilitation Training

In the absence of appropriately programmed hearing aids or speech processors (the external device of a cochlear implant), limited benefit can be gained from ongoing aural habilitation/rehabilitation. Therefore, periodic audiologic assessments are warranted to monitor the auditory status and to make changes in the device programming for a child with hearing loss (Johnson & Seaton, 2012). During the early stages of language learning, audiologic testing or device reprogramming is recommended every 3 months (Auditory Verbal International [AVI], 1993). However, to benefit optimally from this ongoing audiologic management, there should be an interactive exchange between the audiologist and the aural habilitation and rehabilitation provider.

Because the SLP or auditory-verbal therapist has many opportunities to closely monitor and document the nature of the child's phonemic confusions, she could and should share this information with the audiologist, who can then optimize modifications to the hearing aid or speech processor. Current digital hearing aids and cochlear implant speech processors have numerous features to enhance specific listening environments. They can be programmed with distinctly differing programs to capitalize on specific acoustic or perceptual features to coincide with or facilitate particular training targets (see Chapters 20, 22, and 24).

Perhaps the most valuable input needed by the audiologist for device programming is a descriptive analysis of any observed positive or negative changes in the child's auditory responsiveness reported by the clinician, including:

- Tolerance to specific sounds or device settings
- Attention-getting responses
- Distance listening
- Phonemic confusions

Therapy Environment

The optimal listening and learning environment for any child acquiring language is a quiet, child-friendly setting that affords a variety of sensory experiences and permits independent exploration. The structured auditory therapy session can occur within a range of environments from natural home environments to quiet or noisy classroom settings or acoustically controlled clinic settings, depending on the purpose of the therapy session. It seems counterintuitive to attempt to facilitate critical listening in a distracting environment with competing background noise; however, such may be the purpose of an advanced listening session.

Equally as critical is that auditory therapy should be a parent-child directive (e.g., actively involving the parent or caregiver in the ongoing training tasks). Regardless of the frequency of training sessions, it is indisputable that the parents will be the most consistent source of auditory and speech-language stimulation to the child. It is, therefore, essential to guide the parents in acquiring skills and strategies for eliciting their child's most optimal listening, comprehension, and production responses within naturally occurring daily routines (Cole & Flexer, 2011; Estabrooks, in press).

Now that the fitting of bilateral devices (two hearing aids or cochlear implants, or one cochlear implant with an appropriate hearing aid on the unimplanted ear) is considered best clinical practice, the structural organization of individual training sessions has been forever altered. Particularly during the adjustment period of having amplification on both ears, some portion of each therapy session should be directed toward listening with each device separately and under bilateral conditions. Realizing that one of the expected benefits of bilateral device use is improved listening in noise, training tasks should be used where the hearing aid or implant user is expected to follow spoken language in the presence of competing background noise. Potential noise sources could be commercially available four-talker babble audiotapes (Carver, 2000) or even talk radio. Over time, the signal-to-noise ratio between the speech and noise should be decreased to afford practice in listening environments that better simulate those encountered in everyday social interactions.

Pitfall

- The national mandate to conduct early intervention sessions within the home environment is sometimes erroneously viewed by clinicians and parents alike as an opportunity for parents to merely observe or opt out of participating in the sessions (e.g., using therapy as a break or opportunity to complete household chores while the child is otherwise engaged).

Direct Intervention Services

The primary objectives of providing hearing habilitation and rehabilitation to pediatric hearing aid or implant users is to develop and expand functional listening skills for the purposes of continued language learning and enhanced communicative interactions. Young children fitted with either conventional amplification or cochlear implants require direct instruction to master the vocabulary and linguistic structure of the language being directed to and around them. Their active involvement in meaningful social-communicative interactions with their typically developing and normal hearing peers significantly enriches their language learning efforts.

However, the increased auditory access afforded by a cochlear implant has been observed to facilitate more incidental learning (e.g., learning from mere exposure) in these children relative to their profoundly hearing-impaired peers fitted with conventional hearing aids. During the critical language-learning period (between birth and 3 years of age), the process of attaching meaning to auditory cues occurs with an ease and naturalness that is not observed when listening and speech are initiated at later ages.

Ongoing parent-child-centered training should be provided to an infant or young child with hearing aids or a cochlear implant at least twice a week for 60-minute sessions. Regardless of how often direct therapy services can be delivered, auditory-verbal intervention is recommended if the family's desired outcome for their child is spoken language. (See Chapter 26 for more information about different communication approaches.) In accordance with the child's age and exhibited skills upon entering the hearing habilitation process, she can be expected to achieve greater auditory performance from those baseline levels if provided with appropriate technology and sufficient auditory-based speech and language training.

Systems like Signed English or Cued Speech (Yoshinaga-Itano, 2000) coupled with auditory training may be the appropriate intervention for some older children who were taught visually in earlier intervention and educational programs or who do not have sufficient auditory access. Yoshinaga-Itano (2000) reported that it is indeed possible to map acoustic cues and speech production cues onto an existing or intact sign language system. Both Signed English (i.e., a manual communication system) and cued speech (i.e., a phonemic-based system that uses hand shapes and body positioning to correspond to speech) would afford an older child who is attempting to advance her auditory skills with the best match between what she hears and what she sees. In contrast, American Sign Language (ASL) is a separate language with its own syntax and grammar; it is not designed to be used with spoken language. If ASL is paired with spoken language, a mismatch is created that may complicate the language-learning process.

Pitfall

- Some teachers and clinicians report that they use ASL with English word order. However, because spoken language and ASL are incompatible communication systems, the child will have incomplete access to both spoken English and ASL as functional and complete language systems if they are to be used together.

Training Strategies

Several published auditory curricula offer parents and professionals hierarchical guidelines for auditory skill emergence and a variety of useful training activities (Moog, Biedenstein, & Davidson, 1995; Koch, 1999, Estabrooks, 2004). Such programs are sometimes inappropriately viewed as cookbooks to address the individual training needs of a child fitted with hearing aids or cochlear implants. However, a thorough understanding of the underlying principles and training strategies of the auditory-verbal/listening and spoken language intervention model best complements the current trend of providing evidence-based intervention to this diverse population. Auditory-verbal/listening and spoken language approaches emphasize the development and reliance upon auditory cues to receive, comprehend, and use spoken language in the context of meaningful, real-life experiences.

◆ Conclusions

Documenting auditory skill emergence and speech-language progress over time is the final component of the comprehensive, communication management of children who are deaf or hard of hearing. The professional literature is expanding with the results from a diverse body of research efforts, directed toward identifying critical prognostic indicators of success or benefit from current technology and training options (Anderson & Arnoldi, 2011; Johnson & Seaton, 2012). As a result, SLPs and auditory-verbal practitioners now have quantifiable evidence with which to determine the effectiveness of the hearing habilitation and rehabilitation programming they afford. However, documentation from ongoing diagnostic training, in combination with regularly scheduled comprehensive assessments, should direct future intervention for an individual child. Information from research and clinical domains, in turn, motivates the manufacturers to improve the programming schemas of digital aids and cochlear implant speech processors to meet the needs of an increasingly younger and more diverse population of spoken language communicators with significant hearing loss.

Appendix

The following diagnostic protocol affords a listing of commercially available tests and how they could be used to meet the requirements of a comprehensive functional listening assessment and speech-language evaluation. This listing is by no means exhaustive or intended to suggest that other test measures might not also be useful. Please see table on next page for more descriptive information about the tests and where they can be obtained. Some are discussed in Chapters 11 and 22.

Auditory perception

Tests	Infants	Preschool	School-aged	Teenage	Bilateral
IT-MAIS (Zimmerman-Phillips, Osberger, & Robbins, 1997)	X	X			
LittlEARS (MED-EL, 2006)	X	X			
FAPI (Stredler-Brown & Johnson, 2003)	X	X	X		
ESP (Moog & Geers, 1990)	X	X	X	X	X
COT (MED-EL, 2004)		X	X		
TAC (Trammell et al, 1981)		X	X	X	X
Mr. Potato Head (Robbins, 1994)		X	X		
Common Phrases (Robbins, Renshaw, & Osberger, 1995)		X	X	X	X
AB List (CASPA) (Boothroyd & Minnear, 2001)		X	X	X	X
PBK (Haskins, 1949)			X	X	X
LNT (Kirk, Pisoni, & Osberger, 1995)			X	X	X
HINT-S (Nilsson, Solli, & Sullivan, 1994)			X	X	X

Language functioning

Tests	Infants	Preschool	School-aged	Teenage	Bilateral
CSBS (Wetherby & Prizant, 1993)	X	X			
MacArthur-Bates (Fenson et al, 2006)	X	X			
CASLLS (Wilkes, 1999)	X	X	X		
Reynell (Reynell & Gruber, 1990)	X	X	X		
PLS-5 (Zimmerman, Steiner, & Pond, 2011)	X		X	X	
PPVT-4 (Dunn & Dunn, 2007)		X	X	X	X
CELF-4 (Semel, Wing, & Secord, 2003)			X	X	X
SPELT-3 (Dawson, Stout, & Eyer, 2003)		X	X	X	X
OWLS (Carrow-Woolfolk, 1995)			X	X	X

Speech production

Tests	Infants	Preschool	School-aged	Teenage	Bilateral
GFTA-2 (Goldman & Fristoe, 2000)		X	X	X	X
Intelligibility Measure			X	X	X

Test	Stimuli	Skill domain	Availability
Infant Toddler-Meaningful Auditory Integration Scale (IT-MAIS)	Detection, discrimination, recognition environmental sound and speech	Speech perception	Advanced Bionics
Meaningful Auditory Integration Scale (MAIS)	Detection, discrimination, recognition environmental sounds and speech	Speech perception	Advanced Bionics
LittlEARS Auditory Questionnaire	Detection, discrimination, recognition, comprehension of environmental sounds, songs, phonemes, words, sentences	Speech perception	MED-EL Worldwide, Innsbruck, Austria
Common Objects Token (COT) Test	Discrimination, identification, comprehension of verbal directions	Speech perception	MED-EL Worldwide, Innsbruck, Austria
Functional Auditory Performance Indicators (FAPI)	Detection, discrimination, recognition, comprehension from sounds to sentences	Speech perception	Colorado Department of Education, Special Education Services Unit
Early Speech Perception Test (ESP)	Suprasegmentals, phonemes, words	Speech perception	Central Institute for the Deaf and Hard of Hearing, St. Louis, MO
Mr. Potato Head Task	Words, sentences	Speech perception	Indiana University School of Medicine, DeVault Otologic Research Laboratory
Common Phrases	Sentences	Speech perception	Indiana University School of Medicine, DeVault Otologic Research Laboratory
AB List (Computer Assessed Speech Assessment)	Phonemes, words	Speech perception	Journal of the American Academy of Audiology
Phonetically Balanced Kindergarten (PBK) List	Phonemes, words	Speech perception	ASHA, Washington, DC
Lexical Neighborhood Test (LNT)	Phonemes, words	Speech perception	Audiotec, St. Louis, MO
Hearing in Noise Test–Sentences (HINT-S)	Sentences	Speech perception	Audiotec, St. Louis, MO
Communication Skills Behavior Scales (CSBS)	Suprasegmentals, phonemes, words, sentences	Receptive/expressive	Paul H. Brookes Publishing Co., Baltimore, MD
MacArthur-Bates Communication Developmental Inventories	Words, phrases	Receptive/expressive	Paul H. Brookes Publishing Co., Baltimore, MD
Cottage Acquisition Scales for Listening, Language & Speech (CASLLS)	Words, phrases, sentences	Speech perception/ production, receptive	Sunshine Cottage, San Antonio, TX
Reynell Developmental Language Scales	Words, sentences	Receptive/expressive	Super Duper Publications, Greenville, SC
Preschool Language Scale-5 (PLS-5)	Words, sentences	Receptive/expressive	Pearson, San Antonio, TX
Peabody Picture Vocabulary Test-4 (PPVT-4)	Words	Receptive language	Pearson, San Antonio, TX
Clinical Evaluation of Language Fundamentals (CELF-4)	Words, sentences, paragraphs	Receptive/expressive	Pearson, San Antonio, TX
Oral & Written Language Scales (OWLS)	Words, sentences, paragraphs	Receptive/expressive	Western Psychological Services, Torrance, CA
Goldman-Fristoe Test of Articulation-2	Phonemes, words, sentences	Articulation	Pearson, San Antonio, TX

Discussion Questions

1. What variables most influence the acquisition of optimal functional listening skill emergence and age-appropriate speech and language skills?

2. What role do realistic expectations and consistent communicative demands play in the emergence of listening, spoken language and literacy skills?

3. How does an SLP or auditory-verbal practitioner identify the present level of functioning and training needs for a child who cannot respond on formal test measures?

4. Why should the teenager be actively involved in the decision-making process regarding her communication management?

References

Anderson, K. (2004). Secondary Screening Instrument for Targeting Educational Risk (Secondary SIFTER). Denver, CO: Behavior Educational Audiology Association.

Anderson, K., & Arnoldi, K. A. (2011). Building skills for success in the fast-paced classroom. Hillsboro, OR: Butte.

Anderson, K., & Smaldino, J. (1998). Listening Inventory for Education (LIFE). Denver, CO: Educational Audiology Association.

Auditory-Verbal International. (1993). Suggested protocol for audiological and hearing evaluation. Easton, PA: AVI.

Boothroyd, A., & Minnear, D. (2001). Evaluation of the computer-assisted speech perception test (CASPA). Journal of the American Academy of Audiology, 27, 134–144.

Carrow-Woolfolk, E. (1995). Oral and written language scales. Torrance, CA: Western Psychological Services.

Carver, W. (2000). Four talker babble audiotape. St. Louis, MO: Auditec of St. Louis.

Cole, E., & Flexer, C. (2011). Children with hearing loss: developing listening and talking, birth to six (2nd ed.). San Diego, CA: Plural.

Dawson, J., Stout, C., & Eyer, J. (2003). Structured photographic expressive language test–3. DeKalb, IL: Janelle Publications.

Disability Education Act. (1991). P.L. No. 102-119, Part H.

Dunn, L., & Dunn, L. (2007). Peabody picture vocabulary test (4th ed.). San Antonio, TX: Pearson.

Estabrooks, W. (2004). Auditory-verbal ages and stages of development. Cochlear implants for kids. Washington, DC: The Alexander Graham Bell Association for the Deaf and Hard of Hearing.

Estabrooks, W. (in press). 101 frequently asked questions about auditory-verbal practice. Washington, DC. The Alexander Graham Bell Association for the Deaf and Hard of Hearing.

Fenson, L., Marchman, V., Thal, D., Dale, P., Reznick, S., & Bates, E. (2006). MacArthur-Bates communicative development inventories (CDIs) (2nd ed.). Baltimore, MD: Brookes.

Geers, A. E., Strube, M. J., Tobey, E. A., Pisoni, D. B., & Moog, J. S. (2011). Epilogue: factors contributing to long-term outcomes of cochlear implantation in early childhood. Ear and Hearing, 32(1, Suppl), 84S–92S.

Goldman, R., & Fristoe, M. (2000). Goldman Fristoe test of articulation 2. Circle Pines, MN: American Guidance Service.

Haskins, H. (1949). A phonetically balanced test of speech discrimination for children. Master's thesis, Northwestern University, Evanston, IL.

Johnson, C. D., & Seaton, J. (2012). Educational audiology handbook (2nd ed.). Clifton Park, NY: Delmar-Cengage Learning.

Kirk, K., Pisoni, D., & Osberger, M. (1995). Lexical neighborhood test (LNT). St. Louis, MO: Audiotec.

Koch, M. (1999). Bringing sounds to life. Parkton, MD: York Press.

Med-El. (2004). Common Objects Token (COT) test. Innsbruck, Austria: Med-El Corporation.

Med-El. (2006). LittlEARS auditory questionnaire. Innsbruck, Austria: Med-El Corporation.

Moeller, M. P. (2000). Early intervention and language development in children who are deaf and hard of hearing. Pediatrics, 106(3), E43. PubMed

Moog, J., & Geers, A. E. (1990). Early speech perception test. St. Louis, MO: Central Institute for the Deaf and Hard of Hearing.

Moog, J., Biedenstein, J., & Davidson, L. (1995). Speech perception instructional curriculum and evaluation (SPICE). St. Louis, MO: Central Institute for the Deaf.

National Council on Disability. (1989). The education of students with disabilities: where do we stand? A report to the President and the Congress of the United States. Washington, DC: National Council on Disability, American Psychological Association.

Nilsson, M., Solli, S., & Sullivan, J. (1994). Hearing in noise test (HINT)–sentences. St. Louis, MO: Audiotec of St. Louis.

Pisoni, D. B., & Geers, A. E. (2000). Working memory of deaf children with cochlear implants: correlations between digit span and measures of spoken language processing. Annals of Otolaryngology, Rhinology, Laryngology, 109, 63–64.

Quittner, A. L., Leibach, P., & Marciel, K. (2004). The impact of cochlear implants on young deaf children: new methods to assess cognitive and behavioral development. Archives of Otolaryngology–Head & Neck Surgery, 130(5), 547–554.

Reynell, J., & Gruber, C. (1990). The Reynell developmental language scales. Los Angeles, CA: Western Psychological Services.

Robbins, A. M. (1994). The Mr. Potato Head task. Indianapolis, IN: Indiana University School of Medicine.

Robbins, A., Renshaw, J., & Osberger, L. (1995). The common phrases test. Indianapolis, IN: Indiana University School of Medicine.

Semel, E., Wing, E., & Secord, W. (2003). Clinical evaluation of language fundamentals (4th ed.). San Antonio, TX: Harcourt Assessment.

Sininger, Y. S., Grimes, A., & Christensen, E. (2010). Auditory development in early amplified children: factors influencing auditory-based communication outcomes in children with hearing loss. Ear and Hearing, 31(2), 166–185.

Stallings, L. M., Kirk, K. I., Chin, S., & Gao, S. (2004). Parent word familiarity and the language development of pediatric cochlear implant users. The Volta Review, 102, 237–257.

Stredler-Brown, A., & Johnson, D. (2003). Functional auditory performance indicators. Colorado Department of Education, Special Education Services Unit. Retrieved from http://www.cde.state.co.us/cdesped/SpecificDisability-Hearing.html

Trammell, J., Farrar, C. M., Francis, J., Owens, S. L., Schepard, D. E., Whitlen, R. P., & Faist, L. H. (1981). Test of auditory comprehension. Portland, OR: Foreworks.

Wetherby, A., & Prizant, B. (1993). The communication and symbolic behavior scale. Baltimore, MD: Brookes.

Wilkes, E. (1999). Cottage acquisition scales for listening, language & speech. San Antonio, TX: Sunshine Cottage School for Deaf Children.

Ying, E. (1990). Speech and language assessment: communication evaluation, in hearing impaired children in the mainstream. Parkton, MD: York Press.

Yoshinaga-Itano, C. (2000). Early intervention and language development in children who are deaf and hard of hearing. Pediatrics, 106, 594–602.

Yoshinaga-Itano, C., Sedey, A., Colter, D., & Mehl, A. (1998). Language of early and late identified hearing loss. Pediatrics, 102, 116–171.

Zimmerman, I., Steiner, V., & Pond, R. (2011). Preschool language scale-5 (5th ed.). San Antonio, TX: Pearson.

Zimmerman-Phillips, S., Osberger, M. J., & Robbins, A. M. (1997). Infant-toddler meaningful auditory integration scale [IT-MAIS]. Sylmar, CA: Advanced Bionics Corporation.

Chapter 29

Educational Placement Options for School-Aged Children with Hearing Loss

Susan Cheffo

Key Points

- There are various educational placement options in the mainstream or in schools for the deaf.
- Related services are provided both in and out of class for students who need them.
- Schools are required to provide assistive technology as needed by students.
- Modifications and testing accommodations must be offered as needed.
- All educational services must be listed on a child's Individualized Education Plan (IEP) or 504 plan.

Numerous educational placement options are available for the school-aged child with hearing loss. With legislative changes and expansion of educational programs, the choices of educational placements for children 3 to 21 years of age have increased. Advances in technology, providing children with hearing loss greater access to sound, have led deaf education from segregated schools for the deaf to traditional school settings. Within these settings, quality support services and classroom modifications are required to help the child with hearing loss succeed. Knowledge of the laws, augmented by a creative school staff experienced in working with children with hearing loss, will enhance the educational opportunities for children in the mainstream (see Chapter 30 for more information about educational laws). For families who opt to keep their children in schools for the deaf, there has been movement from sign language to auditory-oral communication. Whether a mainstream or self-contained placement is chosen, individualization within that setting must occur so that the child's hearing, educational, and social needs are met. This chapter will address the various school placement options for children 3 to 21 years of age. Along with placement options, appropriate services, modifica-

tions, and testing accommodations will be discussed. The IEP/504 plan (see Chapter 30) drives the educational services for the child. All services listed on the IEP/504 must be performed by the school. Therefore, including all services, modifications, and accommodations on the IEP will ensure their implementation. A positive reciprocal relationship between school districts, professionals, and family will help create appropriate school services.

◆ Preschool Options

Preschool is usually the time young children with hearing loss first separate from their parents and attend a full- or part-time program. Youngsters develop their preacademic skills, build their listening and verbal skills, and start socializing in preschool; the foundations for education begin at this time.

When children who are deaf or hard of hearing transition from early intervention (EI) (see Chapter 27), to preschool, they need to be evaluated to select appropriate school placement. These evaluations, scheduled with parental consent, include audiology, speech-language, psychological, motor skills, educational readiness, determination of necessary classroom adaptation, and social history. The Individual Family Service Plan (IFSP) is developed by the team after the evaluations are complete and describes the child's abilities and areas of concern. Preschool educational placement will be decided at the IEP meeting. Parents, ultimately, make final decisions about placement. Finding a good match for preschool should not be difficult when information is available about the child's abilities and when the parents have information about various options (Cole & Flexer, 2011). In spite of having good information, parents may feel insecure about their decisions. It is important to remember that if the placement is not successful, the committee can reconvene to determine whether a different type of placement or additional services might be necessary. There needs to be flexibility in creating the appropriate environment for a young child beginning school.

Pearl

- If a preschool placement is not meeting a child's needs, the IEP team can reconvene, and a change in placement can be arranged.

Mainstream Preschool

The mainstream or traditional preschool is one option for youngsters who are deaf or hard of hearing and who have attained age-appropriate or near-age-appropriate speech and language skills. Many parents and clinicians feel that the mainstream preschool experience provides better language role models offered by children with typical hearing. In addition, placement in the mainstream enhances their child's preparation for the larger world (Zwolan & Sorkin, 2006).

There are private and public preschool options. If a parent chooses a private preschool, payment is out-of-pocket. For a public, universal preschool program, funding is provided by the federal government. For parents seeking a private preschool, finding one close to home is preferable. There are a variety of philosophies for preschool education, all of which need to be carefully evaluated by educators and parents.

Whether public or private, preschools that have served children with hearing loss in the past may be most beneficial. Enthusiasm about having a child with hearing loss and a willingness to collaborate with a team of professionals and parents are positive characteristics. Parents may want to bring an educator from EI, their speech-language pathologist, or a clinician from the audiology center to accompany them when visiting different schools. Professional advice may help them make an informed decision as to which program is the best match for their child.

Schools and Programs for Children Who Are Deaf

Private oral schools (now typically identified as Listening and Spoken Language [LSL] schools) called OPTION schools are located in various cities in the United States for children with hearing loss. These schools provide education to children who are deaf or hard of hearing by training use of residual hearing in an enriched auditory/linguistic environment. Sometimes children are enrolled in these programs for early, intensive development of spoken language in their preschool years. There may be an extension of these programs through elementary grades to establish reading skills (Chute & Nevins, 2002). A certified teacher of the deaf (TOD) is usually the class instructor, although an early childhood educator or speech-language pathologist may be in charge. Knowledge of early childhood education and how typically hearing children develop language is important.

During the last few years, schools or programs for children who are deaf that have traditionally used sign language are developing effective auditory-oral (Listening and Spoken Language) programs for their preschool students, and many State Schools for the Deaf (4201 schools) have begun these programs for their infant/preschool children. State-mandated newborn hearing screening has led to early identification of hearing loss and earlier hearing aid use as well as earlier cochlear implantation. All of these advances have increased children's ability to perceive soft speech at a very early age and to develop speech and language similar to their peers with typical hearing (Boons et al, 2012; Geers, Nicholas, & Sedey, 2003). These programs have become another appropriate listening and spoken language option for early identified children.

Some of these schools/programs for children with hearing loss provide an integrative model, in which typical peers attend classes at the site (reverse mainstreaming), or children with hearing loss attend traditional preschool classes part-time. There is usually a liaison from the school for the deaf to work with the mainstream preschool staff, explaining technology, ramifications of hearing loss, teaching strategies, and providing resources. Having hearing children in class can improve language, communicative interaction, and social skills. The pace of instruction and teacher expectation in integrated classes has been observed to increase compared with programs in which all children are hearing-impaired. For parents who decide to place their children in a self-contained program for children with hearing loss where there is no mainstreaming, it is recommended that their child attend after-school activities with typical peers. This will give children the opportunity to interact socially and enhance auditory and verbal skills. Some activities, such as dance, sports, arts and crafts, gymnastics, or library may be helpful. Not all activities are costly. Family gatherings and play dates should also be encouraged.

Although parents may be faced with various placement alternatives and some difficult decisions, it is important for them to remember they are not alone. Professionals can guide families in making choices and supporting parent decisions. A decision may not be 100% satisfactory, and placements may need changing. The school district supports families and will revisit the IEP to make program modifications as needed. Disagreements between parents and the school district may require resolution through alternative means, such as mediation or due process hearings; however, such proceedings are generally not necessary.

◆ Options for School-Aged Children (5 to 21 Years of Age)

Mainstream Schools

Many children who are deaf or hard of hearing are returning to local school districts to continue their education beyond preschool. The law states that children with disabilities are entitled to a free and appropriate education (FAPE) in the least restrictive environment (LRE) (American Speech-Language-Hearing Association [ASHA], 2006) (see Chapter 30). Attending school in the child's local school district is a goal of many parents and can be a positive and fulfilling experience. Children who are deaf or hard of hearing can attend school with neighborhood friends, while participating in school activities alongside their typical peers. Elementary school is a time when children are generally more sensitive to special needs and accepting of differences. It is also a time when lifelong friendships can be developed. During middle and high school, academics are critical and social interactions can positively or negatively affect the school experience. The following options within school districts are similar for students 5 to 21 years old, although readily available options may vary from district to district.

General Education Class

A general education class usually consists of 25 to 30 children, sometimes more. One teacher is in charge of all the children and teaches all subjects. By fourth or fifth grade, departmentalization may be in effect. This is the first time more than one teacher is introduced, and students move from room to room throughout the day. The children in the class are independent learners and require little support, although acoustic access is always an issue that must be considered and managed. Children with hearing loss who attend general education classes usually have age-appropriate language and cognition. They are motivated, articulate youngsters with excellent communication skills and families who can offer academic practice and support at home.

Inclusion Class

There are ~ 20 to 25 children in class, but a percentage of the youngsters have an IEP that mandates special education support and accommodations. There is a full-time classroom teacher, and, in addition, a special education teacher who may be in the room part or all day. There is usually also a teacher assistant all day. Having the classroom teacher and assistant present in the classroom permits special education

children to have individual support throughout the day. It is important to observe the inclusion class to ensure that the needs of the other classified children do not conflict with the needs of the child who is deaf or hard of hearing. Inclusion classes may be called by other names (blended or collaborative class), but the design of the class is similar.

Self-Contained Class

Children who are unable to participate in a general education or inclusion class may benefit from a self-contained, special education class within the local public school. The class size is small. The teacher is certified in special education and there is usually a full-time teacher assistant. The children reap the benefit of individualization and small group learning. This class is designed to help youngsters develop the necessary skills to eventually attend an inclusion or general education class. As skills improve, the child may be able to move into a regular education class for part of the day. Disruptive behavior of other students may be an issue in this type of class, so observation is important to determine whether the class is appropriate for the child in question.

Collaborative Class

Some schools have the ability to create a collaborative experience similar to inclusion, except all the IEP children have hearing loss. Instead of a special education teacher sharing the class, the special education teacher is a TOD. Having a general education teacher and TOD co-teach can be an ideal teaching situation. The children gain the benefit of appropriate curriculum and expectations, with the specific guidance and support of a TOD. A collaborative class is not common in many areas, but this model has been successful.

Pearl

- Parents seeking a mainstream option for school-aged students have usually enrolled early-amplified infants and toddlers in auditory-oral or mainstream preschool. Family members are active participants during this process.

Schools and Programs for Children Who Are Deaf

Children who attend schools for the deaf from 5 to 21 years of age usually have more severe disabilities, or their parents have chosen these schools for cultural or communication reasons. Many of the children who attend these schools or programs require additional educational support and a more restrictive environment. These schools and programs are usually day classes, but residential placements are still available in some areas. There typically is a nurturing, protective environment and an affiliation with other students and adults who are deaf or hard of hearing. There is no cost to parents for state-sponsored schools or programs for the deaf.

Within these schools are various communication options that include:

- Auditory-oral (listening and spoken language), where children use amplification to listen, including frequency modulation (FM) systems, and speech reading is used to support communication
- Total communication, which incorporates any means to communicate with children who are deaf, including a sign language system that is based on English, finger spelling, gestures, and any other means of helping a child understand English
- American Sign Language, a manual language not based on English syntax, that is used within the deaf community, while English is taught as a second language (BEGINNINGS, 2005a)

◆ Related Services

All students who are deaf or hard of hearing require some level of support service throughout their schooling. Whether a child attends a mainstream program or a school for the deaf, related services are part of his educational plan.

The types of related services offered on the elementary, middle, and high school levels are similar to those provided in preschool. However, the delivery of service to an older child is different because there is greater emphasis on academics once a child turns 5. There is also a need for highly qualified providers to deliver these services; educators who are experienced, receive ongoing training, and achieve good results with their students. Although dedication and a nurturing sensibility are evident characteristics in those working with children who are deaf or hard of hearing, knowledge about how to implement these special services is key. There is a need for ongoing staff development training to keep up with changes in the field, as well as advances in technology. Related service providers must expand their knowledge-base to understand new curriculums, state tests, revisions to the law and school curriculum, and today's deaf or hard of hearing child who may have more subtle hearing needs.

Related services are determined at the child's IEP/504 meeting. The committee decides on the appropriate services, the amount of time the service will be provided, as well as the location of service provision. There is no cost to parents for related services as long as the services appear on the child's IEP or 504 plan. School districts pay for this service, which is reimbursed in part by the state. There are various related services detailed below, the most important ones being TOD, speech-language pathology, and FM assistive technology.

Pearl

- The three most frequently used services in the mainstream for children with cochlear implants are speech-language pathology (75%), FM systems (65%), and deaf education services (54%) (Zwolan & Sorkin, 2006).

Teacher of the Deaf (TOD)

The TOD is state certified and has specific training in working with children who are deaf or hard of hearing. In the mainstream setting, the TOD works individually with a student for a determined amount of time. This individual is a very important person to the child who is deaf or hard of hearing throughout his schooling. The major areas of need to consider when including students with special needs in regular classroom settings are modifying the physical environment, providing appropriate levels of support, and monitoring the child's progress (Anderson & Arnoldi, 2011; Dinnebeil & McInerney, 2000); the TOD performs all these functions.

First, the TOD observes the acoustic environment and suggests modifications where necessary. She ensures that appropriate and consistent use of amplification is provided, performs listening checks to be certain equipment is working properly, performs troubleshooting as needed, and will teach school staff to monitor equipment if the TOD is not in the school on a daily basis. Second, the TOD analyzes the child's language, teaches vocabulary, and encourages verbal interactive communication skills. Behavior and social skills may also need to be addressed. Previewing and reviewing academic material, the crux of TOD sessions, can begin during preschool and continue through high school. Third, by assessing the child's progress through evaluations and reporting on IEP goals, the TOD knows where deficits or successes are and whether services need increasing or decreasing. To make sure all providers and parents collaborate, the TOD also oversees a communication notebook, blog, or e-mail exchange, a system of sharing information with all professionals and the child's family. TOD services are provided as a push-in or pull-out model. Push-in is important in preschool and lower elementary school, since being in the classroom is a good way of monitoring communication interaction, facilitating language when needed, and developing a general overview of the child's ability to advocate for his needs. In addition, being in the classroom gives the TOD hands-on information to share with other service providers and with parents.

As academics and language become more challenging, the pull-out model is preferable so that the TOD can preview and review academic material. TOD services are usually provided three to five times a week.

Speech-Language Pathology Services

The speech-language pathologist is a state-licensed individual who has received generalized speech and language training in graduate school. Because delivering speech services to children who are deaf or hard of hearing requires specialized skills, the school pathologist or therapist usually needs support. There are speech-language pathologists and certified Listening and Spoken Language Specialists—Auditory-Verbal Therapists (LSLS Cert. AVT), who specialize in teaching students who are deaf or hard of hearing (Estabrooks, 2012). This learning helps children develop auditory skills to enable them to use hearing to learn language and who can provide training to the school's speech-language pathologist. A LSLS Cert. AVT is knowledgeable in the application and management of technology, strategies, techniques, and procedures to enable youngsters who are deaf or hard of hearing to learn to listen and understand spoken language, and to use hearing to develop spoken language (Estabrooks, 2012). Providing speech, language, and listening therapy in school will positively impact academic outcomes.

School speech services are usually offered three to five times a week. Most speech services are provided in a pull-out format, usually one on one, in a separate, quiet location. Some students receive group speech, where pragmatic skills are addressed during small-group instruction. Understanding the importance of auditory therapy and helping the child maintain this skill is one of the keys to success in school.

Pitfall

- The TOD is responsible for the preview and review work. Therefore, the school speech therapists should not focus on preview and review during speech sessions. Even though school curriculum is the basis for language and vocabulary, listening therapy is still required, and the speech-language pathologist is typically the professional who offers auditory development.

The following additional related services are less common for the child who is deaf or hard of hearing.

Resource Room

Resource room services are provided by a certified, special education teacher, not a TOD. The resource room addresses fundamental academic skills in a small group setting. Some children receive this service when added support is needed in academic subjects because of additional disabilities that affect learning, or if there are too few TODs in a specific geographic region. Students are pulled out for this service, which will add time out of the classroom. Balancing pull-out time is important so that major classroom academics are not missed.

Teacher Assistant/Aide/Shadow/ Intervention Assistant

This individual may or may not be a certified teacher but is an adult who assists the child and the teacher in the classroom. He helps refocus the student who experiences behavioral issues and addresses academic concerns. Care and training are needed to ensure that the assistant/aide/shadow does not interfere with teacher–student interaction. A child returning to the mainstream who is dependent on the assistant/aide will not have the appropriate student–teacher relationship. The classroom teacher, not the classroom assistant, needs to be the main focus for the child with hearing loss.

Interpreter

The student who participates in the general education setting usually has good communication skills and academic ability; however, group discussion or questions asked by students may require interpreting intervention. The interpreter may be used all day or for clarification purposes.

Sign Language

The sign language interpreter is knowledgeable in sign language and preferably has RID (Registry of Interpreters for the Deaf) certification. Some children require the use of an interpreter consistently, since understanding the teacher is difficult for them. Other children who are developing auditory skills can use the sign language interpreter for clarification as support. The sign language interpreter may also be used to reverse-interpret for the teacher and other pupils in the class if the child who is deaf or hard of hearing has unintelligible speech.

Oral

The oral interpreter can be used with a child who has good lip reading skills. The interpreter sits close to the child and repeats the information spoken in the classroom so that the child can lip read. This type of interpreter may be helpful during group interactions, by repeating comments or questions of peers.

Cued Speech

Cued speech is a visual communication system of eight hand shapes or cues as an assist to lipreading. Although less common, a child trained to use cued speech would need a cued speech interpreter in school full time (BEGINNINGS, 2005b).

Controversial Point

- An educational interpreter needs to be sensitive to the needs of a child who is transitioning from a visual system to an auditory one. If the child uses an FM system and derives auditory benefit, the interpreter should be used for clarification purposes and to interpret questions or comments of classmates. Pointing to the individual who is speaking may be sufficient.

Counseling

Some children benefit from counseling services provided by a school psychologist or social worker. Transitioning to a mainstream environment may require support from a trained individual who is familiar with the social and emotional aspects of hearing loss. Being the only child in school with hearing loss may cause a sense of isolation. For secondary students, social issues are a major source of concern. Feeling different because of their hearing loss is prevalent within the adolescent population. In-school counseling and social skills groups or private therapy are helpful (see Chapter 35). Arranging for regular social activities with other children with hearing loss can also be helpful in dealing with social and emotional issues.

Educational Audiologist

An educational audiologist should be available in every school district where there is a child with hearing loss. If the district has many children with hearing loss, an educational audiologist may be employed by the school district. If there are only a very few children, the educational audiologist may consult as an independent provider or may be hired through the regional board of cooperative educational services (BOCES). The educational audiologist will evaluate audiologic test results, in some districts will perform testing with and without technology, will recommend which FM system is appropriate, will obtain and monitor the systems, will teach school staff to use the systems effectively, and will monitor classroom performance. The educational audiologist will also be involved in management of children with auditory processing disorders. (See Chapter 31, and Madell, 2012.)

Educational Consultant

When a child transitions into elementary school, an educational consultant from an audiology center can provide training to district-based personnel. Consultation will cover assistive technology. In school, all children with hearing loss or auditory processing disorder require the use of an FM system that must be included on the IEP (see Chapter 23 for information about FM systems).

Special Consideration

- The FM system should be evaluated in every class, including specials. What works in one room, or with one type of classroom setup, may not work in another.

Closed Captions

Whenever movies are shown in school, they need to be captioned. Children who are deaf or hard of hearing cannot understand all that is said in movies and therefore should not be held responsible for the information unless the movie is captioned. Closed captions will benefit all children in class.

Classroom Modifications

All students who are deaf or hard of hearing need some modifications to participate in the general education curriculum. Some of these modifications are intended for school use, others are provided at home to enhance school performance. For a student who is deaf or hard of hearing, having modifications will create a means for equal access. The following are some examples of typical modifications listed on the IEP.

Strategic Seating
(Formerly Called "Preferential Seating")

For many years, front and center seating was preferable. Listening up-close to the teacher and reading lips were necessary. Today, in most preschools and elementary schools, children are seated in clusters where collaboration and interaction are part of the learning experience. Strategic seating now becomes a place where the child who is deaf or hard of hearing has access to his peers, both auditorally and visually. The FM system will ensure hearing the teacher from any point in the classroom, so sitting directly in front of the teacher is no longer necessary (American Academy of Audiology [AAA], 2008). Movement from one area of the room to another as activities change is also part of strategic seating. The TOD or educational audiologist should analyze the classroom environment to help decide seat placement.

Acoustic Modifications

Due to poor acoustics, modifications are needed in all classrooms (Smaldino & Flexer, 2012).

Wall-to-wall carpeting: Carpeting is a wonderful means of absorbing sound. However, many schools are concerned about allergens, dirt, and bugs and will not add carpeting as an acoustic modification. For any district that will provide wall-to-wall carpeting, it is a powerful means of reducing impulse sounds.

Area rugs: These can be placed in various parts of the classroom and can be easily cleaned. Impulse sound is reduced in a particular area, such as the block corner, but an area rug does not offer the benefit of wall-to-wall carpeting.

Chair-foot covers: Tennis balls or products such as Hushh-Ups (Sound Living Environments, Mississauga, Ontario, Canada), Quiet Feet (Master Manufacturing, Cleveland, OH), or Quiet Chair Foot Covers (Really Good Stuff, Monroe, CT) are placed on the legs of chairs, desks, and tables to reduce noise levels when there is a tile floor. They are not used to absorb sound but to decrease the loud sounds associated with chair and desk movement.

Acoustic tiles and corkboards: These can be used on ceilings and walls to reduce reverberation (echo). They absorb sound and are relatively inexpensive.

Window covering: Drapes, curtains, blinds, or shades can help reduce reverberation.

Dropped ceilings: Many schools have high, vaulted ceilings that are sources of reverberation. Dropping those ceilings and using acoustic ceiling tile produce a better sound environment and are the single most effective means of acoustic management in a classroom.

Static electricity reducers: Cochlear implants are electronic devices that can be affected by static electricity, although newer models are not as vulnerable to electrostatic discharge (ESD) as are older models. However, when ESD occurs, some cochlear implants are susceptible to damage to the speech processor program (Cochlear Americas, 2002). Static electricity reducers, including antistatic mats and screens for computers, wooden chairs substituted for plastic chairs, humidity control to decrease the possibility of static electricity buildup, and antistatic spray for carpets, mats, and other static-causing materials can be added to the child's IEP.

Modified Homework

Some students require too much time to complete homework assignments because of language, learning, or motor deficits. Modifying homework assignments is a means of eliminating repetitive, rote problems, such as computational examples in math. Extended time for long-term assignments may also be helpful.

An extra set of books at home can be used to preview the next week's assignments in terms of vocabulary and concepts. These help the child with hearing loss and enhance reading skills for all children in class.

Copies of class notes or study guides can be used before or during class, as well as for follow-up during TOD sessions or at home. For older elementary students and secondary students, teachers' notes and study guides are extremely beneficial.

Test Accommodations

Students take tests throughout their school years. These exams may take the form of standardized state tests, schoolwide exams, or tests in school subjects. For youngsters who are deaf or hard of hearing, accommodations are necessary to give them an equal opportunity to demonstrate acquired knowledge and skills (Johnson & Seaton, 2012). The right of students with disabilities to appropriate test access and accommodations is also guaranteed under federal laws and regulations. Test accommodations must be listed on the IEP to be in effect. It is important that these test accommodations be carefully addressed at the IEP meeting for the following year, so that students are guaranteed their accommodation needs as soon as classes begin. Accommodations may include extended test-taking time (up to double time) to allow the student time to process information; administering state assessments over multiple days with state approval; taking tests in separate locations or in a small groups to permit children to get more assistance; special acoustics to be certain the child can hear all directions; reading directions, test passages, questions, items, and multiple-choice responses aloud to the student who is deaf or hard of hearing when that student has difficulty reading for himself.

Note-Taking Systems

There are various note-taking systems for students with hearing loss. A scribe or other adult may be needed for young students who have difficulty writing because of motor issues. A computer-assisted system can help students with hearing loss in the mainstream, allowing the student to take detailed information home (Youdelman & Messerly, 1996).

Computer-Assisted Real Time Translation (CART) is the instant translation of the spoken word into English text using a stenotype machine, a notebook computer, and real-time software. A court reporter types what is said, and the text appears on a computer monitor, TV, or projection screen (National Court Reporters Association [NCRA], 2011). CART is found in upper elementary, middle, and high schools, as well as in colleges and graduate programs.

A remote CART system is similar to CART, except the reporter is off site. The teacher wears a microphone that transmits information directly to the reporter. However, student comments and class discussion will be missed, unless the teacher repeats it all.

C-Print is another computer note-taking system. A trained operator produces text of spoken information in text-condensing strategies. The information may be a summarized translation of the content (National Technical Institute for the Deaf [NTID], 2003).

CAN (Computer Assisted Note Taking) uses two laptop computers. A professional note taker or good typist inputs all classroom interactions, which are transmitted to the student's laptop.

A student note taker who volunteers or is chosen by the teacher can provide notes for the student who is deaf or hard of hearing. Quality note taking is important.

> **Pearl**
>
> • Children with hearing loss have a much easier time in the classroom with appropriate access. Computer note-taking systems work effectively in schools and have given children a better sense of participation.

Anderson and Matkin (2007) have developed a table (**Table 29.1**) describing the possible impact of different degrees of hearing loss on understanding speech and language, social skills and needs, and required educational accommodations. It is a very useful document for all school personnel to use to assist in understanding the effect of hearing loss and to know what services might be needed. It is also very useful for audiologists, speech-language pathologists, and educators in clinical settings when making school recommendations, and for parents, to assist them in knowing what to request at IEP meetings. It offers an excellent summary of required services.

◆ Summary

The movement toward mainstreaming students who are deaf or hard of hearing is evolving. Because of advances in early identification, improved technology, and new legislation, mainstreaming is becoming the choice of many parents and their school districts.

Youngsters who have attended school in the mainstream have reported that using FM systems, advocating for their own needs, being responsible for their learning, and using communication aids in the classroom were of prime importance to a successful outcome. For children to succeed, schools need to have a team approach to learning, including having a TOD, who is the most important provider for students who are deaf or hard of hearing. For many school districts, finding quality service providers is the key to the child's positive educational outcome. TODs, speech-language pathologists, educational audiologists, and mainstream staff must receive ongoing training through conferences, workshops, and networking to maximize the success of the child who is deaf or hard of hearing. Having mainstream teachers who are sensitive to the academic, social, and emotional needs of the child with hearing loss will also make a difference. Willingness on the part of the school administration and staff, as well as creative thinking by everyone, can help provide a positive outcome. Parents need to remain actively involved in their children's educational experience while continuing to advocate for them (Eriks-Brophy, Durieux-Smith, Olds, Fitzpatrick, Duquette, & Whittingham, 2006).

It is important to recognize the positive social and emotional outcomes of listening and spoken language success, and of the ability to hear optimally with amplification and to speak intelligibly. With changes in technology, hearing loss has become a more subtle disorder. A student who is deaf or hard of hearing may be the only such student in a school, and social isolation may be a concern (Luterman, 2006). Creating ways of helping schools to encourage greater inclusion within the mainstream will need to be addressed.

Although mainstreaming is the trend today, schools and programs for children who are deaf is still an option for families whose children require a more restrictive environment, for families who culturally make that choice, and for families who desire a greater peer affiliation for their children.

As educational options increase, parents have multiple choices for their children with hearing loss. With the right support within the chosen school placement, students have the opportunity for a happy, productive, and successful educational experience.

Table 29.1 Relationship of hearing loss to listening and learning needs

16–25 dB hearing loss

Possible impact on the understanding of language and speech	Possible social impact	Potential educational accommodations and services
• Impact of a hearing loss that is ~ 20 dB can be compared with ability to hear when index fingers are placed in your ears. Child may have difficulty hearing faint or distant speech. • At 16 dB, student can miss up to 10% of speech signal when teacher is at a distance greater than 3 feet. • A 20 dB or greater hearing loss in the better ear can result in absent, inconsistent or distorted parts of speech, especially word endings (-s, -ed), and unemphasized sounds. • Percent of speech signal missed will be greater whenever there is background noise in the classroom, especially in the elementary grades, when instruction is primarily verbal and younger children have greater difficulty listening in noise. • Young children have the tendency to watch and copy the movements of other students rather than attending to auditorally fragmented teacher directions.	• May be unaware of subtle conversational cues, which could cause him to be viewed as inappropriate or awkward. • May miss portions of fast-paced peer interactions that could begin to have an impact on socialization and self-concept. • Behavior may be mistaken for immaturity or inattention. • May be more fatigued because of extra effort needed for understanding speech.	• Noise in typical classroom environments impedes child from having full access to teacher instruction. • Will benefit from improved acoustic treatment of classroom and soundfield amplification. • Favorable seating necessary. • May often have difficulty with sound and letter associations and subtle auditory discrimination skills necessary for reading. • May need attention to vocabulary or speech, especially when there has been a long history of middle ear fluid. • Depending on loss configuration, may benefit from low-power hearing aid with personal FM system. • Appropriate medical management necessary for conductive losses. • In-service on impact of "minimal" 15–25 dB hearing loss on language development, listening in noise, and learning required for teacher.

26–40 dB hearing loss

Possible impact on the understanding of language and speech	Possible social impact	Potential educational accommodations and services
• Effect of a hearing loss of ~ 20 dB can be compared with ability to hear when index fingers are placed in ears; therefore, a 26–40 dB hearing loss causes greater listening difficulties than a "plugged ear" loss. Child can "hear" but misses fragments of speech, leading to misunderstanding. Degree of difficulty experienced in school will depend upon noise level in the classroom, distance from the teacher, and configuration of the hearing loss, even with hearing aids. • At 30 dB, can miss 25–40% of the speech signal; at 40 dB may miss 50% of class discussion, especially when voices are faint or speaker is not in line of vision. Will miss unemphasized words and consonants, especially when he has high-frequency hearing loss. Often experiences difficulty learning early reading skills, such as letter and sound associations. Child's ability to understand and succeed in the classroom will be substantially diminished by speaker distance and background noise, especially in the elementary grades.	• Barriers begin to build with negative impact on self-esteem as child is accused of "hearing when he wants to," "daydreaming," or "not paying attention." • May believe he is less capable because of difficulties understanding in class. • Child begins to lose ability for selective listening and has increasing difficulty suppressing background noise, causing the learning environment to be more stressful. • Child is more fatigued from effort needed to listen.	• Noise in typical class will impede child from full access to teacher instruction. Will benefit from hearing aids and use of a desktop or ear-level FM system in the classroom. • Needs favorable acoustics, seating, and lighting. • May need attention to auditory skills, speech, language development, speech reading, and support in reading and self-esteem. Amount of attention needed typically related to the degree of success of intervention before 6 months of age to prevent language and early learning delays. • Teacher in-service training on impact of so-called "mild" hearing loss on listening and learning to convey that it is often greater than expected.

Table 29.1 *(Continued)* Relationship of hearing loss to listening and learning needs

41–55 dB hearing loss

Possible impact on the understanding of language and speech	Possible social impact	Potential educational accommodations and services
• Consistent use of amplification and language intervention before age 6 months increases the probability that the child's speech, language, and learning will develop at a normal rate. • Without amplification, child understands conversation at a distance of 3–5 feet, if sentence structure and vocabulary are known. • The amount of speech signal missed can be 50% or more with 40 dB loss, and 80% or more with 50 dB loss. • Without early amplification the child is likely to have delayed or disordered syntax, limited vocabulary, imperfect speech production, and flat voice quality. • Addition of a visual communication system to supplement audition may be indicated, especially if language delays and/or additional disabilities are present. • Even with hearing aids, child can "hear" but may miss much of what is said if classroom is noisy or reverberant. With personal hearing aids alone, ability to perceive speech and learn effectively in the classroom is at high risk. • A personal FM system to overcome classroom noise and distance is typically necessary.	• Barriers build with negative impact on self-esteem as child is accused of "hearing when he wants to," "daydreaming," or "not paying attention." • Communication will be significantly compromised with this degree of hearing loss if hearing aids are not worn. • Socialization with peers can be difficult, especially in noisy settings, such as cooperative learning situations, lunch, or recess. • May be more fatigued than classmates for effort needed to listen.	• Consistent use of amplification (hearing aids + FM) is essential. • Needs favorable classroom acoustics, seating, and lighting. • Consultation/program supervision by a specialist in childhood hearing impairment to coordinate services is important. • Depending on intervention success in preventing language delays, special academic support necessary if language and academic delays are present. • Attention to growth of oral communication, reading, written language skills, auditory skill development, speech therapy, self-esteem likely. • Teacher in-service training required, with attention to communication access and peer acceptance.

56–70 dB hearing loss

Possible impact on the understanding of language and speech	Possible social impact	Potential educational accommodations and services
• Even with hearing aids, child will typically be aware of people talking around him but will miss parts of words said, resulting in difficulty in situations requiring verbal communication (both one-to-one and in groups). • Without amplification, conversation must be very loud to be understood; a 55 dB loss can cause a child to miss up to 100% of speech information without functioning amplification. • If hearing loss is not identified before 1 year of age and appropriately managed, delayed spoken language, syntax, reduced speech intelligibility, and flat voice quality are likely. • Age when first amplified, consistency of hearing aid use, and success of early language intervention strongly tied to speech, language, and learning development. • Addition of visual communication system often indicated if language delays or additional disabilities are present. • Use of a personal FM system will reduce the effects of noise and distance and allow increased auditory access to verbal instruction. • With hearing aids alone, ability to understand in the classroom is greatly reduced by distance and noise.	• If hearing loss was identified late and language delay was not prevented, communication interaction with peers will be significantly affected. • Child will have greater difficulty socializing, especially in noisy settings, such as lunch, cooperative learning situations, or recess. • Tendency for poorer self-concept and social immaturity may contribute to a sense of rejection; peer in-service training helpful.	• Full-time, consistent use of amplification (hearing aids + FM system) is essential. • May benefit from frequency transposition (frequency compression) hearing aids depending upon loss configuration. • May require intense support in development of auditory, language, speech, reading, and writing skills. • Consultation and supervision by a specialist in childhood hearing impairment to coordinate services is important. • Use of sign language or a visual communication system by child with substantial language delays or additional learning needs may be useful to access linguistically complex instruction. • Note taking, captioned films, and other accommodations often needed. • Requires teacher in-service training.

(Continued on page 330)

Table 29.1 *(Continued)* Relationship of hearing loss to listening and learning needs

71–90 dB and 91+ dB hearing loss

Possible impact on the understanding of language and speech	Possible social impact	Potential educational accommodations and services
• The earlier the child wears amplification consistently, with concentrated efforts by parents and caregivers to provide rich language opportunities throughout everyday activities or provision of intensive language intervention (sign or verbal), the greater the probability that speech, language, and learning will develop at a relatively normal rate. • Without amplification, children with 71–90 dB hearing loss may hear loud noises only about 1 foot from ear. • When amplified optimally, children with hearing ability of 90 dB or better should detect many sounds of speech if presented from close distance or via FM. • Individual ability and intensive intervention prior to 6 months of age will determine the degree that sounds detected will be discriminated and understood by the brain into meaningful input. • Even with hearing aids, children with 71–90 dB loss are typically unable to perceive all high-pitched speech sounds sufficiently to discriminate them or benefit from incidental listening, especially without the use of FM. • The child with hearing loss > 70 dB may be a candidate for cochlear implants, and the child with hearing loss > 90 dB will not be able to perceive most speech sounds with traditional hearing aids. • For full access to language to be available visually through sign language or cued speech, family members must be involved in child's communication mode from a very young age.	• Depending on success of intervention in infancy to address language development, the child's communication may be minimally or significantly affected. • Socialization with hearing peers may be difficult. • Children in general education classrooms may develop greater dependence on adults because of difficulty perceiving or comprehending oral communication. • Children may be more comfortable interacting with peers who are deaf or hard of hearing due to ease of communication. • Relationships with peers and adults who have hearing loss can make positive contributions toward the development of a healthy self-concept and a sense of cultural identity.	• There is no one communication system that is right for all hard of hearing or deaf children and their families. • Whether a visual communication approach or auditory/oral approach is used, extensive language intervention, full-time consistent amplification use, and constant integration of the communication practices into the family by 6 months of age will highly increase the probability that the child will become a successful learner. • Children with late-identified hearing loss (after 6 months of age) will have delayed language. This language gap is difficult to overcome, and the educational program of a child with hearing loss, especially those with language and learning delays secondary to hearing loss, requires the involvement of a consultant or teacher with expertise in teaching children with hearing loss. • Depending on the configuration of the hearing loss and individual speech perception ability, frequency transposition (frequency compression) aids or cochlear implantation may be options for better access to speech. • If an auditory/oral approach is used, early training is needed on auditory skills, spoken language, concept development, and speech. • If culturally deaf emphasis is selected, frequent exposure to deaf, American Sign Language users is important. • Educational placement with other signing deaf or hard of hearing students (special school or classes) may be a more appropriate option to access a language-rich environment and free-flowing communication. • Support services and continual appraisal of access to communication and verbal instruction are required. • Note-taking, captioning, captioned films, and other visual enhancement strategies are necessary. • Training in pragmatic language use and communication repair strategies helpful. In-service training of general education teachers is essential.

Table 29.1 *(Continued)* Relationship of hearing loss to listening and learning needs

Unilateral hearing loss

Possible impact on the understanding of language and speech	Possible social impact	Potential educational accommodations and services
• Child can "hear" but can have difficulty understanding in certain situations, such as hearing faint or distant speech, especially if poor ear is aimed toward the person speaking. • Will typically have difficulty localizing sounds and voices using hearing alone. • The unilateral listener will have greater difficulty understanding speech when environment is noisy or reverberant, especially when normal ear is toward the overhead projector or other competing sound source and poor-hearing ear is toward the teacher. • Exhibits difficulty detecting or understanding soft speech from the side of the poor-hearing ear, especially in a group discussion.	• Child may be accused of selective hearing because of discrepancies in speech understanding in quiet versus noise. • Social problems may arise as child experiences difficulty understanding in noisy cooperative learning or recess situations. • May misconstrue peer conversations and feel rejected or ridiculed. • Child may be more fatigued in classroom from greater effort needed to listen, if class is noisy or has poor acoustics. • May appear inattentive, distractible, or frustrated, with behavior or social problems sometimes evident.	• Allow child to change seat locations to direct the normal-hearing ear toward the primary speaker. • Student is at 10 times the risk for educational difficulties compared to children with two normal-hearing ears, and one-third to one-half of students with unilateral hearing loss experience significant learning problems. • Children often have difficulty learning sound and letter associations in typically noisy kindergarten and first-grade settings. • Educational and audiologic monitoring is warranted. • Teacher in-service training is beneficial. • Typically, the child will benefit from a personal FM system with low gain/power or a soundfield FM system in the classroom, especially in the lower grades. • Depending on the hearing loss, the child may benefit from a hearing aid in the impaired ear.

Mid-frequency hearing loss or reverse slope hearing loss

Possible impact on the understanding of language and speech	Possible social impact	Potential educational accommodations and services
• Child can "hear" whenever speech is present, but will have difficulty understanding faint or distant speech, such as a student with a quiet voice speaking from across the classroom. • The "cookie bite" or reverse slope listener will have greater difficulty understanding speech when environment is noisy or reverberant, such as a typical classroom setting. • A 25–40 dB degree of loss in the low- to mid-frequency range may cause the child to miss ~ 30% of speech information, if unamplified; some consonant and vowel sounds may be heard inconsistently, especially when background noise is present. Speech production of these sounds may be affected.	• Child may be accused of selective hearing or "hearing when he wants to" because of discrepancies in speech understanding in quiet versus noise. • Social problems may arise as child experiences difficulty understanding in noisy cooperative learning situations, lunch, or recess. • May misconstrue peer conversations, believing that other children are talking about him. • Child may be more fatigued in classroom setting due to greater effort needed to listen. • May appear inattentive, distracted, or frustrated.	• Personal hearing aids are important, but must be precisely fitted to hearing loss. • Child likely to benefit from a soundfield FM system, a personal FM system, or assistive listening device in the classroom. • Student is at risk for educational difficulties. Can experience some difficulty learning sound and letter associations in kindergarten and first-grade classes. • Depending on the degree and configuration of loss, child may experience delayed language development and articulation problems. • Educational monitoring and teacher in-service training warranted. • Annual hearing evaluation to monitor for hearing loss progression is important.

(Continued on page 332)

Chapter 30

Education and Access Laws for Children with Hearing Loss

Donna L. Sorkin

Key Points

- Underlying a child's or adult's eligibility for services under U.S. laws is the need to demonstrate a disability that limits one or more major life activities.

- U.S. disability laws support the provision of services needed to enable children and adults to attend school, live, and work in the mainstream with full access to telecommunications; communication access; and other services that support their needs as people with hearing loss.

- Passage of laws does not guarantee access to needed services. Children with hearing loss should be involved in the individualized education plan (IEP) and all discussions of their needs from a young age, so that they can develop the knowledge and skills that they will need to be their own best advocates.

Many parents still experience periodic frustrations when seeking services and appropriate placement options, but overall, families can expect that their children who are deaf or hard of hearing will attend a neighborhood school with their hearing peers and with needed services, go to college with full communication opportunities, enter the workforce supported by whatever accommodations they require, and enjoy meaningful access to a wide range of telecommunications products and services. In the past 30 years there has been a dramatic expansion in the application of federal laws to address the needs of people with disabilities. Children and young adults with hearing loss have benefited from such legislation in diverse and important ways.

We have now moved from an environment in which a child with a significant hearing loss could expect to work in a "deaf" trade (such as typesetting) and spend her life in the deaf community, to a largely open society in which a young person who is motivated and has received appropriate services and support can pursue whatever academic and professional career she chooses, regardless of her level of hearing loss or communication modality. Not long ago, those of us who were deaf relied on telecommunications relay volunteers to call our family members or our business associates. I still vividly remember waiting my turn for a volunteer relay assistant to become available to help me make a telephone call so I could speak to a client. If I happened to find someone who could type quickly without too many errors, I proceeded to make all the calls I needed to make that day in nonstop fashion.

Our perspective now in the United States and in many parts of the world is that services and support should be available to provide full access for a child with hearing loss. The scope of our national disability laws has been broadened to require freedom from discrimination as a result of a disability; full use of available technologies like cell phones and broadcast and cable television; appropriate services and support for families during early intervention and for school-aged children at school; consideration of workplace needs; and communication access in public places, such as theaters, museums, and transportation facilities. By and large, the laws are in place. Still, passage of laws is one thing; ensuring that a child or a young adult has what she is entitled to is another matter entirely.

This chapter is designed to provide the information needed to undertake three important tasks as an audiologist: (1) mentor and coach a family and child to become advocates for the needs of a child with hearing loss; (2) become familiar enough with the laws to help families know what they are entitled to under our legal system; and (3) point them to additional resources—beyond what you can realistically offer—that they can tap into now and as the child ages and her needs progress. With regard to the last task—as with all children—just when we think we have the hang of parenting, our children enter a new phase of their lives and parents are forced to adjust to a whole new set of challenges. Children with hearing loss are no different in this regard. For that reason, it is important to provide families and patients with resources and skills that will aid them over the long term.

◆ The Concept of Disability

Patients today will grow up in a society that views disability very differently than was the case in our country 50 or even 25 years ago. Our new model for disability has been evolving for some time now, but the new thinking is that there is no pity or shame in having a disability. Rather, the stereotyping and fears about disability, and ultimately the discrimination that occurs because of a lack of access to services, are the real problems. We have moved away from trying to hide the fact that someone cannot hear or see. We encourage people to be open about their disabilities and instead focus on what they need to fully participate (Sorkin, 2004a).

A public example of the way this new perspective has played out involves President Franklin Delano Roosevelt (FDR). Roosevelt contracted polio as a young man, before being elected governor of New York, and never walked again after his illness. Although it was widely known that he had difficulty moving about because of the paralysis, the fact that he used a wheelchair and could not walk was little known by the average American. He was never photographed in his wheelchair, and on those occasions when he appeared in public, he wore painful leg braces and was assisted by others when he walked. None of this was publicly discussed until well after his death because of the stigma associated with being confined to a wheelchair and having a significant disability.

In 1997, a national memorial honoring FDR was completed in Washington, DC. The initial design gave no hint that Franklin Roosevelt used a wheelchair. The larger-than-life statue of President Roosevelt at the memorial site (**Fig. 30.1**) shows him seated, with a cape draped over his legs, in such a way that his wheelchair is entirely hidden. Disability advocates were furious that a memorial of this magnitude on the national mall in Washington, D.C. purposely concealed the fact that Roosevelt used a wheelchair. They felt it was a continuation of past practices in which society hid people with disabilities or, in this case, intentionally veiled the fact that a powerful and charismatic person was not able-bodied. Disability organizations successfully argued that an additional statue be added to the memorial, a statue that shows FDR in his wheelchair. Although his disability was never revealed to the public during his lifetime, advocates stated that if he were alive today, Roosevelt would have wanted the public to know that he served as president of the United States—the most

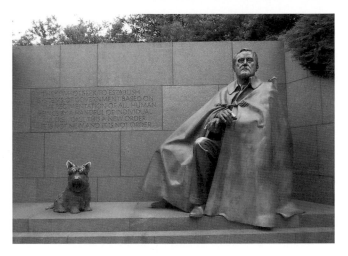

Fig. 30.1 The initial statue of President Franklin Delano Roosevelt at the FDR Memorial in Washington, DC conceals the fact that he was seated in a wheelchair. (Photo by Donna Sorkin.)

powerful position in the world—with a significant disability (Sorkin, 2004b). Another statue of FDR in his wheelchair (**Fig. 30.2**) was added in 2000 to coincide with the 10th anniversary celebration of the passage of the Americans with Disabilities Act and was formally dedicated by President Bill Clinton.

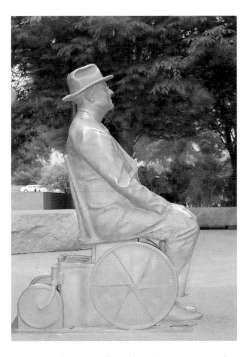

Fig. 30.2 Several years after the FDR Memorial opened, a second statue was added that clearly shows President Roosevelt in his wheelchair. Although no such photographs were published of FDR during his lifetime, 50 years after his death public perspectives dictated a more open approach to his disability. (Photo by Donna Sorkin.)

That viewpoint provides the basis for our federal laws that require nondiscrimination and access. For an individual to be eligible for coverage under most U.S. laws that provide services or accessibility for a child or an adult with hearing loss, the individual must demonstrate a known disability. For example, under the Americans with Disabilities Act (ADA), the definition of disability was construed broadly to include anyone who has a physical or mental impairment that substantially affects one or more major life activities. Hearing loss is considered to be one of these impairments (U.S. Department of Justice, 2006).

But what if assistive technology so improves the individual's condition that he is no longer limited in life activities? There have been several Supreme Court cases in which the definition of an individual with a disability was narrowed. In one case, individuals were denied jobs as commercial airline pilots because they were nearsighted (*Sutton v. American Airlines*, 1999). With eyeglasses, their vision was corrected to 20/20. Those individuals felt that they should have been protected by the ADA because without glasses their vision was a significant limitation. The court ruled in favor of the airline, stating that those individuals had too much sight with corrective glasses to fall within the definition of an individual with a disability to be protected under the ADA.

The *Sutton* decision suggests that an individual who receives substantial benefit from assistive technology such as hearing aids or cochlear implants could also lose the protection (or possibly services) of disability laws if the correction provided by technology provides the equivalent of normal hearing. An audiologist may be asked by families to discuss their child's hearing loss and her need for services. This expertise can be invaluable in demonstrating functional or practical aspects of hearing loss as well as the specific services that a child needs to keep up with her peers. At present, no hearing technology provides the equivalent of normal hearing for a child with hearing loss, so it is important to demonstrate and discuss the impact of a child's hearing loss on listening and learning.

Pearl

- For example, using Hearing in Noise Test (HINT) scores or single words in quiet or noise to demonstrate how much a child is missing may help demonstrate the impact of the hearing loss on her functional performance.

Still another aspect of the issue relates to a reticence by some families to think of their child with a hearing loss as having a disability. Some families so desperately want their child to be normal that they are reluctant to call attention to her hearing loss and consequently do not pursue services, such as a frequency modulation

(FM) system that could help her. Even parents of children with profound hearing loss who use cochlear implants have been known to minimize the impact of the child's deafness and boast that their child does not need services at school. Without delving into the psychological aspect of this kind of thinking and the impact that it could have on the child, it is important to acknowledge and understand that the concept of disability underlies the framework for laws that ensure educational services and accessibility features that allow children and adults to engage in various activities and be included in all of the same opportunities in life as anyone else.

Although the person's disability determines eligibility, our laws in America emphasize the individual's ability and our commitment as a society to provide what is needed to allow inclusion. Within this context, an agency or organization—public or private—is prohibited from discriminating on the basis of a person's disability. It is also expected that organizations will provide reasonable accommodations and services that will make their offerings accessible to children and adults with hearing loss.

Three categories of laws will be covered in this chapter:

- Education
- Telecommunications
- General access in public places and in the workplace

There is some overlap between these categories. For example, some laws that primarily concern general access can be applied to educational settings for children who do not qualify for coverage under the Individuals with Disabilities Education Act (IDEA), and there are general access laws (such as the ADA) that have telecommunications components.

◆ Education Laws

The Individuals with Disabilities Education Act

IDEA is the primary federal program that requires state and local aid to address the requirements of children with disabilities in educational settings. The legislation was originally passed in 1975 because America's educational system was not meeting the needs of children with disabilities. At the time that IDEA was first signed into law by President Gerald Ford, only one in five children with disabilities attended public school. After passage of IDEA, school attendance and matriculation rates for children with disabilities dramatically increased (U.S. Department of Education, 2006b).

IDEA was most recently updated as the 2004 Reauthorization of the Individuals with Disabilities Education Improvement Act of 2004. The 2004 law maintains the basic structure and civil rights guarantees of the original IDEA law. As with all federal legislation, IDEA was passed by Congress and signed into law by the president. Regulations explaining how the IDEA law is to be implemented by states and local school districts were then developed by the U.S. Department of Education with input from diverse organizations. At this writing in 2012, the most recent regulations were published in the *Federal Register* on August 14, 2006 (U. S. Department of Education, 2006a), and include revised language relating specifically to children with hearing loss. Since IDEA is a funding statute, states and local school districts must follow these procedures to receive federal funds for public education.

An audiologist's expertise is vital to the families he serves in helping to demonstrate the importance of specific and appropriate services for a child who is deaf or hard of hearing. Like most federal programs, IDEA has its share of jargon, and even experienced audiologists can be intimidated by the alphabet soup of acronyms that fills the pages of the regulations. Nonetheless, the audiologist's expertise is in understanding the audiologic needs of patients, and such information is invaluable in helping children receive the early intervention or school-based services they need to excel.

Part B of the Individuals with Disabilities Education Act

Part B of IDEA focuses on school-based services and covers children 3 to 21 years of age. The cornerstone of the law, since its initial passage, has been the concept of a free and appropriate public education (FAPE) that provides for special education and related services that are specifically designed to meet the needs of a child with a disability. The legal intent is to allow children with disabilities full access to an education while addressing their special learning or access needs. The following glossary of terms covering FAPE and other key concepts is intended to help best understand terms within the IDEA framework.

Free and Appropriate Public Education

A free and appropriate public education (FAPE) is to be provided to the child with a disability as described in the IEP (the document that describes how the child's needs will be met). The services to be provided are free. Families cannot be charged if the services are identified in the child's IEP. The word *appropriate* is important and emphasizes that the school district must consider the individual needs of the child.

Individualized Education Plan

The IEP is a written legal document that provides detail on the special education and related services that a child needs to receive an education. The IEP should be developed in a collaborative way between the family and school personnel. It should outline both the child's needs and how his school placement and services will address his unique needs. An IEP should include: (1) the child's current educational performance; (2) goals for the school year and how these goals will be met with specific educational or related services; (3) whether and how the child will participate in regular education programs; and (4) criteria for evaluating the child's progress against the goals. It is very important to have the IEP provisions in writing. Although we generally think of the IEP process as being an annual event, if there is significant change in the child's status (such as undergoing cochlear implant surgery over winter break, or experiencing a decline in hearing, or any occurrence that affects the child's ability to access her educational program), parents can ask for a review of the IEP and this can be done at any time.

Least Restrictive Environment

Least restrictive environment (LRE) emphasizes that the child will be educated, to the extent possible, with children who do not have disabilities. IDEA emphasizes that children should be removed from the regular classroom only to the extent needed to provide special services. LRE requirements, as described in the 2006 regulations, are "a strong preference, not a mandate, for educating children with disabilities alongside their peers without disabilities" (U.S. Department of Education, 2006a).

The LRE concept can be a source of controversy when families and school personnel disagree on what placement is best for the child. There are many instances in which a school district's perspective on LRE for a child is driven by what programs or options are already in place, rather than by what placement would best serve the child. School districts are required by the law to offer a continuum of alternative placements to meet the needs of students, but the reality is that a continuum of placements is not available in some areas of the country.

It is helpful to think of LRE and the continuum of placements as a line along which the student may move according to his needs, usually (though not always) from a more restrictive environment to a lesser one. See **Fig. 30.3** for an example of the continuum of public school placements. One child might best be served by an initial placement in a resource room (or self-contained classroom with other children who are hearing impaired) for most of the day. Over the course of his school career, he might spend less time in the resource room and eventually he might be better served in a mainstream classroom with accommodations for his hearing loss (such as an FM system). Another child might spend his entire public school time in a state school for the deaf. Still another child might be best served by a 100% mainstreamed placement from first

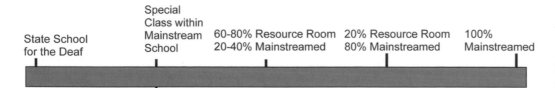

Fig. 30.3 Continuum of public school placements.

grade onward. IDEA requires that the child's needs drive the placement. As the child's hearing care expert, the audiologist has a key role in helping the child and her family work with the school district to ensure she has a placement (and services) that is determined by her unique needs and not a placement that is driven by the too frequently used adage, "This is what we offer."

Mainstreaming

Mainstreaming is sometimes equated with the LRE. It is not the same; rather, mainstreaming is one example of how the LRE concept can be applied (Tucker, 1998). For many families, the goal is eventually to have their children who are deaf or hard of hearing attend school with their normally hearing peers in a mainstream classroom. Other families believe that their children are best served in a classroom with other children with hearing loss. When and whether a child is ready for a mainstream placement should be a function of the child's readiness, both academically and socially. Some school districts discourage mainstream placement because they do not offer itinerant services, so it is difficult to serve children with hearing loss who are not clustered in one location.

Special Education

Schools must design and provide instruction that is specially designed to meet the unique needs of the individual child.

Related Services

These are services that help the child benefit from special education and may include speech and audiology services, physical or occupational therapy, and psychological services. The most recent version of the IDEA regulations specifies that routine checking of hearing aids and cochlear implants is appropriately covered as a related service, although replacement of the cochlear implant device and mapping is not the responsibility of the local school district (U.S. Department of Education, 2006a).

Helping a Family with the Individualized Education Plan

A child's audiologist and the other hearing care professionals who serve her and her family (including the teacher for hearing-impaired children, the speech pathologist, and the auditory-verbal therapist) should provide guidance and documentation to support the development of the IEP. Such materials might include information on the child's communication skills, hearing status, and cognitive abilities; assessment of the listening environment she will be placed in and whether acoustical improvements are needed; assistive technology needs (i.e., hearing aid, cochlear implant, FM system); social and emotional factors; related services required (speech, educational audiologist, listening therapy); communication access needs, such as interpreters, note-taking, or captioning; in-service training for teachers and others, including classmates; and provision for daily troubleshooting of the child's technology (hearing aids, cochlear implant, FM). Keep in mind that the IEP is a binding document, but services will be provided only if they are written into the IEP. If the audiologist feels that the child is ready and would benefit from the mainstream, she has a key role in helping the family demonstrate the child's readiness and to identify and justify those services she needs in the mainstream to learn and to achieve.

> **Pearl**
>
> - As the expert on your patient's hearing needs, you have a key role in supporting the family to ensure everything the child needs is specified clearly in the written IEP document.

Guidance on Individuals with Disabilities Education Act Regulations

The 2004 IDEA Regulations, published in August 2006, highlighted several topics of note to audiologists. Several legal decisions would have required school districts to provide mapping or programming services for children with cochlear implants as an audiology service. The 2004 Regulations make it clear that schools are not responsible for "post-surgical maintenance, programming, or replacement of the medical device" (U.S. Department of Education, 2006a). The school responsibilities for hearing aids and cochlear implant processors are similar in that schools are required to ensure that hearing aids and external components of surgically implanted medical devices are functioning properly, which includes routine troubleshooting, and assistive technology, such as FM systems, are provided when needed and are maintained.

There has been some question as to whether a student may use school-purchased assistive technology, such as an FM system, at home or in other settings outside of school. The new regulations state that the child's team may approve such use if it is needed to receive FAPE. Children often do have learning opportunities outside of school, so parents could argue that the FM system is needed to access spoken language in those settings.

In the new regulations, interpreting services are identified as a related service. The definition of interpreting services has been expanded to include various forms of captioning and note-taking. Additionally, all of the various types of interpreting are covered, including cued speech, oral transliteration, and sign language interpreting.

Part C of the Individuals with Disabilities Education Act

Part C of IDEA addresses early intervention (EI) services for children up to 3 years. This part of IDEA provides grants to states to develop early intervention programs for infants and toddlers if they have developmental delays or have a diagnosed condition that could impact the child's development. Children with hearing loss often experience language delays and are usually eligible for services under Part C. Unlike Part B, early intervention services are coordinated by a designated state agency, which controls the implementation and provision of services at the local level. The state agency varies by state and may be the state school for the deaf, social services, health department, or a special early intervention agency.

Individualized Family Service Plan

Part C services are provided through the Individualized Family Service Plan (IFSP), which addresses the needs of the child and family members, rather than just the child, as is the case with Part B. IFSP services vary by state and might include

- Speech-language pathology and audiology services
- Auditory therapy by a certified auditory-verbal therapist or by someone who is not certified
- Home-based deaf education services
- Family training, counseling, and home visits
- Occupational or physical therapy
- Hearing aids or FM systems
- Psychology or social work services
- Sign language instruction for the child and family
- Information about, and exposure to, Deaf Culture
- Service coordination
- Transportation

A key role of early intervention professionals in any of these functions is to train the family in how to encourage language development in their child who experiences hearing loss. Since many families are new to hearing loss, and because young children are likely to develop language as part of their family interactions, communication is an appropriate emphasis.

As part of the IFSP, a family will be assigned a service coordinator who will help the family obtain services as a function of the child's needs, the state's offerings, and the resources allocated by the state for early intervention. As the child's audiologist, you have a key role in helping the family and the service coordinator determine services and providers that will address the child's hearing loss, the family's preferences as to the child's language modality, family goals, and any other special needs that the child may have. About 40% of children with hearing loss have an additional disorder (Perigoe & Perigoe, 2005). These other issues can affect a child's ability to develop language and should be considered along with hearing loss.

One final word about the early intervention process is in order. Given that most families will be new to hearing loss and that they are starting on a long journey with their children, it is important that professionals recognize from the start the importance of helping parents develop the skills they will need to negotiate the early intervention (and later the school system) as well as the medical and psychosocial aspects of raising a child who is deaf or hard of hearing. IDEA recognizes that parents have the right to make key choices for their children. Some states have recognized the need to provide encouragement by establishing parent mentoring programs, such as Wisconsin's Guide by Your Side, which is also offered by the parent organization Hands and Voices (Hands and Voices, 2006). If the state early intervention (EI) agency does not provide such mentors for parents, they should be encouraged to do so.

Pearl

- You might also assist parents by establishing your own informal mentor network, linking parents of newly identified children with more experienced families.

No Child Left Behind Act of 2001

IDEA focuses on providing access to an educational program; No Child Left Behind (NCLB) spotlights academic achievement. The law holds schools accountable for ensuring that all students, including those with disabilities, meet specific standards. NCLB highlights the responsibility of states, school districts, and individual schools to target resources to improve the achievement of students with disabilities and to monitor closely the quality and impact of services provided under IDEA.

In the past, students with disabilities were often excluded from assessments and accountability systems. NCLB is a useful mechanism to further highlight and address the needs of pediatric patients in those instances in which the audiologist, other service providers, or the family feels that the child's IEP is not sufficiently providing quality services that allow her to meet the same high standards as her peers. The law authorized new federal monies to states and districts for activities designed to strengthen teacher quality in areas like reading, math, science, and English fluency. The extra support and attention that can be applied due to NCLB can translate into greater emphasis on gaining a high level of performance for students with hearing loss.

Section 504 of the Rehabilitation Act and the Americans with Disabilities Act

Section 504 mandates that all entities receiving federal funds must not discriminate and must offer services that provide access to their programs. Since all public schools and most colleges and universities receive federal funds, they are subject to the requirements of Section 504. Some children with hearing loss who are performing at grade level have been categorized by their school districts as not having an educationally significant hearing loss and thus are not eligible for an IEP. If this is the case, Section 504 can be used to provide related services, such as FM systems, interpreters, and captioning.

Colleges and universities (receiving federal funds) are not required to modify their academic programs for students with disabilities substantially, but under Section 504 they are required to make adjustments that will allow equal opportunity. For example, an art course might be substituted for music or a student may need to be provided with more time to complete academic requirements than is customary. The college student will not have an IEP team to help her, so she must request and work out such adjustments that allow her access to her college program.

The ADA can be applied similarly because the ADA requires that programs open to the public be communications accessible. The ADA's Title III (Public Facilities) applies to public schools (K-12) as well as to college and universities, regardless of whether or not they receive federal funding.

A summary of provisions of IDEA and the three other laws covered in this section is provided in **Table 30.1**.

◆ Telecommunication Laws

Before the telecommunications revolution, a lack of telephone access was one of the most limiting aspects of having a hearing loss. I can clearly remember what it was like before the ready availability of all of the telecommunications options we now have, including landline and wireless telephones with volume control and telecoil compatibility, telecommunications relay services provided by state agencies (rather than volunteers), email and instant messaging, and captioned television and video programming. This set of services has made an extraordinary difference in the lives of young people who are deaf or hard of hearing, regardless of their level of hearing loss or mode of communication. A child with a hearing loss today will make heavy use of text messaging and email, putting her on a par with her hearing peers who are using the same technology.

A bit of history is in order as we review the framework for today's telecommunications laws. Ironically, the telephone was invented by Alexander Graham Bell, a teacher of the deaf, in part because of his abiding concern about augmenting communication opportunities for people who are deaf and his related interest in acoustics. Bell's mother and wife Mabel were both hard of hearing. He was interested in teletype machines as a mechanism for providing reliable messaging options for people with hearing loss, an interest that eventually led to his invention of the telephone. How ironic that his discovery actually produced extraordinary frustration and isolation for people with hearing loss for nearly a century, until relatively recent federal legislation mandated that telephone equipment and services provide access for people with hearing loss.

Hearing Aid Compatibility Act

Wireline Telephones

The Hearing Aid Compatibility (HAC) Act of 1988 required that all wireline and cordless (not wireless) telephones manufactured after 1989 incorporate the ability to connect internally with the telecoil in hearing aids. (Wireless telephones were originally exempt from the HAC rules; see below for the 2003 rules, which later were expanded to include wireless.) A negotiated rulemaking completed in 1996 added the requirement that all wireline and cordless phones manufactured after 1998 also provide volume control with minimum gain of 12 dB and additional boost options up to 18 dB; there is also an option to provide even more gain if the phone has an automatic reset mechanism. The rulemaking also

Table 30.1 Laws pertaining to education for children with hearing loss

Education laws	Coverage	Relevant federal agency	Web resources
IDEA Public Law 108-446	This is the primary federal law addressing the educational needs of children with disabilities. It requires that states and local school districts provide free and appropriate early intervention and educational services that address the child's specific needs.	Department of Education	
Part B	This part focuses on school-based services and covers children 3 to 21 years of age.	Department of Education	http://www.ed.gov/legislation/FedRegister/finrule/2006-3/081406a.pdf http://www.ed.gov/policy/speced/guid/idea/modelform-iep.pdf
Part C	Part C of IDEA addresses EI services for children up to 3 years. It provides grants to states to develop EI programs for young children who have a diagnosed condition that could impact on the child's development.	Department of Education	http://www.nectac.org/idea/idea.asp
NCLB, 2001	By focusing on academic achievement, this law's intent is to hold schools accountable for ensuring that all students—including those with disabilities—meet specific standards. IDEA focuses on access to the child's educational program, whereas NCLB provides a mechanism for monitoring the quality and impact of services provided under IDEA.	Department of Education	http://www.ed.gov/policy/el-sec/guid/edpicks.jhtml?src=fp htttp://www.whitehouse.gov/news/releases/2002/01/20020108.html
Section 504 of the Rehabilitation Act	For children who do not qualify for special education services under IDEA, Section 504 can be utilized to provide related services, such as FM systems or captioning. See "General Access" below on other § 504 elements.	Relevant Federal Agency	www.usdoj.gov/crt/ada/cguide.htm#anchor 65610 www.section508.gov/index.cfm?FuseAction=Content&ID=15
ADA, Title II (public schools) and Title III (private schools)	ADA can be applied in similar fashion to § 504. Private schools and higher education institutions are required to make their programs communications accessible.	Access Board (guidelines) Department of Justice (enforcement)	See "General Access"

Abbreviations: ADA, Americans with Disabilities Act; EI, early intervention; FM. Frequency modulation; IDEA, Individuals with Disabilities Education Act; NCLB, No Child Left Behind Act.

specified public locations where wireline phones were required to be HAC. These include

- The workplace
- Hospitals and residential health care facilities
- Coin-operated and credit-card–operated telephones
- Emergency telephones (i.e., elevators, tunnels, highways)
- Hotel rooms

Having this requirement in place has greatly expanded the likelihood that people using hearing technology will have the telephones they need when they are in various familiar or unfamiliar environments.

There are large variations in how well various telephones work for different individuals. In a setting such as a hotel room or a phone at rest stop on the high-

way, where one does not expect to be using a given telephone again, one does the best one can. But if the setting is one's regular workplace (where one will be relying on a particular piece of equipment regularly) and the individual finds that the phone does not work well, she should take the initiative to request that her employer work with her to find equipment that provides acceptable access. Individuals of all ages should be encouraged to advocate for themselves and search for other telephones if one particular technology does not work well for them.

Wireless Telephones

The first wireless telephones were analog and did not create major accessibility problems for people using hearing technology, although few (if any) of these first wireless phones were HAC (i.e., included a method internally to connect with a telecoil). When Congress passed HAC 1989, it exempted wireless telephones, though it left the door open for inclusion of some phones in the future if specific criteria were met (i.e., if removing the exemption was in the public interest).

In 1995, a new type of digital wireless telephone technology began appearing in the United States, some years after its introduction in Europe and other parts of the world. The reported experiences of hearing aid wearers in those regions where digital wireless phones were being used were not promising. Before long, digital wireless technology took the country by storm. Advocates for people with hearing loss quickly realized that this was a significant problem that needed to be addressed within the federal regulatory framework. As a result of ongoing advocacy by consumers and their organizations over a period of almost 10 years, the Federal Communications Commission (FCC) eventually did agree to lift the wireless exemption for hearing aids under HAC. The FCC established technical standards set forth in the American National Standards Institute (ANSI) Standard C63.19. The FCC further required that each manufacturer or mobile service provider offer at least two digital wireless handset models that meet a specific interference standard by September 16, 2005, and that at least 50% of their offerings comply with the standard by February 18, 2008. Additionally, each manufacturer or service provider was required to offer at least two models that met the standard for inductive coupling (with the telecoil of a hearing aid) by September 18, 2006 (Federal Communications Commission [FCC], 2003a, 2003b).

In providing guidance to patients, it is helpful to explain and reference the ratings that telephone handset manufacturers are required to include with the written materials about their products in stores and on their Web sites. Handsets that receive a compatibility rating of M3 or M4 have met (M3) or surpassed (M4) the ANSI compatibility standard for hearing aids set in microphone mode, as adopted by FCC. The higher the M-rating, the higher the signal quality (and the lower the interference level) the handset will have. Handsets that receive a telecoil rating of T3 or T4 have met (T3) or surpassed (T4) the required standard as adopted by the FCC. The higher T4 rating will generally provide a better result for the user.

Although this rating scheme was specifically developed for hearing aid users, because it is a measure of radiofrequency interference, it is also appropriate as a guide for cochlear implant or bone-anchored implant users. Patients should be advised to use these ratings to assist in their selection of telephone models, but always to test a telephone before buying, because what works for one person may not work for another.

Telecommunications Act of 1996

Section 255

Section 255 of the Act required that telecommunications products and services be accessible to, and usable by, people with disabilities, if readily achievable to do so. The law covers wide-ranging products and services, including telephones (wireline, cordless, wireless); answering machines; pagers; and services such as call waiting, voice mail, and interactive voice response systems, that have implications for people with hearing loss. The legislation was important in that it brought attention to the importance of thinking about the diverse needs of people with disabilities as part of the design of new products, a concept known as universal design.

Pearl

- The universal design paradigm will be important to children of today as new products that have not been offered before are conceptualized and developed for our use.

There is some overlap between the Telecommunications Act and HAC. HAC is absolute, whereas the Telecommunications Act allows companies to fall back on the "readily achievable" language as grounds for not providing access. Section 255 has been important in requiring manufacturers to address the compatibility of their products with specialized equipment used by consumers who are deaf or hard of hearing. A good example of this is the compatibility of wireless telephones with teletypes (TTYs) and assistive listening devices.

Section 713 (Closed Captioning)

Closed captioning of television programming enables children and adults with hearing loss to view the audio portion of a TV program as text on the television screen. (**Fig. 30.4** demonstrates captioning of the children's TV program *Arthur*.) All televisions sold in the United States with screens larger than 13 inches include the capability to display captions, a consequence of a 1990 federal law—The Television Decoder Circuitry Act. Section 713 of the Telecommunications Act made captioning a reality in America by mandating that all television programming, including broadcast, cable, and satellite, follow a specific schedule for implementing captioning. Although there are some exemptions (such as overnight programs that air between 2:00 am and 6:00 am), 100% of all new English-language TV programming must now

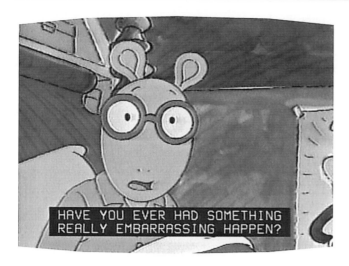

Fig. 30.4 The children's television program *Arthur* with closed captions, as mandated by the Telecommunications Act. (Image by Marc Brown and WGBH/Boston.)

be closed-captioned and 75% of previously developed programming (first shown before January 1, 1998) must be captioned as of 2008. Spanish-language programming follows a different schedule. As a result of this important legislation, people with hearing loss of all ages have nearly full access to television programming.

Unless paid for by the federal government (see the following discussion of Section 508), videos (DVD or VHS format) developed by private companies are not required to be closed-captioned, although most entertainment videos produced today are captioned.

Pearl

- Ironically, most educational videos developed for use in school settings are not captioned.

Section 508 of the Rehabilitation Act

Section 508 establishes requirements for electronic and information technology developed, maintained, procured, or used by the federal government. Section 508 requires federal electronic and information technology to be accessible to people with disabilities, including employees and members of the public. Federal agencies must comply with specific accessibility requirements when they procure or develop electronic and information technology. This requirement has important implications for employees or potential employees with hearing loss, as the standards effectively address key areas that often present barriers for people with hearing loss: telephones,

TVs, videotapes, DVDs, multimedia Web sites, interactive voice response systems, and information kiosks. Although Section 508 applies only to those who are federal employees or those using federal programs, it also serves as a model that other employers can emulate in providing accessible workplaces.

Americans with Disabilities Act, Title IV

Title IV of the ADA requires that telephone companies provide interstate and intrastate telecommunications relay services 24 hours a day, 7 days a week at no cost to the caller. Telephone relay services enable a person with hearing loss, who cannot understand speech on the telephone, to communicate with others through a relay assistant who types (or signs) what the hearing person is saying. A variety of options are available to relay users, including captioned telephone, in which a computer, PDA, or wireless device can be used to make a call, without special telephone equipment. Captions provided on a computer screen can accommodate persons with low vision because they can take advantage of the large text, variable fonts, and colors that are available. Relay services continue to evolve and improve.

A summary of telecommunications laws reviewed in this section is provided in **Table 30.2**.

◆ General Access

Section 504 of the Rehabilitation Act

Section 504 of the Rehabilitation Act forbids organizations and employers from excluding or denying individuals with disabilities an equal opportunity to receive program benefits and services. The act applies to any federal agency or entity or program receiving federal funds, and it broadly defines discrimination as not being accessible to someone with a disability. Any grant, loan, or contract to a public or private entity or program requires that entity to follow the regulations of the act. It applies to employers, hospitals, human service programs, public schools, colleges, and universities—that receive federal funds.

Section 504 can be used to ensure that a child (or a person of any age) receives the accommodations she needs to participate fully in a program. It can be used to access services like FM systems, interpreting, captioning, and note-taking. It may even be possible to use the act to obtain acoustical improvements in the built environment. Like most federal laws, Section 504 has a specific complaint process. What is a bit different is that this law allows each federal agency to have its own set of Section 504 regulations that apply to its own programs and the entities that receive aid from them.

Table 30.2 Telecommunications laws pertaining to people with hearing loss

Telecommunication laws	Coverage	Relevant federal agencies	Web resources
HAC of 1988 Final Negotiated Rulemaking 1996	Requires all new wireline and cordless (not wireless) phones to provide both coupling with the telecoil in a hearing aid and volume control. Wireless phones were initially exempted from HAC rules (see below).	FCC	www.fcc.gov/Bureaus/ common_carrier/FAQ/ faq_hac.html www.access-board.gov/ telecomm/marketrep/ guidelines/43i.htm
Hearing Aid Compatibility Rules for Wireless Telephones, 2003	The FCC later broadened HAC definition to include usability by people without telecoils via acoustic coupling. The rules directed digital wireless manufacturers to develop phones that are usable with hearing aids and to provide labeling and information about usability.	FCC	www.fcc.gov/cgb/consumerfacts/ hac.html www.aboutus.vzw.com/ accessibility/digitalPhones.htm www.ce-mag.com/archive/01/ Spring/Hollihan.html
Telecommunications Act of 1996 Section 255	This act requires that companies make products and services accessible to, and usable by, people with disabilities, if readily achievable. It covers telephones (wireless, cordless, wireline), answering machines, pagers, and services such as call waiting, voice mail, and interactive voice response.	FCC	www.fcc.gov/cgbl/dro/ section255.html www.fcc.gov/telecom.html
Telecommunications Act of 1996 Section 713	As of 2006, 100% of all new English-language television programming must be closed-captioned; 75% of programming first shown before 1/1/1998 must be captioned as of 2008. Spanish-language programming follows a different schedule. Some exceptions exist, such as overnight programs (2:00 am–6:00 am) and for those for whom captioning would constitute an undue burden.	FCC	www.fcc.gov/cgb/ consumerfacts/ closedcaption.html
Section 508 of the Rehabilitation Act of 1973	Federal agencies must comply with specific accessibility requirements when they procure or develop electronic and information technology. Impacts telephones, televisions, DVDs, videotapes, multimedia Web sites, interactive voice response systems, information kiosks, pagers.	Relevant federal agency	www.access-board.gov/ 508.htm www.section508.gov www.opm.gov/disability
ADA, Title IV (Telephone Relay Services)	Requires telephone companies to provide interstate and intrastate telecommunications relay services 24 hours a day, 7 days a week, at no cost to the caller.	FCC	www.fcc.gov/cgb/dro/ title4.html

Abbreviations: ADA, Americans with Disabilities Act; FCC, Federal Communications Commission; HAC, Hearing Aid Compatibility Act.

Although we tend to think of applying Section 504 at school, the law may also be used to gain access to any educational or cultural program that a child might wish to participate in outside the usual school setting. As the child ages, Section 504 also applies to the workplace and to other institutions. The child's audiologist should encourage the child and his family to develop the skills and knowledge to seek whatever accommodations he needs to participate. This kind of thinking will serve the child now and throughout his life.

The Americans with Disabilities Act

The ADA was intended to provide people with protection from discrimination in all aspects of their lives. The four parts of the ADA address access to (1) employment; (2) state and local government services (which include educational institutions) and transportation; (3) public accommodations, which means anywhere the public goes (stores, theaters, places of entertainment, hotels and motels, health care facilities); and (4) telecommunications relay services (see the foregoing discussion of telecommunications laws). The overriding goal of all these parts ensures that people with hearing loss can use, benefit from, and enjoy the same services and opportunities as everyone else.

Title I: Employment Provisions

Title I, employment provisions of the ADA, requires any employer with 15 or more employees not to discriminate on the basis of a person's disability and further to remove barriers that prevent a qualified person from performing a job. The ADA does not say that an employer is required to hire someone who could not perform the essential functions of the job. For example, if a person cannot hear well enough to respond reliably to questions on the telephone, an employer would not be legally required to hire that person as a telephone receptionist. However, if an employee is qualified for a job and can do everything relating to her job except access spoken information during large group training activities, the employer would be required to provide communication access (such as a FM system, captioning, or interpreter) as a reasonable accommodation to meet the employee's needs. An employer is required to provide such accommodations unless they are deemed burdensome. The courts have generally viewed accommodations like these access services as reasonable and not burdensome. As with all parts of the ADA, there is a specific process for lodging complaints should that be necessary.

Title II: State and Local Governments

Title II requires that state and local governments give people with disabilities equal access to the programs, services, and activities they sponsor. This part of the ADA is similar to Section 504; the main difference is that Section 504 applies to recipients of federal government monies, whereas Title II of the ADA pertains to all state and local governments regardless of size. For a child with hearing loss, this means that all offerings accessed by the child and her family—library, recreation, social services, and so forth—must be made accessible unless doing so would result in an undue financial or administrative burden.

Classroom acoustics is an issue that has been discussed for inclusion in the ADA since 1997. With the publication and 2010 revision of the ANSI/ASA S12.60 Classroom Acoustics Standard, parents, audiologists and others strongly urged inclusion of acoustical requirements in the ADA (Acoustical Society of America [ASA], 2010). A proposed rule is planned for fiscal year 2013 that would make the provisions manda-

tory in all new construction as well as in substantial renovations of public school buildings. It is proposed that the acoustic standard would also apply to private schools (under Title III of the ADA). The standard can also be used to guide acoustical improvements for students under IDEA.

Title II also addresses public transportation, such as city buses or rail transit. Both the service and the communication systems that support the service (i.e., information kiosks, telephone information lines) are to be made accessible. In theory, this means that voice announcements on transit systems should also be provided in a text format.

Title III: Public Accommodations

Title III, public accommodations, covers businesses and nonprofit organizations that offer services to the general public. Any entity that normally conducts business with the public, including restaurants, hotels, stores, movies, theaters, convention centers, doctors' offices, sports stadiums, fitness clubs, and private schools, is subject to the ADA Title III provisions. One area where there has been considerable effort by advocates is captioning at the movies and at live theater offerings. Although movie theaters are required to provide assistive listening devices, including a means to link to the telecoil of a hearing aid, movies were exempt in the original ADA language from being required to show open-captioned movies. Several court cases upheld advocates' position that although theaters are not required by the ADA to provide open captioning, closed captioning is a needed and appropriate method of providing communications access. Many live theaters now provide one or two sign-interpreted or captioned showings per run for a particular show. **Fig. 30.5** demonstrates one technology for providing closed captioning in movie theaters and other places of entertainment.

The definition of "places of public accommodation" continues to evolve. A 2012 court case brought by the National Association of the Deaf against Netflix argues that providers of streaming video entertainment on the Internet should provide captioning. Courts in two states, Massachusetts and California, came up with two very different decisions on the matter. By consent decree of a federal court in Massachusetts, Netflix agreed to caption 100% of its streaming content within two years (U.S. District Court for the State of Massachusetts, Western Division, 2012).

The specifics of how the ADA is to be implemented are described in detail in the revised Americans with Disabilities Act Standards for Accessible Design, which were adopted in 2010 and took effect March 15, 2012. The following changes (U.S. Access Board,

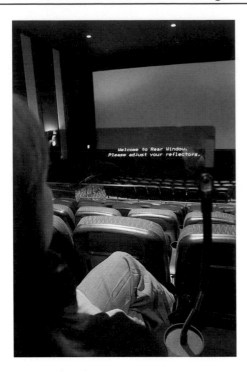

Fig. 30.5 Rear Window is a closed captioning technology developed by WGBH National Center for Accessible Media in Boston and used in movie theaters around the country and at select attractions at Walt Disney World and other theme parks. Rear Window displays reversed captions on a light-emitting diode text display that is mounted in the rear of the theater. Transparent acrylic panels, which attach to the seat in a theater, reflect the captions for people with hearing loss. (Photo by Jeffrey Dunn for WGBH.)

2010) in the regulations are of interest to children and adults with hearing loss:

- Technical standards for assistive listening systems (ALS) used in public places are required (for the first time) to ensure consistency in the quality and strength of the auditory signal.
- Neckloop attachments must be provided to allow inductive coupling between the ALS receiver and the telecoil in hearing aids or cochlear implants.
- Public telephones must have volume control with gain up to 20 dB.
- The number of required TTYs in public places was increased.
- Fire alarm alerts, audible and visual, shall be permanently installed in a specific percentage of hotel rooms.

A summary of Section 504 provisions as well as general access provisions under the ADA appears in **Table 30.3**.

◆ Helping the Child Become Her Own Best Advocate

One of the most important lessons we can teach our children with hearing loss is that they must learn to be their own best advocates. We should help them understand that the laws are there to help them fully ben-

Table 30.3 General access laws pertaining to people with hearing loss

General access	Coverage	Relevant federal agency	Web resources
Section 504 of the Rehabilitation Act of 1973 (Non-Discrimination under Federal Grants and Programs)	Requires that any federal agency, organization, or program receiving federal funds not discriminate based on disability. Nondiscrimination means that such organizations must be fully accessible to people with disabilities. Any grant, loan, or contract to an entity or program—public or private—requires that entity to follow the regulations of the act. Applies to employers, hospitals, human service programs, public schools, colleges, and universities—if they receive federal funds.	Relevant federal agency	www.section508.gov/ index.cfm?FuseAction= content&ID=15 www.usdoj.gov/crt/ada/ cguide.htm
ADA, 1990	Title I: Employment Title II: State & Local Government & Transportation Title III: Public Facilities (private and nonprofit services open to the general public) Title IV: Telephone relay (see above)	Title I: EEOC Title II: Transportation complaints to Federal Transit Administration Title II–IV: Access Board (for guidelines and standards), Department of Justice (enforcement)	www.access-board.gov/ ada-aba/index.htm www.jan.wvu.edu/links/ ADAtam1.html www.usdoj.gov/crt/ada/ cguide.htm www.access-board.gov/ Adaag/about/index.htm www.ada.gov/pcatoolkit/ chap1toolkit.htm

Abbreviation: ADA, Americans with Disabilities Act

efit from all life has to offer, and the accommodations that we reviewed here—at school, in the workplace, at the movies, when traveling, for telecommunications access—are basic rights in America. From an early age, we should involve children in the IEP process. The IEP should not be something that is done for the child; rather it should be a collaboration that allows the child to eventually become a full participant. The child's involvement can be something very simple to start. For example, the child might serve punch to the IEP team and discuss how his technology helps him. The next year, he would be expected to contribute a bit more. As time goes on, we want our children to transition into being full partners in the IEP process, articulating their own needs and helping formulate their goals. In some cases, we are seeing teens who are running the meeting, which is highly desirable and will serve those adolescents well as they begin their college careers in a different setting without the support of their teams. This does not happen overnight, so we need to begin the process of teaching children to advocate for themselves while they are still young. In so doing, we are instilling in our children the understanding that laws are there to help address their needs. However, to enjoy the benefits of our federal laws, we must (1) know and understand our rights; (2) speak up about what we need; and (3) know how to negotiate the system politely but firmly. Whether we are talking about hiring the type of interpreter we want at school or ensuring that a facility is providing an assistive listening system, our children will benefit from the wide-ranging laws reviewed here only if they know how to advocate for themselves.

Many parents have difficulty resisting the temptation to do everything for their children. When the child has a disability, the urge to do it for her is even more likely to take over. As the child's audiologist, you can make a positive contribution to your patients' success beyond the hearing loss by coaching families in the importance of helping children develop their own advocacy skills. Many resources are available to help you accomplish that.

Discussion Questions

1. Children with hearing loss are now being identified at birth and fitted early with technology that is considerably improved from what was available 10, or even 5, years ago. Regardless of their level of hearing loss, many children are learning language at a level equivalent to their hearing peers. What kinds of issues does this create in terms of eligibility under various disability laws, and what is your role in advising parents and school professionals?

2. What are the differences between legal intent and practice as it applies to each of the three categories of laws reviewed in the chapter?

3. How should we teach a child to advocate for herself, and at what age should that process begin?

4. What if you do not agree with the school district's decision about placement and services for a patient? What is your role vis-à-vis the child, her family, and the school-based personnel?

5. Does your role as a hearing health professional include or exclude being an advocate for the child and her family? What are the boundaries?

References

Acoustical Society of America. (2010). ANSI/ASA S12.60–2010/Part 1 American National Standard acoustical performance criteria, design requirements, and guidelines for schools, Part 1: permanent schools and Part 2: relocatable classroom factors. Retrieved from http://asastore.aip.org

Federal Communications Commission. (2003a). Hearing aid compatibility order. 18 FCC Red at 16780 Paragraph 65; 47 C.F.R. Section 20.19(c).

Federal Communications Commission. (2003b). In the matter of Section 68.4 of the commission's rules governing hearing aid-compatible telephones, WT Docket 01-309, RM-8658. Report and Order. FCC 03-168. Retrieved from http://hraunfoss.fcc.gov/edocs_public/attachmatch/FCC-03-168A1.pdf

Hands and Voices. (2006). Guide-by-your-side program. Retrieved from http://www.handsandvoices.org/services/guide.htm

No Child Left Behind Act. (Act of 2001). P.L. 107-110, 115 Stat. 1425.

Perigoe, C., & Perigoe, R. (2005). Multiple challenges—multiple solutions: children with hearing loss and special needs. The Volta Review, 104(4), 211.

Sorkin, D. L. (2004a). Disability law and people with hearing loss: we've come a long way (but we're not there yet). Hearing Loss, 25, 13–17.

Sorkin, D. L. (2004b). FM technology: reimbursement and the law. In D. A. Fabry & C. D. Johnson (Eds.), ACCESS: achieving clear communication, employing sound solutions. Proceedings of the first international FM conference (pp. 239–243). Warrenville, IL: Phonak. Retrieved from http://www.phonakpro.com/content/dam/phonak/b2b/Events/conference_proceedings/1st_fm_conference_2003/2003proceedings_chapter25.pdf

Sutton v. United Airlines (1999). 527 U.S. 471.

Tucker, B. (1998). IDEA advocacy for children who are deaf or hard of hearing. San Diego, CA: Singular.

U.S. Access Board. (2010). Americans with Disabilities Act (ADA) guidelines for accessible design. Retrieved from http://www.access-board.gov/ada-aba/ada-standards-doj.cfm

U.S. Department of Education. (2006a). Assistance to states for the education of children with disabilities and preschool grants for children with disabilities, final rule. Federal Register, 2006(August 14), 46540–46845.

U.S. Department of Education. (2006b). Raising the achievement of students with disabilities: new ideas for IDEA. Retrieved from http://www2.ed.gov/admins/lead/speced/ideafactsheet.html

U.S. Department of Justice. (2006). ADA tool kit. Retrieved from http://www.ada.gov/pcatoolkit/chap1toolkit.htm

U.S. District Court for the State of Massachusetts, Western Division. (2012). National Association of the Deaf, Western Massachusetts Association of the Deaf and Hearing Impaired, and Lee Nettles v. Netflix, Inc., Civil Action No. 11-30168-MAP, consent decree. Retrieved from http://dredf.org/captioning/netflix-consent-decree-10-10-12.pdf

Additional Readings

Breslin, M., & Silvia, Y. (2002). Disability rights law and policy: international and national perspectives. Ardsley, NY: Transnational.

Strauss, K. P. (2006). A new civil right: telecommunications equality for deaf and hard of hearing Americans. Washington, DC: Gallaudet University.

Tucker, B. (1998). IDEA advocacy for children who are deaf or hard of hearing. San Diego, CA: Singular.

Resources and Helpful Web Sites

1. Alexander Graham Bell Association for the Deaf and Hard of Hearing provides books and other resources on education and advocacy for people with hearing loss with a focus on children: http://www.agbell.org. Last accessed October 18, 2012.

2. Listening and Spoken Language Knowledge Center is a comprehensive resource for parents and professionals addressing parent advocacy training, negotiating the IEP, IDEA Part C, training opportunities for professionals, auditory learning, and more: http://www.listeningandspokenlanguage.org. Last accessed October 18, 2012.

3. Hands and Voices is a parent organization that emphasizes unbiased advisement on options, parent information and support: http://www.handsandvoices.org. Last accessed October 18, 2012.

4. Hearing Loss Association of America provides materials on advocacy, access laws, and telecommunications: http://www.hearingloss.org. Last accessed October 18, 2012.

5. National Dissemination Center for Children with Disabilities (NICHCY) has technical assistance materials relating to the education of children with disabilities of all ages, including state resource sheets listing agencies in each state: http://www.nichcy.org. Last accessed October 18, 2012.

6. The No Child Left Behind (NCLB) Act has the following explanatory Web site: http://www.ed.gov/nclb/landing.jhtml. Last accessed October 18, 2012.

7. National Parent Technical Assistance Center (NTPAC). http://www.parentcenternetwork.org/national/aboutus.html. Last accessed October 18, 2012.

8. The U.S. Access Board has extensive online guidance materials on the ADA and Section 504: http://www.access-board.gov. Last accessed October 18, 2012.

9. Wrightslaw provides materials on education law for attorneys and advocates: http://www.wrightslaw.org. Last accessed October 18, 2012.

Chapter 31

Screening, Evaluation, and Management of Auditory Disorders in the School-Aged Child

Rebecca Kooper

Key Points

- Screening programs should be designed to separate children who are at risk for hearing loss or middle ear disorders from children with normal hearing.

- Audiologists must develop screening protocols to meet the needs of their specific populations.

- Assessment of the hearing status of school-aged children is similar to the assessment of adults, with added emphasis on speech audiometry to determine how the hearing loss is affecting the development of speech and language skills.

- Educational audiologists play an integral role in the assessment and management of hearing loss in the school-aged child.

◆ Hearing Screening

The goal of a hearing screening program is to identify children who may have hearing loss and therefore require further testing. It is important to identify these children as early as possible, since hearing loss can adversely affect educational performance (Anderson & Arnoldi, 2011). The early identification and subsequent management of hearing loss in children can help improve academic achievement (Apuzzo & Yoshinaga-Itano, 1995; Bess, Dodd-Murphy, & Parker, 1998). Fortunately, the acceptance of universal newborn hearing screening in most states has lowered the age of identification of congenital hearing loss. However, there remains a need to screen the school-aged child, because later-onset hearing loss may occur.

Later-onset and progressive hearing loss can occur in children for a variety of reasons, including (see Chapter 2):

- Syndromes like Usher or Hunter syndrome (Sprintzen, 2001)

- Disorders like enlarged vestibular aqueduct
- Genetic disorders, such as connexin 26 mutations
- Nonsyndromic progressive sensorineural hearing loss
- Infectious diseases, such as meningitis or measles
- Ototoxicity from chemotherapy (Berg, Spitzer, & Garvin, 1999)
- Exposure to high-intensity levels of noise and music (Shafer, 2006)

Fluctuating conductive hearing loss resulting from otitis media can also disrupt the learning process. Therefore, screening children for middle ear disorders is an important step in minimizing the negative effects of chronic otitis media (Gravel et al, 2006).

When developing a screening program for school districts, audiologists need to consider the following issues:

- Who should be screened?
- How often should children be screened?
- Where will the screening take place?
- Should the screening program be limited to identifying those at risk for hearing loss or should it also identify those at risk for middle ear disorders?
- What tests should be included in the screening program?
- Who will perform the tests?
- What is the follow-up protocol for those who fail the screening tests?

The Individuals with Disabilities Education Act (IDEA) (1990) is a federal law that requires states to identify children with disabilities, including children with hearing loss. Therefore, many states have promulgated legal regulations to identify these children. Screening protocols vary from state to state, and audiologists must contact their state agencies to determine if there is a mandated screening protocol.

Who Should Be Screened for Hearing Loss?

State regulations dictate who should be included in a hearing screening program. Audiologists may also consider guidelines offered by the American Academy of Audiology (AAA) (2011) when developing a screening program. These guidelines suggest screening:

- All children enrolling in school for the first time.
- All children in specific grades. Targeted grades that are recommended include grades 1, 3, 5, and either 7 or 9.
- Referral students, which includes students who are in the Response to Intervention (RtI) process or in the special education eligibility process.

Parents or school personnel can complete screening checklists, such as the Screening Instrument for Targeting Educational Risk (SIFTER) (Anderson, 1989), Fisher's Auditory Problems Checklist (Fisher, 1985) or Children's Auditory Processing Performance Scale (CHAPPS) (Smoski, 1990), or they can alert school personnel to the need for screening. Chapter 23 has a more detailed discussion of functional assessments.

Who Should Be Screened for Middle Ear Disorders?

A decision must be made whether to include a screening for middle ear disorders as part of the hearing screening program. Since chronic middle ear dysfunction and subsequent fluctuating hearing loss can adversely affect academic performance, screening for these disorders may be recommended for children who are at risk for middle ear problems. The AAA (1997) includes the following children in the "at risk" category:

- Children with craniofacial anomalies
- Children of Native American heritage
- Children with known histories of chronic otitis media
- Children who have had middle ear effusion that persists for 3 months
- Children diagnosed with learning disabilities
- Children diagnosed with speech and language delays
- Children who were diagnosed with sensorineural hearing loss
- Children who have failed the pure tone screening

Where Will the Screening Take Place?

Screening must take place in a quiet environment; it must be quiet enough for a student with normal hearing to be able to hear the test frequencies at 20 dB hearing level (HL). If ambient noise levels are too high to hear test signals at 20 dB, it is not acceptable to raise the intensity level of the stimuli. Rather, it is recommended that the environment be modified to improve the acoustics. These acoustic recommendations may include installing carpeting or acoustic ceiling tiles. Selecting a test room that is away from known noise sources, such as heating systems, gymnasiums, cafeterias, and playgrounds, is essential.

Equipment Specifications

Audiometers should be calibrated to current standards developed and adopted by the American National Standards Institute (ANSI) (2004). Specifications and appropriate corrections should be made when using insert earphones (AAA, 2011).

What Tests Are Recommended?

Pure tone screening is the basic component of a hearing screening program. Immittance testing may be added to screen for middle ear disorders. The decision to include immittance testing would be based on the population in the school. It would be wise to include it in kindergarten centers or special education school programs. Tympanometry is the most common immittance measure used in schools. If tympanometry is to be included in the screening protocol, it must be preceded by an otoscopic evaluation of the external ear canal to ensure that the ear canal is free from obstructions, such as debris and cerumen. The presence of pressure equalizing (PE) tubes should be noted at this time. The AAA (2011) recommends tympanometry only in conjunction with pure tone screening in young children in communities where medical health care providers and school systems are looking to identify children with otitis media with effusion.

Otoacoustic emissions (OAEs) testing is recommended only for school-aged children for whom pure tone screening is not developmentally appropriate. Pure tone tests continue to be the most effective screening tool (Krueger & Ferguson, 2002).

What Are the Testing Protocols?

A hearing screening should be performed at the frequencies 1000, 2000, and 4000 Hz at 20 dB HL. A child must respond to all frequencies in both ears to pass the screening. Testing can be performed using routine test procedures or conditioned play audiometry if needed. Referral for a rescreening is recommended if the child fails to respond to any frequency in either ear. The rescreening should take place as soon as possible, preferably within 24 to 48 hours. Children who fail the rescreening should be referred for a complete audiologic evaluation.

More comprehensive screening protocols may be instituted. The Colorado Department of Education (2004) recommends including 500 Hz for children from preschool through fifth grade if tympanometry is not available.

Some studies have noted the increased prevalence of noise-induced hearing loss in children. To identify these children, it has been suggested that screening frequencies include 6000 and 8000 Hz, because these frequencies are sensitive to noise-induced hearing loss (Montgomery & Fujikawa, 1992).

If tympanometry is performed, a rescreen is recommended for children 7 years and older if peak admittance is less than 0.4 mmho or tympanometric width is greater than 400 daPa. Children 6 years and younger should be rescreened if they exhibit static admittance less than 0.3 mmho or tympanomteric width greater than 200 daPa. Rescreening should take place within 4 to 6 weeks. If the child fails the screening again, a medical referral is warranted (AAA, 2011).

To identify those at risk for tympanic membrane perforation, refer immediately if tympanometric volume is greater than 1.0 cm³ and is accompanied by a flat (type B) tympanogram. However, do not refer if PE tubes can be visualized through otoscopy.

Acoustic reflex tests and tympanometric peak pressure are not considered appropriate screening procedures.

Controversial Point

- With the increase of noise-induced hearing loss in younger children, should the more comprehensive screening protocols that include frequencies higher than 4000 Hz become the accepted procedure for all to use?

Who Will Administer the Screening?

Personnel conducting the screenings usually include audiologists, speech-language pathologists, and school nurses. Individual state regulations may allow additional people to be placed on this list. All who are conducting the hearing screenings should have knowledge of the following topics:

- Goal of hearing screenings
- Familiarity with audiologic equipment
- Requirements for an appropriate test environment
- How to instruct students on screening procedures
- Criteria for passing and failing the hearing screening
- How to report results
- How to follow up with parents and school personnel
- How to test the very young or difficult-to-test child

What Is the Follow-up Protocol?

Parents should be notified about the results of the screening and the need for further evaluation. Children who are referred for a complete audiologic evaluation should be seen within 3 months of the referral. It is important for personnel to follow up to ensure that the audiologic diagnostic evaluation was performed. The strength of a screening program is only as good as its follow-up procedures (Johnson & Seaton, 2012). If children who fail the screening are not seen for a full audiologic evaluation, the screening program has failed. Diligent follow-up procedures need to be in place as part of the program.

Screening the Difficult-to-Test Child

Some children cannot be tested with standard pure tone screening methods. These children may have significant developmental delays or substantial physical problems that prevent them physically from being able to respond to the test stimulus. Some of these children respond well to conditioned play audiometry. Others are unable to perform that technique. A notation of "CNT" (cannot test) on the screening form does not mean that the screening requirement has been fulfilled. Merely "trying" to administer the test is not sufficient. Other screening tools, such as OAEs, may be used (Lyons, Kei, & Driscoll, 2004). However, screening using OAE tests should be performed only by a licensed audiologist (AAA, 2011). If other screening tests are not available, a complete audiologic evaluation must be recommended. Follow-up protocols need to ensure that every child is screened with some test measure that concludes with a definitive statement regarding hearing status.

Pearl

- No matter how difficult it is to test a child, it is possible to screen everyone. Audiologists need to diligently identify the correct screening tool to meet each individual child's specific needs.

Audiologic Evaluation

The standard audiologic evaluation typically includes case history, otoscopy, immittance measures (tympanometry, static immittance, and acoustic reflexes), pure tone air and bone conduction thresholds, speech audiometry, and OAEs. This evaluation is usually completed by the child's pediatric audiologist. However, once children enter the public school arena, they may receive audiologic services provided by the school district. To qualify to receive these services, they must be included in the child's Individualized Education Plan (IEP). (For more information on IEP development, see Chapter 30.) The following services may be included in the IEP:

- A complete unaided audiologic evaluation and aided evaluation with the child's hearing aid or cochlear implant and frequency modulation (FM) system
- Provision and use of an FM system in the classroom
- Management plan for monitoring personal and classroom amplification
- In-service workshops for school staff

The Responsibilities of the Educational Audiologist

For specific information on audiologic procedures, see Chapters 7–11.

Identifying Students in Need of Services

Educational audiologists are responsible for developing and implementing hearing screenings in the schools. (See the preceding section on hearing screening for more details.)

The Educational Audiologist as a Member of an Educational Team

Educational audiologists should be part of the team that manages the cases of students who have been identified in the school as having a hearing impairment that adversely impacts educational performance (Johnson & Seaton, 2012). Once a student is identified, the school district should convene a meeting to develop an IEP that will make recommendations regarding placement, services, and need for assistive technology. Services often considered for these students include speech-language/auditory therapy and support by a Teacher of the Deaf (TOD) if the student is placed in a general education class.

Regularly scheduled team meetings to monitor the progress of these students should be recommended.

Pearl

- When sharing test results with school personnel, it is especially important to perform a speech recognition test at average conversational levels (50 dB HL) and also at soft conversational levels (35 dB HL) to help the teacher understand how the child is performing in the classroom.

Educational audiologists provide audiologic services in the school district. They have a unique perspective, as they can observe the child in his school environment and collaborate with school staff. While the audiologic assessment usually includes the standard battery just described, educational audiologists often expand their assessment to include a more in-depth evaluation of speech recognition skills.

Speech audiometry provides information about how a child functions in the real world. Although the degree of hearing loss has a significant impact on speech scores, hearing sensitivity is not the sole determinant of speech reception skills. Some children with good access to the auditory signal, as indicated by pure tone testing, may have great difficulty following conversational speech. Conversely, children with hearing loss may have excellent speech reception skills. Speech audiometry includes speech reception thresholds (SRTs), speech detection thresholds (SDTs), and speech recognition testing. An evaluation of speech in noise is essential to determine how the child will function in the classroom. (For a complete discussion of speech audiometry, see Chapter 11.) Sometimes an educational audiologist can administer an evaluation in the classroom to provide information about how the child performs in his daily environment. The Functional Listening Evaluation (Johnson & Seaton, 2012) is performed in the classroom and demonstrates how noise and distance may have an adverse effect on the speech recognition abilities of students with hearing loss.

Some educational audiologists administer auditory skills assessments that are components of an auditory training curriculum. Curriculums such as the Developmental Approach to Successful Listening II (DASL II) (Stout & Windle, 1994) or Speech Perception Instructional Curriculum and Evaluation (SPICE) (Moog, Biedenstein, & Davidson, 1995) include these assessments. Other tests, such as the Test of Auditory Comprehension (Trammell & Owens, 1981), provide information on auditory memory and speech-in-noise and auditory comprehension. This information could help the TOD or SLP develop appropriate auditory training goals.

FM System Evaluation

FM systems are assistive listening devices that are commonly used in the schools. Children with various auditory needs have benefited from the use of FM in the classroom. With the advent of different types and models, it is essential to evaluate the child to ensure that maximum benefit is derived from the device (AAA, 2008). It has become necessary for the educational audiologist to make sure that personal FM devices can interface with technology used in the school (e.g., SMART Boards, SMART Technologies, Calgary, Canada). Some districts have installed classroom audio distribution systems (CADS) in many of the classrooms in their schools. When connecting FM systems to existing CADS, it is imperative that the educational audiologist verify that the sound being delivered to the ear is appropriate and has not been distorted by the use of the two systems together. For more information on FM systems, see Chapter 23.

Report Writing

When writing audiologic reports, clinical audiologists often use terminology that is unfamiliar to school personnel. To help teachers meet the needs of the child with hearing loss, educational audiologists create reports that will explain how hearing loss will affect communication (Anderson & Arnoldi, 2011). Reports should include information like: "With hearing aids, the student will not detect the softer speech sounds such as 's,' 'sh,' 'f' and therefore may have difficulty understanding concepts of plurals and possessives" or "The student will have difficulty understanding speech at a distance of 6 ft or more from the speaker."

Plotting audiologic results on a familiar sounds audiogram is also helpful. This graphically depicts the sounds that are inaudible to the student and may help the educational staff understand the effects of the hearing loss on communication (**Fig. 31.1**).

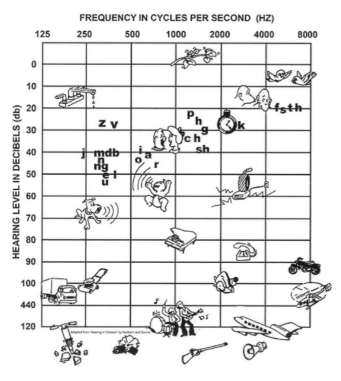

Fig. 31.1 Speech sounds audiogram. From Northern, J., & Downs, M. (2002). Hearing in children (5th ed., p. 18). Baltimore, MD: Lippincott Williams & Wilkins. Used with permission.

Classroom Acoustics

Classrooms have become noisy environments. Gone are the days when children sat quietly in rows listening to their teacher. Today's classrooms often have many "Learning Areas" where small groups of children go to work on projects together. There are also many different technologies used in today's rooms, including SMART Boards and computers. Together these factors have increased the noise level in the classroom. The educational audiologist needs to:

- Explain to school personnel the role that good classroom acoustics can play in enhancing learning (Flexer, 2004)
- Determine noise levels by taking measurements with a sound level meter or with a sound level meter app on a smart phone (Smaldino & Flexer, 2012)
- Identify noise sources in the classroom and recommend ways to reduce this noise and reverberation (please see Chapter 23 for more information)

Monitoring Amplification

Plans for the monitoring and maintenance of personal and classroom amplification should be created for each child. This plan should include a statement of who will provide the amplification check, how often it will be done, and what steps will be taken when equipment malfunctions (AAA, 2008).

In-Service Workshops

Educational audiologists should provide in-service workshops to school personnel. Topics of these workshops should include:

- Hearing loss: How hearing loss affects learning, communication, and language development in the classroom. Tapes, CDs, or apps that simulate hearing loss are especially useful to help school personnel understand the effect of hearing loss on communication. Techniques to maximize communication in the classroom should be reviewed as well as techniques to minimize noise in the classroom. The student's audiologic report should be reviewed and interpreted to staff.
- Hearing aids and cochlear implants: How a hearing aid or cochlear implant works should be reviewed. A description of how to perform a daily listening check should be detailed.
- FM systems:
  – Reasons FM is needed in the classroom. This topic includes a review of classroom acoustics and the limitations of personal amplification in the classroom.

- How an FM system works. It is helpful when reviewing how an FM system works to provide the teachers with an opportunity to listen through an FM system.
- Effective use of FM in the classroom. It is important to review when to use FM and when not to use FM. Proper microphone placement should be demonstrated at this time.
- Daily listening check of FM and troubleshooting techniques

Counseling

When children with a hearing loss attend school in the regular education environment, they often feel there is no one in the school who understands their challenges. Many of these children have no one to talk to and often feel different from peers with normal hearing. Educational audiologists can counsel these children about the nature of their loss and about the benefits and limitations of personal amplification. The need for FM use in the classroom should also be explained. Besides learning about hearing loss, the child often needs help exploring the emotions that accompany the realization that one is "different." With counseling, the child can be helped to integrate hearing loss into the rest of the child's total personality. For more information, see Chapter 35.

Collaborating with School Personnel

Educational audiologists must collaborate with school personnel to design a program of services that best suits each child's specific needs. The TOD and the speech language pathologist are two people who often have the greatest contact with the student. If equipment malfunctions, it is important that these staff members know who to call to help reduce equipment down time.

◆ Summary

Since hearing loss can negatively affect a child's academic performance, a complete audiologic evaluation needs to be performed on all children who fail a hearing screening or on all children for whom hearing loss is suspected. The accuracy of the assessment depends on the evaluation and comparison of various test procedures. When evaluating the school-aged child, it is important to determine her auditory and speech perception skills with tests that can be performed in the sound booth and in the classroom. Educational audiologists work with school personnel to ensure that the children's auditory needs are met and to maximize their access to audition in the classroom. Proper assessment and management can increase the child's chances of success, academically and socially (Anderson & Arnoldi, 2011).

Discussion Questions

1. What would be the hearing screening recommendations for a class of kindergarten children, and for a class of high school students?

2. Excessively high noise levels in the room where hearing screening is performed may cause school personnel to want to raise the intensity of the test stimulus. They come to you, the audiologist, for advice. How do you solve this problem?

3. A second-grade student is doing poorly in school. The speech-language pathologist notes that this child seems to have great difficulty hearing in noise. The child passes the hearing screening test. What is the next recommendation?

4. A first-grade student with a moderate sensorineural hearing loss is entering public school for the first time. What steps should the educational audiologist take to help this child have a successful school year?

References

American Academy of Audiology. (1997). Identification of hearing loss and middle-ear dysfunction in preschool and school-age children. McLean, VA: American Academy of Audiology.

American Academy of Audiology. (2008). Clinical practice guidelines for remote microphone hearing assistance technologies for children and youth birth–21 years. Retrieved from http://www.audiology.org/resources/document library/Documents/HATGuideline.pdf

American Academy of Audiology. (2011). Childhood Hearing Screening Guidelines. Retrieved from http://www.audiology .org/resources/documentlibrary/Documents/20110926_ ChildhoodHearingScreeningGuidelines.pdf

American National Standards Institute. (2004). Specifications for audiometers (ANSI S3.6–2004). New York, NY: ANSI.

Anderson, K. (1989). Screening Instrument for Targeting Educational Risk (SIFTER). Tampa, FL: Educational Audiology Association.

Anderson, K., & Arnoldi, K. A. (2011). Building skills for success in the fast-paced classroom. Hillsboro, OR: Butte.

Apuzzo, M. L., & Yoshinaga-Itano, C. (1995). Early identification of infants with significant hearing loss and the Minnesota Child Development Inventory. Seminars in Hearing, 16, 124–139.

Berg, A. L., Spitzer, J. B., & Garvin, J. H., Jr (1999). Ototoxic impact of cisplatin in pediatric oncology patients. The Laryngoscope, 109(11), 1806–1814.

Bess, F. H., Dodd-Murphy, J., & Parker, R. A. (1998). Children with minimal sensorineural hearing loss: prevalence, educational performance, and functional status. Ear and Hearing, 19(5), 339–354.

Colorado Department of Education. (2004). Standards of practice for audiology services in the schools. Retrieved from http://www.cde.state.co.us/HealthAndWellness/ download/Stndrs_Practice_Audiology_Svcs.pdf

Fisher, L. I. (1985). Learning disabilities and auditory processing. In R. J. Van Hattam (Ed.), Administration of speech language services in schools: a manual (pp. 231–290). San Diego: College-Hill.

Flexer, C. (2004). The impact of classroom acoustics: listening, learning, and literacy. Seminars in Hearing, 25(2), 131–140.

Gravel, J. S., Roberts, J. E., Roush, J., Grose, J., Besing, J., Burchinal, M., . . . Zeisel, S. (2006). Early otitis media with effusion, hearing loss, and auditory processes at school age. Ear and Hearing, 27(4), 353–368.

Individuals with Disabilities Education Act. (1990). PL 101-476. Title 20, U.S.C. 1400 et seq. United States Statutes at Large, 104, 1103–1151.

Johnson, C. D., & Seaton, J. (2012). Educational audiology handbook (2nd ed.). Clifton Park, NY: Delmar–Cengage Learning.

Krueger, W. W., & Ferguson, L. (2002). A comparison of screening methods in school-aged children. Otolaryngology-Head and Neck Surgery, 127(6), 516–519.

Lyons, A., Kei, J., & Driscoll, C. (2004). Distortion product otoacoustic emissions in children at school entry: a comparison with pure-tone screening and tympanometry results. Journal of the American Academy of Audiology, 15(10), 702–715.

Montgomery, J. K., & Fujikawa, S. (1992). Hearing thresholds of students in the second, eighth and twelfth grades. Language, Speech, and Hearing Services in Schools, 23, 61–63.

Moog, J., Biedenstein, J., & Davidson, L. (1995). The SPICE, St Louis, MO: Central Institute for the Deaf.

Shafer, D. N. (2006, April 11). Noise-induced hearing loss hits teens. The ASHA Leader.

Smaldino, J., & Flexer, C. (2012). Handbook of acoustic accessibility: best practices for listening, learning and literacy in the classroom. New York, NY: Thieme.

Smoski, W. (1990). Use of CHAPPS in a children's audiology clinic. Ear and Hearing, 11, 53S–56S.

Sprintzen, R. (2001). Syndrome identification for audiology. San Diego, CA: Singular.

Stout, G., & Windle, J. (1994). Developmental approach to successful listening II. Englewood, CO: Resource Point, Inc.

Trammell, J., & Owens, S. L. (1981). The auditory skills instructional planning system at the secondary level. Journal of the Academy of Rehabilitative Audiology, 14, 198–207.

Chapter 32

Managing Infants and Children with Auditory Neuropathy Spectrum Disorder (ANSD)

Marilyn W. Neault

Key Points

- Three advances enabled audiologists to observe ANSD in infants: otoacoustic emissions (OAEs), insert earphones for auditory brainstem response (ABR) testing, and multifrequency tympanometry.

- Cochlear microphonics (CM) at 70 dB HL and higher followed by flat or nonreplicable waves support the diagnosis of ANSD.

- The audiologist must counsel parents carefully about predictions for auditory development and effectiveness of hearing aids and cochlear implants for their child with ANSD.

- In addition to ABR information, it is important to observe the child's listening skills and to gather observation data from parents and other caregivers about the child's benefit from technology and progression in language development.

- Never say "never" or "always" in the realm of ANSD.

Audiologists are forever in training, refining and mastering new tests for hearing and balance. New tests can add enough pixels to the grainy picture of a poorly understood disorder to define it, and thus begin to help those who have it. Auditory neuropathy spectrum disorder (ANSD) epitomizes such developments in audiology. ANSD is a class of hearing disorders characterized by active outer hair cells but reduced generation of synchronous auditory neuronal firing, resulting in smeared or absent auditory percepts.

Three advances enabled audiologists to observe ANSD in infants: otoacoustic emissions (OAEs), insert earphones for auditory brainstem response (ABR) testing, and multifrequency tympanometry. Many contributors to this book began to practice pediatric audiology before these tests were launched. The emergence of evoked otoacoustic emission (OAE) tests (Kemp, 1978) unearthed surprising cases of robust hair cell activity with little or no functional audition.

Another indicator of hair cell function, the cochlear microphonic (CM), became observable in the clinic when insert earphones began to replace supraaural earphones to record auditory brainstem response (ABR) waves (Beauchaine, Kaminski, & Gorga, 1987). Using insert earphones, single-polarity (all rarefaction or all condensation) clicks can yield response tracings that are free of signal artifact even at high intensities. Use of supraaural earphones in the earlier days of ABR testing required the use of alternating-polarity signals at high intensities to reduce signal artifact, which also obscured the CM response. However, observation of hair cell activity using OAE and CM measures requires normal middle ear transduction. Normative data for multifrequency tympanometry (Calandruccio, Fitzgerald, & Prieve, 2006) became necessary to assess middle ear status in infants on the day of the audiological evaluation, as the OAE and CM can be reduced by conductive overlay. In addition, use of multifrequency tympanometry contributes to the recording of an infant's middle ear muscle reflex (MEMR), which is absent or has a greatly elevated threshold in ANSD. Armed with new understanding from description of existing cases (Starr, Picton, Sininger, Hood, & Berlin, 1996) and with tools (Berlin et al, 1998), audiologists could think back on prior perplexing cases who probably had ANSD (Worthington & Peters, 1980) and think forward to incorporate the assessment for ANSD into routine test batteries. By 2008, sufficient experience with assessment and management existed that a consensus conference held in Como, Italy, could result in agreement on a name for the class of disorders (ANSD, inclusive of auditory neuropathy, auditory dyssynchrony, and neural hearing loss) and a statement of clinical guidelines (Bill Daniels Center for Children's Hearing, 2008).

In ANSD, outer hair cells show activity, evidenced by the presence of a cochlear microphonic (CM) response in the ABR that persists, and by the presence of evoked OAEs that may, however, disappear over time and in fact may not be present when first assessed. ABR waves following the CM are absent, or are present only at high intensities and grossly abnormal. Middle ear muscle reflexes (MEMRs) are absent or have greatly elevated thresholds. These findings, recorded when the middle ears are clear, are sufficient to state that a child has a pattern of test results consistent with ANSD. Beyond this initial constellation of findings, however, children having ANSD diverge widely on other auditory measures over time. Children with ANSD who show seemingly identical audiological profiles on the routine test battery (normal tympanograms with probe tone frequency appropriate for age, MEMRs absent, ABR showing only the CM with no subsequent waves, and OAEs present) may have pure tone audiograms ranging from the normal to profound hearing loss range, and speech recognition ability ranging from functional to nil. Because of the lack of correlation between today's commonly used physiological measures and the variety of functional outcomes, close monitoring of the child's auditory behavior and vigilant attention to any improvements in physiological measures are interdependent with case management decisions.

◆ Looking for ANSD in Right and Wrong Places

Recognizing a large polarity-inverting cochlear microphonic response in the ABR, a signature finding in ANSD, can be bewildering to an audiologist without proper training and mentoring. Two clinicians at the start of their learning curves stated: "Because the ABR response did not show polarity inversion when ipsilaterally and contralaterally recorded tracings were superimposed, there is no evidence of auditory neuropathy" and "A polarity-inverting cochlear microphonic response was seen on superimposed rarefaction and condensation click tracings, indicating absence of auditory neuropathy." Both drew erroneous conclusions and needed education and validation. **Fig. 32.1a-c** depicts proper recording and superimposition of ABR tracings when evaluating ANSD, while **Fig. 32.1d–f** depicts three types of recordings that often are confused with ANSD.

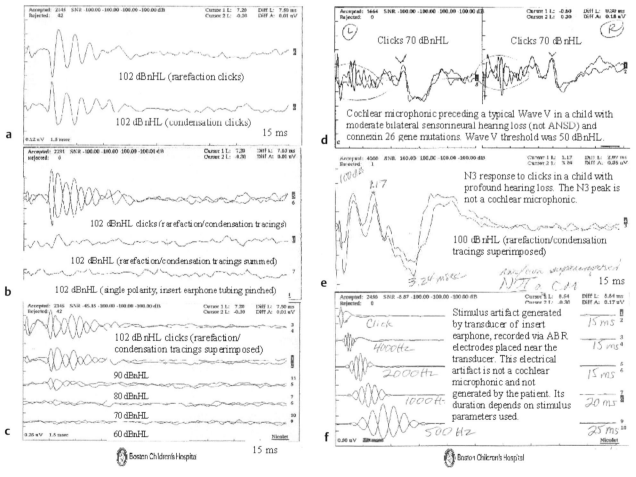

Fig. 32.1a–f **(a–c)** ABR findings in a 9-month-old, born premature, who passed newborn hearing screening by OAEs but parents suspected hearing loss. Note that a single-polarity trace **(a)** showing a lengthy cochlear microphonic can mimic an ABR, until rarefaction and condensation tracings are superimposed **(b)** and the CM's stability in latency with changes in signal intensity are shown **(c)**. **(d–f)** show three types of tracings that should not be confused with ANSD: CM followed by a typical ABR wave **(d)**, N3 peak **(e)**, and electrical artifact from the insert earphone **(f)**.

The click-evoked ABR tracings in **Fig. 32.1a–c** can be recorded efficiently, once the audiologist has documented lack of response to weaker signals and proceeded to test higher intensities. Although the audiologist may be tempted to proceed with the presentation of tone bursts at several frequencies in each ear, following the usual procedure with non-ANSD cases, it happens that when the click fails to elicit ABR waves in ANSD, the ABR to tone bursts is likely to be noncontributory to the initial diagnosis of ANSD. In addition, the auditory steady state response (ASSR) is unlikely to assist in predicting the audiogram in ANSD (Rance, et al, 2005). The audiologist's time is much better spent counseling the family than recording the ABR to tone bursts or ASSR at the initial session. Visual aids such as those depicted in **Fig. 32.2a,b** and acoustic simulations of ANSD help to demonstrate that a child may hear, but the new words he needs to learn are blurred because of poor timing of firing in the auditory nerve.

◆ How Children with ANSD Present to the Audiologist

As many as 10% of children who have permanent hearing loss have a pattern of test results consistent with ANSD (Roush, Frymark, Venediktov, & Wang, 2011). If a child who has ANSD does not have a newborn hearing screen, passes an OAE-only screen, or is misdiagnosed with a more typical sensorineural hearing loss, the child's listening behavior and language development are vulnerable to confusion and delay. The audiologist must be alert to children with undiagnosed ANSD who may present in four different ways, described in **Table 32.1** along with suggested protocols for testing, intervention, and counseling.

Most cases present as referrals from newborn hearing screening programs, having shown no response on automated ABR tests. Of these cases, roughly half spent time in a neonatal intensive care nursery. **Fig. 32.3a–c** (Case1) shows the auditory journey of a neonatal in-

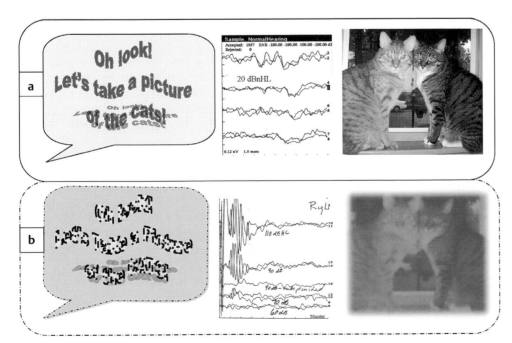

Fig. 32.2a,b **(a)** To the child with normal hearing, words stand out easily against modest amounts of noise and reverberation. Because auditory neurons are firing synchronously, the auditory "picture" retains details accurately enough for language learning. **(b)** The child with ANSD who has partial hearing receives a distorted signal with blurred edges between sounds. Without synchronous neural firing and without prior experience with the words, the child who is acquiring language can detect but not recognize or understand the utterance. Recognizing a blurred image depends upon having accurate sensory input during prior experiences with the nondistorted image. The use of the blurred image of the cats is a visual analogy, not intended to suggest blurred vision.

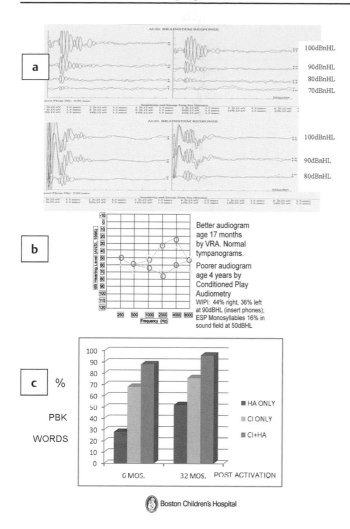

Fig. 32.3a–c Case 1 shows test results and outcome data from a child with a history of premature birth, neonatal complications, and cerebral palsy. **(a)** ABR tracings at age 4 months and 33 months. **(b)** Pure tone audiograms at age 17 months and 4 years. **(c)** Word recognition scores at 6 months and 32 months post left cochlear implant activation, with continued right hearing aid use. Cochlear implantation occurred at age 5 years.

How can a parent move forward without knowing whether the child will hear unassisted by technology, whether hearing aids will help, or whether cochlear implants are indicated? The audiologist is challenged to listen closely to parental observations, explain what is known and what the baby has yet to share over time, connect the parents to other families with children who have varying outcomes, enlist the parents as co-captains of their child's planning team, and develop a plan of action with parental buy-in to the importance of refining the plan based on the child's progress.

Pearl

- When a newborn presents with ANSD, the audiologist acknowledges with compassion the difficulty of receiving the diagnosis and begins to educate and enlist the parents as co-experts in observing responses, choosing and revising interventions, and monitoring progress, just as the audiologist should do for any child with a hearing loss. The specific prediction for the utility of hearing aids or cochlear implants, however, is postponed until the baby's audiogram and auditory-based language progress can be estimated.

---

tensive care unit (NICU) graduate with ANSD, partial hearing, and benefit from both a hearing aid and a cochlear implant.

As is the case with any newborn baby referred by screening, parents may not have had the opportunity to suspect their child's hearing disorder and may be shocked and confused by the diagnosis. Their confusion may be compounded by the audiologist's inability to describe the baby's auditory future. At our present level of ability to predict outcomes, test battery results consistent with ANSD in a newborn present the audiologist with a monumental counseling challenge. How can a parent accept that the audiologist cannot predict whether the child has sufficiently useful audition to support spoken language?

An interdisciplinary team approach is necessary to help the family keep the child's language development on target by planning timely interventions based on coordinated assessments. The audiologist and speech-language pathologist communicate closely so that the audiologist knows the receptive and expressive language status and modalities, as well as any changes tied to interventions like hearing aids. The otolaryngologist ensures that the middle ear status and inner-ear anatomy are assessed and determines whether there is a normal appearance of the cochlear nerves on magnetic resonance imaging (MRI), which is critical to know for predicting cochlear implant benefit (Huang, Roche, Buchman, & Castillo, 2010). The MRI may include the brain as well as the inner ears, to assist the neurologist in assessing the child's neurological status. Over time, the neurologist checks for signs of other peripheral neuropathies or concomitant conditions, such as Charcot-Marie-Tooth disease or Friedreich ataxia. Genetic workup may include clinically available tests for gene mutations known to be associated with the profile of audiological findings seen in ANSD—at this time, notably, mutations in the *OTOF* gene, which has an autosomal recessive pattern of inheritance and which codes for otoferlin, a protein that participates at the level of the inner hair cell synapse (Rodrígues-Ballesteros et al, 2008).

Table 32.1 Four clinical presentations of previously undiagnosed ANSD and suggested protocols

Group	Description	Test protocol	Counseling and management
1 and 2	Group 1: Newborn, referred by ABR screen Group 2: Infant or toddler, passed OAE screen but parent suspects hearing loss	• Record parental observations. • Otoscopy, tympanometry using 1000 Hz probe tone, MEMR, OAE. • ABR evaluation. When ABR thresholds to clicks are elevated, proceed to 90 dB nHL clicks, rarefaction and condensation series to observe CM. Intensity series 100–90–80–70–60 dB nHL, rarefaction and condensation, to observe threshold for CM and absence of latency-intensity function. At least one run is needed at a slowed stimulation rate < 20/sec at the weakest intensity at which the CM was seen, to see whether noninverting ABR waves emerge. • Repeat ABR, MEMR, and OAE at 3–6 months of age and at decision points, such as changes in language intervention strategies, hearing aid fitting, or cochlear implant candidacy • Behavioral audiometry by 6–8 months, then every 3 months to age 2 years, then every 6 months if stable. Use insert earphones and pulsed tones. For soundfield testing, use pulsed warbled tones and very quiet test background in the room (advise parent and audiology assistant not to vocalize). Note that narrowband noise may elicit responses at a weaker level than tones in ANSD, and soundfield thresholds may be better than either ear separately. • Separate-ear speech recognition testing when child is able. Note whether score improves at elevated versus conversational intensity for each ear. • Encourage use of functional listening evaluation as tool(s) by parents and early intervention provider.	• Monitor and discuss parental observations. • Counsel re: progressive assessment of auditory capacity, fostering auditory development, advisability of visual language. • Encourage parent-to-parent contacts. • Explain early intervention program options, the same as for infants with typical hearing loss. • Hearing aid fitting: Wait until behavioral thresholds of audibility can be estimated or established. Mild to severe audibility loss with OAEs present or absent: fit hearing aids (to targets). Exception: if audiogram has been improving, parent reports good responses, and OAEs are present, defer hearing aid fitting. • With or without hearing aids, try FM system to improve hearing in group/noise. • CI candidacy for those with mild to moderately severe loss depends on lack of sufficient hearing aid benefit and lack of sufficient progress in spoken language development. If OAEs remain robustly normal, observe potential improvement in functional hearing, behavioral audiogram, and possible development of synchronous ABR waves and MEMR particularly closely if cochlear implant candidacy is being considered • Profound loss, OAEs present or absent: confirm cochlear nerves present by MRI, prior to fitting hearing aids. • If cochlear nerves are present, counsel re: cochlear implant candidacy. If child never responds to sound, even during tests, consider not fitting hearing aids. If cochlear nerves are absent or severely dysplastic, counsel re: visual language and current status/outcomes of auditory brainstem implantation.

◆ Identification of ANSD after Newborn Screening

The presence of a CM or OAE with unilateral profound hearing loss often signals the presence of unilateral cochlear nerve dysplasia (Laury, Casey, McKay, & Germiller, 2009; Neault, Kenna, Prabhu, & Licameli, 2010), to be assessed by MRI. The OAEs and CM may disappear in time. Auditory management is the same as for a typical profound unilateral sensorineural hearing loss.

Although the most common path for an infant with ANSD to reach the audiologist is by not passing a newborn hearing screening test using automated

ABR, a second clinical presentation of ANSD is that of infants in the well-baby nursery who may have been screened or rescreened using only OAEs and passed the screen. Parents may, however, suspect hearing loss even before delayed language development can be observed and may bring the baby for audiological evaluation as an infant or toddler. The baby may be old enough for the parents to give a detailed description of auditory response patterns and to start with behavioral audiometric measures prior to the ABR. Parental observations can be extremely valuable in guiding the order of sounds to present during the behavioral audiological evaluation. One might start with a low-frequency stimulus if the child responds

Table 32.1 (*Continued*) Four clinical presentations of previously undiagnosed ANSD and suggested protocols

Group	Description	Test protocol	Counseling and management
Groups 3 and 4	Group 3: Older child, audiometrically hard of hearing, ANSD not previously diagnosed, aided benefit and spoken language development poorer than expected for degree of hearing loss Group 4: Persistent parental concern about hearing despite good hearing on pure tone audiograms, with speech and language delay (may include older child presenting with concerns about auditory processing or specific concerns about hearing in noise)	• Record history of parental observations of child's listening behavior with or without hearing aids. • Pure tone audiogram, speech recognition tests in quiet and noise. • Perform MEMR test to determine whether the MEMR is absent or elevated > 100 dB HL. • Perform OAE test. • Review past ABR. Repeat ABR to high-intensity clicks if the original ABR was not done in such a way as to observe a CM.	• Advise introduction of visual language for Group 3; possibly for Group 4 to boost reception, if spoken language ability insufficient. • Consider cochlear implantation if speech and language are delayed despite intensive intervention. • If hearing was better in the past and ANSD has developed, neurological exam is especially important.

All groups	• Acknowledge difficulty for parents in accepting confusing diagnosis and prognosis.
	• Referral to otolaryngologist, with consideration of:
	  – MRI to assess status of cochlear nerves and brain
	  – Referral to neurologist
	  – Referral for genetic testing
	  – Referral to ophthalmologist
	• Speech-language evaluation and monitoring.
	• Early consultation by team psychologist and/or teacher of the deaf re: raising a child with hearing disorder, communication options, need for support.
	• Provide handouts and guided Internet resources.
	• Educate early intervention provider(s) or teachers regarding ANSD and establish frequent communication with them.
	• Encourage language nurturing activities in quiet area with acoustic highlighting of spoken utterances.
	• Counsel that child is likely to hear speech poorly in noisy places and may act irritable in noisy places.
	• If early hearing aid trial failed, try hearing aids again later, especially if child has some word recognition skills that improve at high-intensity presentation level versus conversational intensity.
	• Revisit implant candidacy consideration frequently, particularly if hearing status is holding communication development back instead of pushing it forward (if hearing is not sufficient to meet the child's developmental needs).
	• Functional listening evaluation tools and watching (with parents) a recorded video sample of the child's language interaction can foster commitment to appropriate interventions.		

Abbreviations: ABR = auditory brainstem response, MEMR = middle ear muscle reflex, OAE = otoacoustic emissions, CM = cochlear microphonic, CI = cochlear implant.

better to male voices, or with a high-frequency stimulus if the child's best response at home is elicited by the hissing of a soda bottle opening or to a particular squeak toy. Separate-ear testing is the goal, but if sounds are presented in the soundfield, keeping the signals and reinforcement to one side (whichever way the child turns first) and keeping a very quiet background increases the chances of determining the child's thresholds of audibility.

A third way in which a child with ANSD may present to the audiologist is the preschool or school-aged child with hearing aids who baffles deaf educators because his speech recognition ability and auditory comprehension skills are poorer than would be predicted from his audiogram. This child's ANSD is easy to miss, because one might not consider doing an ABR for a child who can perform conditioned play audiometry. Presence of OAEs or absence of MEMRs would be clues to the ANSD, but OAEs may have disappeared and MEMRs may be absent due to the severity of the hearing loss or to myringotomy tubes. Careful questioning and review of past ABR waveforms should lead the way to the ANSD diagnosis in this type of case. The child may be able to lie still for a high-intensity click-evoked ABR without sedation. If a CM is observed without subsequent ABR waves, the diagnosis of ANSD is supported and the child's language development will be better understood and better served, and cochlear implant candidacy can be considered if an optimized hearing aid fitting and expert auditory therapy by a speech-language pathologist do not result in appropriate progress in spoken language development.

Pearl

- Watch not only the wiggly lines on the screen but also the child. Listen to the child. Watch the child listen. Listen to the parents and other caregivers. Is the child's hearing helping to push language development forward, or holding it back? Even a child with ANSD who receives some benefit from hearing aids and who has good expressive language skills may be frustrated by inability to understand speech outside, on the phone, in the car, and in a group; this child may prove to be a good candidate for the additional benefit provided by cochlear implantation.

The fourth way in which a child with ANSD may present to the audiologist is the child with a near-normal audiogram and difficulty hearing in noise. This child may appear with a question of central auditory processing disorder. A measurement that should be included in all auditory processing evaluations is the MEMR, as an absent MEMR with a near-normal audiogram would be a red flag for the need to evaluate the child for ANSD. If the child does prove to have present or past test results showing ANSD, it is possible that the child is one of the minority of children with ANSD whose hearing improves to a truly functional range, as did Case 3 and Case 4 in **Fig. 32.4a–e**.

Pitfall

- Never say "never" or "always" in the realm of ANSD. Early hypotheses that children with ANSD "never" benefit from hearing aids, "always" need a certain communication modality, or "always" have typical cochlear implant outcomes have crumbled with experience and evidence. Outcome predictions for children with ANSD who have known genetic mutations or electrocochleographic patterns should remain open for observations, pending further study.

◆ The Team Approach

The interdisciplinary team approach does not end after the radiological, genetic, and speech-language status have been explored, nor after a decision has been reached to use hearing aids or cochlear implants. On the contrary, children with ANSD continue to need interdisciplinary follow-up over time, particularly those with additional challenges. **Fig. 32.5** shows a child with ANSD who has spastic quadriparesis and good cognitive potential. He cannot speak or sign and needs frequent team interaction to maintain optimal seating for communication, to provide feedback to the audiologist that is needed to optimize his cochlear implant program, and to couple the output of his augmentative communication device to his cochlear implant processor.

While clinicians and parents thirst for guidelines (e.g., that children with ANSD and *OTOF* mutations will remain deaf and can be implanted very early, that those with a history of hyperbilirubinemia will show improved hearing over time, or that a child who has auditory nerves but has a postsynaptic site of lesion on electrocochleography could not benefit from a cochlear implant), clear links to outcome measures in these cases have yet to be forged. An issue needing creative attention is whether synchronous neuronal firing may be elicited only by some patches along the cochlear partition and not by others in some individuals, and if so, what these "live zones" mean for benefit from amplification.

The "black box" of the cochlea has opened to reveal ANSD as a variety of sensorineural hearing loss. With higher levels of investigations, varieties within ANSD may become better defined, each with its own signature test results and its own body of evidence to assist in counseling and intervention. Electrocochleography shows promise as a tool to distinguish presynaptic versus postsynaptic site of lesion in children with ANSD (McMahon, Patuzzi, Gibson, & Sanli, 2008). While logically one would predict that a child with ANSD who has a postsynaptic site of lesion may not benefit from a cochlear implant, sufficient outcome data do not exist to rule out candidacy for such a child. Cortical auditory evoked potentials (CAEPs), beginning to find their way into comprehensive pediatric audiology services, also show great promise to distinguish children with ANSD who have functional speech recognition ability and benefit from hearing aids from those who do not (Rance, Cone-Wesson, Wunderlich, & Dowell, 2002). Correlation of temporal processing measures, such as gap detection, should be explored as clinical measures related to speech perception outcomes, because individuals with ANSD have disrupted temporal processing with impaired detection of brief gaps in auditory stimulation (Zeng, Kong, Michalewski, & Starr, 2005).

Figure 32.4 (A-C). Case 2. Normalization of ABR waves following neonatal ANSD with peak bilirubin of 44.
A. CM with no ABR waves at age 2 weeks. OAEs were present.
B. CM remained unusually large at 17 months but ABR had developed.
C. At 17 months, clear ABR responses to clicks and tone bursts at 20dBnHL were present. Child responsive to sound but localized poorly.

Figure 32.4 (D-E). Case 3. ABR at 2 months (**D**) and audiogram at 6 years (**E**) for a child whose older sibling showed a similar pattern. Neither required newborn intensive care. Both had robust OAEs; acoustic reflexes and word recognition developed over time. Each has the same two novel mutations in the otoferlin (OTOF, DFNB9) gene.

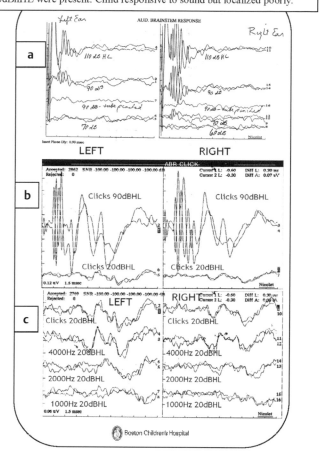

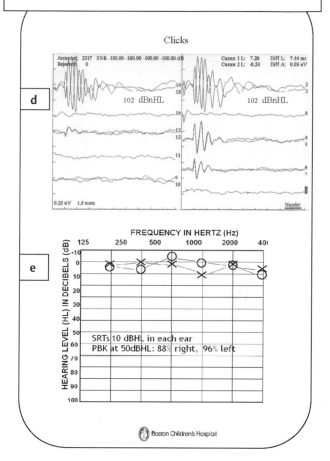

Fig. 32.4a–e Development of functional audition after findings of ANSD in infancy. The left column **(a–c)** shows Case 2, an infant with hyperbilirubinemia. Initial results **(a)** showed a pattern consistent with ANSD. Subsequent ABR at 17 months showed clear repeatable responses to clicks and to tone bursts at 4000, 2000, and 1000 Hz at 20 dB nHL. Functional hearing ability without hearing aids or cochlear implants could be predicted with confidence on the basis of the ABR results in **(b)** and **(c)**. The right column shows Case 3, a child with an initially absent ABR, prominent CM and OAEs, and absent MEMRs, who developed a normal audiogram, MEMRs, and speech recognition ability over time.

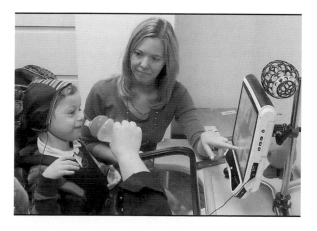

Fig. 32.5 Example of teamwork needed to foster communication in a child with ANSD and other challenges, representing many NICU graduates. This 3-year-old boy has a history of premature birth, hypoxemia, twin-to-twin transfusion, and ANSD. He has functional word recognition ability using a right cochlear implant. Unable to speak, sign, or point because of cerebral palsy, he has requested "drink" using eye gaze technology from picture choices on the computer screen. The audio output of the augmentative communication device is connected by a cable to his cochlear implant processor, which is under his cap. Two speech-language pathologists, an occupational therapist, and an audiologist participate routinely in his care. (Photo courtesy of Center for Communication Enhancement, Boston Children's Hospital.)

The nonauditory developmental challenges faced by some intensive care nursery graduates with ANSD, along with multicultural backgrounds, linguistic diversity, and socioeconomic disparities, do complicate the plan of care, as for children with typical sensorineural hearing loss. However, the available test protocols, bulk of experience, and outcome data for children with ANSD should give the audiologist competence and confidence in guiding families and supporting these children to achieve good language skills.

Discussion Questions

1. What diagnostic tests and observations are required to elicit a diagnosis of ANSD?

2. A three-year-old comes to see a pediatric audiologist for an audiologic evaluation. What factors would lead you to suspect a possible ANSD diagnosis for this child?

3. What are the roles and responsibilities of the professionals involved in managing children who have a diagnosis of ANSD?

4. When would you consider moving a child with ANSD from a hearing aid to a cochlear implant?

5. What school services might a child with ANSD require?

References

Beauchaine, K. A., Kaminski, J. R., & Gorga, M. P. (1987). Comparison of Beyer DT48 and Etymotic insert earphones: auditory brain stem response measurements. Ear and Hearing, 8(5), 292–297.

Berlin, C. I., Bordelon, J., St John, P., Wilensky, D., Hurley, A., Kluka, E., & Hood, L. J. (1998). Reversing click polarity may uncover auditory neuropathy in infants. Ear and Hearing, 19(1), 37–47.

Bill Daniels Center for Children's Hearing. (2008). Guidelines for identification and management of infants and young children with auditory neuropathy spectrum disorder. Aurora, CO: Children's Hospital Colorado.

Calandruccio, L., Fitzgerald, T. S., & Prieve, B. A. (2006). Normative multifrequency tympanometry in infants and toddlers. Journal of the American Academy of Audiology, 17(7), 470–480.

Huang, B. Y., Roche, J. P., Buchman, C. A., & Castillo, M. (2010). Brain stem and inner ear abnormalities in children with auditory neuropathy spectrum disorder and cochlear nerve deficiency. AJNR. American Journal of Neuroradiology, 31(10), 1972–1979.

Kemp, D. T. (1978). Stimulated acoustic emissions from within the human auditory system. The Journal of the Acoustical Society of America, 64(5), 1386–1391.

Laury, A. M., Casey, S., McKay, S., & Germiller, J. A. (2009). Etiology of unilateral neural hearing loss in children. International Journal of Pediatric Otorhinolaryngology, 73(3), 417–427.

McMahon, C. M., Patuzzi, R. B., Gibson, W. P., & Sanli, H. (2008). Frequency-specific electrocochleography indicates that presynaptic and postsynaptic mechanisms of auditory neuropathy exist. Ear and Hearing, 29(3), 314–325.

Neault, M., Kenna, M., Prabhu, S., & Licameli, G. (2010). Unilateral ANSD: audiological and radiological findings. Podium presentation, American Academy of Audiology, Annual Convention, Featured Session, April 16, 2010. In preparation, 2012.

Rance, G., Roper, R., Symons, L., Moody, L. J., Poulis, C., Dourlay, M., & Kelly, T. (2005). Hearing threshold estimation in infants using auditory steady-state responses. Journal of the American Academy of Audiology, 16(5), 291–300.

Rance, G., Cone-Wesson, B., Wunderlich, J., & Dowell, R. (2002). Speech perception and cortical event related potentials in children with auditory neuropathy. Ear and Hearing, 23(3), 239–253.

Rodríguez-Ballesteros, M., Reynoso, R., Olarte, M., Villamar, M., Morera, C., Santarelli, R., . . . del Castillo, I. (2008). A multicenter study on the prevalence and spectrum of mutations in the otoferlin gene (OTOF) in subjects with nonsyndromic hearing impairment and auditory neuropathy. Human Mutation, 29(6), 823–831.

Roush, P., Frymark, T., Venediktov, R., & Wang, B. (2011). Audiologic management of auditory neuropathy spectrum disorder in children: a systematic review of the literature. American Journal of Audiology, 20(2), 159–170.

Starr, A., Picton, T. W., Sininger, Y., Hood, L. J., & Berlin, C. I. (1996). Auditory neuropathy. Brain, 119(Pt 3), 741–753.

Worthington, D. W., & Peters, J. F. (1980). Quantifiable hearing and no ABR: paradox or error? Ear and Hearing, 1(5), 281–285.

Zeng, F.-G., Kong, Y.-Y., Michalewski, H. J., & Starr, A. (2005). Perceptual consequences of disrupted auditory nerve activity. Journal of Neurophysiology, 93(6), 3050–3063.

Chapter 33

Working with Multicultural and Multilingual Families of Young Children with Hearing Loss

Ellen A. Rhoades

Key Points

- Prejudices negatively affect the children we serve.
- A multicultural outlook pervades the delivery of all clinical services.
- Audiologists strive to develop an effective alliance with parents.
- Each child is actively encouraged to learn the language spoken at home.
- Interpreters are chosen with care.
- Audiologists learn about each child's family culture.
- With parent commitment and consistent boundaries, children with hearing loss can become bilingual.

During the last decade of the 20th and the first decade of the 21st centuries, immigration trends created dramatic changes in developed countries (Migration Policy Institute, 2006); this phenomenon has significantly influenced services provided by audiologists and other auditory-based practitioners. A traditional family in Anglo-Western culture had a dual-parent egalitarian structure stereotypically defined by the self-sufficient family's individualistic, competitive nature (Foster et al, 2003), but social changes have resulted in minority groups collectively becoming the majority in some parts of Anglo-Western countries (Maines, Abbady, & Benedick, 2006). Profound family-related changes have occurred with respect to women in the labor force, living arrangements, social expectations, and cultural values (Farrell, VandeVusse, & Ocobock, 2012; Gibson-Davis & Gassman-Pines, 2010). Approximately half of America's children younger than 5 years are currently considered racial or ethnic minorities (U.S. Census Bureau, 2009), and that segment is rapidly increasing. Consequently, there is no dominant form against which families can now be measured or judged; family diversity is the 21st century norm (Baca Zinn & Eitzen, 2004; Farrell et al, 2012).

Racism still prevails within majority Anglo-Western countries, negatively affecting children of color (Dunn, 2003; Lemos, 2005; Shifrer, Muller, & Callahan, 2011). Stereotypes drive prejudices, which cause discrimination that is unjustified or harmful behavior (Rhoades, 2010a, 2010b). Even when implicit, racism has a deleterious effect on the health, education, and psychosocial growth of children (Caughy, Nettles, O'Campo, & Lohrfink, 2006; Guarino, Buddin, Pham, & Cho, 2010; McKenzie, 2003; Tyler, Boykin, & Walton, 2006). On the whole, Anglo-Western cultures, including America, still tend to be disrespectful of diversity (Stepanova & Strube, 2012; Vasquez & Wetzel, 2009).

And yet, multiculturalism, a social, intellectual, and moral movement, is an ethical force based on the goals of inclusion, social justice, and mutual respect (Fowers & Davidov, 2006). As such, multiculturalism is extraordinarily influential in psychology, child development, education, and various allied health professions (Hwang, 2006; Todd & Galinsky, 2012; Tyler, Boykin, & Walton, 2006). Linguistic, religious, racial, ethnic, and socioeconomic characteristics of each family have direct relevance to understanding specific domains of child development (Hughes et al, 2006; Kraus, Piff, & Keltner, 2011). Such characteristics influence adult–child interactions, the way children are raised and educated, and long-term goals for them (Cabrera, Shannon, West, & Brooks-Gunn, 2006; Cosier & Causton-Theoharis, 2011; Gibson-Davis & Gassman-Pines, 2010; Halgunseth, Ispa, & Rudy, 2006; Rodriguez & Olswang, 2003). Moreover, the ways that children play, socialize, learn, problem solve, communicate, and perceive the world are culturally grounded (Cole, Tamang, & Shrestha, 2006; Goneu, Mistry, & Mosier, 2000; Kobayashi, Glover, & Temple, 2006; Nisbett & Miyamoto, 2005; Qi, Kaiser, Marley, & Milan, 2011; Suzuki & Aronson, 2003; Tudge et al, 2006). When practitioners better understand cultural differences, miscommunications and overrepresentation of minority students receiving special services are likely to decrease (Crago, Eriks-Brophy, Pesco, & McAlpine, 1997).

Family relationships are dramatically altered in single-parent households, within financially impoverished families, and in those families whose children have disabilities (Naseef, 2001; Powers, Elliott, Patterson, Shaw, & Taylor, 1995). At least 10% of parents and their children have at least one disability. Children with disabilities are more likely to live with single women (Cohen & Petrescu-Prahova, 2006). Some parents are unemployed or in poor health; some children are abused or have many special needs. Nearly three quarters of America's children live in low-income or impoverished families, mostly with at least one employed parent. The majority of these children live in single-parent households, most of them children of color younger than 6 years of age (Chau, 2006). Young children from impoverished homes are at greater risk of having delays in communication and other behaviors (Guarino et al, 2010; Koblinsky, Kuvalanka, & Randolph, 2006; Nelson, Welsh, Trup, & Greenberg, 2011; Peterson et al, 2011; Watamura, Phillips, Morrissey, McCartney, & Bub, 2011), which, in turn, affect academic performance (Schiff & Lotem, 2011).

A review of the literature indicates that diagnosis of hearing loss in a child confers parental stress in just about any family (Phillips, Worley, & Rhoades, 2010). Unfortunately, minority status accorded to any family that includes a child with hearing loss places all its family members at even greater risk (Solem, Christophersen, & Martinussen, 2011; Wilkens, 2009). Data show that families of children with hearing loss are more likely to report poorer health status, have Medicaid, live in single-mother households, and reside below the poverty level (Boss, Niparko, Gaskin, & Levinson, 2011). Moreover, children with cochlear implants in families of low socioeconomic backgrounds tend to have higher rates of postoperative complications, worse follow-up compliance, and lower rates of bilateral implantation (Chang, Ko, Murray, Arnold, & Megerian, 2010). Audiologists report that socioeconomic status seems to affect speech and language outcomes with children who received cochlear implants (Kirkham et al, 2009).

In spite of the trend toward multicultural families in American schools, audiologists and other practitioners serving families and their children with hearing loss remain overwhelmingly white English-speakers from traditional Anglo-Western culture (American Speech-Language-Hearing Association [ASHA], 2008; Rhoades, Price, & Perigoe, 2004). Although there have been concerted nationwide efforts in culturally sensitizing practitioners since the last decade of the 20th century (Dennis & Giangreco, 1996; Lynch & Hanson, 1992; Sanchez, 1995), the reality is that diversity continues to present considerable challenges.

Pediatric audiologists and other practitioners strive to provide *family-centered* services (Kargina, 2004; Rhoades, 2010c), necessitating the development of skills to optimally meet the needs of diverse learners within diverse family contexts. To accomplish this level of intervention, it follows that audiologists must be knowledgeable and supportive of many family systems, cultures, and languages. Audiologists must first value diversity that is free from intolerance for people of varied cultural and financial backgrounds as well as different sexual orientations and persons with disabilities. Only then can the strengths of each child's family be viewed as cultural capital (Woodrow, 2001); a deficit perspective is untenable.

Following is a discussion of three steps that practitioners can take to develop a minimal level of competency in diversity: engage in introspection, adopt a family systems approach, and make a commitment to diversity.

◆ Step 1: Engage in Introspection

The initial step toward developing a minimal level of competency in diversity necessitates that audiologists first look within to better understand themselves, and to strive toward becoming nonjudgmental with all individuals from minority groups. Overcoming implicit racial biases and cultural attitudes requires that we first understand these attitudes for what they are (Dunham, Baron, & Banaji, 2006). Diversity-sensitive counseling challenges us to confront personal fears, myths, stereotypes, faulty assumptions, and negative attitudes and to redefine whiteness and the Eurocentric perspective (Watt, Maio, Rees, & Hewstone, 2006). Awareness of our ignorance and subconscious beliefs can, in turn, cause us to be vigilant and to consciously refuse to act on them. An ongoing concerted effort, facilitated by knowledge and understanding, must be made to develop tolerance.

Beyond self-analysis, interracial contact can be highly effective for reducing inherent biases (McGlothlin & Killen, 2006). Audiologists are encouraged to actively seek minority individuals to inquire about issues that directly bear on inherent biases. For example, to understand others' experiences better, ask people of different races and cultures what racism means to them. Shadow a minority child for at least a school day (Almarza, 2005). Read books by and about minority persons. Attend local cultural festivals and other celebratory events as well as those places of worship frequented by minority families (Rhoades et al, 2004).

Pitfall

- A professional's inherent racial biases and cultural misperceptions can negatively affect the delivery of services.

◆ Step 2: Adopt a Family Systems Approach

The second step toward developing a minimal level of competency in diversity is for audiologists to develop a family systems perspective (Rambo, Rhoades, Boyd, & Bello, 2010). Family systems theory has to do with the complex interrelationships and negotiations of each family member with others. An invisible web of complementary demands and expectations regulates family behavior (Rhoades, 2010d). The family provides the primary context in which to view the young child who inhabits that context along with other social factors; all are products and producers of culture (Tudge et al, 2000).

It is helpful when core terminology pertaining to the dynamics of family relationships is understood (Christian, 2006; Kaczmarek, 2006). Reading a basic textbook on family systems theory can enable audiologists to at least recognize families that are clearly dysfunctional so that appropriate referrals to family therapists can be made (Graham, 2004; Minuchin & Fishman, 2004; Walker & Akister, 2004). Moreover, when audiologists are able to implement simple family-supportive strategies, optimizing child potential and minimizing the secondary effects of hearing loss are more likely to occur (Rhoades, 2010d). Alternately stated, it is essential that audiologists demonstrate counseling competence during their interactions with caregivers; facilitating positive change mandates good counseling skills.

There are many simple strategies that audiologists can incorporate into their communications with the child's caregivers. One very effective strategy is that of *mimicry*, also known as mimesis, because it tends to facilitate families' perceiving practitioners as being allies (Leighton, Bird, Orsini, & Heyes, 2010; Stel & Harinck, 2011), and practitioners are more likely to empathize with a family (Inzlicht, Gutsell, & Legault, 2012). Mimicry occurs when an audiologist, while addressing a family, adopts that family's language level, mannerisms, communicative style, speech patterns, and familial colloquialisms; practitioners mimic appropriate behaviors (Kavanagh, Suhler, Churchland, & Winkielman, 2011; Leander, Chartrand, & Bargh, 2012). When the practitioner conforms to the family's affective range, joining the family system and mutual rapport tend to occur (Bailenson & Yee, 2005; Graham, 2004; Robbins and Szapocznik, 2000; van Baaren, Holland, Steenaert, & van Knippenberg, 2003). Developing trustworthy practitioner–parent collaborations benefits children with hearing loss; this involves identifying parents as experts on their children (Kummerer, 2012),

Financially impoverished at-risk families are likely to be driven by survival above and beyond any special needs, and they typically need a much stronger supportive network (Rhoades et al, 2004). Given that multicultural families are part of this mix, a huge variety of childrearing practices presents to audiologists, who must then seek an even wider base of practitioner and community collaboration. Services for these families are more frequent and intensive as well as more convenient for them—all without sacrificing the quality of services being delivered. It is important that service providers reflect greater diversity of disciplines as well as cultural backgrounds. More attention is given to facilitating parental self-efficacy; this includes expanding the parental knowledge base and providing them with a culturally similar peer support network as well as improving dyadic communications within the family system (Kirkham et al, 2009; Bernstein & Eriks-Brophy, 2010). Data show that many effects of financial impoverishment on children are mitigated when the support of extended families and peers are enlisted (Lees, Stackhouse, & Grant, 2009; Wager et al, 2010).

◆ Step 3: Make a Commitment to Diversity

Beyond developing an awareness of and sensitivity to cultural differences, effective audiologists operatively demonstrate cultural responsiveness (Association for Supervision and Curriculum Development, 2006). Just as there are differences in learning assumptions and principles between cultures (Woodrow, 2001), teaching strategies that are believed to promote learning in children from the Anglo-Western culture do not necessarily result in greater gains among children from minority cultures (Kolobe, 2004). Viewpoints as to whether audiologists and other practitioners are guardians of knowledge or facilitators of learning are culturally based.

As soon as all minority groups and languages represented in a possible caseload are identified, a pool of consultants and trained peer advocates from minority groups is established (Turner & Lynas, 2000). Be nonjudgmental and show empathy when listening to parents; try to see the world as they see it. Communication obstacles are often culturally controlled and not in one's normal awareness. For example, before informing parents of a child's hearing loss, culturally responsive audiologists inquire about each family's belief system regarding disabilities (Salas-Provance, Erickson, & Reed, 2002). Learning about each child's family background can affect choice of words in speech perception assessments; for example, some immigrant children might not understand football, but those same children might understand soccer.

Furthermore, audiologists and other practitioners who provide culturally relevant services can facilitate multicultural knowledge among all families, including those who are Anglo-Western. In addition to promoting interracial contact (Rutland, Cameron, Bennett, & Ferrell, 2005), a simple technique for reducing prejudice and developing appreciation of diversity includes the consciously consistent use of pictures and availability of children's books that positively feature children of color and multicultural folklore and holidays (Cameron, Rutland, Brown, & Douch, 2006). Children and their families are more likely to thrive when practitioners demonstrate cross-cultural competence in how they think, feel, and behave. Ultimately, audiologists and other practitioners understand that the goal of becoming sensitive and knowledgeable across many cultures is a lifelong quest.

◆ Anchor Language Differences

Language, a culturally based activity (Genesee, Paradis, & Crago, 2004), serves as an anchor for family cohesion, facilitates literacy, promotes bilingualism (Macrory, 2006), and influences human interactions (Chen, Kennedy, & Zhou, 2012). Early auditory exposure to the mother tongue is critical for the development of speech perception (Kuhl, 2010). The home language should be the child's native language (Kohnert, Yim, Nett, Kan, & Duran, 2005). When parents communicate with their young children in a language in which they do not feel comfortable, the child's language experiences are more restricted and emotional distancing can occur, which, in turn, affects the child's social cognition and executive capacities (Chen et al, 2012). Young children who have a strong grounding in their home language tend to perform better in school (Dunbar, 2009). Furthermore, abandoning a heritage language may have extensive personal, familial, religious, cultural, and academic implications that prove unfavorable for the child (Tabors, 1997; Eilers, Pearson, & Cobo-Lewis, 2006).

Approximately one fifth of America's population speaks a language other than English at home (Shin & Kominski, 2010). According to a recent survey, many practitioners do not feel competent when working with linguistic minorities (Guiberson & Atkins, 2012). Although language interpreters are used more frequently than in past decades, they are used with less confidence. Assessment challenges primarily involved a shortage of appropriate assessment tools as well as a lack of normative information about language development in linguistically diverse children (Guiberson & Atkins, 2012).

Assessing performance in the child's home language can be problematic if no normative-referenced standardized tests are available in that language (Peña & Halle, 2011). A parent report instrument that is available in several languages (e.g., Fenson et al, 1993), a culturally anchored parent–child interaction assessment (e.g., Bernstein, Harris, Long, Iida, & Hans, 2005), as well as developmental scales of functional communication can be used to monitor language progress and serve as yardsticks for typical development. Norm-referenced language assessment scores translated from English are invalid; thus, they should not be used as the basis for a child's Family Service or Individual Education Plan (IEP), but they can be used as approximate guidelines to gather information along with the use of informal language samples and parent reports. When necessary, an interpreter can translate a test in advance and provide assistance in implementing alternative assessment procedures (Laing & Kamhi, 2003). All modifications, including use of an interpreter, are important to note when reporting test outcomes.

◆ Interpreters

Because most practitioners in America speak only English (ASHA, 2008; Rhoades et al, 2004), the great linguistic diversity caused by the demographic shift of the past two decades results in daunting challenges for most audiologists and other practitioners. Although family members are often used as interpreters when professional interpreters are unavailable, using them, especially children, in this capacity, is not a good idea, because real and potential family biases and relationships can negatively affect the audiologic session.

If children with hearing loss are to be optimally served, interpreters are needed for parents who speak another language (Karliner, Jacobs, Chen, & Mutha, 2007; Moreno & Morales, 2010). When enlisting the assistance of an interpreter, try to use the same one for the same family so that an ongoing relationship can be developed. Interpreters are selected for a variety of attributes, including honesty, reliability, neutrality, confidentiality, cultural proficiency, and consistency in availability. These are in addition to the highly critical attribute of bilingual proficiency (Tzou, Eslami, Chen, & Vaid, 2012). Ideally, interpreters are of the same ethnicity as that of the family and are also familiar with the family's heritage culture (Turner & Lynas, 2000); cultural and language concordance are of the essence.

Before using interpretive services, the audiologist meets with the interpreter to reiterate the need for confidentiality, to gain rapport, and to set some ground rules, such as the provision of exact translations for parents. Interpreters are advised to avoid gestures and other cues that could unfairly assist the child during administration of audiologic tests. Audiologists spend a few minutes orienting interpreters to the subject matter, procedures, and goals of audiologic services and to review all technical terms. These consultations, completed prior to meeting with child or family, also involve discussion of the relevance of materials and language expressions to be used. Interpreters are asked to speak in the first person and to carry a notepad so that they can take notes as needed. Interpreters are encouraged to ask questions when they are unsure of a term or phrase that was used. Interpreters are also encouraged to project clearly and to mirror the audiologist's overall tone and vocal stresses. Finally, interpreters are advised to refrain from engaging in tangent dialogues with families and from attempting to serve as advocates or mediators in the practitioner–parent dialogue.

During each actual interpreted session, the audiologist faces parents while talking to them; the interpreter is asked to sit next to and slightly behind the audiologist, so that parents are more likely to make eye contact with the audiologist (Lopez, 2002). Audiologists make concerted efforts to avoid using slang, idioms, and metaphors while casually monitoring the process of interpreting, particularly watching that interpreters do not appear to be offering their own thoughts to parents.

Subsequent to each meeting with child or family, the audiologist has a debriefing session with the interpreter. The primary purpose of each post-treatment session is to ensure that the interpreter's perceptions are shared with the audiologist. The audiologist reviews notes and progress, discussing any interpreting issues with the interpreter. In short, the time and effort expended by audiologists in learning how to use interpreters effectively can reap great benefits for families and their children (McEvoy, Santos, Marzan, Green, & Milan, 2009).

◆ Caregiver Intake Interview

From the outset, there needs to be a framework of information relevant to audiologic diagnosis and treatment that involves ascertaining the family's cultural and linguistic status as well as identifying the com-

municative style within the family system (Hughes et al, 2006). The best place to observe a child's proficiency in the home language is within the context of the home, where the child is most comfortable and can interact with family members. At the very least, the audiologist who does not speak the child's home language can observe the family's communicative style in the office or waiting room, noting fluency and variety of communication skills used by child and caregivers.

During the interview process, regardless of whether an interpreter is present, the audiologist demonstrates warmth while initially avoiding prolonged eye or physical contact. In a trustworthy, compassionate, and personable manner, both closed-ended and open-ended questions are asked of caregivers, using sufficient pauses to enable them time to think and respond (Rhoades, 2007).

Pearl
• Language is rooted in culture. Diversity is good.

◆ Learning a Second Spoken Language

Bilingualism, referring to proficient conversational fluency in at least two languages, is a treasured asset for child, family, and society. Bilingualism easily confers many advantages on children and adults that include improved spoken language processing, attention, working memory, and many other cognitive capacities (Barac & Bialystok, 2012; Bialystok, Craik, & Luk, 2012; Hernández, Costa, & Humphreys, 2012; Kroll, Dussias, Bogulski, & Kroff, 2012; Tsukada, 2012). Alternatively, conceptual knowledge and skills transfer across languages (Naqvi et al, 2012). When bilingual children discover commonalities and differences in two languages, they tend to have improved phonological awareness in comparison to monolingual children (Naqvi, McKeough, Thorne, & Pfitscher, 2012). Bilingualism changes how the brain processes sound; hence, it facilitates perceptual learning (Krizman, Marian, Shook, Skoe, & Kraus, 2012; Wattendorf et al, 2012; Werker, 2012). Furthermore, bilingualism facilitates multicultural understanding (López, 2012). On a global level, bilingualism is the rule rather than the exception. All languages are equal; that is, no one spoken language is harder for children to learn than another (Pearson, 2007).

When two learned languages are spoken, it is referred to as *unimodal bilingualism*; this, in turn, means that both languages are typically perceived through the auditory sense (Emmorey, Borinstein,

Thompson, & Gollan, 2008). Early auditory exposure to home and second languages is important for the development of bilingualism (Tsai, Park, Liu, & Lau, 2012) as well as speech perception (Dietrich, Swingley, & Werker, 2007; Montrul & Foote, 2012).

The notion that confusion or delays occur when typically hearing children learn two languages at the same time is a myth (Petitto, 2006). When children learn two languages during the first 3 years of life, the process is known as simultaneous bilingualism or bilingual first-language acquisition (Genesee and Nicoladis, 2009). Although young bilingual children typically engage in some language mixing, it is quite normal and transitory, soon stabilizing into what is called code switching, which, more often than not, involves nouns (Holowka, Brosseau-Lapre, & Petitto 2002). This often serves social and discourse functions that include the signaling of topic changes, establishing linguistic proficiency, and creating identity or cultural emphasis (Zentella, 1997). This language mixing is rule-governed and responsive to nonlinguistic social requirements in bilingual conversations (Holowka et al, 2002; Petitto et al, 2001; Yumoto, 1996).

A critical realization is that, within English-majority countries, the key to raising bilingual children is in establishing the minority language (Pearson, 2007; Eilers et al, 2006). Quality and quantity of minority home language use as well as home literacy resources, such as effective use of dual-language children's books, are predictors of successful bilingualism (Quiroz, Snow, & Zhao, 2010; Naqvi et al, 2012). Furthermore, children speaking minority languages are better served when school environments and intervention programs support each parent-child minority language (Quiroz & Dixon, 2012).

The number of American children with hearing loss being raised in homes where a minority language is spoken is increasing from year to year (Gallaudet Research Institute, 2011); there is a great need for more detailed recordkeeping with these children for purposes of planning intervention and developing inclusion strategies (Mahon et al, 2011). Many children with hearing loss and consistent access to soft conversational sound as a result of hearing technology can become unimodally bilingual; that is, they can become conversationally fluent in at least two spoken languages to a degree approximating that of typically hearing peers (Francis & Ho, 2003; Guiberson, 2005; Phillips, 1999; Rhoades, 2009a; Rhoades, Perusse, Douglas, & Zarate, 2008; Thomas, El-Kashlan, & Zwolan, 2008; Waltzman, Robbins, Green, & Cohen, 2003). However, there are also data showing that some children with hearing loss do not benefit from unimodal bilingualism; some perform worse in spoken language than do monolingual children with hearing loss (Boons et al, 2012; Teschendorf, Janeschik, Bagus, Lang, & Arweiler-Harbeck, 2011). Communication mode and variables within the home,

school, and community influence whether or not bilingualism can be attained (Dixon, Zhao, Quiroz, & Shin, 2012; Yim, 2012).

The younger the child, the more likely progress in learning English will be rapid (Petitto, 2006). However, it is imperative that the home language be continuously valued and strengthened; this is important for social and emotional growth and has benefits for intellectual growth as well (Pearson, 2007). Learning one language system can provide a template for a second spoken language; likewise, promoting literacy development in the child's first language can facilitate second-language learning (Naqvi et al, 2012). With sufficient linguistic input in both languages from caregivers and clear linguistic or situational boundaries between school and home, the young child can become fluent in two languages prior to kindergarten.

Special Consideration

- Parents' commitment must be active and consistent to have their bilingual child retain a minority language over time.

Second-language learning by children older than 3 years is known as the sequential or successive bilingual process. Undoubtedly, increasing age upon initiation of learning a second language necessitates greater commitment and effort from school and primary caregivers (Pearson, 2007). Moreover, the older the child when learning a second language, the less likely that the child will speak the second language like a native (Kuhl, Tsao, & Liu, 2003). However, that difficulty does not preclude having bilingualism as a goal for children taking advantage of optimal hearing technology.

Conversational fluency in any spoken language does not necessarily mean the child is ready for academic learning in that language. Typically, children need to master a language at least at the 4-year age equivalency level before they can begin grade school academic learning (Rhoades, 2003). Academic learning will best occur in the child's dominant language. If at all possible, it is important to assess the child in both English and the home language, even when one seems clearly more dominant than the other (Thordardottir, 2006). If the home language remains the child's dominant language, the child may be best served in a bilingual class or dual-language school where code switching is encouraged (Macrory, 2006).

There are some circumstances, however, when initiating the process toward bilingualism may not be an appropriate goal for older children with hearing loss. Neither the child's age nor the intelligence quotient are the decisive variables. Instead, much depends on these critical factors: (1) the child's accessibility to soft conversational sound; (2) the level of consistently effective support of primary caregivers toward facilitating bilingualism; (3) the presence of significant neurophysiologic dysfunction; and (4) the intactness of the child's working memory (Ardila, 2003; Swanson, Sáez, & Gerber, 2006).

Controversial Point

- A child with profound deafness can simultaneously learn two spoken languages.

Second-spoken-language learners, particularly those engaged in the sequential bilingual process, may have greater difficulty listening in noisy environments (Mayo, Florentine, & Buus, 1997; Nelson, Welsh, Trup, & Greenberg, 2005; van Wijngaarden, Steeneken, & Houtgast, 2002; van Wijngaarden, 2001). Therefore, audiologists and other practitioners working with these children take special care to minimize classroom noise and to ensure the availability of effective assistive hearing technologies that improve access to spoken language.

◆ Becoming Bimodal Bilingual

Families with deaf parents may use a signed language such as American Sign Language (ASL) as their primary home language. Bimodal bilinguals—those who know both a signed and spoken language—represent a considerably less explored form of bilingualism. Instead of code switching, bimodal bilingual children typically produce code blends; that is, simultaneously produced spoken and signed words (van den Bogaerde & Baker, 2006; Emmorey et al, 2008). Code blending seems to occur more often with verbs rather than nouns, which tend to differ in combinatorial structure (Emmorey at al, 2008). Some code blending may persist into adulthood (Bishop & Hicks, 2005).

Although there are relatively sparse data pertaining to bimodal bilingualism, it may confer neurobiological advantages, such as improved executive capacities (Kushalnagar, Hannay, & Hernandez, 2010), similar to those conferred upon unimodal bilingual children. However, there are equivocal data as to whether bimodal bilingual children attain a degree of literacy commensurate with typically hearing peers (Marschark & Spencer, 2005; Mayer & Akamatsu, 2003). Learning a spoken language via the printed word may not be a sufficient route to either literacy or spoken language mastery (Mayer & Leigh, 2010). It

remains debatable whether most bimodal bilingual children with hearing loss can attain literacy, particularly if they have typically hearing parents (Swanwick & Watson, 2005).

For young children in the process of learning spoken language, evidence is lacking that learning ASL facilitates the acquisition of spoken language (Nittrouer, 2008). Recent data indicate that infants with hearing loss may find speech perception more difficult when signs are presented simultaneously (Ting, Bergeson, & Miyamoto, 2012). Moreover, accumulating data show that, over the long term, bimodal bilingual children with access to soft conversational sound tend not to perform as well in speech perception (Geers, 2002; Jiménez, Pino, & Herruzo, 2009; Kos, Deriaz, Guyot, & Pelizzone, 2009; Sarant, Blamey, Dowell, Clark, & Gibson, 2001), speech production (Dillon, Pisoni, Cleary, & Carter, 2004; Geers et al, 2002; Jiménez et al 2009; Tobey, Rekart, Buckley, & Geers, 2004), and spoken language (Geers, Nicholas, & Sedey, 2003; Jiménez et al, 2009; Nittrouer, 2009) as do those relying exclusively on spoken language and similar access to soft conversational sound. Such findings seem to occur regardless of whether implantation occurred during toddlerhood (Nittrouer, 2009), across childhood (Tobey et al, 2004), or in adolescence (Caposecco, Hickson, & Pedley, 2012; Kos et al, 2009). Furthermore, subsequent to cochlear implantation, changing from a signed language to a spoken one may be difficult (Kos et al, 2009). In addition, risk of academic delay may be greater in bimodal bilingual children (Nittrouer, 2009; Venail, Vieu, Artieres, Mondain, & Uziel, 2010).

It is widely understood that many children with hearing loss have additional special needs with compromised learning capacities (Edwards & Crocker, 2008; Rhoades, 2009b). Already at risk for relative efficiency in learning one spoken language (Cruz et al., 2012; Gérard et al, 2010; Britz, Fry, & Owston, 2010), these children are at greater risk for not learning two languages, spoken and/or signed (Boons et al, 2012; Nittrouer, 2009; Venail et al, 2010). If children with complex needs are learning a signed language at home and will eventually receive a cochlear implant with the hopes of transitioning to a spoken language, they may benefit the most from learning Signing Exact English (Rhoades, 2011). There are insufficient data pertaining to languageless children simultaneously learning two languages after three years of age and then becoming conversationally fluent in both languages, regardless of whether the languages are signed or spoken.

Children with typical hearing who grow up in homes where ASL is the primary language will hear the language of the larger community and typically become natural bimodal bilingual communicators (Petitto & Kovelman, 2003), often translating for their parents. However, children with severe to pro-

Geers, A. E., Nicholas, J. G., & Sedey, A. L. (2003). Language skills of children with early cochlear implantation. Ear and Hearing, 24(1, Suppl), 46S–58S.

Genesee, F., & Nicoladis, E. (2009). Bilingual first language acquisition. In E. Hoff & M. Shatz (Eds.), Blackwell handbook of language development (pp. 324–341). Oxford, UK: Wiley-Blackwell.

Genesee, F., Paradis, J., & Crago, M. B. (2004). Dual language development and disorders. Baltimore, MD: Brookes.

Gérard, J.-M., Deggouj, N., Hupin, C., Buisson, A.-L., Monteyne, V., Lavis, C., . . . Gersdorff, M. (2010). Evolution of communication abilities after cochlear implantation in prelingually deaf children. International Journal of Pediatric Otorhinolaryngology, 74(6), 642–648.

Gibson-Davis, C. M., & Gassman-Pines, A. (2010). Early childhood family structure and mother-child interactions: variation by race and ethnicity. Developmental Psychology, 46(1), 151–164.

Goneu, A., Mistry, J., & Mosier, C. (2000). Cultural variations in the play of toddlers. International Journal of Behavioral Development, 24, 321–329.

Graham, P. J. (2004). Cognitive behaviour therapy for children and families. Cambridge, UK: Cambridge University Press.

Guarino, C. M., Buddin, R., Pham, C., & Cho, M. (2010). Demographic factors associated with the early identification of children with special needs. Topics in Early Childhood Special Education, 30, 162–175.

Guiberson, M. M. (2005). Children with cochlear implants from bilingual families: considerations for intervention and a case study. The Volta Review, 105, 29–40.

Guiberson, M., & Atkins, J. (2012). Speech-language pathologists' preparation, practices, and perspectives on serving culturally and linguistically diverse children. Communication Disorders Quarterly, 33, 169–180.

Halgunseth, L. C., Ispa, J. M., & Rudy, D. (2006). Parental control in Latino families: an integrated review of the literature. Child Development, 77(5), 1282–1297.

Hernández, M., Costa, A., & Humphreys, G. W. (2012). Escaping capture: bilingualism modulates distraction from working memory. Cognition, 122(1), 37–50.

Holowka, S., Brosseau-Lapre, F., & Petitto, L. A. (2002). Semantic and conceptual knowledge underlying bilingual babies' first signs and words. Language Learning, 52, 205–254.

Hughes, D., Rodriguez, J., Smith, E. P., Johnson, D. J., Stevenson, H. C., & Spicer, P. (2006). Parents' ethnic-racial socialization practices: a review of research and directions for future study. Developmental Psychology, 42(5), 747–770.

Hwang, W. C. (2006). The psychotherapy adaptation and modification framework: application to Asian Americans. The American Psychologist, 61(7), 702–715.

Hyde, M., & Punch, R. (2011). The modes of communication used by children with cochlear implants and the role of sign in their lives. American Annals of the Deaf, 155(5), 535–549.

Inzlicht, M., Gutsell, J. N., & Legault, L. (2012). Mimicry reduces racial prejudice. Journal of Experimental Social Psychology, 48, 361–365.

Jiménez, M. S., Pino, M. J., & Herruzo, J. (2009). A comparative study of speech development between deaf children with cochlear implants who have been educated with spoken or spoken+sign language. International Journal of Pediatric Otorhinolaryngology, 73(1), 109–114.

Kaczmarek, L. A. (2006). A team approach: supporting families of children with disabilities in inclusive programs. Young Children on the Web, January, 1–10. Retrieved from http://www.journal.naeyc.org/btj/200601/KaczmarekBTJ.pdf

Kargina, T. (2004). Effectiveness of a family-focused early intervention program in the education of children with hearing impairments living in rural areas. International Journal of Disability Development and Education, 51, 401–418.

Karliner, L. S., Jacobs, E. A., Chen, A. H., & Mutha, S. (2007). Do professional interpreters improve clinical care for patients with limited English proficiency? A systematic review of the literature. Health Services Research, 42(2), 727–754.

Kavanagh, L. C., Suhler, C. L., Churchland, P. S., & Winkielman, P. (2011). When it's an error to mirror: the surprising reputational costs of mimicry. Psychological Science, 22(10), 1274–1276.

Kirkham, E., Sacks, C., Baroody, F., Siddique, J., Nevins, M. E., Woolley, A., & Suskind, D. (2009). Health disparities in pediatric cochlear implantation: an audiologic perspective. Ear and Hearing, 30(5), 515–525.

Kobayashi, C., Glover, G. H., & Temple, E. (2006). Cultural and linguistic influence on neural bases of 'Theory of Mind': an fMRI study with Japanese bilinguals. Brain and Language, 98(2), 210–220.

Koblinsky, S. A., Kuvalanka, K. A., & Randolph, S. M. (2006). Social skills and behavior problems of urban, African American preschoolers: role of parenting practices, family conflict, and maternal depression. The American Journal of Orthopsychiatry, 76(4), 554–563.

Kohnert, K., Yim, D., Nett, K., Kan, P. F., & Duran, L. (2005, Jul). Intervention with linguistically diverse preschool children: a focus on developing home language(s). Language, Speech, and Hearing Services in Schools, 36(3), 251–263.

Kolobe, T. H. A. (2004). Childrearing practices and developmental expectations for Mexican-American mothers and the developmental status of their infants. Physical Therapy, 84(5), 439–453.

Kos, M.-I., Deriaz, M., Guyot, J.-P., & Pelizzone, M. (2009). What can be expected from a late cochlear implantation? International Journal of Pediatric Otorhinolaryngology, 73(2), 189–193.

Kraus, M. W., Piff, P. K., & Keltner, D. (2011). Social class as culture: The convergence of resources and rank in the social realm. Current Directions in Psychological Science, 20, 246–250.

Kroll, J. F., Dussias, P. E., Bogulski, C. A., & Kroff, J. R. V. (2012). Juggling two languages in one mind: What bilinguals tell us about language processing and its consequences for cognition. Psychology of Learning and Motivation, 56, 229–262.

Krizman, J., Marian, V., Shook, A., Skoe, E., & Kraus, N. (2012). Subcortical encoding of sound is enhanced in bilinguals and relates to executive function advantages. Proc. Natl. Acad. Sci. USA, 109(20), 7877–7881.

Kuhl, P. K. (2010). Brain mechanisms in early language acquisition. Neuron, 67(5), 713–727.

Kuhl, P. K., Tsao, F. M., & Liu, H. M. (2003). Foreign-language experience in infancy: effects of short-term exposure and social interaction on phonetic learning. Proc. Natl. Acad. Sci. USA, 100(15), 9096–9101.

Kummerer, S. E. (2012). Promising strategies for collaborating with Hispanic parents during family-centered speech-language intervention. Communication Disorders Quarterly, 33, 84–95.

Kushalnagar, P., Hannay, H. J., & Hernandez, A. E. (2010). Bilingualism and attention: a study of balanced and unbalanced bilingual deaf users of American Sign Language and English. Journal of Deaf Studies and Deaf Education, 15(3), 263–273.

Laing, S. P., & Kamhi, A. (2003). Alternative assessment of language and literacy in culturally and linguistically diverse populations. Language, Speech, and Hearing Services in Schools, 34, 44–45.

Leander, N. P., Chartrand, T. L., & Bargh, J. A. (2012). You give me the chills: embodied reactions to inappropriate amounts of behavioral mimicry. Psychological Science, 23(7), 772–779.

Lees, J., Stackhouse, J., & Grant, G. (2009). Learning to talk: community support and views of parents from socially disadvantaged families. Journal of Research in Special Educational Needs, 9, 91–99.

Leighton, J., Bird, G., Orsini, C., & Heyes, C. (2010). Social attitudes modulate automatic imitation. Journal of Experimental Social Psychology, 46, 905–910.

Lemos, G. (2005). The search for tolerance: challenging and changing racist attitudes and behaviour among young people. York, UK: Joseph Rountree Foundation.

Lopez, E. C. (2002). Recommended practices in working with school interpreters to deliver psychological services to children and families. In A. Thomas & J. Grimes (Eds.), Best practices in school psychology IV (pp. 1419–1432). Bethesda, MD: National Association of School Psychologists.

López, V. G. (2012). Spanish and English word-initial voiceless stop production in code-switched vs. monolingual structures. Second Language Research, 28, 243–263.

Lynch, E. W., & Hanson, M. J. (1992). Developing cross-cultural competence: A guide for working with young children and their families. Baltimore, MD: Brookes.

Macrory, G. D. (2006). Bilingual language development: what do early years practitioners need to know? Early Years, 26, 159–169.

Mahon, M., Vickers, D., McCarthy, K., Barker, R., Merritt, R., Szagun, G., . . . Rajput, K. (2011). Cochlear-implanted children from homes where English is an additional language: findings from a recent audit in one London centre. Cochlear Implants International, 12(2), 105–113.

Maines, J., Abbady, T., & Benedick, R. (2006, August 15). Broward County is more diverse. Fort Lauderdale Sun-Sentinel.

Marschark, M., & Spencer, P. E. (2005). Oxford handbook of deaf studies, language, and education. New York, NY: Oxford University Press.

Mayer, C., & Akamatsu, C. T. (2003). Bilingualism and literacy. In M. Marschark & P. Spencer (Eds.), Oxford handbook of deaf studies, language, and education (pp. 136–147). New York, NY: Oxford University Press.

Mayer, C., & Leigh, G. (2010). The changing context for sign bilingual education programs: issues in language and the development of literacy. International Journal of Bilingual Education and Bilingualism, 13, 175–186.

Mayo, L. H., Florentine, M., & Buus, S. (1997). Age of second-language acquisition and perception of speech in noise. Journal of Speech and Hearing Research, 40(3), 686–693.

McEvoy, M., Santos, M. T., Marzan, M., Green, E. H., & Milan, F. B. (2009). Teaching medical students how to use interpreters: a three year experience. Medical Education Online, 14, 12.

McGlothlin, H., & Killen, M. (2006). Intergroup attitudes of European American children attending ethnically homogeneous schools. Child Development, 77(5), 1375–1386.

McKenzie, K. (2003). Racism and health. British Medical Journal, 326(7380), 65–66.

Migration Policy Institute. (2006). Migration information source. http://www.migrationinformation.org/GlobalData

Minuchin, S., & Fishman, H. C. (2004). Family therapy techniques. Cambridge, MA: Harvard University Press.

Montrul, S., & Foote, R. (2012). Age of acquisition interactions in bilingual lexical access: A study of the weaker language of L2 learners and heritage speakers. International Journal of Bilingualism, OnlineFirst, May 8. DOI:10.1177/1367006912443431

Moreno, G., & Morales, L. S. (2010i). Hablamos juntos (together we speak): interpreters, provider communication, and satisfaction with care. Journal of General Internal Medicine, 25(12), 1282–1288.

Naqvi, R., McKeough, A., Thorne, K., & Pfitscher, C. (2012). Dual-language books as an emergent literacy resource: culturally and linguistically responsive teaching and learning. Journal of Early Childhood Literacy, OnlineFirst, July 2. DOI: 10.1177/1468798412442886

Naseef, R. A. (2001). Special children, challenged parents. Baltimore, MD: Brookes.

Nelson, P., Kohnert, K., Sabur, S., & Shaw, D. (2005, Jul). Classroom noise and children learning through a second language: double jeopardy? Language, Speech, and Hearing Services in Schools, 36(3), 219–229.

Nelson, K. E., Welsh, J. A., Trup, E. M. V., & Greenberg, M. T. (2011). Language delays of impoverished preschool children in relation to early academic and emotion recognition skills. First Language, 31, 164–194.

Nisbett, R. E., & Miyamoto, Y. (2005). The influence of culture: holistic versus analytic perception. Trends in Cognitive Sciences, 9(10), 467–473.

Nittrouer, S. (2008). Outcomes for children with HL: Effects of age of ID, sign support, and auditory prosthesis. Perspectives on Hearing and Hearing Disorders in Childhood, 18, 74–82.

Nittrouer, S. (2009). Early development of children with hearing loss. San Diego, CA: Plural.

Pearson, B. Z. (2007). Social factors in childhood bilingualism in the U.S. Applied Psycholinguistics, 28(3), 399–410. DOI: 10.1017/S014271640707021X

Peña, E. D., & Halle, T. G. (2011). Assessing preschool dual language learners: Traveling a multiforked road. Child Development Perspectives, 5, 28–32.

Peterson, C. A., Wall, S., Jeon, H-J., Swanson, M. E., Carta, J. J., Luze, G. J., & Eshbaugh, E. (2011). Identification of disabilities and service receipt among preschool children living in poverty. Journal of Special Education, OnlineFirst, 28 April. DOI:10.1177/0022466911407073

Petitto, L. A. (2006). How young monolingual and bilingual children acquire language. Presentation at Office of English Language Acquisition Summit, November 13, 2002, Washington, DC.

Petitto, L. A. (2009). Educational neuroscience: New discoveries from bilingual brains, scientific brains, and the educated mind. Mind, Brain, and Education, 3(4), 185–197.

Petitto, L. A., & Kovelman, I. (2003). The bilingual paradox: how signing-speaking bilingual children help us resolve bilingual issues and teach us about the brain's mechanisms underlying all language acquisition. Learning Languages, 8, 5–18.

Petitto, L. A., Katerelos, M., Levy, B. G., Gauna, K., Tétreault, K., & Ferraro, V. (2001). Bilingual signed and spoken language acquisition from birth: implications for the mechanisms underlying early bilingual language acquisition. Journal of Child Language, 28(2), 453–496.

Phillips, A. H. (1999). Retrospective study of 48 hearing impaired children who participated in MOSD parent infant and/or nursery programs (birth dates 1987–1993). In A. H. Phillips et al (Eds.), Early intervention at the Montreal Oral School for the Deaf: Five companion studies. Quebec, Canada: Research Reports presented to Interministerial Committee for the Health and Education Ministries, Government du Quebec.

Phillips, R., Worley, L., & Rhoades, E. A. (2010). Socioemotional considerations. In E. A. Rhoades & J. Duncan (Eds.), Auditory-verbal practice: toward a family-centered approach (pp. 187–223). Springfield, IL: Charles C. Thomas.

Powers, A. R., Elliott, R. N., Patterson, D., Shaw, S., & Taylor, C. (1995). Family environment and deaf and hard-of-hearing students with mild additional disabilities. Journal of Childhood Communication Disorders, 17, 15–19.

Qi, C. H., Kaiser, A. P., Marley, S. C., & Milan, S. (2011). Performance of African American preschool children from low-income families on expressive language measures. Topics in Early Childhood Special Education, 32(3), 175–184.

Quiroz, B., & Dixon, Q. (2012). Mother-child interactions during shared literacy activities: Education in a fractured bilingual environment. Journal of Early Childhood Literacy, 12, 139–175.

Quiroz, B. G., Snow, C. E., & Zhao, J. (2010). Vocabulary skills of Spanish-English bilinguals: impact of mother-child language interactions and home language and literacy support. The International Journal of Bilingualism, 14, 379–399.

Rambo, A. H., Rhoades, E. A., Boyd, T. V., & Bello, N. (2010). Introduction to systemic family therapy. In E. A. Rhoades & J. Duncan (Eds.), Auditory-verbal practice: Toward a family-centered approach (pp. 113–136). Springfield IL: Charles C. Thomas.

Rhoades, E. A. (2003). Lexical-semantic and morpho-syntactic language assessment in auditory-verbal intervention: a position paper. The Volta Review, 103, 169–184.

Rhoades, E. A. (2007). Setting the stage for culturally responsive intervention. Volta Voices, 14(4), 10–13.

Rhoades, E. A. (2009a). Learning a second language: potentials and diverse possibilities. Hearing Loss, 30(2), 20–22.

Rhoades, E. A. (2009b). What the neurosciences tell us about adolescence. Volta Voices, 16(1), 16–21.

Rhoades, E. A. (2010a). Revisiting labels: Hearing or not? The Volta Review, 110, 55–67.

Rhoades, E. A. (2010b). Enablement and environment. In E. A. Rhoades & J. Duncan (Eds.), Auditory-verbal practice: toward a family-centered approach (pp. 81–96). Springfield, IL: Charles C. Thomas.

Rhoades, E. A. (2010c). Toward family-centered practice. In E. A. Rhoades & J. Duncan (Eds.), Auditory-verbal practice: toward a family-centered approach (pp.167–186). Springfield, IL: Charles C. Thomas

Rhoades, E. A. (2010d). Core constructs of family therapy. In E. A. Rhoades & J. Duncan (Eds.), Auditory-verbal practice: toward a family-centered approach (pp. 137–163). Springfield, IL: Charles C. Thomas.

Rhoades, E. A. (2011). Listening strategies to facilitate spoken language learning among signing children with cochlear implants. In R. Paludneviciene & I. W. Leigh (Eds.). Cochlear implants: shifting perspectives (pp. 142–171). Washington DC: Gallaudet University.

Rhoades, E. A., Perusse, M., Douglas, W. M., & Zarate, C. (2008). Auditory-based bilingual children in North America: Differences and choices. Volta Voices, 15(5), 20–22.

Rhoades, E. A., Price, F., & Perigoe, C. B. (2004). The changing American family and ethnically diverse children with multiple needs. The Volta Review, 104, 285–305.

Robbins, M. S., & Szapocznik, J. (2000). Brief strategic family therapy. Juvenile Justice Bulletin, April, 1–11.

Rodriguez, B. L., & Olswang, L. B. (2003). Mexican-American and Anglo-American mothers' beliefs and values about child rearing, education, and language impairment. American Journal of Speech-Language Pathology, 12(4), 452–462.

Rutland, A., Cameron, L., Bennett, L., & Ferrell, J. (2005). Interracial contact and racial constancy: a multi-site study of racial intergroup bias in 3–5 year old Anglo-British children. Journal of Applied Developmental Psychology, 26, 699–713.

Salas-Provance, M. B., Erickson, J. G., & Reed, J. (2002). Disabilities as viewed by four generations of one Hispanic family. American Journal of Speech-Language Pathology, 11, 151–162.

Sanchez, W. (1995). Working with diverse learners and school staff in a multicultural society. ERIC Digest 390018.

Sarant, J. Z., Blamey, P. J., Dowell, R. C., Clark, G. M., & Gibson, W. P. R. (2001). Variation in speech perception scores among children with cochlear implants. Ear and Hearing, 22(1), 18–28.

Schiff, R., & Lotem, E. (2011). Effects of phonological and morphological awareness on children's word reading development from two socioeconomic backgrounds. First Language, 31, 139–163.

Seal, B. C., & Hammett, L. A. (1995). Language intervention with a child with hearing whose parents are deaf. American Journal of Speech-Language Pathology, 4, 15–21.

Shifrer, D., Muller, C., & Callahan, R. (2011). Disproportionality and learning disabilities: parsing apart race, socioeconomic status, and language. Journal of Learning Disabilities, 44(3), 246–257.

Shin, H. B., & Kominski, R. A. (2010). Language use in the United States: 2007 (American Community Survey Reports, ACS-12). Washington, DC: U.S. Census Bureau.

Solem, M.-B., Christophersen, K.-A., & Martinussen, M. (2011). Predicting parenting stress: Children's behavioural problems and parents' coping. Infant and Child Development, 20, 162–180.

Stel, M., & Harinck, F. (2011). Being mimicked makes you a prosocial voter. Experimental Psychology, 58(1), 79–84.

Stepanova, E. V., & Strube, M. J. (2012). The role of skin color and facial physiognomy in racial categorization: Moderation by implicit racial attitudes. Journal of Experimental Social Psychology, 48, 867–878.

Suzuki, L., & Aronson, J. (2003). The cultural malleability of intelligence and its impact on the racial/ethnic hierarchy. Psychology, Public Policy, and Law, 31, 320–327.

Swanson, H. L., Sáez, L., & Gerber, M. (2006). Growth in literacy and cognition in bilingual children at risk or not at risk for reading disabilities. Journal of Educational Psychology, 98, 247–264.

Swanwick, R., & Watson, L. (2005). Literacy in the homes of young deaf children: Common and distinct features of spoken language and sign bilingual environments. Journal of Early Childhood Literacy, 5, 53–78.

Tabors, P. O. (1997). One child, two languages: a guide for preschool educators of children learning English as a second language. Baltimore: Brookes.

Teschendorf, M., Janeschik, S., Bagus, H., Lang, S., & Arweiler-Harbeck, D. (2011). Speech development after cochlear implantation in children from bilingual homes. Otology & Neurotology, 32(2), 229–235.

Thomas, E., El-Kashlan, H., & Zwolan, T. A. (2008). Children with cochlear implants who live in monolingual and bilingual homes. Otology & Neurotology, 29(2), 230–234.

Thordardottir, E. (2006). Language intervention from a bilingual mindset. ASHA Leader, 11, 20–21.

Ting, J. Y., Bergeson, T. R., & Miyamoto, R. T. (2012). Effects of simultaneous speech and sign on infants' attention to spoken language. The Laryngoscope,122(12), 2808–2812.

Tobey, E. A., Rekart, D., Buckley, K., & Geers, A. E. (2004). Mode of communication and classroom placement impact on speech intelligibility. Archives of Otolaryngology–Head & Neck Surgery, 130(5), 639–643.

Todd, A. R., & Galinsky, A. D. (2012). The reciprocal link between multiculturalism and perspective-taking: How ideological and self-regulatory approaches to managing diversity reinforce each other. Journal of Experimental Social Psychology, 48, 1394–1398.

Tsai, K. M., Park, H., Liu, L. L., & Lau, A. S. (2012). Distinct pathways from parental cultural orientation to young children's bilingual development. Journal of Applied Developmental Psychology, 33, 219–226.

Tsukada, K. (2012). Non-native Japanese listeners' perception of vowel length contrasts in Japanese and Modern Standard Arabic (MSA). Second Language Research, 28, 151–168.

Tudge, J., Doucet, F., Hayes, S., Odero, D., Kulakova, N., Tammeveski, P., & Meltsas, M. (2000). Parents' participation in cultural practices with their preschoolers. Psicologia, Teoria e Pesquisa, 16, 1–11.

Tudge, J. R. H., Doucet, F., Odero, D., Sperb, T. M., Piccinini, C. A., & Lopes, R. S. (2006). A window into different cultural worlds: young children's everyday activities in the United States, Brazil, and Kenya. Child Development, 77(5), 1446–1469.

Turner, S., & Lynas, W. (2000). Teachers' perspectives on support for under-fives in families of ethnic minority origin. Deafness & Education International, 2, 152–164.

Tyler, K. M., Boykin, A. W., & Walton, T. R. (2006). Cultural considerations in teachers' perceptions of student classroom behavior and achievement. Teaching and Teacher Education, 22, 998–1005.

Tzou, Y.-Z., Eslami, Z. R., Chen, H.-C., & Vaid, J. (2012). Effect of language proficiency and degree of formal training in simultaneous interpreting on working memory and interpreting performance: Evidence from Mandarin–English speakers. The International Journal of Bilingualism, 16, 213–227.

U.S. Census Bureau. (2009). http://www.census.gov/compendia/statab/2012/tables/12s0010.pdf

van Baaren, R. B., Holland, R. W., Steenaert, B., & van Knippenberg, A. (2003). Mimicry for money: behavioral consequences of imitation. Journal of Experimental Social Psychology, 39, 393–398.

van den Bogaerde, B., & Baker, A. E. (2006). Code mixing in mother-child interaction in deaf families. Sign Language and Linguistics, 8, 155–178.

van Wijngaarden, S. J. (2001). Intelligibility of native and non-native Dutch speech. Speech Communication, 35, 103–113.

van Wijngaarden, S. J., Steeneken, H. J., & Houtgast, T. (2002). Quantifying the intelligibility of speech in noise for non-native listeners. The Journal of the Acoustical Society of America, 111(4), 1906–1916.

Vasquez, J. M., & Wetzel, C. (2009). Tradition and the invention of racial selves: symbolic boundaries, collective authenticity, and contemporary struggles for racial equality. Ethnic and Racial Studies, 32, 1557–1575.

Venail, F., Vieu, A., Artieres, F., Mondain, M., & Uziel, A. (2010). Educational and employment achievements in prelingually deaf children who receive cochlear implants. Archives of Otolaryngology–Head & Neck Surgery, 136(4), 366–372.

Wager, F., Hill, M., Bailey, N., Day, R., Hamilton, D., & King, C. (2010). The impact of poverty on children and young people's use of services. Children & Society, 24, 400–412.

Walker, S., & Akister, J. (2004). Applying family therapy: a guide for caring professionals in the community. Lyme Regis, UK: Russell House.

Waltzman, S. B., Robbins, A. M., Green, J. E., & Cohen, N. L. (2003). Second oral language capabilities in children with cochlear implants. Journal of Otology and Neurotology, 24(5), 757–763.

Watamura, S. E., Phillips, D. A., Morrissey, T. W., McCartney, K., & Bub, K. (2011,). Double jeopardy: poorer social-emotional outcomes for children in the NICHD SECCYD experiencing home and child-care environments that confer risk. Child Development, 82(1), 48–65.

Watson, L. M., Hardie, T., Archbold, S. M., & Wheeler, A. (2008). Parents' views on changing communication after cochlear implantation. Journal of Deaf Studies and Deaf Education, 13(1), 104–116.

Watt, S. E., Maio, G. R., Rees, K., & Hewstone, M. (2006). Functions of attitudes towards ethnic groups: effects of level of abstraction. Journal of Experimental Social Psychology, 43, 441–449.

Wattendorf, E., Festman, J., Westermann, B., Keil, U., Zappatore, D., Franceschini, R., . . . Nitsch, C. (2012). Early bilingualism influences early and subsequently later acquired languages in cortical regions representing control functions. International Journal of Bilingualism, OnlineFirst, 28 August. DOI:10.1177/1367006912456590

Werker, J. (2012). Perceptual foundations of bilingual acquisition in infancy. Annals of the New York Academy of Sciences, 1251, 50–61.

Wheeler, A., Archbold, S., Gregory, S., & Skipp, A. (2007). Cochlear implants: the young people's perspective. Journal of Deaf Studies and Deaf Education, 12(3), 303–316.

Wilkens, C. P. (2009). Elementary school placements of African American students who are profoundly deaf. Journal of Disability Policy Studies, 20, 155–161.

Woodrow, D. (2001). Cultural determination of curricula, theories and practices. Pedagogy, Culture & Society, 9, 5–27.

Yim, D. (2012). Spanish and English language performance in bilingual children with cochlear implants. Otology & Neurotology, 33(1), 20–25.

Yumoto, K. (1996). Bilingualism, code-switching, language mixing, transfer and borrowing: clarifying terminologies in the literature. Kanagawa Prefectural College of Foreign Studies, Working Papers, 17, 49–60.

Zentella, A. C. (1997). Growing up bilingual: Puerto Rican children in New York. Oxford, UK: Blackwell Publishers.

Chapter 34

Counseling and Collaboration with Parents of Children with Hearing Loss

Jackson Roush and Garima Kamo

Key Points

- The stress and anxiety experienced by most parents at the time of diagnosis are a normal reaction to unfamiliar and unforeseen circumstances.

- Interactions between the audiologist and the family at the time of diagnosis can set the tone for future interactions.

- Identification of hearing loss in infancy puts parents in the position of receiving a diagnosis without the benefit of direct observation.

- Delivering difficult news requires careful consideration of how information is presented and the dialogue that follows.

- Parents' initial level of concern or emotional upheaval is usually unrelated to their child's type or degree of hearing loss.

- Audiologists need to be forthright in providing information to parents, but also to be willing to listen and to reflect on their concerns and priorities.

- Inexperienced clinicians may provide more information than a family can comprehend, especially at the time of diagnosis.

- The support of other parents is vital to many families.

- Parents may experience ambivalent feelings throughout their child's early years, especially during periods of transition.

- It is important to consider the educational preparation of future clinicians and ways to provide meaningful learning opportunities while ensuring that families are not harmed by an inexperienced clinician who has not acquired proficiency as a counselor.

Historically, the diagnosis of hearing loss was a confirmation of what parents had suspected over a period of weeks or months. Now, with the widespread implementation of newborn screening, hearing loss is often identified in early infancy. Counseling at the time of diagnosis has always been important, but the role of the audiologist has been made more challenging by the need to address these issues soon after birth. Furthermore, identification of hearing loss in infancy puts parents in the difficult position of needing to accept the diagnosis without the benefit of direct observation. These realities, combined with the remarkable expansion of information available to many families through the Internet and other sources, require the audiologist to consider the emotional aspects of parent counseling while providing the information families need to be well-informed consumers and decision makers.

This chapter explores the audiologist's dual role of counselor and information provider within a family-centered framework. From the shared perspectives of a pediatric audiologist (JR) and the parent of a child with hearing loss (GK), we examine successful models for counseling and informing families as well as challenges and potential pitfalls.

◆ The Audiologist as Counselor and Informant

The early weeks and months following diagnosis are a time of conflict and emotional upheaval for most families. Not surprisingly, parents and family members differ in their reactions to these events. For some parents, the diagnosis is a call to immediate action; for others, time and space are needed to reflect on the diagnosis and recommendations. Regardless of the families' initial reaction, it is important for the audiologist to recognize that most parents and family members are not emotionally disturbed but emotionally upset. Indeed, Luterman (1979, 1991, 2008) describes the distress and anxiety experienced by most parents as a normal response to unfamiliar and unforeseen circumstances. Consistent with that assumption, Clark and English (2004) characterize the audiologist's counseling role as one that is based on a well-patient model, with the goal of helping parents and family members acquire the support and information needed to attain a positive and constructive outlook.

What Does It Mean to Be Family-Centered and Why Does It Matter?

Early intervention was, for many years, a child-focused endeavor designed to enhance developmental outcomes for young children with disabilities. The origin of the term "family-centered" has been attributed to the field of health care in the 1960s as professionals attempted to provide a greater decision-making role for families (Trivette, Dunst, Boyd, & Hamby, 1995). Bronfenbrenner (1977) was among the first to apply the term to early intervention at a time when he and others sought to increase the level of parent participation in early education. Public Law 99-457, which was passed in the mid-1980s, established the Individualized Family Service Plan (IFSP), which, for the first time, required documentation of a family's strengths and needs, services to be provided, and specification of intended outcomes.

The years following implementation of PL 99-457, although better for families in many ways, have been characterized by inconsistency in how family-centered practices are defined and implemented. Since the 1990s, many professionals have advocated for a family-centered approach that focuses on the development of collaborative relationships between families and professionals (Trivette et al, 1995). Bailey et al (1998) emphasized the importance of examining family outcomes as well as those intended for the child, and Trivette, Dunst, and Hamby (2010) proposed an expanded service-delivery model focusing on the social systems and environmental variables associated with development-enhancing and family-strengthening consequences. This model includes children's learning opportunities, supports for parenting, and community supports provided within a family-centered framework. As suggested by Crais, Roy, and Free (2006), providing successful family-centered services does not require identification of the ideal or perfect set of practices. Rather, it requires recognition of the family's role in deciding and implementing those practices. With each reauthorization of what is now known as the Individuals with Disabilities Education Act (IDEA), a fundamental principle has been maintained: the importance of parental decision making and individualized choices for families throughout the delivery of assessment and intervention services.

Support for this tenet can be found in the growing evidence of how family participation affects child outcomes. For families whose children are deaf or hard of hearing, there is no better example than the work of Moeller (2000), who explored the relationship between age of enrollment in intervention and language outcomes at 5 years of age. Moeller also studied the relationships between performance and various factors, including family involvement, degree of hearing loss, and nonverbal intelligence. Her findings indicated that children enrolled earliest in intervention programs demonstrated significantly better vocabulary and verbal reasoning than later-enrolled children. Interestingly, only two factors explained a significant amount of the variance: age of enrollment and the level of family involvement. In fact, family involvement explained the most variance after accounting for other variables.

Pearl

- High levels of family involvement are associated with greater benefits from early intervention.

Applying Family-Centered Principles to Clinical Audiology

A family-centered approach requires careful examination of parent–professional communication and the dynamics of each context that brings parents and professionals together (Roush, 2001). Simeonsson et al (1996) describe the early services provided to families as an intervention cycle composed of discrete components that include referral, assessment, intervention planning, service implementation, and follow-up. Each component involves a succession of encounters that children and families have with professionals, and each encounter is defined by mutual expectations, roles, and activities for families and service providers. Ideally, our encounters with children who are deaf or hard of hearing and their families will be a continuous process of family-centered service delivery where audiologists are simultaneously engaged in overseeing early identification programs, establishing an accurate diagnosis of hearing loss, coordinating timely audiologic service, and providing effective family support and counseling (American Speech-Language-Hearing Association [ASHA], 2008). Initially, the encounters revolve around the screening and diagnostic process and later with the selection and fitting of hearing instruments and the delivery of early intervention services. Along the way, professionals counsel families, provide information, and offer choices. For the audiologist, the parent–professional relationship often begins when an infant is referred from new-born screening. Other encounters include decisions regarding hearing aids or cochlear implants and options for early intervention and school placement. The initial contacts during the early weeks and months following diagnosis may set the tone for future encounters and create a foundation for the interactions that follow (Roush, 2001).

Informing Families of Diagnostic Results

The audiologist's ever-increasing technological capability, combined with the remarkable expansion of universal infant hearing screening, has brought fundamental changes in how and when the diagnosis occurs. In contrast to earlier times, when the audiologic assessment confirmed parental suspicions, the news now comes unexpectedly to many families. It is important to remember that physiologic evidence, such as auditory brainstem response (ABR) test results, may be unequivocal to the audiologist. But in the absence of behavioral evidence, families may have difficulty comprehending or accepting the diagnosis. Clinicians must be prepared to respond to a broad range of questions and a variety of reactions to the news. There is no easy way to impart the diagnosis to families when testing reveals permanent hearing loss, but advice from other disciplines can be helpful. In his book *How To Break Bad News*, Robert Buckman, an oncologist, characterizes the patient interaction as having two components: a divulging of information at the time of diagnosis and a therapeutic dialogue that follows (Buckman, 1992). Divulging information, according to Buckman, requires careful consideration and preparation of how the diagnosis will be presented. The therapeutic dialogue requires the clinician to listen carefully and respond appropriately to how information is received. Buckman offers a protocol that attempts to balance the inevitable limitations of time in most clinical settings with the need to consider, in a sensitive way, the impact of the news. The following strategies are adapted from Buckman (1992) and influenced by other authors cited here. They are also shaped by the authors' own experiences as bearers and recipients of difficult news.

Preparation

The physical setting should be arranged to minimize physical discomfort and to ensure privacy. This generally requires a quiet, comfortable room with phones off and the door closed for privacy and to ensure that the counseling session can proceed without interruption. Once seated, it is important to make introductions and establish who is present and their relationship to the family. Buckman recommends starting with a question (e.g., "How are you doing?") to convey concern about the parents' feelings and to encourage a conversational tone. Tye-Murray emphasizes the importance of eye contact, slowed or softened speaking, and attention to the parents' body language in conveying compassion and empathy.

Find Out What the Family Already Knows

Most families come with at least some knowledge or expectation regarding their children's hearing status. This may be based on previous audiologic assessments or information they have acquired on their own.

> **Pearl**
>
> - Allowing the family to talk first not only sets a tone that encourages conversational interaction; it also gives the clinician an opportunity to assess the family's level of understanding and communicative style.

Again, it is important for the clinician to listen carefully, making appropriate eye contact and showing a genuine interest in what parents say, even if their knowledge is incomplete or incorrect. This is also an opportunity to evaluate how they seem to be feeling emotionally.

Determine What the Family Wants to Know

Luterman (1979) emphasizes the importance of meeting parents where they are at each point in time. In addition to delivering information clearly and accurately with sensitivity to the impact of this news, it is important to remember that the parents' level of emotional upheaval is unrelated to the child's degree of hearing loss. For some families the diagnosis of mild or even unilateral hearing loss may be emotionally traumatic. Parents typically have many questions regarding the cause of hearing loss, and how they should proceed with intervention (Roush, 2000a).

> **Pitfall**
>
> - Inexperienced clinicians may be inclined to provide more information than the family can comprehend, especially at the time of diagnosis.

Share Information

Although many parents are emotionally upset at the time of diagnosis, most want a forthright explanation of the findings, a preliminary treatment plan, the prognosis, and services available to them (Buckman, 1992; Roush, 2000a, 2000b, Tye-Murray, 2012). Luterman (1979, 2008) and English (2002) emphasize the importance of differentiating content versus affect-level questions. Both are important, but the latter require careful listening and reflection. At the time of diagnosis and during the early weeks and months, many of the questions asked by parents may appear on the surface to be seeking content information when, in fact, there is an underlying concern (Clark & English, 2004).

Special Consideration

Listening for Affect

- Carl Rogers was an influential 20th-century psychologist and founder of the humanist approach to psychology. Over time he moved away from traditional psychotherapy aimed at changing or curing patients to an approach that sought ways to facilitate personal growth. He encouraged "listening for affect" in an effort to identify underlying intent and feelings. As we apply these principles to counseling in pediatric audiology, it is important to remember that a parent's questions and concerns at the time of diagnosis may be unpredictable. For example, at our medical center a young mother's only question at the time of diagnosis for her three-month-old infant was about the implications of deafness when she reaches adolescence. The best response in a case like this might be to simply acknowledge that "it must be difficult not knowing what this will mean for her," and recognizing that "it's hard to predict how the hearing loss will affect her so far into the future," but then assuring the family that much can and will be done to assist them along the way. The clinician is not forced to choose between an informational versus an affective response. Often the best approach is to acknowledge the question while recognizing the feelings that may be underlying the parent's concern.

Although it is important for the clinician to listen for affect, it is also important to recognize that parents want and need information, and the nature of the information they seek can change over time. At the time of diagnosis, Harrison and Roush (2002) found that many parents of a newly identified child are especially interested in the etiology of the child's hearing loss and issues related to coping with the emotional aspects of the diagnosis. Many parents also want information about how and when their children will learn to listen and speak. However, the same respondents indicated somewhat different needs for information a few months following the diagnosis, with many turning greater attention to communication options, timelines for developing speech and language, responsibilities of early intervention providers, and legal rights of children with hearing loss (Harrison & Roush, 2002). Still, it is important to remember that each family is unique. Asking them what they want to know and what they hope to accomplish at each visit ensures that counseling and information are relevant to their current goals and priorities.

Pediatric audiologists face a variety of counseling situations, but in many ways the first meeting at the time of diagnosis is the most challenging. Buckman (1992) suggests that the initial session include content related to diagnosis, treatment, prognosis, and support. As a starting point, the audiologist can use the information provided by the parents about what they already know to reinforce what was accurate in their interpretation. Recognizing that many people retain few details once confronted with serious news, information must be delivered in small increments consisting of a frank but sincere statement of the facts followed by elaboration and explanation. Applied to the diagnostic audiology visit, the clinician might say: "Our testing indicates that Ben has a hearing loss in both ears. We were able to obtain reliable test results and I believe our diagnosis is accurate." This candid appraisal might be followed by a reassuring statement that indicates what can be done to help the child and family. Buckman emphasizes the importance of using plain English, avoiding technical language, and frequently checking on reception and understanding: "Am I making sense?" "Does this seem clear to you?" Important points need to be restated to ensure comprehension, and the clinician must remember that the primary concerns of a parent at the time of diagnosis may be difficult to predict. It is also possible that parents will not believe or will disagree with the diagnosis. While it may be possible to "demonstrate" the hearing loss when the child is older, delivering news at this early stage relies on clear, careful explanations conveyed at an appropriate level of complexity.

Pearl

- Clinicians can blend the patient's agenda with their own, respecting the parents' issues and concerns but highlighting the most important recommendations and carefully checking for comprehension of the information provided.

Respond to the Parents' Feelings

There is considerable variability in how parents respond to news about their child's hearing loss. Reactions may be shaped by many factors, including the knowledge they bring with them, but their response to the diagnosis may also be affected by social or cultural factors. It is sometimes informative to ask the family whether they have ever met a person who is deaf, or whether they know someone with congenital hearing loss. There can be mistaken beliefs or unwarranted concerns based on limited contact with a person who is deaf or hard of hearing; conversely, there may be a more optimistic attitude if past experiences have been positive.

Most families do not have prior experience with congenital hearing loss, and for many the diagnosis is profoundly disturbing. Several authors have examined initial reactions and various stages that follow a serious diagnosis, including disbelief, shock, anger, guilt, denial, and displacement or diversion of activities (Luterman, 1985, 2008; Moses, 1987; Buckman, 1992; Clark & English, 2004; Tye-Murray, 2012). Feelings of guilt may be especially acute and enduring, even if the etiology is beyond the parents' control. Most parents eventually come to some level of acceptance, although these feelings can reappear as new challenges arise. In the first few weeks following diagnosis, emotions may fluctuate between hope and despair. When parents appear distraught, and most are, Buckman (1992) advises adherence to three principles, adapted here for application to a parent/child with hearing loss:

1. Don't promise anything you can't deliver. Over-assurance about the implications of hearing loss is misleading and condescending to families. It is important to be realistic, but also to assure families that much can and will be done.
2. Allow the parent to express his/her concerns and feelings. Encouraging an honest expression of emotions gives parents permission to be themselves. They will remember and appreciate this later.
3. Let them know your relationship will continue—they're not in this alone. More than anything at this early stage, families want to know they are in capable hands and that you will help guide them through the process.

The inexperienced clinician should not be surprised if some parents respond with tears to the diagnosis of hearing loss. A crying parent can be unsettling even to the experienced clinician, but it is important to recognize that for many people this is a natural reaction and often a beneficial one. Pausing in the dialogue and providing a tissue lets them know it is okay to express their feelings. Years later most parents will still remember that encounter. They will not recall the specific information conveyed, but most will remember how they were treated and whether the audiologist expressed genuine concern and compassion (Luterman, 2008).

Follow-Up and Follow-Through

The most successful counseling session is incomplete without a well-articulated plan based on mutual understanding of what needs to happen next. This includes the specific action items from the clinician's perspective, but it must also acknowledge questions or concerns raised by the parents. Remembering again that most parents do not recall everything they are told the first time, it is important for them to leave with information to take home: carefully selected handouts and literature, contact information for professional service providers and other families, and an appointment card for the next visit. At the conclusion it is important to confirm that everyone is in agreement on the next steps. If it is a new diagnosis, some pediatric audiologists will invite parents to call if they have further questions before the next appointment. Many will.

◆ Decisions about Amplification and Cochlear Implantation

Providing information at the time of diagnosis is emotionally demanding for parents and clinicians. Adding to the pressure is a need to make important decisions soon after the diagnosis. Position statements of the Joint Committee on Infant Hearing (JCIH) (2007) recommend that infants without medical contraindications, and whose families concur, begin use of amplification within 1 month after confirmation of the hearing loss. For nearly all parents, this is a stressful and uncertain period, with implications for the entire family. Most families are ready to proceed with amplification at the time of diagnosis, and many appear to gain a sense of relief knowing that an intervention plan is under way. But some families are not ready to proceed at that pace and may require additional time. Indeed, when parents were asked to indicate the optimal time interval from diagnosis to hearing aid fitting, Sjoblad, Harrison, Roush, and McWilliam (2001) found that nearly three-fourths of the parents surveyed said 3 to 4 weeks, but approximately one-fourth believed that 1 to 3 months was optimal. This finding illustrates the natural variability among families and the importance of not assuming that all will want to proceed at the same pace. However, it may also reflect the need for better counseling or peer support at the time of diagnosis. It may be that families who favored a longer delay lacked the information and support needed to proceed comfortably with hearing aid selection and fitting (Roush, 2001).

An issue rarely discussed but on the minds of most parents is the issue of appearance. Deafness is often described as an invisible handicap. This changes once the child is fitted with hearing aids. Sjoblad et al (2001) reported that more than half of the parent respondents expressed concern about the appearance of the devices. Nearly two-thirds also expressed concerns about the perceived benefits of amplification. Fortunately, for more than half the respondents, perceptions about both appearance and benefit became more positive over time, and only a small number (fewer than 5%) felt less positive over time.

When acoustic amplification proves to be unsuccessful or of limited value, families are faced with decisions about cochlear implantation. In recent years the decision has expanded to include the issue of unilateral versus bilateral implantation. As criteria for cochlear implantation have become more flexible, implanting ears with usable residual hearing occurs more frequently. Audiologists can support families by staying current with cochlear implant technology and candidacy to provide accurate information and to ensure timely referral when consideration of implantation is appropriate. For children who already have one implant, the issue of bilateral implantation may be stressful for some parents, especially if it means losing an ear with aidable residual hearing. Bilateral implantation is no longer uncommon, and there is evidence of beneficial outcomes, but there are also anecdotal reports of older children and adults who do well with "bimodal hearing," the simultaneous use of a cochlear implant on one side and amplification on the other. Considering the complexity of preselection, assessment, surgical intervention, and unilateral versus bilateral implantation, families will be best served by a team of professionals who specialize in cochlear implants.

◆ Decisions about Early Intervention

Maximizing developmental language outcomes for young children with hearing loss requires that children be fitted with appropriate technology and provided with early intervention services soon after the hearing loss has been identified (Yoshinaga-Itano, Sedey, Coulter, & Mehl, 1998; Carney & Moeller, 1998; Moeller, 2000). But to make informed decisions about therapeutic intervention or special services, families need information that is objective, culturally sensitive, and considerate of their emotional state (Luterman, 1985; Luterman & Kurtzer-White, 1999; JCIH, 2007; Barrera & Corso, 2002). Audiologists who work

with infants and their families must be familiar with legislative mandates as well as state and local referral procedures. Moreover, they must provide unbiased information regarding options for intervention.

Pearl

- The most important issue is not necessarily the initial decisions made by families, but how freely they can modify their service and intervention plans as they acquire more information and greater confidence.

This entails a philosophical orientation that encourages families to make their own decisions and for professionals to support them in this process. Parents often seek advice from audiologists in making decisions regarding available intervention services. It is important for audiologists to recognize that legal and regulatory issues are unfamiliar to most parents. The audiologist must be well informed about eligibility criteria and know where to refer families for accurate and unbiased information. Reports intended for those agencies must be written in a manner that will facilitate eligibility for special services, environmental modifications, and provision of FM or other assistive technologies.

◆ Counseling Parents as Their Children Get Older

Transitions in life can be stressful for any family, but they may be especially difficult when they involve a child with special needs. Important transitions for a child with hearing loss include home- to center-based services, early intervention to preschool, preschool to kindergarten, elementary to middle or high school, and transition at any age from a self-contained program to mainstream settings. The inevitable changes that occur with routines and personnel can bring anxiety to even the most experienced and self-confident parent. Many parents report recycling previous emotions (grief, worry, frustration) as they face new challenges or confront new milestones (Tye-Murray, 2012). When, at age 3, their child is transitioning from early intervention to school-based services, parents are often concerned about maintaining the quality and quantity of services they have had during the first 3 years. They are also anxious about life skills in a new setting. The transition to preschool or from preschool to kindergarten often entails noisy environments and teachers with little or no experience managing hearing aids and FM systems. Parents may worry about their children being left behind as classes move from room to room, or left out when children interact socially. As children progress through the elementary grades, the work is more challenging academically, and many families feel the need for additional services. Children with hearing loss may get so focused on listening that comprehension lags. And the need to listen and learn is not limited to academic material. Cole and Flexer (2011) emphasize the importance of overhearing pragmatic transactions as well as the incidental conversations that occur among children.

In middle school, most children seek conformity. Although this can be a challenging time for the child and family, optimal communication is the key to maximizing academic and social success. Good acoustic environments rarely exist in the educational setting, so it becomes imperative for the audiologist to collaborate effectively with parents and with school personnel to advocate for assistive technology and support systems. Once provided, there needs to be ongoing management of the acoustic environment, appropriate microphone use, and modifications of communication style to optimize the child's receptive communication (Madell, 2012). The clinic-based audiologist can play a key role by ensuring that parents are aware of school-based services and by providing the documentation needed to qualify the child for assistive technology and special services. This is especially important as states revise eligibility criteria. The audiologist can assist parents in their advocacy efforts by helping them understand the legal and regulatory issues that determine eligibility and maintenance of special services. This can be accomplished by the audiologist's providing information directly or referring the family to an appropriate agency, institution, or resource person. In this context, the relationship between the parent and the audiologist is a collaborative one, based on informational counseling essential to the acquisition of hearing instruments, assistive technologies, or support services. As new challenges arise, the audiologist can alert parents to the obstacles they may encounter, helping them anticipate issues associated with each transition and working closely with them to minimize the frustrations.

◆ Other Sources of Information for Families

Audiologists and professional service providers were at one time the primary sources of information available to families. Today, many have access to information via the Internet, advocacy organizations, and other resources. Communication with other parents has expanded considerably in recent years and, for many families, represents a vital resource. There is also a growing number of programs that provide family-centered information and advocacy services.

Professional Support for New Families

For more than 20 years, a program based in North Carolina, Beginnings for Parents of Children who are Deaf or Hard of Hearing (http://www.ncbegin.org/), has provided emotional support, unbiased information about communication and educational options, and technical assistance to parents whose children range in age from birth to 21 (Alberg, Wilson, & Roush, 2006). Beginnings also supports parents who are deaf or hard of hearing and whose children may or may not have hearing loss. The belief that parents should be the primary decision makers for their child is a guiding principle for Beginnings. When a child in North Carolina is diagnosed with a hearing loss, parents are informed about Beginnings and invited to talk with a parent educator. Audiologists are the primary source of referral, although anyone can make a referral. A parent educator is assigned to each family referred to Beginnings. Parents provide informed consent for parent educators to first contact the referral source to gain additional information regarding the family and their needs. The parent educator then meets with the family at a convenient time and place, usually in the family's home. Initially, home visits are intended to ensure that parents understand their child's hearing loss and to provide information regarding financial assistance, language development, communication options and early intervention services. Beginnings parent educators emphasize the importance of keeping appointments with the audiologist, and they encourage parents to enroll their child as soon as possible in North Carolina's early intervention program, offering assistance if needed with the logistics of scheduling and transportation. The Beginnings model, which provides a bridge between the pediatric audiologist and early intervention providers, has been so successful that it is now being replicated in several other states (Alberg et al, 2006).

Parent-to-Parent Support

Among the greatest gifts the pediatric audiologist can give to families is a direct link to other parents who have a child who is deaf or hard of hearing. Many experienced parents are willing to be available by phone or in person, and some are willing to initiate contact if desired by the family. Once parents are ready to connect with a larger circle of families, parent support groups can become an invaluable resource. In North Carolina a volunteer organization called HITCH-UP (Hearing Impaired Toddlers and Children Have Unlimited Potential), founded by parents and now active in several regions within the state, organizes monthly support groups for families. Operated entirely by parents without public support, HITCH-UP plays an important role in providing peer support, exchange of information, and advice to professional organizations for improving and expanding services to families with children who are deaf or hard of hearing. Often, the most effective support groups are informal organizations that meet regularly, invite professionals to speak on topics of interest, and organize social functions throughout the year. It is comforting for families to know they are not alone and that they can interact with other families facing similar circumstances. One of the authors (GK) has drawn considerable strength from other families as well as satisfaction in seeing new families join and benefit from the collective experiences of many.

Internet Resources

Every year the Internet becomes a more important source of information for families. For many it is a primary resource for personal and health-related issues. An Internet search using the terms *hearing loss in children* will produce hundreds of Web sites offering information on every aspect of hearing loss and its management. Needless to say, information from the Web varies in complexity and accuracy. A Web-based resource we have found to be especially helpful to families is http://www.babyhearing.org, developed at Boys Town National Research Hospital with a grant from the National Institutes of Health. The site provides accurate, up-to-date information in English or Spanish, at a level most families can comprehend. In addition there are several user groups available to families on the Internet. These groups allow members to ask questions, and all members have the opportunity to share their knowledge or experiences. Many of the user groups are maintained by dedicated and supportive volunteers. Some of the groups are specific; for example, there is an active Yahoo! group on large vestibular aqueducts syndrome (LVAS) and several related to cochlear implantation.

Preparing Future Clinicians

Audiology students must be thoroughly prepared to apply the instrumentation and technology needed to assess and treat hearing loss. Equally important is guidance and experience in counseling and communication with families. But how do we create meaningful learning opportunities for students while ensuring that families are not harmed by an inexperienced clinician who has not yet acquired profi-

ciency as a counselor? This is a challenging area in health care education. For decades, medical schools in the United States have used "simulated" or "standardized" patients for educational purposes; that is, actors who engage in role playing designed to simulate various patient–physician scenarios that provide opportunities for students to acquire experience and feedback on their communication and listening skills (Davidson, Duerson, Rathe, Pauly, & Watson, 2001; Rosenbaum, Ferguson, & Lobas, 2004). Tharpe and Rokuson (2010) describe the use of standardized patients with audiology students, noting that students acquire counseling experiences that are rarely possible in traditional clinical practicum. These include opportunities to apply communication skills with challenging patients or in difficult situations; to review their own clinical behavior as often as necessary; and to make mistakes without interruption by the supervising clinician. For programs that do not have access to standardized patients, Flasher and Fogle (2012) describe role-playing exercises that engage the students themselves in various counseling roles.

Whether using standardized patients or informal role-playing exercises, simulated counseling sessions are most effective when video is recorded for later analysis using an evaluation instrument designed to assess the clinician's performance. Miller, Hope, and Talbot (1999) developed the "Breaking Bad News Assessment Schedule" (BAS) to evaluate medical practitioners' skill at delivering patient information related to a cancer diagnosis. The tool is designed to identify areas where further mentoring is needed or to evaluate the effectiveness of counselor training. English, Naeve-Velguth, Rall, Uyehara-Isono, and Pittman (2007) adapted the BAS for use with audiology students learning to deliver news to parents regarding the diagnosis of hearing loss. Their adapted instrument, called the Audiologic Counseling Evaluation (ACE), was first evaluated for content validity by experienced clinicians. A revised version was then assessed to determine internal consistency and inter-rater reliability (English et al, 2007). The ACE is now available online (http://gozips.uakron.edu/~ke3/ACE.pdf) and is used by several university training programs in the United States. Although intended primarily for evaluating students, the ACE can also serve as a valuable summary and self-assessment tool for practicing clinicians.

◆ Conclusion

Pediatric audiologists, especially those who work with newly identified infants and young children and their families, are called upon to serve as information providers and counselors. The role of informant often begins with an explanation of the diagnosis and options for audiologic intervention with amplification or cochlear implantation. In these technical matters, families want and need an audiologist who is confident, self-assured, and willing and able to provide an accurate but understandable explanation of the findings and recommendations. But it is equally important for the audiologist to listen to families, their questions, their priorities, and their needs at each point in time. This requires the audiologist to serve as both counselor and confidant: roles that require, in addition to effective expressive communication, careful listening and reflection.

Families have access to a tremendous amount of information about their child's hearing loss. The pediatric audiologist can assist families by staying current with available resources, by identifying information that is accurate and up to date, and by making recommendations for how families can access and use available resources. Connecting parents with other parents is especially important. Where family resources are unsatisfactory or insufficient, audiologists can work with parents to establish better mechanisms for peer support and advocacy. They can empower families by promoting partnerships that encourage parents to assume responsibility for decisions that impact their children's educational and audiologic management. A few parents will be interested in working to make improvements at a systems level, and some may take on roles that influence public policies and procedures. For all families, the audiologist can provide consultation, informational resources, and referral to advocacy groups. By recognizing the dual responsibility of information provider and counselor, and the importance of working collaboratively, the audiologist can facilitate the most important outcome: confident, well-informed families capable of determining what is best for their child and comfortable knowing they will be supported and encouraged by their professional service providers.

Summary Pearls

- Families need hope based on the knowledge that much can and will be done to help them and their child.
- When delivering difficult news, give families an opportunity to respond and express their feelings; don't be afraid of a little silence.
- At the outset of each clinic appointment ask families what they are hoping to accomplish at that visit. Return to their priorities at the conclusion of the visit to determine if their goals were met and to confirm agreement on next steps.
- Observe parents interacting with their child and praise their efforts. Simple phrases, such as "Look how he responds to you!" are encouraging and empowering to parents.

Summary Pitfalls

- Providing parents with too much information at one time can be overwhelming to them.
- Delivering news in a manner that is overly positive fails to consider the seriousness of the situation.
- Delivering news in a manner that is negative or pessimistic can hinder the families' progress toward achieving a hopeful outlook for the future.
- Clinicians should not assume that they know how a family feels or what they want for their child. Trusting and collaborative relationships develop slowly over time.

Discussion Questions

1. What does it mean to be family-centered? What if the parent's priorities or decisions differ from those of the audiologist?

2. Some families are slow to accept the diagnosis and reluctant to move forward with the audiologist's recommendations. Although it is important to recognize that families need to move at their own pace, what factors might account for lack of acceptance and what might you do to help them?

References

Alberg, J., Wilson, K., & Roush, J. (2006). Statewide collaboration in the delivery of EHDI services. The Volta Review, 106, 259–274.

American Speech-Language-Hearing Association. (2008). Guidelines for audiologists providing informational and adjustment counseling to families of infants and young children with hearing loss birth to 5 years of age [Guidelines]. Retrieved from http://www.asha.org/policy

Bailey, D. B., McWilliam, R. A., Darkes, A., Hebbeler, K., Simeonsson, R. J., Spiker, D., & Wagner, M. (1998). Family outcomes in early intervention: a framework for program evaluation and efficacy research. Exceptional Children, 64, 313–328.

Barrera, I., & Corso, R. (2002). Cultural competency as skilled dialogue. Topics in Early Childhood Special Education, 22(2), 103–113.

Bronfenbrenner, U. (1977). Toward an experimental ecology of human development. The American Psychologist, 32, 513–521.

Buckman, R. (1992). How to break bad news: a guide for health care professionals. Baltimore, MD: Johns Hopkins University Press.

Carney, A. E., & Moeller, M. P. (1998). Treatment efficacy: hearing loss in children. Journal of Speech, Language, and Hearing Research: JSLHR, 41(1), S61–S84.

Clark, J., & English, K. (2004). Counseling in audiologic practice. Boston, MA: Allyn and Bacon.

Cole, E., & Flexer, C. (2011). Children with hearing loss: Developing listening and talking, birth to six (2nd ed.). San Diego, CA: Plural.

Crais, E. R., Roy, V. P., & Free, K. (2006). Parents' and professionals' perceptions of the implementation of family-centered practices in child assessments. American Journal of Speech-Language Pathology, 15(4), 365–377.

Davidson, R., Duerson, M., Rathe, R., Pauly, R., & Watson, R. T. (2001). Using standardized patients as teachers: a concurrent controlled trial. Academic Medicine, 76(8), 840–843.

English, K. (2002). Counseling children with hearing impairment and their families. Boston, MA: Allyn and Bacon.

English, K., Naeve-Velguth, S., Rall, E., Uyehara-Isono, J., & Pittman, A. (2007). Development of an instrument to evaluate audiologic counseling skills. Journal of the American Academy of Audiology, 18(8), 675–687.

Flasher, L., & Fogle, P. (2012). Counseling skills for speech-language pathologists and audiologists. Clifton Park, NY: Delmar–Cengage Learning.

Harrison, M., & Roush, J. (2002). Information for families with young deaf and hard-of-hearing children: reports from parents and pediatric audiologists. In R. Seewald & J. Gravel (Eds.), A sound foundation through early amplification, Proceedings of the Second International Conference (pp. 233–251). Bury St Edmunds, UK: St. Edmundsbury Press.

Joint Committee on Infant Hearing. (2007). 2000 Position Statement: Principles and Guidelines for Early Hearing Detection and Intervention Programs. Pediatrics, 120(4), 898–921.

Luterman, D. (1979). Counseling parents of hearing impaired children. Boston, MA: Little, Brown.

Luterman, D. (1985). The denial mechanism. Ear and Hearing, 6(1), 57–58.

Luterman, D. (1991). Counseling the communicatively disordered and their families. Austin, TX: Pro-Ed.

Luterman, D. (2008). Counseling persons with communication disorders and their families (4th ed.). Austin, TX: Pro-Ed.

Luterman, D., & Kurtzer-White, E. (1999). Identifying hearing loss: parents' needs. American Journal of Audiology, 8(1), 13–18.

Madell, J. R. (2012), Acoustic accessibility: the role of the clinical audiologist. In J. J. Smaldino & C. Flexer (Eds.), Handbook of acoustic accessibility: best practices for listening, learning, and literacy in the classroom (pp. 128–142). New York, NY: Thieme.

Miller, S. J., Hope, T., & Talbot, D. C. (1999). The development of a structured rating schedule (the BAS) to assess skills in breaking bad news. British Journal of Cancer, 80(5-6), 792–800.

Moses, K. (1987). The impact of childhood disability: the parent's struggle. Ways Magazine, (Spring issue).

Moeller, M. P. (2000). Early intervention and language development in children who are deaf and hard of hearing. Pediatrics, 106(E43), 1–9.

Rosenbaum, M. E., Ferguson, K. J., & Lobas, J. G. (2004). Teaching medical students and residents skills for delivering bad news: a review of strategies. Academic Medicine, 79(2), 107–117.

Roush, J. (2000a). Implementing parent–infant services: advice from families. In R. Seewald & J. Gravel (Eds.), A sound foundation through early amplification (pp. 159–165). Stäfa, Switzerland: Phonak, AG.

Roush, J. (2000b) What happens after screening? Hearing Journal, 53(Special Issue), 56–60.

Roush, J. (2001). Staying family centered. In E. Kurtzer-White & D. Luterman (Eds.), Early childhood deafness (pp. 49–62). Timonium, MD: York Press.

Simeonsson, R. J., Huntington, G. S., Sturtz-McMillen, J., Haugh-Dodds, A., Halperin, D., & Zipper, I. (1996). Services for young children and families: evaluating intervention cycles. Infants and Young Children, 9, 31–42.

Sjoblad, S., Harrison, M., Roush, J., & McWilliam, R. A. (2001). Parents' reactions and recommendations after diagnosis and hearing aid fitting. American Journal of Audiology, 10(1), 24–31.

Tharpe, A. M. & Rokuson, J. M. (2010, August 31). Simulated patients enhance clinical education: Vanderbilt offers unique program for audiology students. The ASHA Leader.

Trivette, C. M., Dunst, C. J., Boyd, K., & Hamby, D. W. (1995). Family-oriented program models, helpgiving practices, and parental control appraisals. Exceptional Children, 62, 237–248.

Trivette, C., Dunst, C., & Hamby, D. (2010). Influences of family-systems intervention practices on parent-child interactions and child development. Topics in Early Childhood Special Education, 30, 3.

Tye-Murray, N. (2012). Counseling for adults and children who have hearing loss. In L. Flasher & P. Fogle (Eds), Counseling skills for speech-language pathologists and audiologists (pp. 313–340). Clifton Park, NY: Delmar–Cengage Learning.

Yoshinaga-Itano, C., Sedey, A. L., Coulter, D. K., & Mehl, A. L. (1998). Language of early- and later-identified children with hearing loss. Pediatrics, 102(5), 1161–1171.

Chapter 35

Educating and Counseling Children and Teens with Hearing Loss

Kris English

Key Points

- Educating children about hearing loss requires an updated understanding of how people learn.

- Counseling children and teens about living with hearing loss requires audiologists to know the answer to the question, "Who owns this hearing loss?"

- Most materials designed to teach children about hearing loss can also be used as a springboard to counseling conversations about their reactions and concerns about living with hearing loss.

- If the audiologist suspects that a child has a more complicated learning or emotional problem than a hearing loss can account for, the audiologist must convey those concerns to parents and to an appropriate specialist.

Audiologists are uniquely qualified to teach children and teens about their hearing loss and to provide counseling support for psychological or emotional reactions associated with hearing loss. This chapter will describe how audiologists can educate and counsel children with hearing loss from elementary school age to the teen years.

◆ Teaching and Counseling in the 21st Century

Audiologists as Teachers

Before we begin, it is important to update our thinking about "teaching." Traditionally, this process implies that the adult talks while the child listens. This approach is based on a set of assumptions—specifically, that when an adult speaks, the child will understand and remember what was said and translate words into meaningful concepts (i.e., will learn).

However, research indicates that these assumptions are flawed. When measured by outcomes, the "teaching-by-telling/learning-by-listening" approach tends to yield unimpressive results. Children who merely listen to lectures or directions will soon forget most of what was said and usually will not generalize what they do remember to other situations (Medina, 2008).

On the other hand, when learners are actively engaged in their own learning, they demonstrate more desirable outcomes. When learners participate in problem solving, discussion, role playing, research, "thinking out loud" activities, building, creating, or writing, they are more likely to understand new content because they discover connections to previously learned content. Those connections help them remember the new content longer and apply that content to novel situations. Although not a new idea (e.g., see Dewey, 1938), recent neurological evidence now supports the use of active learning: compared with listening only, "learning by doing" results in more neural activity and the creation of more synaptic connections, which allow the brain to function more efficiently (Zull, 2011).

Being actively engaged also provides children meaningful and tangible evidence that they are indeed learning and mastering skills. Without clear evidence and feedback, the learner becomes doubtful and discouraged and is at risk of abandoning the learning process altogether. In other words, active engagement in the learning process not only helps the brain create new neural pathways but also provides the necessary encouragement each learner needs to stay focused and motivated (English, 2010). These conditions contribute to the development of *self-efficacy*, defined by Bandura (1977) as the belief in one's abilities to control achievement outcomes. Audiologists do not generally pay much attention to beliefs, but we need to be aware of the truism that if a child does not believe he can learn something, he will not learn it. As we engage in teaching, we need to keep the concept of self-efficacy in mind: Are we providing consistent and meaningful evidence to learners that they are indeed expanding their knowledge base, improving a skill, becoming more sophisticated thinkers? Are we helping the learner recognize progress and growth?

These issues are important because, of course, we are not providing information merely for information's sake. Our goal is to help children and teens not only understand and remember the information but also use it to make decisions that are in their best interests. This goal may seem obvious, but recently Falvo (2011) felt it necessary to explain that while "many people think of patient education as the transfer of information . . . the real goal is *patient learning*, in which patients are not only provided with information, but helped to incorporate it into their daily lives" (p. 21).

Later in this chapter, we will consider examples of how to engage the school-aged child and the teen as active learners. Audiologists will note that this approach will require them to reconsider their role as teacher, here held to be less a "sage on the stage" and more a "guide on the side." First, however, let us evaluate our role as audiologic counselors.

Audiologists as Counselors

Until recently, counseling and explaining were considered to be synonymous terms. However, counseling actually has two dimensions: patient education (discussed in the foregoing paragraphs as "providing information") and personal adjustment counseling (Kennedy & Charles, 2001). Neither dimension was effectively addressed in audiology training in the past, but, as audiology has evolved into a doctoral-level profession, most graduate programs now include counseling in their curricula (English & Weist, 2005).

Personal support counseling in pediatric settings attempts to help children understand their reactions to living with hearing loss and to accept themselves as persons with impaired hearing. The principles of audiologic counseling have much in common with active learning: Rather than telling children how they should feel or act or think or believe, audiologists should develop strategies to help children explain to themselves how they perceive the world and their lives. By describing out loud (by voice or sign) how she thinks and feels, a child is now better able to understand those thoughts and feelings and, thus, takes the first step in learning how to handle them.

During this process, audiologists-as-counselors must resist playing the role of rescuer. It is very tempting to take over with advice and action plans or try to help children feel better. In all aspects of counseling, practitioners are reminded to ask themselves, "Who owns this problem?" Individuals with a problem must assume responsibility of owning that problem before they are able to address it. In audiology,

we must routinely ask ourselves, "Who owns this hearing loss?" (Clark & English, 2013). For the population under consideration, the answer for younger children is, "The child and parents." As children become teens, the ownership of their hearing loss must gradually transition from their parents to them.

This chapter will therefore also include a discussion on how to help children and teens own their hearing loss as they acquire new information about hearing. Blending education and personal adjustment counseling into the same activities is not only efficient; it is also a natural process. All learners have emotional and psychological reactions to the material they are learning, particularly when the instructional material is about themselves. It is both expeditious and logical to discuss what one is learning, and how one thinks, feels, and believes about that learning, at the same time.

Pearl

- It may seem more efficient to an audiologist to assume a directive (telling) role rather than a facilitative one when teaching or counseling children. Consider the time spent as an investment in the future: the long-term goal is to help the child develop independence, confidence, and strategies to succeed, and these goals are acquired only with practice and support. They cannot be taught by telling.

◆ Teaching and Counseling Younger Children

One of the most useful materials available to the audiologist is a curriculum called "Knowledge Is Power" (KIP) (Martilla & Mills, 2009). This program provides lessons designed to help children understand their hearing loss, hearing aids, assistive devices, and more. Lessons are written in both an introductory and an advanced level, so that the audiologist can present the same material in more depth as the child becomes older.

Each lesson has specific learning objectives to reflect increasing interest in obtaining measurable outcomes. The curriculum contains crisp graphics to explain the function of hearing aids and cochlear implants, Web pages for assistive devices and legislation information, information about telephone relay services, and auditory testing, including otoacoustic emissions and auditory brainstem response.

Each lesson also includes pretests and posttests to measure learning and take-home letters asking parents or caregivers to review content with their child. This review surely helps the parent as well as the child and hopefully helps both parent and child feel comfortable talking about hearing problems. In addition, a page on hearing aid care is provided to serve as a stand-alone handout for a child who would like to develop a presentation for her class.

Earlier it was mentioned that we might strive to combine instruction and counseling into the same activities. The KIP curriculum provides resources to do just that. A section called "Our Stories" has contributions from children and young adults with hearing loss, and their own words are used. No editing was done to clean up syntax and grammar. Children can be encouraged to read "Our Stories" and either write their own stories or discuss the stories in KIP: Are there similarities to their own experiences? Are there lessons to learn? What would they want to ask the author? What would they want to add to the stories?

The section titled "Coping, Part 1" asks children to consider big questions such as "How do you feel about your hearing loss?" "Does your family accept your hearing loss?" "Who do you talk to when you have a problem?" Topics about responsibility for communication problems and friendships are open for consideration, and KIP gives a framework for the audiologist to bring them to the fore.

The section called "Coping, Part 2" provides a helpful introduction about how audiologists might help children recognize that negative beliefs ("I should not have to wear this hearing aid") can create barriers for themselves, affecting how they feel and ultimately how they act. A set of activities is provided to help children identify how they do think about circumstances and then how they can change those thoughts.

Pitfall

- Although counseling is now part of most audiology training programs, it is not uncommon for an audiologist to feel unprepared for these kinds of conversations. In that situation, it is recommended that an appropriate professional be contacted for help. A school counselor, social worker, or psychologist could provide invaluable support but may also need specialized information from the audiologist to meet children's needs.

Additional Resources for Younger Children

Following are other materials we can use to teach and counsel younger children about hearing loss and related topics. These materials provide opportunities to share new information as well as to listen for a child's thoughts and feelings.

Time Out! I Didn't Hear You! (Palmer, Butts, Lindley, & Snyder, 1996) is a handbook developed to help children with hearing loss participate in sports. This manual presents a range of listening challenges, with solutions that can focus on both teaching/learning and personal adjustment concepts. For example, while reviewing the range of accommodations available, we can also ask about the process: when arranging for accommodations in sports, does one feel confident, uncomfortable, unsure? Are these reactions understandable, insurmountable, manageable? Would it help to rehearse beforehand?

I Start/You Finish (Clark & English, 2013) is an open-ended activity that gives children an open forum. We start by providing "stem phrases" such as "I am happy when . . . ," "I am sad when . . . ," "The thing I like most in the world is . . . ," "The thing I would most like to change is . . ." "Because I have a hearing loss . . ." Children are asked to complete the phrase and expand on their answer as they choose.

◆ Teaching and Counseling Middle- and High-School Teens

It may surprise the reader to learn that few materials are available for the audiologist who wants to continue teaching and counseling children as they reach their teen years. However, one tool has been expressly designed for this purpose. It is called the Self-Assessment of Communication—Adolescents (SAC-A) (Elkayam & English, 2003), and it was modified from an instrument originally designed for adults. The original SAC (Schow & Nerbonne, 1982) is a popular self-assessment tool because it is short, addresses multiple domains, and has a version that a significant other (SO) can complete. A comparison of the two reports leads to insights regarding the stressors, thoughts, and feelings of both patient and significant other. The SO version of the SAC-A is to be completed by a good friend (the Significant Other Assessment of Communication—Adolescent [SOAC-A]).

Both instruments have 12 questions about how the teen with hearing loss functions, how the teen feels about her hearing loss, and what others might have mentioned about her hearing loss. For example, are there problems communicating with one person? A small group? Listening to entertainment? Does the teen feel left out or upset when it's hard to hear, or does it seem people often get the wrong impression because of the hearing loss?

To use the SAC-A and the SOAC-A as a teaching and counseling tool, the audiologist would first ask whether the teen is interested in completing the SAC-A, and have a friend complete the SOAC-A. As with most self-assessment administrations, the two parties are not likely to be in full agreement with their answers. Depending on the teen's preference, the audiologist can ask the teen to expand on answers in the friend's presence, or in private. The audiologist can learn if the teen is experiencing problems, understands the problems, or needs help solving them. Is the problem something technology can improve? Is the teen aware of the technology (or relevant communication repair strategy)? Is the teen aware of a solution but unwilling to make a change at this time?

Special Consideration

- The audiologist can be mindful of a counseling maxim: "Help is defined by the recipient." Although it is tempting to provide every solution possible to the teen, the teen must declare what help is desired. The audiologist's first role is to serve as a sounding board, then to convey trust in the teen's own ability to find solutions to many of these problems, before "leapfrogging" into problem-solving mode (Stone, Patton, & Heen, 1999).

Anecdotal evidence indicates that many teens do not have a friend they can approach to help with this activity. If this is the case, the audiologist should take extra care to be readily available to the teen and to watch for the possible need to refer to a professional counselor (Stepp, 2000).

The SAC-A has been found to be a reliable tool (Wright, English, & Elkayam, 2010) and can help audiologists find a starting point for conversations with teens. The conversation is often the first time both parties communicate with each other about specific challenges associated with hearing loss.

Teaching and Counseling in a Group Format

The counseling activity described above is likely to be a one-on-one conversation between teen and audiologist. However, there are many benefits of group and peer interaction, including the fact that learning is enhanced by social interaction (Suter & Suter, 2008). The audiologist may decide to capitalize on the dynamics of a group format to help teens tackle the challenges of living with hearing loss.

In keeping with the philosophy expressed throughout this chapter that help is defined by the recipient, it is recommended that the audiologist conduct a teen education/counseling group in a format similar to that described by Hickson (2007). Rather than pre-developing a lecture or presenting packaged material, the audiologist allows the members of the group to set the agenda. The audiologist might feel uncomfortable about releasing this kind of control, so she

should be clear that the goals are to help teens (1) express their thoughts and reactions to living with hearing loss; (2) develop some insights about their thoughts and reactions; (3) learn a helpful strategy or two; and (4) obtain a sense of support from others who have the same experiences. These are teen-centered goals and, therefore, not goals that an audiologist can teach. Teens need to engage in the process actively to achieve those goals.

How would such a program be managed? A basic overview would include these steps: Once teens are seated and introductions are made, the audiologist models a teen-centered approach from the beginning by informing the group members that they will determine the topics for discussion. To keep the focus on hearing, they can be asked to complete a statement such as "Because I have hearing loss . . ." The audiologist writes each response on a chalkboard or big piece of paper. If teens do not know and trust each other yet, they may prefer to write their thoughts on a piece of paper; these are then read aloud but anonymously. When responses are similar or overlapping, they can be clustered together thematically. The audiologist then directs the group to consider all the responses and ask, "As a group, what are our top three concerns today?" The group must prioritize from the choices and acknowledge that not all topics will be addressed.

When the top three topics are identified, the audiologist facilitates the discussion with the following three prompts:

- As a group, what do we know about each topic (i.e., develop common ground)?
- What might explain the situation (develop group insights)?
- What would help the situation (problem solving)?

Note that problem solving is not attempted until teens feel understood and until they are given the opportunity to understand the underlying concerns.

Case Study

A group of teens indicates that Topic #1 was "Because I have hearing loss . . . I feel left out most of the time." The audiologist first asks, "As a group, what do we know about feeling left out? What does it look like, what does it feel like?" Possible answers might be never being asked for a date; not receiving any text messages or phone calls; rarely being included in trips to the movies; having only one friend when most people seem to have several, and so on. As the teens describe their observations and experiences, the audiologist will give teens the floor as much as possible. To ensure that outcome, when each teen is finished speaking, it is particularly helpful to ask the teen to call on the next speaker, rather than the audiologist doing so. This strategy helps the teens talk to each other instead of only to the expert adult.

When it is clear that the group has fully addressed the first question, the audiologist asks the second question: "What might explain why teens with hearing loss feel left out?" Possible answers might be that persons with normal hearing do not understand hearing loss; that people with hearing loss have less energy for socializing; that teens with hearing loss may be self-conscious about making social mistakes and that could make others uncomfortable; and so on.

When all possible insights are expressed, the final question is, "There is much agreement in this group about the experiences of feeling left out and why that might happen. What would help the situation?" Some teens are natural problem solvers; other teens benefit from observing that skill. Each group member should describe one strategy they will try to improve their situation.

Now the group moves on. Topic #2 is "Because I have a hearing loss . . . I have to work 10 times harder at schoolwork than other kids." The audiologist again facilitates the discussion with the same questions: What do we know about learning with hearing loss? What might explain the situation? What would help the situation? And so on.

Analysis

Were the goals of this teen group met? Let's review: The goals were to help teens (1) express their thoughts and reactions to living with hearing loss; (2) develop some insights about their thoughts and reactions; (3) learn a helpful strategy or two; and (4) obtain a sense of support from others who have the same experiences. In this case study, the audiologist organized the teen meeting in such a way that all teens had the chance to talk, share, vent, commiserate, learn, and engage in problem solving. If the teens were polled after the session, it is likely they would affirm that these goals were indeed met.

Additional Resources for Teens

The following materials are available on the Internet at no cost. They are designed specifically to provide both information and support to middle- and high-school students with hearing loss.

- The *Guide to Access Planning* (GAP) is an online resource that contains self-assessments, informational materials, and learning activities for teens, young adults, professionals, and parents (Guide to Access Planning, n.d.).
- *Self-Advocacy for Students Who Are Deaf or Hard of Hearing* (English, 2012) is a 12-unit curriculum that addresses transition issues that arise

during the high school grades. The four units provide opportunities to learn information about transitioning while discussing how to develop a support system and work with others who may not know much about hearing loss.

◆ Do We See Any Red Flags?

Clearly, the interactions described above take the audiologist and child beyond the superficial "Are your hearing aids working OK?" relationship. Now that we are genuinely talking and listening, we may realize that a child's learning style is affected not only by the hearing loss but by other traits as well (attention span, logic, knowledge base, memory skills, for instance). The audiologist should discuss these observations with the classroom teacher, since that professional may have attributed all learning challenges to the hearing loss alone.

Bullying

Additionally, during these interactions, conversations are inherently more personal and may lead to new self-disclosures. A relatively new concern is the apparent increase in bullying occurring in school, out of school, and online. The Centers for Disease Control and Prevention (CDC) report that one in three children in the United States reports being bullied, and that children who have disabilities are up to 63% more likely to be bullied than other children (Hamburger, Basile, & Vivolo, 2011). However, children often choose not to tell adults when they are being bullied, usually confusing telling with "tattling." They may also be embarrassed to acknowledge that other children don't like them or that they can't stop the bullying themselves, or they worry that adults will make the situation worse. "Not telling" could contribute to an escalation of problems, potentially resulting in harm to self or others.

To discuss this sensitive topic and "help kids tell," health care providers are developing protocols to screen for bullying problems. For instance, pediatricians are encouraged to include screening questions during wellness exams and patient visits, such as "I'd like to hear about how school is going. Do you ever feel afraid to go to school? Do other kids ever bully you at school, in your neighborhood, or online? Who can you go to for help if you or someone you know is being bullied?" (StopBullying.gov, n.d.). Readers are encouraged to research how audiologists are addressing this health and safety issue.

More than ever before, children with hearing loss need someone to talk to. More than ever before, we have a professional responsibility to make ourselves approachable, trustworthy, and available to children's concerns about safety and security. These issues also highlight our responsibility in working with local referral processes and community resources when we are aware of a child who is experiencing more than the expected problems of living with hearing loss. Even when the audiologist is not completely sure about the concerns, she must ensure that professional counsellors are informed and follow up.

◆ Conclusion

When adults plan their teaching, they often ask themselves, "What am I going to cover (talk about)?" Although typical, this approach gives no attention to the learner's role in the process. Instead of that question, audiologists involved with instruction and counseling should ask themselves, "What is the child going to do?" If the answer is, "Listen and take notes," the instruction must be redesigned! A learner-centered approach will result in more learning, so the answer needs to be, "The child will do" something, such as

- Write a story
- Describe anatomy to a parent
- Find information on new devices and share it with friends
- Conduct a survey
- Interview a peer about friendships

The time available to teach and counsel children is usually limited, so the audiologist will want to use that time as effectively as possible. Audiologists who engage in this level of support will find it to be a highlight of their career.

Discussion Questions

1. Describe a time when you participated in an exceptionally positive learning experience. Why was that experience memorable? What did the designer of that instruction do to ensure that you understood and remembered the content? Describe your emotional or psychological response to that learning experience. Was that response important?

2. Children must feel a sense of safety before they open up to (learn) new information. Are children with hearing loss comfortable talking to their audiologists? What barriers might exist, and what can audiologists do to remove those barriers?

3. Stepp (2000) wrote that teens need support from three groups: peers, parents, and other adults, such as youth group leaders, coaches, and teachers. The role of other adults is to endow teens with confidence so that they can gradually disconnect from parents and develop autonomy with increasing self-direction. Do audiologists typically relate to teens with hearing loss as influential other adults? Why or why not?

References

Bandura, A. (1977). Self-efficacy: toward a unifying theory of behavioral change. Psychological Review, 84(2), 191–215.

Clark, J. G., & English, K. (2013). Counseling-infused audiologic care. Boston, MA: Allyn & Bacon.

Dewey, J. (1938). Experience and education. New York, NY: Macmillan & Co.

Elkayam, J., & English, K. (2003). Counseling adolescents with hearing loss with the use of self-assessment/significant other questionnaires. Journal of the American Academy of Audiology, 14(9), 485–499. Retrieved from http://gozips.uakron.ed/~ke3/SAC-A-0311.pdf

English, K. (2010). Child and teen education and counseling. In R. C. Seewald & J. M. Bamford (Eds.), Proceedings from the Phonak 2010 Sound Foundations Conference (p. 307–313). Chicago, IL: Phonak.

English, K. (2012). Self-advocacy for students who are deaf or hard of hearing (2nd ed.). Retrieved from http://gozips.uakron.edu/~ke3/Self-Advocacy.pdf

English, K., & Weist, D. (2005). Proliferation of AuD degrees found to increase training in counseling. Hearing Journal, 58, 54–58.

Falvo, D. (2011). Effective patient education: A guide to increased adherence (4th ed.). Sudbury, MA: Jones & Bartlett.

Guide to Access Planning. (n.d.). Retrieved from http://www.phonakonline.com/MyGap/GapMain.html

Hamburger, M. E., Basile, K. C., & Vivolo, A. M. (2011). Measuring bullying victimization, perpetration, and bystander experiences: A compendium of assessment tools. Atlanta, GA: Centers for Disease Control and Prevention, National Center for Injury Prevention and Control.

Hickson, L. (2007). Pull out an "ACE" to help your patients become better communicators. Hearing Journal, 60, 10–16.

Kennedy, E., & Charles, S. (2001). On becoming a counselor: a basic guide for nonprofessional counselors. New York, NY: Consortium.

Martilla, J., & Mills, M. (2009). Knowledge is power. Educational Audiology Association. Retrieved from http://www.edaud.org

Medina, J. 2008. The brain rules. Seattle, WA: Pear Press.

Palmer, C., Butts, C., Lindley, G., & Snyder, S. (1996). Time out! I didn't hear you. Retrieved from http://www.pitt.edu/~cvp/timeout.pdf

Schow, R. L., & Nerbonne, M. A. (1982). Communication screening profile: use with elderly clients. Ear and Hearing, 3(3), 135–147.

Stepp, L. (2000). Our last best shot: guiding our children through early adolescence. New York, NY: Riverhead.

Stone, D., Patton, B., & Heen, S. (1999). Difficult conversations: how to discuss what matters most. New York, NY: Viking.

StopBullying.gov. (n.d). Roles for pediatricians in bullying prevention and intervention. Retrieved from http://www.stopbullying.gov/resources-files/roles-for-pediatricians-tipsheet.pdf

Suter, P. M., & Suter, W. N. (2008). Patient education. Timeless principles of learning: a solid foundation for enhancing chronic disease self-management. Home Healthcare Nurse, 26(2), 82–88, quiz 89–90.

Wright, K., English, K., & Elkayam, J. (2010). Reliability of the Self-Assessment of Communication—Adolescent. Journal of Educational Audiology, 16, 30–36.

Zull, J. (2011). From brain to mind: using neuroscience to guide change in education. Sterling, VA: Stylus Publishing.

Index

Note: Page numbers followed by *f* and *t* indicate figures and tables, respectively.